Musculoskeletal Disorders

Musculoskeletal Disorders

The Fatigue Failure Mechanism

Sean Gallagher
Auburn University, Auburn, AL, USA

Mary F. Barbe
Temple University, Philadelphia, PA, USA

WILEY

This edition first published 2022

Registered Office
John Wiley & Sons, Inc., 111 River Street, Hoboken, NJ 07030, USA

Editorial Office
John Wiley & Sons, Inc., 111 River Street, Hoboken, NJ 07030, USA

For details of our global editorial offices, customer services, and more information about Wiley products visit us at www.wiley.com.

Wiley also publishes its books in a variety of electronic formats and by print-on-demand. Some content that appears in standard print versions of this book may not be available in other formats.

Library of Congress Cataloging-in-Publication Data applied for:

ISBN: 9781119640042

Cover image: © MDGRPHCS/Shutterstock
Cover design by Wiley

Set in 9.5/12.5pt STIXTwoText by Straive, Pondicherry, India

To Dad and Mom, who set a high bar; to Nancie for her constant love and support; and to Drew and Brendon for being wonderful and thoughtful sons.

Sean Gallagher

To my parents, who taught me how to dream; to Hugh, the love of my life, for his continued aid and support; and to Susan, my twin and other half of my soul, for always being my best friend, companion, and muse.

Mary F. Barbe

Contents

Preface

During the course of my [SG's] doctoral work with Dr. William S. Marras, I became familiar with the work of researchers such as Adams, Cyron, Hutton, and Brinckmann who had performed *ex vivo* studies examining the effects of repeated stress on fatigue failure of spinal motion segments (Adams & Hutton, 1985; Brinckmann, Biggemann, & Hilweg, 1988; Cyron & Hutton, 1978). When the time came to select a dissertation topic, the option of performing an *ex vivo* fatigue failure study on spines at different levels of forward flexion was offered and I accepted the opportunity. The results of our research showed once again that spines subjected to repeated stress exhibited a classic fatigue failure response, and that the relationship is also affected by the degree of flexion of the motion segments adopted (Gallagher et al., 2007).

This research added to the existing body of evidence that cadaveric spinal motion segments fail in accordance with the mechanism of fatigue failure. However, though *ex vivo* fatigue failure data (on various musculoskeletal tissues) had been accumulating for some time, the implications of this mechanism regarding tissue damage were generally neither reflected in the development of musculoskeletal risk assessment tools nor in epidemiological studies examining musculoskeletal disorder risk factors. It is not entirely clear why this is the case, but it is the author's belief that researchers were reluctant to assume that this process would work in a similar manner in the setting of a complex biological system. This is understandable as no real evidence existed at that time that such a process was actually taking place *in vivo*.

One day in 2011, I had just finished giving a fatigue-based presentation to some of my NIOSH colleagues in Pittsburgh and was walking out of the conference room door when I suddenly realized that the *S–N* curve (which governs the fatigue failure response of materials) would predict a specific pattern of interaction between the risk factors of force and repetition and that the interaction predicted would look exactly like the interaction observed in the classic studies by Silverstein et al. for carpal tunnel syndrome and by Armstrong et al. for hand-wrist tendinitis (Armstrong, Fine, Goldstein, Lifshitz, & Silverstein, 1987; Silverstein, Fine, & Armstrong, 1987).

This result strongly suggested that a fatigue failure process might indeed be occurring *in vivo*. This finding piqued my curiosity and I then performed (with my NIOSH collaborator John Heberger) a systematic review of epidemiology studies in the ergonomics literature that had tested for a force-repetition interaction. The goal was to examine whether studies that had tested the interaction found a pattern indicative of a fatigue failure process (like the aforementioned studies). Results of this review showed only twelve studies in the literature that reported results of a statistical test for the interaction of force and repetition (or which provided data by which such an interaction could be examined). Of these, ten provided data indicative of the predicted pattern, one that tested for such an interaction consisted only high force tasks (where the test for interaction was meaningless), and in the other, the relationship was not present (Gallagher & Heberger, 2013). Overall, the results of this systematic review provided compelling evidence that many musculoskeletal disorder (MSD) outcomes exhibited a pattern of force and repetition that would suggest that a fatigue failure process might be an important etiological factor. This appeared to be the case across a wide range of disorders and joints.

Concurrent with the development of this paper, I met Mary Barbe, whose novel rat model provided additional support that fatigue failure of musculoskeletal tissues occurs *in vivo*. Her research demonstrated that damage to tendons, bone, and cartilage all followed the fatigue failure predicted force-repetition pattern (Barbe et al., 2013). The same was true for many cytokines, whose expression appears to be tied to the amount of damage occurring in musculoskeletal tissues (Barr, Barbe, & Clark, 2004). Since that time, we have continued to collaborate on numerous papers and projects.

In 2018, I asked Mary if she would be willing to collaborate on a book dealing with the fatigue failure model of MSD development. The idea was to provide evidence that fatigue failure was occurring in musculoskeletal tissues and to examine the diverse implications of fatigue failure occurring in a complex biological setting. As will be seen in this book, this process (a *modified* fatigue failure process) is likely influenced by numerous physiological and psychological factors, all of which would be expected to play important roles in maintaining musculoskeletal health.

This book is the result of our examination of the impact of the fatigue failure process and its interactions with biological and physiological mechanisms affecting musculoskeletal health. The book provides considerable information on the musculoskeletal and nervous systems; the epidemiology of MSDs; evidence that musculoskeletal tissues fail via a fatigue failure process; implications in terms of MSD etiology; remodeling and healing processes; use of fatigue failure methods in risk assessment; and numerous other topics. We hope that our readers will find this book helpful in understanding the etiology of MSDs and, conversely, the importance of the fatigue failure process in the maintenance of musculoskeletal health.

Bibliography

Adams, M., & Hutton, W. (1985). Gradual disc prolapse. *Spine, 10*, 524–531.

Armstrong, T., Fine, L., Goldstein, S., Lifshitz, Y., & Silverstein, B. (1987). Ergonomics considerations in hand and wrist tendinitis. *The Journal of Hand Surgery, 12A*, 830–837.

Barbe, M., Gallagher, S., Massicotte, V., Tytell, M., Popoff, S., & Barr-Gillespie, A. (2013). The interaction of force and repetition on musculoskeletal and neural tissue responses and sensorimotor behavior in a rat model of work-related musculoskeletal disorders. *BMC Musculoskskeletal Disorders, 14*, 303.

Barr, A., Barbe, M., & Clark, B. (2004). Work-related musculoskeletal disorders of the hand and wrist: epidemiology, pathophysiology, and sensorimotor changes. *Journal of Orthopaedic & Sports Physical Therapy., 34*, 610–627.

Brinckmann, P., Biggemann, M., & Hilweg, D. (1988). Fatigue fracture of human lumbar vertebrae. *Clinical Biomechanics, 3*(Suppl. 1), S1–S23.

Cyron, B., & Hutton, W. (1978). The fatigue strength of the lumbar neural arch in spondylolysis. *Journal of Bone and Joint Surgery, 60B*, 234–238.

Gallagher, S., & Heberger, J. (2013). Examining the interaction of force and repetition on musculoskeletal disorder risk: A systematic literature review. *Human Factors, 14*, 108–124.

Gallagher, S., Marras, W., Litsky, A., Burr, D., Landoll, J., & Matkovic, V. (2007). A comparison of fatigue failure responses of old versus middle-aged lumbar motion segments in simulated flexed lifting. *Spine, 32*, 1832–1839.

Silverstein, B., Fine, L., & Armstrong, T. (1987). Occupational factors and carpal tunnel syndrome. *American Journal of Industrial Medicine, 11*, 343–358.

Acknowledgments

The authors wish to acknowledge the following individuals who have aided in the process of writing this book:

First, we would like to acknowledge our spouses, Nancie and Hugh, respectively, for their support and tolerance during the development of this book. The demands of writing have unfortunately required them to put up with longish periods of our absence.

Acknowledgment is also due to the Center for Occupational Safety, Ergonomics, and Injury Prevention (COSEIP) team at Auburn University (both faculty and students), who have been integral in the development of the fatigue failure-based risk assessment tools presented in this book. We would like to thank faculty members Dr. Richard F. Sesek, Dr. Mark C. Schall, Jr., and Dr. Jerry Davis, along with former students (notably Dr. Rong Huangfu and Dr. Dania Bani Hani) for their critical contributions to risk assessment tool development. Other former and current students have contributed to this research including Dr. Tenchi Smith, Dr. Nick Smith, Ivan Nail, Nathan Pool, Bob Sesek, and Yuting Ma.

We would also like to acknowledge the National Institute for Occupational Safety and Health (NIOSH) for the long-standing funding provided in support of the Deep South Center for Occupational Health and Safety, along with other extramural funding. We also thank the National Institute of Arthritis and Musculoskeletal and Skin Diseases (NIAMS) and the National Center for Complementary and Integrative Health (NCCIH), which have helped advance our research in this area.

Great thanks is also due to our colleagues who have taken the time to review draft chapters of this book. In particular, we would like to thank Dr. Michael Zabala and Dr. Sa'd Hamasha (both of Auburn University) for their valuable time and assistance rendered in reviewing draft chapters in this book.

Finally, we would like to acknowledge the Wiley book team (especially Summers Scholl, Judy Howarth, Veerabaghu Nagarajan, Judit Anbu Hena Daniel, Rajalakshmi Venkatesaperumal, and Stefani Volk) for their support and patience during the development of this book. Their commitment is deeply appreciated as is their care and attention in the book's production.

Sean Gallagher
Mary F. Barbe

Acknowledgments

About the Authors

Sean Gallagher, PhD, CPE, FAIHA, is the Hal N. and Peggy S. Pennington Professor of Industrial and Systems Engineering at Auburn University. Dr. Gallagher has over 35 years of experience in the field of ergonomics, including having worked for the US Bureau of Mines, the National Institute for Occupational Safety and Health (NIOSH), and Auburn University. He is a Fellow of both the Human Factors and Ergonomics Society and the American Industrial Hygiene Association. Dr. Gallagher is a two-time recipient of the International Ergonomics Association/Liberty Mutual Medal in Occupational Safety and Ergonomics (2013 and 2018) and a recipient of the 2020 Paper of the Year Award by the journal *Ergonomics*. He has received various other team-based awards, including the 2009 Alice Hamilton Award for Excellence in Occupational Safety and Health (Educational Materials Category) and the 2011 HHS Innovates Award (Secretary's Pick).

Mary F. Barbe, PhD, FAAA, is currently a Full Professor at the Center for Translational Medicine at Lewis Katz School of Medicine of Temple University in Philadelphia. She has over 212 peer-reviewed publications to her credit. She has been involved in research investigating mechanisms and treatments for pain and work-related musculoskeletal disorders (repetitive strain injuries) in humans and using rat models. She is a Fellow of the American Association of Anatomists (FAAA) and of the American Society of Bone and Mineral Research. She is also the president of the Advances in Mineral Metabolism society for 2021–2023. She is the recipient of the Senior Faculty Research Excellence Award from the Lewis Katz School of Medicine in 2017, the Temple University Faculty Research Award from Temple University in 2019, the Educator Award from the Philadelphia Chapter of the Society for Neuroscience in 2008, the Christian R. and Mary F. Lindback Foundation Award from Temple University for Distinguished Teaching in 2008, and the Excellence in Teaching Award from College of Allied Health Professions in 1997 and 2007. Other awards that she has received include various team-based awards, including The ISSLS Prize for Lumbar Spine Research 2018 from the International Society for the Study of the Lumbar Spine.

1

Introduction

The ability to move about freely can be easily taken for granted, but if one stops to consider the finely tuned coordination of the multiple intricate systems necessary to accomplish even simple movements, both the beauty and remarkable complexity of the musculoskeletal system can be appreciated. Movement requires careful synchronization of a complex structure made of muscle, bone, cartilage, tendon, ligament, and nerve to permit specific movement goals to be achieved. Not only is the musculoskeletal system itself complex, but it is also dependent on other complex systems to supply the resources necessary to accomplish desired movement objectives. These other supporting systems (e.g., nervous, cardiovascular, respiratory, and gastrointestinal) provide nutrition and other resources required by musculoskeletal tissues that allow us to perform tasks or activities that we desire to accomplish (or which may be required of us), and otherwise live our everyday lives. However, despite the remarkable capabilities of the musculoskeletal system, each system component is made of materials that will experience damage when exposed to repeated stress. The accumulation of damage that can result may lead to tissue injury, pain, disability, and/or system dysfunction.

Injuries to the musculoskeletal system result in extraordinary societal impacts and economic costs. In the United States alone, over 73 million adults suffer from chronic low back pain, and the annual cost of treatment and lost wages associated with back pain was estimated at $315 billion (United States Bone and Joint Initiative, 2021). Musculoskeletal disorders (MSDs) also account for a substantial loss of productivity in the workplace. For example, back and neck disorders were associated with 264 million annual lost workdays according to data from 2015 (United States Bone and Joint Initiative, 2021). However, back pain is but one of the many MSDs that lead to these substantial economic, societal, and individual costs. An analysis of work-related upper extremity disorders in US workers indicated that the 30-day prevalence of these disorders was 8.2% but ranged as high as 9.9% in the construction industry (Ma et al., 2018). Workers experiencing these disorders typically require more time to recuperate than those experiencing other work-related illnesses and injuries. For example, US workers with carpal tunnel syndrome (CTS) took a median of 32 days to return to work and those with tendonitis required a median of 15 days of recuperation compared to the median of nine days off for all work-related injuries and illnesses in the United States for 2014 (Ma et al., 2018).

If we are to effectively combat the enormous societal burden associated with these disorders, it is essential to gain a better understanding of the processes involved with MSD development. Over the past several decades, considerable research has been performed, and a great deal learned about these disorders. However, despite these important advances in our understanding, the identification of specific causal mechanisms that explain exactly *how* and *why* these disorders develop

Musculoskeletal Disorders: The Fatigue Failure Mechanism, First Edition. Sean Gallagher and Mary F. Barbe.

has been lacking. To better understand the development of MSDs, we must identify the specific processes that possess causal powers or capacities to bring about changes in the state of musculoskeletal tissues. Identification of such processes or pathways is a central ambition of science and can confer numerous benefits. In the case of MSDs, benefits may include improved risk assessment methods, better injury prevention strategies, and greater insight into physiological and biomechanical processes affecting the development of damage in musculoskeletal tissues.

The purpose of this book is to evaluate a prospective causal mechanism of musculoskeletal tissue damage recently promoted by the authors, to provide evidence in support of this mechanism, and to discuss its rather substantial implications in terms of musculoskeletal tissue damage development, healing, and overall musculoskeletal health (Barbe et al., 2013; Gallagher & Heberger, 2013; Gallagher & Schall, 2017). This mechanism is known as *fatigue failure* and is the theory that explains *how* and *why* damage development occurs in materials subjected to repeated stress. Fatigue failure is not a new theory; in fact, it has a history going back well over a century and a half (Rankine, 1843). However, the application of fatigue failure principles and their role in the development of MSDs have not received much attention until recently. Given that musculoskeletal tissues are materials that are known to experience exposure to repeated stress and that musculoskeletal tissues exhibit damage development, fatigue failure would seem a natural candidate as a causal mechanism to explain the initiation and propagation of damage in musculoskeletal tissues (and the consequent development of MSDs).

The evidence that fatigue failure is a causal mechanism by which inert (i.e., nonbiological) materials experience cumulative damage is by now beyond dispute (Stephens, Fatemi, Stephens, & Fuchs, 2001). This process is observed in all materials exposed to repeated stress, with each exhibiting the distinctive exponential relationship between stress magnitude and the number of cycles to failure. As we will discuss in this book, there is abundant evidence to suggest the same process occurs in musculoskeletal tissues. However, there are some important differences between inert materials and biological tissues in the response to damage invoked by the fatigue failure process. For example, biological tissues possess the remarkable capacity to sense mechanical loading and to remodel (to a degree) tissues to help them adapt to the stresses they experience. Furthermore, when damage is experienced, there is a healing process by which such damage might be repaired. Thus, the fatigue failure process in living tissues may be considered a *modified* fatigue failure process in which the competing processes of damage and healing will both be important to the health status of the tissue. Having remodeling and healing processes is quite fortunate as they would be expected to extend the *fatigue life* of musculoskeletal tissues (i.e., the number of loading cycles that can be experienced prior to failure) well beyond what would be possible in the absence of these processes.

Over the past few decades, numerous methods have been developed to assess the risk of developing various types of MSDs. Some of the more popular methods include the National Institute for Occupational Safety and Health (NIOSH) Lifting Equation (Waters, Putz-Anderson, Garg, & Fine, 1993), The Liberty Mutual Psychophysical tables (Potvin, Ciriello, Snook, Maynard, & Brogmus, 2021; Snook, 1978; Snook & Ciriello, 1991), The Strain Index (Moore & Garg, 1995), and the Threshold Limit Value for Hand Activity (Rempel, 2018). These methods are discussed in greater detail in Chapter 8. As discussed in that chapter, these MSD models have been validated against MSD prevalence and incidence in several epidemiology studies and have provided much knowledge in terms of improving the risk assessment of MSDs. These risk assessment tools have unquestionably aided in the prevention of untold injuries and disability in workers.

Despite the benefits of these methods, however, there appears much to be gained in applying fatigue failure principles to assess MSD risk. As will be discussed in this book, there are many validated fatigue failure techniques that provide ready solutions to challenging problems that have long been faced by musculoskeletal researchers. The following text provides some of the benefits of applying fatigue failure methods to MSD risk assessment.

- *Validated Methods of Cumulative Exposure Assessment*. It has been a general assumption of musculoskeletal researchers that it is the totality of exposure that an individual experiences (often involving exposure to several tasks with highly variable loading profiles) that determines the risk of developing MSDs. However, not all current models provide methods of combining the risk associated with the performance of multiple tasks during a workday. Fortunately, the fatigue failure theory has validated methods for assessing the cumulative effects associated with highly variable loading histories, as might be experienced in multitask jobs (Miner, 1945; Palmgren, 1924). This technique (described in detail in Chapter 9) not only allows assessment of the cumulative effects of loading but can also evaluate the proportion of risk associated with each individual task. This provides the ability to identify work tasks most responsible for the overall risk (and most in need of ergonomic intervention). These cumulative exposure techniques have been shown to correlate well with MSD outcomes in fatigue failure-based risk assessment tools (Gallagher, Sesek, Schall Jr, & Huangfu, 2017; Bani Hani et al., 2021; Gallagher, Schall Jr, Sesek, & Huangfu, 2018).
- *Biomechanics and Injury Risk*. Biomechanical analysis is an important method of evaluating the forces and moments acting on the body due to the performance of physically demanding tasks. However, while this technique allows for the quantification of stresses on the musculoskeletal system, the relationship of calculated forces and moments to actual injury risk has often been missing. For example, a traditional introductory biomechanical problem asks the student to calculate the force required of the elbow flexor muscles to hold a certain load in the hands. For example, it might be calculated that holding a 11.3 kg (25 lbs) weight, the upper arm perpendicular to the floor, and the elbow flexed at 90° require an elbow flexor muscle force of approximately 1,000 N (225 lbs). It is, of course, interesting in itself that the muscle forces required are vastly greater than the load being held. But what if we are interested in estimating the probability of an injury outcome to the elbow flexor tendons if such a load was handled 100 times in a workday? And what if this task were combined with another where 500 repetitions of handling a load of 5 kg (11.0 lbs.) in the same posture? Biomechanical modeling techniques alone cannot answer these questions. However, when used in conjunction with fatigue failure techniques, one can use biomechanical estimates of tissue stress to estimate injury probabilities associated with either mono-task jobs or combinations of tasks. Chapter 5 discusses the benefits of applying fatigue failure principles to biomechanical analyses to help estimate the fatigue life of tissues experiencing repeated biomechanical stress.
- *Damage versus Healing*. As indicated earlier, musculoskeletal health is expected to be dependent upon both damage development (due to repeated stress) and healing. As noted long ago by Nash, despite the additional complexity of the presence of a healing component, it is relatively easy to develop an injury model that incorporates both cumulative damage development and healing using a fatigue failure approach (Nash, 1966). This simply involves use of the Palmgren–Miner method (Chapter 9) to ascertain the cumulative damage associated with the experienced variable magnitude loading, and then subtracting out the damage healed over the same time frame. If the rate of cumulative damage is greater than the healing rate, damage will occur; in contrast, if the healing rate equals or exceeds the rate of damage development, no damage would be expected to occur. This model can also be employed to assess risk in conditions associated with impaired healing (such as psychological stress, aging, and obesity), as discussed in Chapter 10. Thus, in contrast to previous models, fatigue failure techniques are well positioned to address important

complexities of the biological environment that are important in maintaining musculoskeletal health. This "damage and healing" model may be useful, for example, in assessing the MSD risk associated with factors known to impair the healing process, such as psychological stress, obesity, and aging (Guo & DiPietro, 2010). These and other implications are discussed further in Chapter 10.

- *Real-Time Risk Assessment*. The fatigue failure theory also has techniques that could be used as real-time exposure assessment methods continue to develop and mature (Radwin, 2011). Due to the variable amplitude loading histories experienced by humans in the performance of physical work, a method will be needed to evaluate the risk associated with complex and irregular loading curves. Fortunately, this situation is also encountered in the loading of other materials and methods have been developed to deconstruct complex loading curves into cycles that can then be assessed by fatigue failure models. The consensus technique is known as *rainflow analysis* (Matsuishi & Endo, 1968). This technique evaluates stress "reversals" (half-cycles) associated with complex loading histories and derives full cycles for analysis while accounting for the entire load history (Chapter 9). Thus, the fatigue failure approach is well positioned for the future of risk assessment in which complex loading curves derived from real-time exposure assessment can be rapidly analyzed using validated techniques as discussed further in Chapter 13.
- *Cumulative Risk from Different Loading Modalities*. Fatigue failure methods also hold the promise of combining the risks associated with diverse loading modalities. For example, imagine a delivery driver who experiences whole-body vibration from driving across rough roads and then must carry heavy boxes to complete the delivery. Fatigue failure methods hold the promise to combine these two types of repetitive stress into a single measure of risk and provide an estimate of cumulative damage associated with both exposures. Whole-body vibration is known to be an exposure that imposes repeated stress on the low back (Gallagher & Schall, 2017) as does repetitive compressive loading due to lifting (Brinckmann, Biggemann, & Hilweg, 1988). Since both can be expressed in terms of cumulative damage, fatigue failure techniques could be used to combine these disparate loading modalities to obtain a cumulative measure of overall risk not previously available (Chapter 9).
- *Combining Static and Cyclic Loading*. MSDs may also be the result of both static and/or dynamic activities. Thus, it would be helpful to have a method of calculating the combined risk associated with a combination of creep (static) loading and cyclic (dynamic) loading. Fortunately, the fatigue failure theory also has a validated method of evaluating the cumulative effects associated with combined static and dynamic loading (Wright, Carroll, Sham, Lybeck, & Wright, 2016). This method allows estimating the proportion of risk associated with dynamic versus static loads overall, as well as the proportion of individual task risks for both types of loading (See Chapters 9 and 13).
- *Assessing Risks of Job Rotation*. Job rotation is a technique sometimes used in industry in an attempt to balance the biomechanical demands associated with different jobs. However, a recent award-winning article in the journal *Ergonomics* using fatigue failure techniques demonstrated that job rotation may be more harmful than helpful in terms of the overall MSD risk to a pool of workers (Mehdizadeh et al., 2020). Due to the nature of the fatigue failure risk function, any reduction in risk for higher risk jobs is guaranteed to be smaller than the increase in risk experienced by those in lower-risk jobs (See Chapter 13). The magnitude of this effect will vary from extremely large, if a single high-risk job is present in the pool, to small if all jobs are fairly low risk. Such an analysis would be difficult to achieve with some prior models but is straightforward using fatigue failure principles.
- *Influence of Personal Characteristics on MSD Risk*. Fatigue failure also offers the potential to incorporate certain personal characteristics into risk assessment. As an example, fatigue failure theory stipulates that the ultimate strength of a material determines the number of cycles to

failure at different percentages of that strength. If an individual performs a lifting task resulting in a 2,500 N compressive load on the spine, they will incur damage more quickly if they have a spine ultimate strength of 6,000 N (say at age 60) as opposed to 8,000 N (at age 30). Factors such as age, anthropometry, sex, bone mineral density, and others could be considered to develop "personalized" risk assessments that may be more protective for workers based on their individual characteristics. Risks associated with personal characteristics are discussed in Chapter 12.

The preceding examples provide a sampling of the opportunities that may be realized with the use of the fatigue failure approach to MSD risk, many of which would be difficult to realize with previous approaches. There are numerous other useful applications of this model as will be described in detail later in the book.

In summary, fatigue failure is a universally accepted causal mechanism of damage nucleation and propagation for nonbiological materials, and there is ample evidence to suggest that the same process occurs in musculoskeletal tissues. Much of what has been learned regarding the process of material damage resulting from repeated stress appears applicable to the assessment of musculoskeletal risk, and many techniques developed in this theory appear to provide ready solutions to challenging problems faced by musculoskeletal researchers. These include simple methods of estimating the cumulative impact of multiple tasks having highly variable loading conditions. Techniques are also available for assessing cumulative damage associated with complex loading curves that will be useful soon as real-time exposure assessment methods for MSDs become available. Furthermore, models incorporating the effects of healing and other biological processes critical to musculoskeletal health have been put forth, thus allowing the complexity of the fatigue failure process in the biological environment to be more fully understood.

As indicated by the earlier discussion, there are many topics to be discussed and implications to be addressed when evaluating the effects of a fatigue failure process in a biological environment and the roles of damage and healing in overall musculoskeletal health. We have structured the 16 chapters in a logical order, and the chapters are grouped into four general themes. Chapters 2–5 provide detailed information regarding common MSDs and the components of the musculoskeletal system, including the structure and function of musculoskeletal structures, the material properties of these tissues, and the important role of nerves and the nervous system in the musculoskeletal system. Chapters 6–9 cover fundamental concepts of biomechanics, evidence of fatigue failure processes in musculoskeletal tissues, and fundamental concepts in fatigue failure analytical methods relevant to the assessment of MSD risk. Chapters 10–12 discuss concepts related to the unique aspects of fatigue failure in a biological environment, addressing the body's healing capacity and the influence of personal characteristics and psychosocial stress on MSD risk. The final four chapters (Chapters 13–16) provide methods for assessing risk using fatigue failure methods, implications for MSD prevention, suggestions for optimizing musculoskeletal health, and assessment of the status of knowledge and the need for future research in this area. We would note that the book need not be necessarily consumed in the order in which it was written, as many chapters can be read on their own without loss of meaning.

Bibliography

Bani Hani, D., Huangfu, R., Sesek, R., Schall, M. C., Jr., Davis, G. A., & Gallagher, S. (2021). Development and validation of a cumulative exposure shoulder risk assessment tool based on fatigue failure theory. *Ergonomics*, *64*(1), 39–54.

Barbe, M. F., Gallagher, S., Massicotte, V. S., Tytell, M., Popoff, S. N., & Barr-Gillespie, A. E. (2013). The interaction of force and repetition on musculoskeletal and neural tissue responses and sensorimotor behavior in a rat model of work-related musculoskeletal disorders. *BMC Musculoskskeletal Disorders*, *14*, 303. https://doi.org/10.1186/1471-2474-14-303. PMID: 24156755; PMCID: PMC3924406

Brinckmann, P., Biggemann, M., & Hilweg, D. (1988). Fatigue fracture of human lumbar vertebrae. *Clinical Biomechanics*, *3*(Suppl. 1), S1–S23.

Carter, D., & Hayes, W. (1976). Fatigue life of compact bone—I. Effects of stress amplitude, temperature and density. *Journal of Biomechanics*, *9*, 27–34.

Dong, R., Wu, J., Xu, X., Welcome, D., & Krajnak, K. (2021). A Review of Hand–Arm Vibration Studies Conducted by US NIOSH since 2000. *Vibration*, *4*, 482–528.

Gallagher, S., & Heberger, J. (2013). Examining the interaction of force and repetition on musculoskeletal disorder risk: A systematic literature review. *Human Factors*, *14*, 108–124.

Gallagher, S., Marras, W., Litsky, A., Burr, D., Landoll, J., & Matkovic, V. (2007). A Comparison of fatigue failure responses of old versus middle-aged lumbar motion segments in simulated flexed lifting. *Spine*, *32*, 1832–1839.

Gallagher, S., & Schall, J. M. (2017). Musculoskeletal disorders as a fatigue failure process: Evidence, implications and research needs. *Ergonomics*, *60*, 255–269.

Gallagher, S., Schall, M., Jr., Sesek, R., & Huangfu, R. (2018). An upper extremity risk assessment tool based on material fatigue failure theory: The distal upper extremity tool (DUET). *Human Factors*, *60*, 1146–1162.

Gallagher, S., Sesek, R., Schall, M., Jr., & Huangfu, R. (2017). Development and validation of an easy-to-use risk assessment tool for cumulative low back loading: The Lifting Fatigue Failure Tool (LiFFT). *Applied Ergonomics*, *63*, 142–150.

Gosain, A., & DiPietro, L. (2004). Aging and wound healing. *World Journal of Surgery*, *28*, 321–326.

Guo, S., & DiPietro, L. (2010). Factors affecting wound healing. *Journal of Dental Research*, *89*, 219–229.

Kiecolt-Glaser, J., Marucha, P., Malarkey, W., Mercado, A., & Glaser, R. (1995). Slowing of wound healing by psychological stress. *Lancet*, *346*, 1194–1196.

Kumar, S. (2001). Theories of musculoskeletal injury causation. *Ergonomics*, *44*, 17–47.

Ma, C., Gu, J., Charles, L., Andrew, M., Dong, R., & Burchfiel, C. (2018). Work-related upper extremity musculoskeletal disorders in the United States: 2006, 2009, and 2014 National Health Interview Survey. *Work*, *60*, 623–634.

Matsuishi, M., & Endo, T. (1968). Fatigue of metals subjected to varying stress. *Paper presented to the Japanese Society of Mechanical Engineers*. Fukuoka, Japan: Japanese Society of Mechanical Engineers.

McEwan, B. (1998). Stress, adaptation, and disease: Allostasis and allostatic load. *Annals of the New York Academy of Sciences*, *840*, 33–44.

Mehdizadeh, A., Vinel, A., Hu, Q., Schall, M., Jr., Gallagher, S., & Sesek, R. (2020). Job rotation and work-related musculoskeletal disorders: A fatigue-failure perspective. *Ergonomics*, *63*, 461–476.

Miner, M. A. (1945). Cumulative damage in fatigue. *Journal of Applied Mechanics*, *16*, A159–A164.

Moore, J., & Garg, A. (1995). The strain index: A proposed method to analyze jobs for risk of distal upper extremity disorders. *American Industrial Hygiene Association Journal*, *56*, 443–458.

Nash, J. C. (1966). *Fatigue of self-healing structure: A generalized theory of fatigue failure*. New York: American Society of Mechanical Engineers.

Palmgren, A. (1924). Die Lebebsdaue rvon Kugellagern. *Zeitschrift des Vereines Deutscher Ingenieure*, *68*, 339–341.

Potvin, J., Ciriello, V., Snook, S., Maynard, W., & Brogmus, G. (2021). The Liberty Mutual manual materials handling (LM-MMH) equations. *Ergonomics*. https://doi.org/10.1080/00140139.2021.1891297

Radwin, R. G. (2011, September). Automated video exposure assessment of repetitive motion. In *Proceedings of the human factors and ergonomics society annual meeting* (Vol. 55, No. 1, pp. 995–996). Sage CA: Los Angeles, CA: SAGE Publications.

Rankine, W. (1843). On the causes of the unexpected breakage of the journals of railway axles, and on the means of preventing such accidents by observing the law of continuity in their construction. *Minutes of the Proceedings of the Institution of the Institution of Civil Engineers* (pp. 105–107). London: Institution of Civil Engineers.

Rempel, D. (2018). 1631c Recent changes to the ACGIH hand activity level TLV. *Occupational and Environmental Medicine, 75*(Suppl 2), A258–A258.

Schechtman, H., & Bader, D. (1997). In vitro fatigue of human tendons. *Journal of Biomechanics*, 829–835.

Snook, S. (1978). The design of manual handling tasks. *Ergonomics, 21*, 963–985.

Snook, S., & Ciriello, V. (1991). The design of manual handling tasks: Revised tables of maximum acceptable weights and forces. *Ergonomics, 34*, 1197–1213.

Stephens, R., Fatemi, A., Stephens, R., & Fuchs, H. (2001). *Metal fatigue in engineering* (2nd ed.). New York: John Wiley & Sons.

Sun, H., Andarawis-Puri, N., Li, Y., Fung, D., Lee, J., Wang, V., . . . Flatow, E. L. (2010). Cycle-dependent matric remodeling gene expression response in fatigue-loaded rat patellar tendons. *Journal of Orthopaedic Research, 28*, 1380–1386.

Thornton, G., Schwab, T., & Oxland, T. R. (2007). Cyclic loading causes faster rupture and strain rate than static loading in medial collateral ligament at high stress. *Clinical Biomechanics, 22*, 932–940.

United States Bone and Joint Initiative. (2021, January). *The burden of musculoskeletal diseases in the United States (BMUS)*, (3rd ed.), 2014. Rosemont, IL. Retrieved from http://www.boneandjointburden.org.

Waters, T., Putz-Anderson, V., Garg, A., & Fine, L. (1993). Revised NIOSH equation for the design and evaluation of manual lifting tasks. *Ergonomics, 36*, 749–776.

Weightman, B., Chappell, D., & Jenkins, E. (1978). A second study of tensile fatigue properties of human articular cartilage. *Annals of the Rheumatic Diseases, 37*, 58–63.

Wright, J., Carroll, L., Sham, T.-L., Lybeck, N., & Wright, R. (2016). Determination of the creep–fatigue interaction diagram for alloy 617. *Proceedings of the ASME 2016 Pressure Vessels and Piping Conference (PVP2016)* (p. 10). Vancouver, British Columbia, Canada: EPRI 2016 Creep Fatigue Workshop In Collaboration with ASME PVP.

2

Common Musculoskeletal Disorders

Overview

For the purpose of this book, the term "musculoskeletal disorders" (MSDs) refers to "conditions involving the experience of pain, discomfort, and/or disability in the human musculoskeletal system, usually as the result of cumulative damage to one or more of the components of this system, including muscles, tendons, ligaments, nerves, cartilage, ligaments, bone, and/or fascia." Note that this definition excludes musculoskeletal injuries that might occur due to slips, trips, or falls (acute injuries). Instead, MSDs are viewed to be the consequence of exposure to repetitive stress resulting from occupational tasks, athletic pursuits, and other physical activities.

Terms used to describe MSDs over the past several decades include "repetitive stress injuries," "repetitive strain injuries," "cumulative trauma disorders," and "cumulative trauma injuries" (National Research Council – Institute of Medicine, 2001). These labels seem to imply that musculoskeletal injuries/disorders result from (a) exposure of musculoskeletal tissues to stress/strain, (b) the stress/strain application is repetitive in nature, and (c) that the repetitive stress/strain results in the development of cumulative trauma to the tissues. Thus, the very terms used to describe these disorders over the years seem to intuit the presence of a fatigue failure process in the development of MSDs. In fact, the terms above may actually be better descriptors of the actual injury process, as opposed to the all-encompassing (but vague) term "MSDs." However, in this book, we will use the latter term due to its standard current usage.

Burden of MSDs

MSDs account for a large societal and economic burden throughout the world. The burden associated with low back pain (LBP) was particularly notable, as its prevalence can be up to 20% in some countries (Fatoye, Gebrye, & Odeyemi, 2019). MSDs, as a whole, accounted for an average of 16% of years lived with disability (YLDs) worldwide in 2017 (Global Burden of Disease 2017 Disease and Injury Incidence and Prevalence Collaborators, 2018). These disorders were seen as a major reason for rising YLD rates per person in this analysis. These increases were attributed to tendencies toward greater age, obesity, and physical inactivity. MSDs were also seen to be an important driver of health care expenditures in middle- to high-income countries (Global Burden of Disease 2017 Disease and Injury Incidence and Prevalence Collaborators, 2018).

In an earlier analysis, a considerable proportion of LBP worldwide was attributed to occupational exposure (Punnett, 2005). On average, 37% of LBP was determined to be workplace related,

Musculoskeletal Disorders: The Fatigue Failure Mechanism, First Edition. Sean Gallagher and Mary F. Barbe.

with considerable variation across different regions of the world. Men had a higher attributable proportion than women, ostensibly due to higher exposure to occupations involving occupational lifting tasks and whole-body vibration. Approximately 818,000 disability-adjusted life years were lost annually due to the occupationally related LBP (Punnett, 2005).

The global burden associated with upper extremity MSDs is somewhat less clear due to the lack of a systematic method of defining cases. Studies have shown that the percentage of office workers who suffer from MSDs ranges from 20 to 60% worldwide (Global Burden of Disease 2017 Disease and Injury Incidence and Prevalence Collaborators, 2018). One older study from the United States reported lifetime prevalence of upper extremity (UE) MSDs of 29% in dentists (Stockstill, Harn, Strickland, & Hruska, 1993). Unfortunately, case definitions used by different researchers differed dramatically; thus, global estimates were not possible (Huisstede, Bierma-Zeinstra, Koes, & Verhaar, 2006). In Europe, MSDs are the leading cause of loss of productivity, sickness absence, and work disability across all European Union (EU) member states. Lost productivity due to MSDs is estimated to represent approximately 2% of the EU gross domestic product (Bevan, 2015).

Clearly, MSDs exact a significant toll on individuals throughout the globe. Not only do these afflictions result in terrible burdens with respect to human disability and suffering, but there are also enormous economic and societal prices to be paid. Any attempt to reduce the effects of these MSD sequelae is clearly more than just a formidable challenge. It should be apparent that the complete control of these disorders, or even a sizable portion of them, is currently well beyond our grasp. Gaining a better understanding of the processes associated with the development of damage in musculoskeletal tissues and physiological mechanisms associated with both damage and repair of these tissues may help our ability to exert some modest degree of control over injury risk (or improved healing) in some circumstances. However, we clearly need to understand our adversary better. To start this process, we will begin by providing a brief review of some of the more common MSDs, providing descriptions and characteristic features of the disorders, prevalence and incidence data, relevant anatomy and pathology, and the risk factors or activities associated with the development of the disorders.

As can be seen below, this review focuses on MSDs affecting the low back, hands/wrists, elbows, and shoulders. While disorders affecting the hips, knees, and ankles are of interest to many musculoskeletal researchers, our emphasis is on the occupational setting, in which the former disorders tend to predominate.

Common Musculoskeletal Disorders

Low Back Pain

Description/characteristic features

LBP is a typically benign condition, though one of the most expensive conditions in industrialized countries (Mayer & Gatchel, 1988). It is associated with substantial loss in the quality of life (Punnett, 2005). LBP is characterized by pain that can range from a dull ache to a sharp, intense, and disabling pain. The focus of this pain is generally in and around the lumbar portion of the spinal column. The lumbar spine is a complex structure, consisting of vertebral bones, intervertebral discs, cartilage endplates, and nerves, and with all of these structures, there are many possible sources of pain.

LBP is often episodic, with most cases being relatively short-lived. In fact, 40–90% of people obtain complete relief after 6 weeks (Manchikanti, 2000). LBP is often classified by duration as acute (pain lasting less than 6 weeks), sub-chronic (6–12 weeks), or chronic (more than 12 weeks) (Koes et al., 2010). The condition may be further classified by the underlying cause as mechanical, nonmechanical, or referred pain (Manusov, 2012). While most pain is self-limited, pain continuing after 3 months of LBP is considered chronic, as this is well beyond the 6- to 12-week time period that normal connective tissues take to heal (Chawla, 2018).

Recent data suggest that approximately 38.5% of work-related MSDs in the United States in 2016 involved the lower back (Bureau of Labor Statistics, 2018). Many occupational tasks have been associated with a higher prevalence of recurrent LBP, including lifting and/or carrying heavy weight and adoption of awkward postures such as bending, twisting, squatting, and kneeling (Amorim et al., 2019; Hoogendoorn, Poppel, Bongers, Koes, & Bouter, 1999). Exposure to whole-body vibration in drivers (e.g., tractor drivers, taxi drivers, and helicopter pilots) appears to contribute heavily to LBP risk (Bovenzi, Schust, & Mauro, 2017), as does adoption of awkward postures when driving (Bovenzi, Schust, Menzel, Prodi, & Mauro, 2015). In the professional driving occupations cited earlier, there is also an exposure-dependent increase in the development of degenerative changes in the spinal column, resulting in spondylolisthesis (Byeon et al., 2013; Chen, Chan, Katz, Chang, & Christian, 2004; Christ & Dupuis, 1966; Froom et al., 1984). The degenerative changes referenced earlier are thought to be due to repetitive mechanical loading and shock to the spinal column that lead to damage accumulation and degeneration (Bovenzi et al., 2017). Individual differences likely impact the effects of loading due to differences in muscle mass and strength as well as due to differences in kinematic and muscle recruitment strategies (Gallagher & Heberger, 2015; Marras et al., 2006).

Prevalence/incidence

LBP is the most common MSD with lifetime prevalence estimates ranging from 65 to 80% (Manchikanti, 2000). Approximately 9–12% of people (632 million) have LBP at any given point in time, and nearly 25% report having it at some point over a 1-month period (Mayer & Gatchel, 1988; Waddell, 1987). Estimates of the annual prevalence of LBP range from 15 to 45% with a point prevalence of approximately 30% (Andersson, 1999). Sixty percent of those who suffer from acute LBP recover in 6 weeks and up to 80–90% recover within 12 weeks; however, the recovery of the remaining patients with LBP is less certain (Andersson, 1999).

Historical data suggest that in Americans less than 45 years of age, chronic LBP is the commonest cause of disability (Kelsey & White 3rd, 1980; Waddell, 1987). Each year, 3–4% of the US population is temporarily disabled, and 1% of the working-age population is totally and permanently disabled by LBP (Andersson, 1999; Cunningham & Kelsey, 1984; Mayer & Gatchel, 1988). Difficulty most often begins between 20 and 40 years of age (Casazza, 2012). Men and women are approximately equally affected ("Back Pain Fact Sheet", NINDS, 2014). LBP is more common among people aged between 40 and 80 years, with the overall number of individuals affected expected to increase as the population ages (Hoy, 2012).

Although common in the general population, there is considerable evidence that LBP risk is exacerbated by the performance of occupational tasks, and account for a significant portion of morbidity in occupational settings. A great deal of evidence suggests that heavy physical work, repetitive lifting, prolonged static work postures, bending and twisting, and exposure to whole-body vibration likely contribute to the development of LBP (National Institute for Occupational Safety and Health [NIOSH], 1997; National Research Council – Institute of Medicine, 2001). Jobs that are highly demanding, that involve prolonged standing, and that require awkward lifting are among work-related physical risk factors for LBP (Sterud & Tynes, 2013).

Anatomy/pathology

The lumbar spine is a complex structure composed of several different materials (see Figures 2.1–2.3), many of which have been touted as potential sources of LBP. Some of the

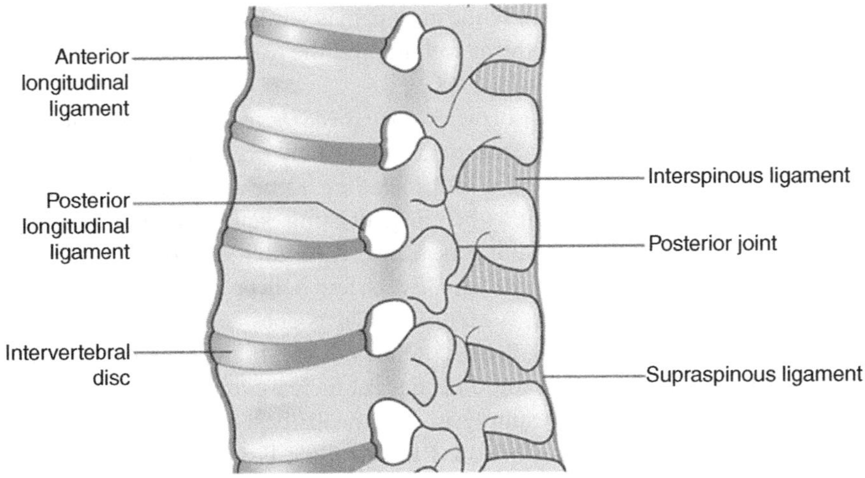

Figure 2.1 A motion segment of the lumbar spine. Duckworth, T. & Blundell, C. M. (2010). *Lecture notes: Orthopaedics and fractures*, 4th ed., Wiley. ISBN: 978-1-405-13329-6.

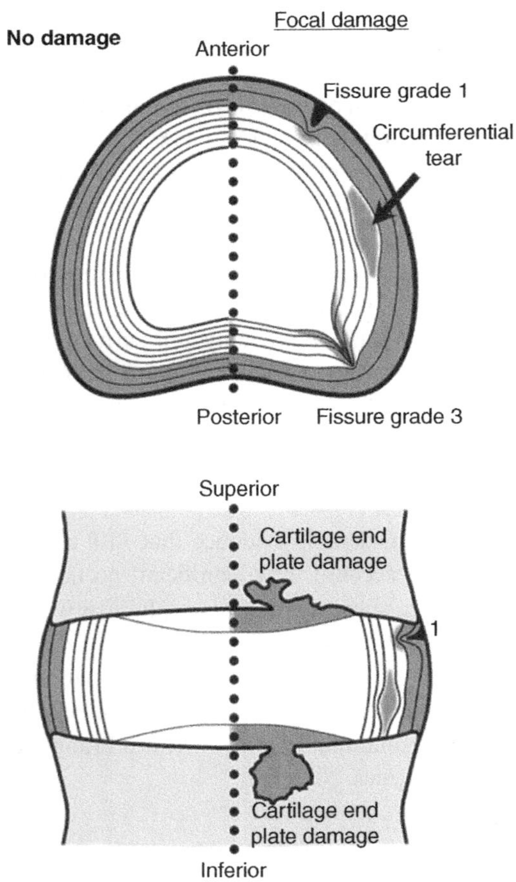

Figure 2.2 Focal damage in the intervertebral disc. Fissures of grade 1 (grade 2 not shown) and circumferential tears are not likely to be symptomatic. However, grade 3 fissures are highly associated with chronic back pain. Cartilage endplate damage is also shown. Fournier, D.E., Kiser P.K., Shoemaker, J.K., Battié, M.C., & Séguin, C.A. (2020). Vascularization of the human intervertebral disc: a scoping review. *JOR Spine, 3(4):* e1123. doi: 10.1002/jsp2.1123 / John Wiley & Sons / CC BY-4.0.

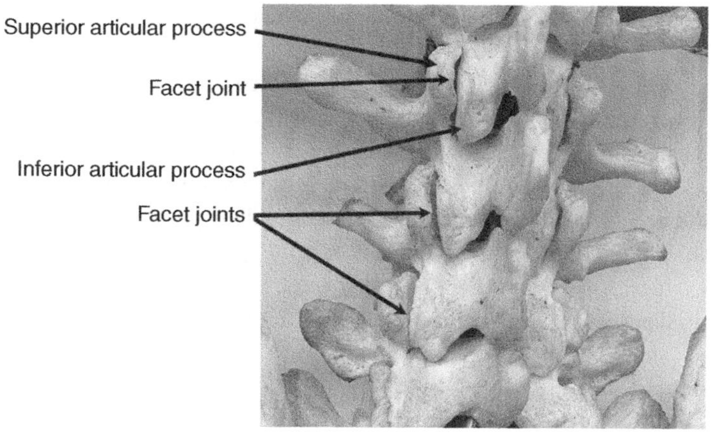

Figure 2.3 Lumbar vertebrae and their facet (zygopophyseal) joints, which are the articulation of superior and inferior processes.

potential pain-generating structures include the intervertebral disk, facet (zygopophyseal) and sacroiliac joints, spinal nerve roots, and the muscles that attach to the bony processes of the vertebra (Chawla, 2018).

The intervertebral disc has been shown to be a structure capable of causing pain. Kuslich, Ulstrom, and Michael (1991) demonstrated that pain could be elicited by the use of surgical instruments or a low voltage electrical current stimulating the annulus fibrosis of the disc. The process of internal degeneration of the disc has also been implicated in the development of pain (Bogduk, Aprill, & Derby, 2013). Specifically, fissures radiating outward from the nucleus pulposus as the disc degenerates appear to be highly correlated with pain report from patients, especially as these fissures move into the outer third of the disc, where pain fibers are known to exist (Figure 2.2). The action of proinflammatory cytokines has also been implicated in the development of intervertebral disc pain (Zhang, 2016). The slow rate of tissue repair in the poorly perfused intervertebral disc has been suggested as a possible factor in patients experiencing chronic LBP (Chawla, 2018).

Facet joints (Figure 2.3), or more properly zygopophyseal joints, are a small set of joints formed by the superior and inferior articular processes of adjacent vertebrae. These joints are believed, when loaded, to develop wear and tear of the gliding surfaces of the joint, which may lead to arthritis over time (Eisenstein & Parry, 1987; Farfan, 1973). Bending forward and/or side-to-side bending is believed to place damaging stress concentrations on the cartilage surface of the joints, leading to degeneration (Farfan, 1973). As the facet joint begins to degenerate, small defects in the joint surfaces appear. As with the disc, the cartilage surfaces of the facet joints have limited blood supply, which impedes the body's ability to repair the damage. This limited repair capacity makes the facet joint susceptible to degeneration. In fact, degeneration of the facet joints is believed by some to be a result of disc degeneration (Vernon-Roberts & Pirie, 1977). This is because when a disc degenerates, it loses height. When this occurs, it causes the bone and cartilage of the facet joint (normally separated) to come into contact and grind against each other, causing degeneration of the surfaces. Studies have suggested that up to 45% of patients with back pain demonstrate facet pain and that approximately 15% of chronic LBP cases may be due to facet joint pain (Schwarzer, Aprill, & Bogduk, 1995).

The sacroiliac joint is formed where the sacrum of the spine joins the iliac bone in the pelvis, is innervated by the first four sacral nerves, and is a demonstrated source of LBP (Schwarzer et al., 1995). Data from studies involving nerve-blocking agents suggest the prevalence of sacroiliac pain to be 2–30% in chronic LBP sufferers (Chawla, 2018).

Pathological mechanisms associated with spinal nerve root pain (or radicular pain) are not well understood. It has been hypothesized that spinal nerve roots may be vulnerable to compression, potentially leading to pain. Some early studies found that nerve roots might exhibit an inflammatory response when exposed to viable nucleus pulposus material from an intervertebral disc (McCarron, Wimpee, Hudkins, & Laros, 1987). However, degenerated nucleus pulposus material appears not to provoke such an inflammatory response (Chawla, 2018). Exposure of spinal nerve roots to the proinflammatory cytokine TNF-α is another suggested cause, as it would be expected to provoke neuropathic pain in spinal nerves (Klyne, Barbe, & Hodges, 2017; Klyne & Hodges, 2020).

Physical risk factors/activities associated with LBP

Most experts agree that heavy physical work, lifting, prolonged static work postures, frequent bending and twisting, and exposure to vibration may contribute to back injuries. A systematic review of physical work factors performed by the NIOSH found strong evidence of a causal relationship between both lifting/forceful movements and exposure to whole-body vibration and LBP. Evidence suggesting a causal relationship to LBP was also found for adoption of awkward postures and heavy physical work (NIOSH, 1997). A further systematic review performed by the (National Research Council–Institute of Medicine, 2001) demonstrated that activities such as manual materials handling, frequent twisting and bending, heavy physical load, and exposure to whole-body vibration demonstrated positive association to risk of low back disorders in the preponderance of studies investigating such factors. These findings have been supported by more recent data on the relationship between LBP and occupational activities, in which tasks such as carrying, lifting heavy weight while in trunk flexion, and adoption of awkward postures (including bending, squatting, twisting, and kneeling) demonstrated higher LBP risk (Amorim et al., 2019).

UE Tendon and Muscle Disorders

MSDs of the distal UE are prevalent in the working world and have substantial economic costs (Dale et al., 2013; Descatha, Leclerc, Chastang, & Roquelaure, 2003; Gerr et al., 2002; Silverstein et al., 2010; Tanaka, Petersen, & Cameron, 2001). These MSDs can affect each segment of the upper extremity, from the shoulder to the hand. Risk factors for wrist and hand MSDs include repetitive pushing, hand force, combined exposure to both force and repetition, sustained gripping (e.g., computer or hand tool use), repetitive redundant movement of the thumb and digits (e.g., typing or texting), sustained or repeated static loading of the weight of an instrument or tool, and use of vibrating tools (Barr, Barbe, & Clark, 2004; Fry, 1986; Gold, Mohamed, Ali, & Barbe, 2014; Gupta & Mahalanabis, 2006; Kakosy, Nemeth, Kiss, Laszloffy, & Kardos, 2006).

Hand-intensive jobs that feature forceful and repetitive activities are associated with both the onset and severity of hand and wrist MSDs (Barr et al., 2004; Viikari-Juntura & Silverstein, 1999). Other physical risk factors shown to exacerbate risk include adoption of non-neutral wrist and forearm postures, sustained gripping, sustained or repeated static loading of the weight of an instrument or tool, high impact jolting, exposure to hand-arm vibration (HAV), and exposure to cold temperatures (NIOSH, 1997; NRC-IOM, 2001). Continuous movement of a joint into end of range, for example, with repeated hyperextension of metacarpophalangeal joints, may be another causative factor due to enhanced inflammation in joint and tendon tissues (Gold et al., 2014;

Walsh, Delahunt, & McCarthy, 2011). Individuals with prolonged heavy or one-sided hand workloads or increased high impact "jolting" of the hand show increased incidence of hand osteoarthritis, with higher incidence in females (Bernard, Wilder, Aluoch, & Leaverton, 2010; Blumenfeld et al., 2014; Rossignol et al., 2005). The following sections discuss some of the more common UE disorders, their characteristics, prevalence and incidence, anatomy and pathology, and risk factors.

Hand-wrist tendinopathy

Description/characteristic features Wrist tendinopathy is a broad term used to characterize disorders involving damage or irritation to tendons and/or their synovial sheaths located in and around the wrist joint. Such disorders comprise the most common complaints evaluated by hand care professionals (McCauliffe, 2010). These disorders were formerly characterized as wrist tendinitis; however, recent research has demonstrated that these disorders demonstrate relatively few inflammatory cells (McCauliffe, 2010). Instead, these tendon disorders often appear to be the result of a disruption in the structural integrity of the tendon. This has led some to prefer use of the term *tendinosis* (implying a breakdown in the collagen structure of a tendon) or the broader and more clinically used term *tendinopathy* (a term implying a general disease process of the tendon).

Wrist tendinopathy usually affects a single tendon, but in some cases, it involves two or more tendons. Symptoms may start with a mild pain that progressively worsens with continued activity. The pain often presents as diffuse, as opposed to a localized, and may extend up to the forearm or into the fingers. Pain may be variously described as a dull ache, a burning sensation, or a sharp stabbing pain. Symptoms may be so painful that they may result in significant adverse effects on the activities of daily living. Even common tasks such as turning doorknobs or lifting a coffee cup may prove painful. Symptoms more rarely observed include numbness, loss of motion, or pain at rest. Often, wrist tendinopathy occurs at points where the tendons cross each other or pass over a bony prominence. These are possible sites of irritation and can lead to discomfort when moving the wrist joint. De Quervain's disease is often characterized by the development of pain on palpation, stiffness, and a decrease in strength capacity in the affected areas. Other similar conditions are trigger thumb and triggering of the middle and ring fingers, characterized by pain with motion of the affected tendon.

Epidemiology (prevalence/incidence) MSDs involving the arm and hand account for only 5.1% of all work-related MSDs (Bureau of Labor Statistics, 2018), and disorders of the hand and wrist constitute 40% and 13%, respectively, of such cases (Bureau of Labor Statistics, 2015). Hand complaints are common among manual workers with self-reported prevalence generally around 30–45% (Thomsen et al., 2007). Symptoms are not always accompanied by clinical findings. Several studies found very low prevalence of wrist tendinopathy with swelling and/or crepitation but with a considerable variation—from no cases of clinical tenosynovitis at all, up to more than 18%, apparently with more or less the same case definition (Thomsen et al., 2007).

Tendinopathy cases of the hand and wrist (e.g., de Quervain's tenosynovitis) or fingers (e.g., trigger finger) numbered 4,896 in 2001 (Bureau of Labor Statistics, 2001). Evaluation of the incidence of de Quervain's disease among U.S. military personnel from 1998 through 2006 demonstrated that women had a significantly ($p < 0.0001$) higher rate of this disorder (2.8 cases per 1,000 person-years) compared to men (0.6 cases per 1,000 person-years). Other risk factors for de Quervain's disease in this population included age greater than 40 and greater incidence among blacks (Wolf, Sturdivant, & Owens, 2009).

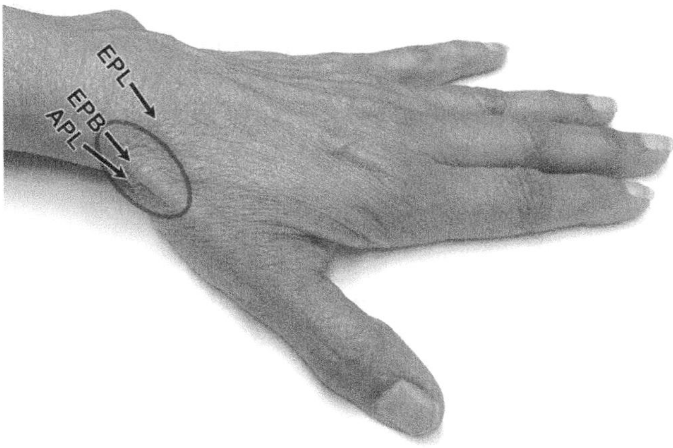

Figure 2.4 The site of de Quervain's syndrome is encircled. APL: abductor pollicis longus; EPB: extensor pollicis brevis; EPL: extensor pollicis longus.

Anatomy/pathology De Quervain's disease is a specific wrist tendinopathy involving the entrapment of the tendons of the extensor pollicis brevis and abductor pollicis longus. Figure 2.4 illustrates the region associated with the development of de Quervain's syndrome. Patients with de Quervain's disease (as well as trigger finger) tend to exhibit a lack of inflammation in the affected region (Clarke, 1998; Sbernardori & Bandiera, 2007). Instead, there appears to be a breakdown of tissues of the gliding layer of the tendon sheath. Examination of tendons tends to reveal nodularity and tendon fraying, which is thought to be secondary to impingement by the damaged sheath. Both disorders often exhibit the development of fibrotic tissue. In the case of de Quervain's syndrome, deposition of fibrotic tissue in the extensor retinaculum can be thickened up to five times greater than the thickness in control tissues (Clarke, 1998). Overall, signs point to a process of tissue degeneration as opposed to an inflammatory response, with the degeneration resulting from abnormal mechanical stress being imposed on the tendon and the tendon sheath (McCauliffe, 2010).

Risk factors/activities associated with hand-wrist tendinopathy Tendinopathy of the hand, wrist, and forearm has long been associated with performance of forceful and repetitive hand activities as potential causal factors (e.g., Armstrong, 1987). Studies assessing risk factors associated with hand-wrist tendinopathy demonstrate that exposure to force, repetition, and non-neutral postures all demonstrate positive associations; however, the combination of force and repetition demonstrate the strongest relationship with these hand-wrist disorders (Armstrong, 1987; Barbe et al., 2013; Byström, Hall, Welander, & Kilbom, 1995; Kurrpa, Viikari-Juntura, Kuosma, Huuskonen, & Kivi, 1991; Luopajärvi, Kuorinka, Virolainen, & Holmberg, 1979; Roto & Kivi, 1984). The study by Kurrpa et al. (1991) was prospective in nature and found that greater time on the job was associated with increased risk of hand-wrist disorders, demonstrating temporality. Repetitive forceful activity of the thumb is often associated with the development of de Quervain's syndrome (Freivalds, 2004).

Lateral tendinopathy of the elbow

Characteristics/description Lateral epicondylitis (commonly referred to as "tennis elbow") is a disorder characterized by pain at or near the lateral epicondyle of the humerus. The pain may be localized to this region, may radiate down the extensor muscle group of the forearm, and occasionally may radiate proximally to the upper arm (Vaquero-Picado, Barco, & Antuña, 2017). This pain can be triggered or exacerbated by contraction of the common extensor mass in response to a variety of activities (Ahmad et al., 2013). Tenderness is most often exhibited at the site of the attachment of the extensor carpi radialis brevis (ECRB) tendon; however, pain and tenderness on palpation can also be experienced around the prominence of the lateral epicondyle. Pain intensity can be quite variable and manifest as intermittent and mild to constant and severe. The latter can affect a wide range of daily activities and may even occur at night, thereby causing a disturbance in sleep.

Epidemiology Studies suggest that the prevalence of lateral epicondylitis in the general population in the United Kingdom is approximately 1–3% and is more common in adults aged 35–55 years. Gender does not appear to play a significant role as to prevalence (Smidt & van der Windt, 2006). However, the examination of the prevalence rates of lateral epicondylitis in working populations provides a different picture. A study of the prevalence of lateral epicondylitis among workers at 12 worksites indicated a prevalence rate of 5.2% in the dominant arm (Fan et al., 2009). A Finnish study found that the true incidence of lateral epicondylitis was due to the overuse of or change in biomechanics as a result of elbow pain (Shiri, Viikari-Juntura, Varonen, & Heliövaara, 2006). Incidence was found to be variable depending on the criteria used to confirm the diagnosis. They found it to be definitely present in 1.3% of the population between the ages of 30 and 65 years and likely present in a further 2.98%.

Anatomy/pathology In lateral epicondylitis, it is believed that a common extensor tendon (a conglomeration of the tendons of the extensor carpi radialis brevis, the extensor digitorum, the extensor digiti minimi, and the extensor carpi ulnaris) is affected by progressive process of inflammation and then degeneration (Figure 2.5). The degeneration of the tendon is the result of repetitive application of stress, leading to the microtear development in the common tendon (Kraushaar & Nirschl, 1999). The accumulation and growth of microtears is the process by which tendinosis initiates and propagates in the tendon. If the tendon continues to experience stress in this region, these pathologic changes may ultimately lead to partial or complete rupture of the tendon (Kraushaar & Nirschl, 1999).

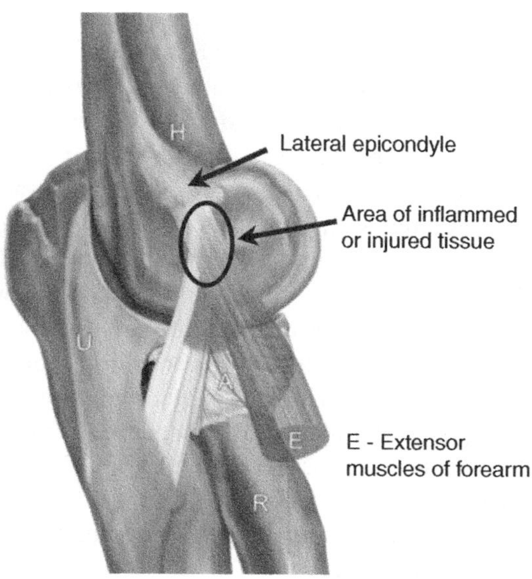

Figure 2.5 Location of inflamed or injured tissues in the extensor carpi radialis brevis (ECRB) tendon. Jacobson, J. A., Chiavaras, M. M., Lawton, J. M., Downie, B., Yablon, C.M., & Lawton, J. (2014). Radial collateral ligament of the elbow: Sonographic characterization with cadaveric dissection correlation and magnetic resonance arthrography. *Journal of Ultrasound in Medicine*, *33*(6), 1041–1048. DOI: 10.7863/ultra.33.6.1041. Wiley.

Risk factors/activities associated with lateral epicondylitis As the nickname "tennis elbow" suggests, this disorder is often associated with activities that require repetitive or prolonged gripping activities (such as a tennis racquet when playing tennis). Occupationally, tasks that require forceful, prolonged, or repetitive use of hand tools are often associated with the development of lateral epicondylitis. This disorder is also associated with the use of powered hand tools, such as hand drills or other powered drivers requiring repetitive and forceful exertions involving the forearm extensor muscles, especially if such activities are required of the worker throughout an entire workday. In addition, handling tools greater than 1 kg, weights in excess of 20 kg (more than 10 times per day), and repetitive activities greater than 2 hour/day have been implicated as occupational risk factors for lateral epicondylitis (Ahmad et al., 2013).

Medial elbow tendinopathy

Characteristics/description Medial epicondylitis is an overuse tendinopathy due to chronic repetitive concentric or eccentric loading of the wrist flexors and pronator teres, resulting in angiogenic and fibroblastic changes (Kiel & Kaiser, 2019). Although epicondylitis is most commonly experienced on the lateral side of the elbow, certain activities (often occupational tasks) that cause repeated stress on the elbow can lead to pain and discomfort affecting the medial epicondyle. Pain associated with medial epicondylitis is often localized to the medial epicondyle, sometimes with radiation to the proximal forearm (Amin, 2015). Pain associated with medial epicondylitis is often increased in activities involving wrist flexion or pronation (Kiel & Kaiser, 2019) This pathology is due to the development of microtrauma and degeneration of the common flexor tendon and is most commonly seen in patients above 40 years of age (Amin, 2015). The prognosis for medial epicondylitis is generally quite favorable. Most patients can return to work or athletic activities after activity modification and/or physical therapy treatment (Kiel & Kaiser, 2019).

Epidemiology Medial epicondylitis is much less prevalent than lateral epicondylitis; however, this disorder still accounts for approximately 10–20% of all epicondylitis (Shiri et al., 2006). According to one study, the prevalence in the general population is quite low, with only 0.4% afflicted. A significantly higher prevalence can be found in individuals participating in activities that repeatedly stress the tendons making up the common flexor tendon (i.e., the pronator teres, flexor carpi radialis, palmaris longus, flexor carpi ulnaris, and the flexor digitorum superficialis) (Kiel & Kaiser, 2019). In some occupational settings, the prevalence of medial epicondylitis has been found to range from 3.8 to 8.2% (Shiri et al., 2006; Descatha et al., 2003; Wolf et al., 2010). Three out of four cases are in the dominant arm. Medial epicondylitis is highest among subjects aged 45–64. Some studies suggest that the prevalence of this disorder in men and women appears roughly equivalent (Amin, 2015), but others have suggested greater prevalence in women (Kiel & Kaiser, 2019).

A study examining the prevalence of medial epicondylitis across five industrial sectors was reported by Descatha et al. (2003). This study indicated prevalence between 4 and 5%, with annual incidence estimated at 1.5% for this disorder. Forceful work was found to be a risk factor for medial epicondylitis but not exposure to repetitive work. Risk factors differed for medial and lateral epicondylitis. The prognosis for medial epicondylitis in this population was good with a 3-year recovery rate of 81% (Descatha et al., 2003). A later study suggested that forceful and repetitive wrist bending, forceful gripping, and rotating/twisting actions of the forearm were significantly associated with medial epicondylitis (Descatha, Dale, Jaegers, Herquelot, & Evanoff, 2013). Odds ratios for these three physical factors were not significant for exposures less than 2 hr/day, but all were significant for exposures greater than 4 hr/day. These findings suggest that repetition (in combination with force) was an important factor in the development of medial epicondylitis in these workers.

Anatomy/pathology The pathology associated with medial epicondylitis is similar to that of lateral epicondylitis; however, different activities may provide the requisite stress on the flexor tendons compared to those affecting the extensor tendons. As with medial epicondylitis repetitive activity leads exposure to forceful and repetitive activities is thought to lead to recurrent microtears in the tendon leading to the development of tendinosis. Although it was thought that the pronator teres and flexor carpi radialis were originally thought to be most commonly affected, more recent literature suggests all muscles may be equally affected, with the possible exception of the palmaris longus (Kiel & Kaiser, 2019). As the tendon undergoes repetitive microtears, there is remodeling of the collagen fibers and increased mucoid ground substance. Focal necrosis or calcification can occur. Subsequently, collagen strength decreases leading to increased fragility, scar tissue formation, and thickening of the tendon. Although less common, acute trauma can also cause medial epicondylitis from a sudden violent contraction of the muscles (Kiel & Kaiser, 2019).

Risk factors/activities associated with medial epicondylitis Medial epicondylitis is sometimes referred to as "Golfers Elbow"; however, numerous other repetitive athletic activities such as overhead throwing, bowling, and weightlifting have also been associated with the development of medial epicondylitis. However, 90% of cases appear not to be associated with athletic activities (Kiel & Kaiser, 2019). Studies have demonstrated that occupational risk factors include activities repeatedly stressing the flexor tendons including wrist bending, rotational motions of the forearm, and forceful gripping are associated with medial epicondylitis.

Shoulder tendinopathy (rotator cuff)

Characteristics/description Shoulder disorders are a common cause of occupational pain and disability in working populations. Rotator cuff disorders (RC) emerge as the dominant source of shoulder pain, accounting for an estimated 65–70% of all shoulder pain (Hales & Bernard, 1996). Symptoms of RC tendinopathy commonly include pain situated at the top and front of the shoulder or outer portion of the upper arm. Shoulder pain can progress from the anterolateral shoulder margin and lateral surface of the arm down to the elbow (Gumina et al., 2014). Pain can be exacerbated if the afflicted individual raises the arm or reaches back behind the body. These disorders are most commonly observed in middle-aged to older patients. Injuries to the shoulder are associated with longer than average recovery times compared to other occupational MSDs with a median of 26 days of lost work. Night pain can occur in 83% patients, and 41% may experience muscle weakness (van Kampen et al., 2014).

Epidemiology Several studies have been performed to assess the overall prevalence of shoulder pain in the general population. In general, prevalence rates tend to suggest overall prevalence rates of approximately 7–20% (Breivik, Collett, Ventafridda, & R., C., & Gallacher, D., 2005; Hasvold & Johnsen, 1993; Parsons et al., 2007; Pope, Croft, Pritchard, & Silman, 1997). In the workforce, MSDs involving the shoulder accounted for 14.9% of all work-related MSDs in the United States in 2016, with heavy tractor-trailer truck drivers and laborers/material movers having a greater proportion of injuries affecting the shoulder than other occupations (Bureau of Labor Statistics, 2018). However, certain personal characteristics have been shown to be influential in the experience of shoulder pain, particularly sex and age. Breakdown by sex show a consistently higher prevalence of shoulder pain in females than in males. Females typically have an approximately 10% higher prevalence than that reported in males (Breivik et al., 2005; Picavet & Schouten, 2003; Treaster & Burr, 2004). Age is another significant factor, with an increased general prevalence in older individuals and a notable increase of shoulder pain prevalence in the 45–64 age-group

(Pribicevik, 2012). In addition, adolescents aged 12–18 years appear to have a greater than average shoulder pain prevalence. In 2014, 88,980 nonfatal shoulder injuries and illnesses occurred that involved days away from work (Bureau of Labor Statistics, 2015).

A systematic review examining physical occupational risk factors for shoulder pain disclosed that jobs involving high force demands, highly repetitive work activities, adoption of non-neutral shoulder postures, and exposure to vibration and duration of employment were observed to be common physical occupational risk factors (Van der Windt, Thomas, & Pope, 2000). This review also examined psychosocial factors (e.g., job dissatisfaction, lack of control at work, poor social support, and/or psychological demands); however, while certain psychophysical factors were found to be significant, these factors were assessed to be inconsistent across the studies examined. Moderate to high levels of physical demand have commonly been associated with the development of shoulder pain (Ariens et al., 2000; Bergenudd, 1987; Devereux, Vlachonikolis, & Buckle, 2002; Malchaire, Cock, & Vergracht, 2001; Miranda, Punnett, Viikari-Juntura, Heliövaara, & Knekt, 2008). Exposure to vibration has also been implicated in the development of shoulder pain (Ariens et al., 2000; Miranda et al., 2008; Stenlund, Goldie, & Hagberg, 1993; van der Windt et al., 2000). Continuous low-intensity muscle contractions also increase the prevalence of neck-shoulder complaints and syndromes, including acromioclavicular syndrome (Balogh et al., 2019; Huysmans, Blatter, & Beek, 2012; Visser & van Dieen, 2006). Finally, the adoption of non-neutral shoulder postures has been associated with shoulder outcomes in a number of studies (Larsson, Sogaard, & Rosendal, 2007; Miranda et al., 2008; Pope et al., 1997; van der Windt et al., 2000). Many studies have failed to examine potential interactions between these physical risk factors; however, Frost and Andersen (1999) provide data suggestive of an interaction between force and repetition and shoulder tendinitis.

Anatomy/pathology Rotator cuff (RC) injuries are generally considered to be the result of a degenerative disorder of the RC tendons, which begins with acute tendinitis (inflammation) that leads to tendinosis (degeneration), ultimately leading to tendon tears (partial or full), as shown in Figure 2.6 (Neer, 1983). There is mounting evidence of some level of inflammation in all tendon injuries (Abraham, Shah, & Thomopoulos, 2017). Animal models of RC pathology in which the tissue are collected long before a surgical repair endpoint show clear evidence of inflammation in rotator cuff tendon proper, epitendon, or surrounding capsule (Abraham et al., 2017; Kietrys, Barr, & Barbe, 2011; Thomas et al., 2014). Yet, histological studies of the affected RC tendons tend to show a minimal amount of inflammatory cells at the time of surgery (Fukuda, Hamada, & Yamanaka, 1990), and serum biomarker studies of patients with long-term RC injuries show increased levels of circulating markers of enzymes that contribute to tissue degradation (matrix metalloproteinases), angiogenesis (increased production of vascular endothelial growth factor, VEGF), and axonal sprouting that may be related to the enhanced pain associated with RC injuries (summarized in Gold et al., 2016). These inflammation and degeneration changes are typically intrinsic factors that can enhance RC injuries (Seitz, McClure, Finucane, Boardman, & Michener, 2011). Extrinsic factors can also enhance RC injuries and impingement of the RC tendons. Some injuries are also thought to be the result of a combination of extrinsic and intrinsic factors.

Risk factors/activities associated with shoulder tendinopathy The development of RC disorders is associated with a number of factors, including personal characteristics (such as age and gender), occupational exposures, and certain sports-related activities. Among personal characteristics, factors such as gender and age tend to be most highly implicated in RC injuries (details). In terms

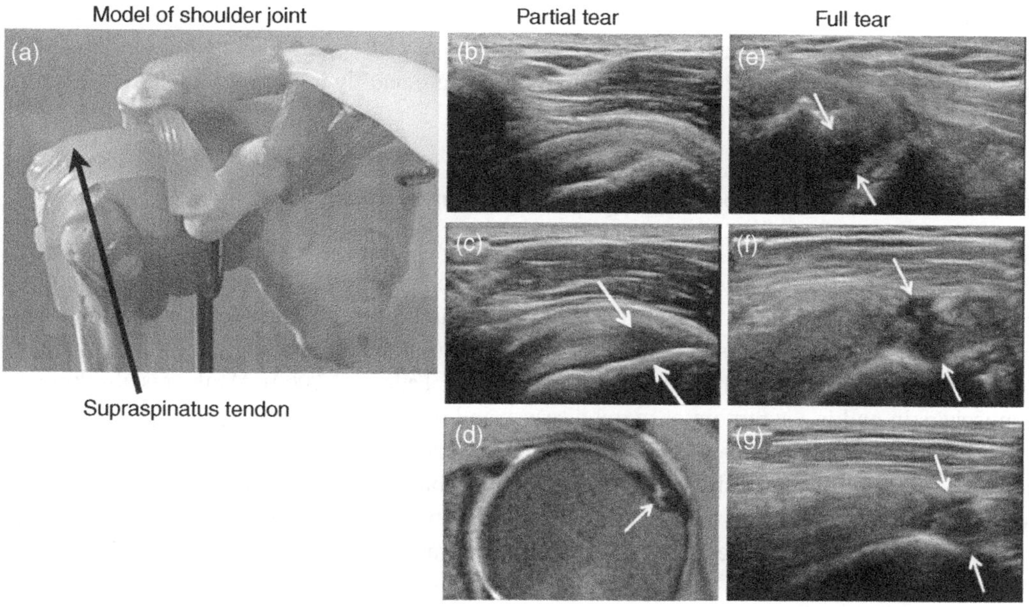

Figure 2.6 Partial and full tears in supraspinatus tendons, a rotator cuff tendon. (a) The location of the supraspinatus tendon. (b–d) X-ray images of a partial-thickness tear in the supraspinatus tendon. In a neutral position (b), a partial tear was not evident; hence, changes were interpreted as tendinosis. Crass position (c) and modified Crass position (d) show a hypoechoic region (arrows) interpreted as a partial tear in a fat-suppressed T2-weighted magnetic resonance image. (e and f) Full-thickness tear (arrows) of a supraspinatus tendon (arrows). Neutral position (e), Crass position (f), and modified Crass position (g). Modified from Shah, N. P., Miller, T. T., Stock, H., & Adler, R. S. (2012). Sonography of supraspinatus tendon abnormalities in the neutral versus Crass and modified Crass positions: A prospective study. *Journal of Ultrasound in Medicine*, *31*(8), 1203–1208. doi: 10.7863/jum.2012.31.8.1203. Wiley.

of physical exposures, a history of occupations involving heavy lifting and/or highly repetitive tasks has been linked to the increased risk of RC disorders, which often result in greater than average lost time from work compared to other MSDs. In terms of physical exposures, a history of occupations involving heavy lifting and/or highly repetitive tasks have been linked to increased risk of RC disorders, which often result in greater than average lost time from work compared to other MSDs. In 2014, 88,980 nonfatal shoulder injuries and illnesses occurred that involved days away from work (Bureau of Labor Statistics, 2015).

High shoulder pain prevalence is often seen in athletic pursuits, particularly those requiring forceful and repetitive motions that involve throwing or other activities where the hands and/or elbows are active above the level of the shoulder. High stresses are placed on the shoulder in activities such as baseball pitching, football throwing, tennis, volleyball, and swimming. These repetitive high-stress activities are likely to result in microdamage and damage propagation that may exceed the repair capacity of shoulder musculoskeletal tissues (Bani Hani et al., 2021).

Subacromial impingement may also occur at the subacromial joint. It is thought to be the result of fatigue in the stabilizing structures of the shoulder (the tendons and ligaments), resulting in humeral subluxation and subsequent impingement of the supraspinatus tendon between the head of the humerus and the inferior surface of the acromion. It has been reported that the most frequent shoulder diagnoses in athletes involve RC dysfunction with signs of supraspinatus tendon impingement (Baring, Emery, & Reilly, 2007; McHardy, Pollard, & Luo, 2007; Pink & Tibone, 2000).

That said, there can also be degenerative changes in the joint structure itself. In one study, the frequency of radiologically detected lesions in shoulders of 152 miners using vibration tools was 40.7% and included degenerative changes (34.5%) that were mainly in the acromioclavicular joint (17.8%) (Kakosy et al., 2006).

Upper Extremity Muscle Disorders: Fatigue, Myalgia, and Fibrosis

Characteristics/description

Muscle fatigue denotes a transient decrease in the force and power capacity of skeletal muscle activity (Enoka & Duchateau, 2008). Repetitive or sustained contraction of skeletal muscle can lead to a progressive and reversible loss in the ability to produce the desired force (Allen, Lamb, & Westerblad, 2008; Ortenblad, Lunde, Levin, Andersen, & Pedersen, 2000). Myalgia is also known as muscle pain and is a symptom of many diseases and disorders, including prolonged repetitive work (Bongers, Ijmker, Heuvel, & Blatter, 2006; Hadrevi et al., 2019; Sjøgaard, Lundberg, & Kadefors, 2000). Muscle fibrosis is characterized by fibroblast and myofibroblast cell proliferation and excessive accumulation of extracellular matrix proteins in fascial tissues, such as collagen and fibronectin (Contreras, Rebolledo, Oyarzun, Olguin, & Brandan, 2016; Fisher et al., 2015). Muscle fibrosis is also associated with increased muscle pain (Fisher et al., 2015; Pavan, Stecco, Stern, & Stecco, 2014), presumably as a secondary consequence of nerve pain receptors becoming enmeshed in the fibrosing fascial tissues (Fisher et al., 2015; Pavan et al., 2014).

Epidemiology

Prolonged standing work and intense training are associated with MSDs and muscle fatigue is considered a precursor to MSDs (Garcia, Laubli, & Martin, 2015; Hadrevi et al., 2019). However, the myriad of underlying possible reasons muscle fatigue discussed in the following section makes epidemiological studies difficult. Work-related muscle pain (myalgia) is considered a public health problem causing otherwise healthy individuals to end up on sick leave (Holtermann, Hansen, Burr, & Sogaard, 2010). Neck pain is one of the more common MSDs, with over 30% of individuals experiencing some degree of discomfort in the neck over a lifetime (Cohen, 2015; Cote, Cassidy, & Carroll, 1998). Most episodes of acute neck pain will resolve with or without treatment, but nearly 50% of individuals will continue to experience some degree of pain or frequent occurrences. A "tissue fibrosis" hypothesis is supported by clinical studies examining biopsies from patients with chronic MSDs (Dennett & Fry, 1988; Ettema, Amadio, Zhao, Wold, & An, 2004; Hirata et al., 2005).

Anatomy/pathology

The origin of muscle fatigue (specifically, a progressive and reversible loss in the ability to produce the desired force) is complex. Muscle fatigue occurs along with physiological changes that reflect changes in the balance between muscular demand and vascular supply (Cote, 2014; Yang, Leitkam, & Cote, 2019). This latter imbalance has also been termed an "energy crisis" (Simons & Travell, 1981). Muscle fatigue can also arise with alterations in neuromuscular junctions, neurotransmitters released from peripheral nerves after tissue damage, and axonal neuropathy if compressive nerve injury develops (Zajac, Chalimoniuk, Maszczyk, Golas, & Lngfort, 2015). Chronic inflammation, which can occur after prolonged high demand tasks, has a direct deleterious effect on skeletal muscles, decreasing force and muscle quality. Persistent elevations of systemic tumor necrosis factor alpha (TNF-α) is a primary endocrine stimulus for contractile dysfunction (Argiles, Campos, Lopez-Pedrosa, Rueda, & Rodriguez-Manas, 2016; Leal, Lopes, & Batista Jr., 2018; So, Kim, Kim, &

Song, 2014). Dependent on the magnitude of mechanical myofiber damage, muscle strength can decline. Substantial muscle damage also induces myofiber apoptosis and a loss of muscle mass. Aging enhances muscle dysfunction due to age-dependent increase in inflammatory responses and cell apoptosis and reduced repair mechanisms (Argiles et al., 2016). Additionally, the Cinderella Hypothesis of a hierarchical recruitment of smaller motor units disproportionately over larger units may provide insight into muscle fatigue (Enoka & Duchateau, 2008). In this hypothesis, the first recruited units are the smallest muscle units, which allow for the fine-tuning of force applied during delicate tasks. These small motor units may also be the last to be relaxed during prolonged muscle contractions. Only as the load reaches the maximum values, larger units are recruited. Thus, the smaller fibers may be more susceptible to an energy crisis of muscle fatigue and pain signaling (Enoka & Duchateau, 2008).

Another cause of physiological muscle fatigue can be altered myocellular calcium [Ca^{2+}] regulation, sarcoplasmic reticulum Ca^{2+} handling, and sarcoplasmic reticulum protein expression, all occurring as a result of chronic muscle overload, as summarized in Figure 2.7. (Allen et al., 2008; Hadrevi et al., 2019; Ortenblad et al., 2000). The process of controlling the production of force within the muscle, known as excitation–contraction–relaxation coupling, requires a tight regulation of the intracellular cytosolic free Ca^{2+} concentration ($[Ca^{2+}]_i$) in muscle enabling activation of the contractile apparatus, while protecting the cell from deleterious $[Ca^{2+}]_i$ overload. This is permitted through an instantaneous release of large amounts of Ca^{2+} through the sarcoplasmic reticulum Ca^{2+} release channel and ryanodine receptor (RyR), thereby increasing $[Ca^{2+}]_i$ and a subsequent, almost simultaneous reuptake of Ca^{2+} into the SR by the SR ATPases (SERCA)

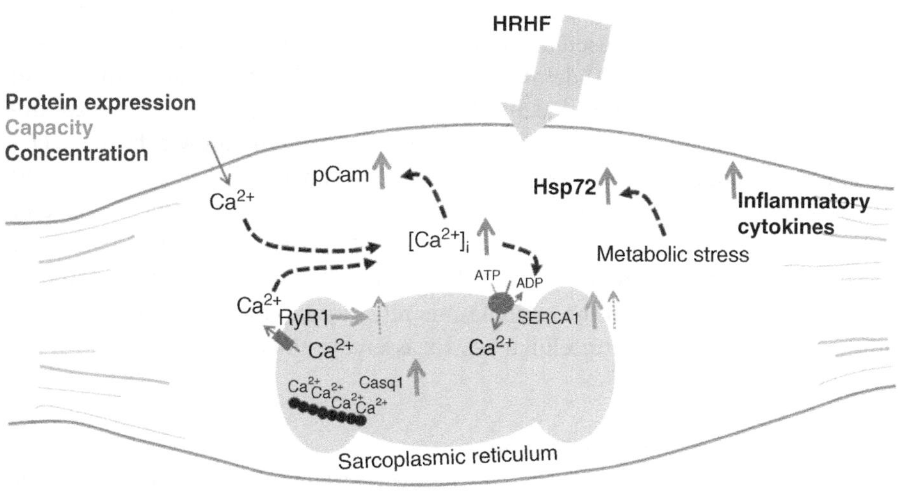

Figure 2.7 A model for possible early and late events in muscle response to a repetitive high repetition high force (HRHF) upper extremity task for 6 weeks. Exposure to the HRHF task induces an impaired muscle Ca^{2+} homeostasis, leading to an increase in $[Ca^{2+}]_i$ as indicated by an increase in pCalmodulin kinase (pCAM). The increased $[Ca^{2+}]_i$ may be mediated by leaky ryanodine receptor 1 (RyR1) with or without an uptake of extracellular Ca^{2+}. Furthermore, HRHF induces muscle metabolic stress indicated by an increase in muscle heat shock protein 72 (Hsp72). The increased $[Ca^{2+}]_i$ is accompanied by an increased sarco/endoplasmic reticulum vesicle Ca^{2+} uptake rate and sarco/endoplasmic reticulum Ca^{2+}-ATPase (SERCA1) together with increased calcequestrin (Casq1), which may lead to an enhanced sarcoplasmic reticulum Ca^{2+} buffering capacity. The model points to an altered myocellular Ca^{2+} handling as an early adaptation to muscle overload. Hadrevi, J., Barbe, M. F., Ortenblad, N., Frandsen, U., Boyle, E., Lazar, S., ... Sogaard, K. (2019). Calcium fluxes in work-related muscle disorder: Implications from a rat model. *BioMed Research International*, 2019, 5040818. doi:10.1155/2019/5040818 / Hindawi / CC BY-4.0.

together with buffering of Ca^{2+} inside the sarcoplasmic reticulum by the protein calcequestrin (Casq1) (Berchtold, Brinkmeier, & Muntener, 2000; Ortenblad & Stephenson, 2003; Periasamy & Kalyanasundaram, 2007).

Muscle myalgia (i.e., muscle pain) is associated with muscle stiffness, weakness, and increased tension (Ohlsson, Attewell, Johnsson, Ahlm, & Skerfving, 1994). Like muscle fatigue, dysfunctional Ca^{2+} homeostasis has been implicated in skeletal muscles of patients suffering from chronic neck and shoulder pain (Hadrevi, Ghafouri, Larsson, Gerdle, & Hellström, 2013). A study of biopsied myalgic muscle from human subjects showed a decreased abundance of calcequestrin (Casq1) together with an increased abundance of sarco/endoplasmic reticulum Ca^{2+}-ATPase (SERCA1) (Hadrevi et al., 2016). This may indicate an increased uptake of Ca^{2+} into the sarcoplasmic reticulum, although with a reduced buffering capacity in that structure. Additionally, increased interstitial concentrations of inflammatory mediators, such as bradykinins, kallidin, lactate, pyruvate, and K^+, have been found in patients with chronic severe trapezius myalgia (Gerdle et al., 2008; Gerdle et al., 2014). Injections of pro-inflammatory cytokines such as tumor necrosis factor alpha have also been shown to increase muscle pain/myalgia by activating the firing of pain-related nerve fibers (i.e., nociceptors) (Kehl, Trempe, & Hargreaves, 2000; Schafers, Sorkin, & Sommer, 2003).

Muscle fibrosis is also hypothesized to be a key factor in motor dysfunction, increased discomfort, and pain observed in patients with MSDs (Backman, Andersson, Wennstig, Forsgren, & Danielson, 2011; Barbe, Gallagher, & Popoff, 2013a; Barbe et al., 2013b; Stauber, 2004). Tissue fibrosis is thought to distort dynamic properties of tissue and contribute to functional declines perhaps due to adherence of adjacent structures or encapsulation of nerve related pain fibers (Driscoll & Blyum, 2011; Fisher et al., 2015; Pavan et al., 2014; Zugel et al., 2018). Fibrotic muscle changes may occur at any point in the musculotendinous unit including within the muscle fibers and at the musculotendinous junction (Abdelmagid et al., 2012; Fedorczyk et al., 2010; Fisher et al., 2015; Hilliard, Amin, Popoff, & Barbe, 2020). There are several possibilities for the continued increase in fibrogenic proteins (which include collagen, transforming growth factor beta 1 (TGF-β1), and connective tissue growth factor/cell communication network factor 2 (CTGF/CCN2) and in the assembly and remodeling of the extracellular matrix with chronic overload or repeated injury, including (a) dysregulation of negative feedback loops and therefore continued translation of fibrogenic proteins from their mRNA; (b) upregulated export of important extracellular matrix proteins, like collagen, from the endoplasmic reticulum to the extracellular matrix; and (c) a shift in the balance between extracellular matrix assembly and degradation to favor the assembly of extracellular matrix.

Risk factors/activities associated with muscle disorders

Repetitive work tasks are known risk factors for causing work-related musculoskeletal chronic muscle pain and fatigue (Bongers et al., 2006; Larsson et al., 2007; Sjøgaard et al., 2000). In normal skeletal muscle, highly repetitive and high force work tasks can independently induce muscle inflammation and fibrosis, concomitant with muscle pain and weakness, with greater pathology when the two risk factors are combined (Barbe, Gallagher, Massicotte, et al., 2013b; Barbe, Gallagher, & Popoff, 2013a; Fisher et al., 2015; Hilliard et al., 2020). Exposure-dependent fibrogenic changes have been observed in an operant rat model of work (repetitive reaching and grasping a varied load levels), with longer duration and higher repetitive and force demand tasks inducing greater tissue fibrosis than shorter or easier tasks, with evidence of inflammation at earlier time points and more fibrosis at later time points after inflammation has resolved (Barbe, Gallagher, Massicotte, et al., 2013b; Barbe, Gallagher, & Popoff, 2013a).

Nerve Disorders

Carpal tunnel syndrome (median nerve entrapment or irritation)

Characteristics/description Carpal tunnel syndrome (CTS) is a hand and wrist disorder caused by nerve entrapment of the median nerve in the wrist (Figure 2.8). Symptoms resulting from the median nerve entrapment include pain, tingling, burning, or numbness in the thumb, index finger, middle finger, and the thumb side of the ring fingers (Burton, 2014). Symptoms generally begin slowly and often first become evident at night. Typical symptoms include numbness, tingling, pain, and/or a burning sensation in the affected regions. Initial symptoms may vary in intensity. However, as symptoms progress, they will often become more consistent and will occur during the daytime hours as well at night. Worsening symptoms may include pain and tingling symptoms radiating to the forearm and shoulder. As the syndrome gets worse, a loss of strength and coordination can be experienced, and many activities of daily living can be severely affected.

Epidemiology CTS is the most common of all the nerve entrapment syndromes (Miller & Reinus, 2010). Estimates of the rate of CTS have been reported to range from 2.3 to 7.5 cases per 100 person-years (Cardona et al., 2019). In a study of 4,321 primarily industrial workers, CTS was observed to afflict 7.8% of the cohort (Dale et al., 2013). Estimates of the prevalence of CTS are generally around 2% of the population (Descatha et al., 2010), with a lifetime incidence of approximately 10–15% (Miller & Reinus, 2010). The higher end of these incidence estimates is generally seen in those having significant occupational exposure (Palmer, Harris, & Coggon, 2007). Women generally exhibit 3–5 times greater incidence rates than men, and cases in women are typically seen between the ages of 30 and 60 years (Miller & Reinus, 2010). Pregnancy is a notable risk factor for CTS in females, thought to be due to increased pressure in the carpal tunnel due to swelling of the structures running through the canal from the additional water retention associated with pregnancy. Cases in men are usually seen between the ages of 35 and 40 years,

Figure 2.8 Location of the carpal tunnel and path of the median nerve in the hand.

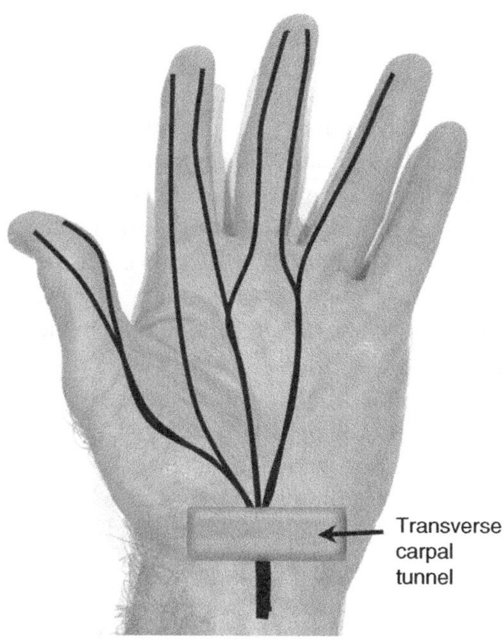

and men's CTS cases are often occupationally related (Palmer et al., 2007). Overall, the dominant hand is the most often affected; however, up to 50% of cases involve bilateral symptoms (Miller & Reinus, 2010).

Medical treatment of CTS has been estimated to cost over $2 billion annually (Dale et al., 2013; Falkiner & Myers, 2002; Stapleton, 2006). Indirect costs such as lost work time and job change may be substantially greater (Faucett, Blanc, & Yelin, 2000; Foley, Silverstein, & Polissar, 2007). Exposure to physical risk factors such as high force, non-neutral working postures, and repetition are well-known risk factors for MSDs (da Costa & Vieira, 2010; National Research Council – Institute of Medicine, 2001; NIOSH, 1997). Recent evidence from a prospective study of 2,474 service and production workers suggests that interactions of these risk factors demonstrate a strong association with incident CTS (Harris-Adamson et al., 2015).

Anatomy/pathology The median nerve is one of the numerous structures passing through the carpal tunnel in the wrist. These include nine tendons (four flexor digitorum superficialis, four flexor digitorum profundus, and the flexor pollicis longus), various blood vessels, and the median nerve. The carpal tunnel is bounded superficially by the flexor retinaculum, has a deep border formed by palmar aspects of several carpal bones, is bounded laterally by the medial surface of the trapezium, and is bounded medially by the lateral surface of the hamate bone.

Various studies have provided findings which suggest that damage development to neural and tendinous tissues may be associated with symptom development (Barbe et al., 2020; Bove et al., 2019; Chikenji, Gingery, Zhao, Passe et al., 2014; Clark, Al-Shatti, Barr, Amin, & Barbe, 2004; Clark et al., 2003; Elliott et al., 2009; Elliott, Barr, Clark, Wade, & Barbe, 2010; Ettema, Zhao, An, & Amadio, 2006; Jain et al., 2014). Studies that have biopsied tissues in CTS cases have suggested that the development of median nerve compression may be the consequence of connective tissues experiencing degeneration due to repeated mechanical stress (Festen-Schrier & Amadio, 2018; Schrier, Vrieze, & Amadio, 2020; Schuind, Ventura, & Pasteels, 1990). Structures affected by repeated stress can include flexor tendons and their synovial sheath (Kerr, Sybert, & Albarracin, 1992). Degenerative noninflammatory fibrosis and thickening of the synovium have been implicated as a factor in median nerve pathology (Chikenji, Gingery, Zhao, Passe et al., 2014; Ettema et al., 2006; Sternbach, 1999). Tendon fibrosis changes may impact the gliding mechanism of the subsynovial connective tissue (SSCT), which moves *en bloc* with the tendons and median nerve (Ghasemi-Rad et al., 2014). Increases in vascularity, fibroblast density, and collagen fiber size have been reported in resected synovial specimens and are also indicative of synovial degeneration (Jinrok et al., 2004). If a decrease in SSCT motion were to result from fibrosis, the movement of the tendons would likely increase shear strain in the SSCT (Ghasemi-Rad et al., 2014). The degree of shear strain would be expected to vary with wrist posture, with the maximum shear predicted at 60 degrees of wrist flexion (Yoshii et al., 2008). High velocity tendon motion has been suggested to place the SSCT at a particularly high risk of shear injury (Yoshii et al., 2011). Hand and finger motions may also result in friction between the flexor digitorum muscles and the median nerve, also potentially leading to cumulative trauma development (Yoshii et al., 2008).

Noninflammatory tendon damage (tendinosis) has also been noted in CTS cases (Kerr et al., 1992). Tendinosis is characterized by microtears in the substance of the tendon and connective tissue, collagen degeneration, and fiber disorientation (Sharma & Maffulli, 2005). These characteristics are also observed during *in vitro* fatigue failure studies of tendons and studies of fatigue failure in animal studies (Barbe et al., 2013b; Schechtman & Bader, 1997; Shepherd & Screen, 2013; Sun et al., 2010). Patients with this syndrome also demonstrate decreased areal bone mineral density (BMD) in distal forearm bones (i.e., radius and ulna) and reduced bone in hand phalanges, as observed using quantitative ultrasound measurements (Erselcan, Topalkara, Nacitarhan, Akyuz, & Dogan, 2001; Kisala, Pluskiewicz, & Adamczyk, 2019).

Risk factors/activities associated with CTS A review undertaken by the NIOSH included over 600 epidemiological studies concerning workplace factors associated with numerous MSDs (including CTS) (NIOSH, 1997). The summary of their review on CTS indicated strong evidence for a relationship between exposure to combinations of force and repetition, or force and posture, and development of CTS. CTS frequently presents in working-aged adults, especially those experiencing prolonged and repetitive flexion and extension of the wrist, especially when combined with forceful gripping (Palmer, 2011). Other potential occupational risk factors may include exposure to HAV and/or exposure to cold conditions. There are several personal risk factors for CTS as well. Of these, being female is one of the strongest (Lee et al., 2019). Females have 2-3 times the risk compared to males (Lee et al., 2019). Other common personal risk factors include increasing age, having a narrow carpal tunnel, previous wrist trauma or injury, diabetes, rheumatoid arthritis, hypothyroidism, and presence of other neurological disorders (Geoghegan, Clark, Bainbridge, Smith, & Hubbard, 2004).

Cubital tunnel syndrome (ulnar nerve entrapment)

Characteristics/description Cubital tunnel syndrome is the second most common mononeuropathy of the upper extremity (Cutts, 2007; Saito et al., 2018). It involves the entrapment of the ulnar nerve within the cubital tunnel at the elbow, which is of clinical significance since the ulnar nerve is one of the primary nerves supplying motor information to many forearm muscles and most of the hand muscles and sensory information from part of the hand. In addition to compression within the cubital tunnel, the ulnar nerve can also be compressed in the neck at cervical level 8 (C8), in the thoracic outlet (thoracic outlet syndrome), and at the wrist in Guyon's canal (Fadel, Lancigu, Raimbeau, Roquelaure, & Descatha, 2017). A double crush syndrome is possible and would mean that the ulnar nerve is compressed in two or more of these various sites. Symptoms of cubital tunnel syndrome at any level of entrapment can lead to an intermittent altered sensation in the little and ring fingers, such as sensory loss (typically the first reported symptom), paresthesia (a burning or prickling sensation), or formication (the sensation of having insects crawling on or under the skin) (Fadel et al., 2017). As the condition progresses, there may be development of pain in the medial elbow and hand weakness, and eventually, atrophy of many of the intrinsic muscles of the hand.

Epidemiology As with all nerve disorders, individuals with diabetes mellitus (diabetes type 2) have increased susceptibility for symptoms of ulnar nerve neuropathy, although these symptoms may occur secondary to a microvascular injury of the nerve, thus causing a local ischemia, or by interfering with local metabolism. Although there have been only a small number of studies examining occupational contributions to cubital tunnel syndrome, its prevalence ranges from 5.9 to 6.9% in workers in the Saint Louis metropolitan area (An, Evanoff, Boyer, & Osei, 2017), Missouri, USA (5.9%), a 6.9% prevalence rate in dock workers in Sao Paulo, Brazil (Saito et al., 2018), and 6.7% in floor cleaners in a systematic review performed in 2009 (van Rijn, Huisstede, Koes, & Burdorf, 2009). It is also reported to be more common in patients whose work involves protracted elbow flexion (e.g., holding a telephone) and flexion of the elbow on hard surfaces, workers who handle vibratory tools, and individuals with past elbow fractures, direct trauma of the ulnar nerve, or marked valgus or varus deformities of the elbow (Cutts, 2007; Saito et al., 2018).

Anatomy/pathology The ulnar nerve is formed from terminal branches of the medial cord of the brachial plexus and contains nerve processes that originate from spinal cord roots located at cervical 8 and thoracic 1 levels. The ulnar nerve descends distally down the arm toward the elbow just anterior to a medially located intermuscular septum (a connective tissue sheath that both divides and provides attachment for the triceps brachial muscles located posteriorly, and brachialis muscle located anteriorly). The ulnar nerve pierces this septum and passes through a fibro-osseous space behind the medial epicondyle of the humus that is known as the *cubital tunnel*. Thereafter, the ulnar nerve passes between the two heads of the flexor carpi ulnaris muscle of the forearm before proceeding distally to the medial wrist and hand. The ulnar nerve innervates several medially located forearm muscles and most of the intrinsic muscles of the hand (such as those acting on the little and ring fingers, the medial two lumbricals, interosseous muscles, and two muscles of the thumb including the adductor pollicis).

This anatomical arrangement places the ulnar nerve posterior to the elbow's axis of motion, so that during elbow flexion, the nerve is required to stretch up to 5 mm longer than its length at rest as well as slide through the cubital tunnel (Cutts, 2007; Fadel et al., 2017). Alterations in the fibro-osseous space and increase in intraneural pressure are believed to be key to the pathogenesis of cubital tunnel syndrome. Flexion of the elbow changes the cubital tunnel's shape from ovoid to ellipse, decreases the cross-sectional area of the space by 55%, and increases intraneural pressure up to 20 times higher than resting pressure (Apfelberg & Larson, 1973; Novak, Lee, Mackinnon, & Lay, 1994). The floor of the tunnel is made up of the elbow joint capsule and a supporting ligament; bones act as walls on either side (the medial epicondyle of the humerus and the olecranon process of the ulna), while the roof is made of elastic connective tissue (a retinaculum). This retinaculum has a variable structure (and may even be missing) with variations in its tightness perhaps also contributing to cubital tunnel syndrome (O'Driscoll, Horii, Carmichael, & Morrey, 1991).

Risk factors/activities associated with cubital tunnel syndrome Although more studies are needed, known risk factors for cubital tunnel syndrome include work that involves holding the elbow in a flexed position for long periods, particularly when on a hard surface (Cutts, 2007), performing repetitive tasks with high force requirements (Fadel et al., 2017), and performing repetitive tasks with vibratory tools (Cutts, 2007). The prevalence for cubital tunnel syndrome is also higher in workers over 50 years of age and in those who have worked for more than 1 year in the job (thus, duration) (Saito et al., 2018; van Rijn et al., 2009). Obesity and presence of diabetes may also increase the risk, particularly for a mechanical double crush of the ulnar nerve (Cutts, 2007).

Hand-arm Vibration Syndrome

Characteristics/description

Hand-arm vibration syndrome (HAVS) is a disorder associated with exposure to HAV, usually as the result of the prolonged use of powered hand tools. HAVS can be a painful and potentially disabling condition, with symptoms including pain, numbness, tingling, and nerve dysfunction. These symptoms can affect the hands, wrists, and forearms and may interfere with sleep. HAVS may also lead to a pallor or cyanosis of the fingers as well as numbness, tingling, and pain. Episodes typically last 5–30 min; however, the duration and severity of symptoms may increase with disease progression. Musculoskeletal symptoms can include decreased grip strength and, in some cases, Dupuytren's contractions—a condition in which fingers in the hand (usually the two fingers farthest from the thumb)—are permanently contracted and cannot be fully straightened out.

Epidemiology

HAV is defined as the transfer of vibration from a tool to a worker's hand and arm. The amount of HAV is characterized by the acceleration level of the tool when grasped by the worker and in use.

The vibration is typically measured on the handle of tool while in use to determine the acceleration levels transferred to the worker. HAVS was first widely recognized as a potential occupational hazard in the mid-1980s. However, the earliest reports of vibration white finger (VWF) were provided in the early 1900s in miners and quarry workers (Laws, 1998). It was only later realized that musculoskeletal and neurologic symptoms were part of the same syndrome. Although the prevalence in the general population is very low, the prevalence in those experiencing prolonged HAV exposure can be as large as 50% and varies with the intensity of the exposure. Risk appears to be increased somewhat in countries with colder climates (Shen & House, 2017). Exposed workers typically exhibit symptoms in middle age, though symptoms can be observed in younger workers with more intensive exposures. The latency period between exposure and symptoms can be quite broad, ranging from less than a year to four decades, depending on the intensity of exposure.

Anatomy/pathology

The tissue damage associated with exposure to HAVS may affect vascular, neurologic, and musculoskeletal structures in the hands, wrist, or forearm. Damage to these various systems may progress at different rates (Pelmear, 2003). The vascular component is also known as VWF and is related to Raynaud's phenomenon, which is the most recognized manifestation of HAVS. The precise pathological mechanism is not totally clear; however, it is believed that vibration exposure causes endothelial damage through mechanical trauma and oxidative stress, leading to vasoconstriction through activation of the sympathetic nervous system. Nerve fibers (both myelinated and nonmyelinated) are thought to be damaged through vibration exposure. Musculoskeletal symptoms may be due to direct damage to musculoskeletal tissues due to the repetitive forces of vibration and/or may be secondary to nerve damage (Shen & House, 2017).

Risk factors/activities associated with HAVS

Sources of vibration that can cause HAVS are varied and include hand drills, chisels, power chain saws, power jigsaws, sanders, riveters, polishing tools, and many others. There is some indication that high-frequency vibration is more relevant to the symptoms of HAVS, as such vibration may be absorbed preferentially by the hand and fingers, whereas lower frequency vibration energy may affect the arms and shoulders to a greater extent (Shen & House, 2017). It is a disorder resulting from prolonged exposure to vibration, specifically to the hands and forearms while using vibrating tools. Symptoms include numbness, tingling, and loss of nerve sensitivity. HAVS is a painful and potentially disabling condition of the fingers, hands, and arms due to vibration. There is initially a tingling sensation with numbness in the fingers. The fingers then become white and swollen when cold and then red and painful when warmed up again. Cold or wet weather may aggravate the condition. Picking up objects such as pins or nails becomes difficult as the feeling in the fingers diminishes, and there is loss of strength and grip in the hands. The pain, tingling, and numbness in the arms, wrists, and hands may interfere with sleep.

Commonalities Among MSDs

If one contemplates the summaries of the various MSDs summarized in Table 2.1, certain commonalities become apparent. One is that all appear to be associated with the development of damage to musculoskeletal tissues (and/or other structures). It should not be surprising that these disorders, all of which result can result in significant pain and dysfunction, would be associated

Table 2.1 Summary of Common MSDs

Disorder	Involved structures
Low back pain	Degeneration and inflammation in many potential tissue sources, including intervertebral discs, facet and sacroiliac joint, spinal roots, and muscles attached to the vertebrae
Hand & wrist tendinopathy	Degenerative changes in extensor pollicis brevis and abductor longus tendons (sheath breakdown, nodularity, tendon fraying)
Lateral tendinopathy of the elbow	Degenerative changes in common extensor tendons at the elbow (microtears that lead to partial or complete rupture)
Medial tendinopathy of the elbow	Degenerative changes in common flexor tendons at the elbow (increased collagen remodeling and mucoid ground substance)
Shoulder tendons (rotator cuff injuries)	Degeneration and inflammation in rotator cuff tendons
Muscle fatigue	Many potential contributors, including physiological changes that lead to an energy crisis, dysfunction in calcium homeostasis, neurological changes (altered neuromuscular junctions), and apoptosis
Myalgia (muscle pain)	Many potential contributors, including dysfunction in calcium homeostasis and increased inflammation
Muscle fibrosis	Increased extracellular matrix production, for example, collagen and fibronectin
Carpal tunnel syndrome (median mononeuropathy)	Median nerve entrapment, irritation, inflammation
Ulnar tunnel syndrome (ulnar mononeuropathy)	Ulnar nerve entrapment
Hand-arm vibration syndrome	Many potential sources, including damage to vascular, neurological, and/or musculoskeletal structures of the hand, wrist, and forearm

with tissue damage. Another consistent refrain is that all of these disorders are associated with exposure to the repetitive application of stress, sometimes expressed in terms of exposure to forceful and repetitive exertions. Adoption of non-neutral postures is another potential source of repeated stress, as such postures generally serve to increase stress on affected tissues in some form or fashion (and may be adopted frequently). Sometimes, the repeated stress comes in the form of vibration exposure, which has been associated with damaging impacts on musculoskeletal tissues, along with other associated tissues.

Whenever one observes damage development in a material exposed to repeated mechanical stress, there is one mechanism that comes to mind that would explain how and why this damage is occurring. This process is, of course, material fatigue failure. Fortunately, the fatigue failure theory has been around since the 1840s, and much is known regarding the response of materials to repeated stress (Stephens, Fatemi, Stephens, & Fuchs, 2001). However, the fact that musculoskeletal tissues are located in a dynamic biological environment, in which exposed materials have a healing capacity, provides an important wrinkle in the development of biological tissue damage. This provides us with competing processes that will control musculoskeletal tissue damage development. Unless some new and unique mechanism of damage development from repeated stress is discovered that applies only to biological materials, we must assume the damage part of the equation is controlled by the mechanism of fatigue failure. We know certain aspects regarding the healing portion of the equation, as well, but much more needs to be learned.

This book examines the development of MSDs as a process of fatigue failure of musculoskeletal tissues, but one modified by complex physiological and biochemical processes (including, but not limited to, tissue healing). To our knowledge, no one has considered such an approach toward understanding the causes of musculoskeletal tissue damage nor for understanding how we might better control MSDs and improve overall musculoskeletal health. We acknowledge at the outset that there is much yet to be learned about this extremely complex process. However, there is much that is known, which may improve our understanding regarding the development and control of MSDs.

Bibliography

Abdelmagid, S. M., Barr, A. E., Rico, M., Amin, M., Litvin, J., Popoff, S. N., . . . Barbe, M. F. (2012). Performance of repetitive tasks induces decreased grip strength and increased fibrogenic proteins in skeletal muscle: Role of force and inflammation. *PloS One*, *7*(5), e38359.

Abraham, A. C., Shah, S. A., & Thomopoulos, S. (2017). Targeting inflammation in rotator cuff tendon degeneration and repair. *Techniques in Shoulder and Elbow Surgery*, *18*(3):84–90.

Ahmad, Z., Siddiqui, N., Malik, S., Abdus-Samee, M., Tytherleigh-Strong, G., & Rushton, N. (2013). Lateral epicondylitis: A review of pathology and management. *Bone and Joint Journal*, *95-B*, 1158–1164.

Allen, D. G., Lamb, G. D., & Westerblad, H. (2008). Skeletal muscle fatigue: Cellular mechanisms. *Physiological Reviews*, *88*(1), 287–332.

Amin, N. K. (2015). Medial epicondylitis: Evaluation and management. *Journal of the American Academy of Orthopaedic Surgeons*, *23*, 348–355.

Amorim, A., Simic, M., Pappas, E., Zadro, J., Carrillo, E., Ordonana, J., & Ferreira, P. (2019). Is occupational or leisure physical activity associated with low back pain? Insights from a cross-sectional study of 1059 participants. *Brazilian Journal of Physical Therapy*, *23*, 257–265.

An, T. W., Evanoff, B. A., Boyer, M. I., & Osei, D. A. (2017). The prevalence of cubital tunnel syndrome: A cross-sectional study in a U.S. metropolitan cohort. *Journal of Bone and Joint Surgery. American Volume*, *99*(5), 408–416. https://doi.org/10.2106/JBJS.15.01162

Andersson, G. (1999). Epidemiologic features of chronic low back pain. *Lancet*, *354*, 581–585.

Apfelberg, D. B., & Larson, S. J. (1973). Dynamic anatomy of the ulnar nerve at the elbow. *Plastic and Reconstructive Surgery*, *51*(1), 76–81.

Argiles, J. M., Campos, N., Lopez-Pedrosa, J. M., Rueda, R., & Rodriguez-Manas, L. (2016). Skeletal muscle regulates metabolism via interorgan crosstalk: Roles in health and disease. *Journal of the American Medical Directors Association*, *17*(9), 789–796. https://doi.org/10.1016/j.jamda.2016.04.019

Ariens, G., Ariens, G. A., Van Mechelen, W., Bongers, P. M., Bouter, L. M., & Van Der Wal, G. (2000). Physical risk factors for neck pain. *Scandinavian Journal of Work, Environment and Health*, *26*, 7–19.

Armstrong, T. J. (1987). Ergonomics considerations in hand and wrist tendinitis. *The Journal of Hand Surgery*, *12A*, 830–837.

"Back Pain Fact Sheet", NINDS, Publication date December 2014. NIH Publication No. 15-5161. Prepared by: Office of Communications and Public Liaison, National Institute of Neurological Disorders and Stroke, National Institutes of Health Bethesda, MD 20892.

Backman, L. J., Andersson, G., Wennstig, G., Forsgren, S., & Danielson, P. (2011). Endogenous substance P production in the Achilles tendon increases with loading in an in vivo model of tendinopathy-peptidergic elevation preceding tendinosis-like tissue changes. *Journal of Musculoskeletal and Neuronal Interactions*, *11*(2), 133–140.

Balogh, I., Arvidsson, I., Bjork, J., Hansson, G. A., Ohlsson, K., Skerfving, S., & Nordander, C. (2019). Work-related neck and upper limb disorders—Quantitative exposure-response relationships adjusted for personal characteristics and psychosocial conditions. *BMC Musculoskeletal Disorders, 20*(1), 139. https://doi.org/10.1186/s12891-019-2491-6

Bani Hani, D., Huangfu, R., Sesek, R., Schall, M. C., Davis, G. A., & Gallagher, S. (2021). Development and validation of a cumulative exposure shoulder risk assessment tool based on fatigue failure theory. *Ergonomics, 64*(1), 39–54.

Barbe, M. F., Gallagher, S., Massicotte, V. S., Tytell, M., Popoff, S. N., & Barr-Gillespie, A. E. (2013b). The interaction of force and repetition on musculoskeletal and neural tissue responses and sensorimotor behavior in a rat model of work-related musculoskeletal disorders. *BMC Musculoskeletal Disorders, 14*(1), 303. https://doi.org/10.1186/1471-2474-14-303

Barbe, M. F., Gallagher, S., & Popoff, S. N. (2013a). Serum biomarkers as predictors of stage of work-related musculoskeletal disorders. *Journal of the American Academy of Orthopaedic Surgeons, 21*(10), 644–646. https://doi.org/10.5435/JAAOS-21-10-644

Barbe, M. F., Hilliard, B. A., Amin, M., Harris, M. Y., Hobson, L. J., Cruz, G. E., & Popoff, S. N. (2020). Blocking CTGF/CCN2 reduces established skeletal muscle fibrosis in a rat model of overuse injury. *FASEB Journal, 34*(5), 6554–6569. https://doi.org/10.1096/fj.202000240RR

Baring, T., Emery, R., & Reilly, P. (2007). Management of rotator cuff disease: Specific treatment for specific disorders. *Best Practice and Research Clinical Rheumatology, 21*, 279–294.

Barr, A., Barbe, M., & Clark, B. (2004). Work-related musculoskeletal disorders of the hand and wrist: Epidemiology, pathophysiology, and sensorimotor changes. *Journal of Orthopaedic and Sports Physical Therapy, 34*, 610–627.

Berchtold, M. W., Brinkmeier, H., & Muntener, M. (2000). Calcium ion in skeletal muscle: Its crucial role for muscle function, plasticity, and disease. *Physiological Reviews, 80*(3), 1215–1265.

Bergenudd, H. L. (1987). Shoulder pain in middle age a study of prevalence and relation to occupational workload and psychosocial factors. *Clinical Orthopaedics and Related Research, 231*, 234–237.

Bernard, T., Wilder, F., Aluoch, M., & Leaverton, P. (2010). Job-related osteoarthritis of the knee, foot, hand, and cervical spine. *Journal of Occupational and Environmental Medicine, 52*, 33–38.

Bevan, S. (2015). Economic impact of musculoskeletal disorders (MSDs) on work in Europe. *Best Practice & Research Clinical Rheumatology, 29*, 356–373.

Blumenfeld, O., Williams, F., Valdes, A., Hart, D. J., Malkin, I., Spector, T. D., & Livshits, G. (2014). Association of interleukin-6 gene polymorphisms with hand osteoarthritis and hand osteoporosis. *Cytokine, 69*, 94–101.

Bogduk, N., Aprill, C., & Derby, R. (2013). Lumbar discogenic pain: State-of-the-art review. *Pain Medicine, 14*, 813–836.

Bongers, P. M., Ijmker, S., Heuvel, S., & Blatter, B. M. (2006). Epidemiology of work related neck and upper limb problems: Psychosocial and personal risk factors (part I) and effective interventions from a bio behavioural perspective (part II). *Journal of Occupational Rehabilitation, 16*(3), 279–302.

Bove, G. M., Delany, S. P., Hobson, L., Cruz, G. E., Harris, M. Y., Amin, M., & Barbe, M. F. (2019). Manual therapy prevents onset of nociceptor activity, sensorimotor dysfunction, and neural fibrosis induced by a volitional repetitive task. *Pain, 160*(3), 632–644. https://doi.org/10.1097/j.pain.0000000000001443

Bovenzi, M., Schust, M., & Mauro, M. (2017). An overview of low back pain and occupational exposures to whole-body vibration and mechanical shocks. *La Medicina Del Lavoro, 108*, 419–433.

Bovenzi, M., Schust, M., Menzel, G., Prodi, A., & Mauro, M. (2015). Relationships of low back outcomes to internal spinal load: A prospective cohort study of professional drivers. *International Archives of Occupational and Environmental Health, 88*, 487–499.

Breivik, H., Collett, B., Ventafridda, V., & R., C., & Gallacher, D. (2005). Survey of chronic pain in Europe: Prevalence, impact on daily life and treatment. *European Journal of Pain, 10*, 287–333.

Bureau of Labor Statistics News, United States Department of Labor (2001). Lost-Worktime Injuries and Illnesses: Characteristics and Resulting Days Away From Work. http://www.bls.gov/iif/home.htm.

Bureau of Labor Statistics (2015). Type of injury or illness and body parts affected by nonfatal injuries and illnesses in 2014. *The Economics Daily*. https://www.bls.gov/opub/ted/2015/type-of-injury-or-illness-and-body-parts-affected-by-nonfatal-injuries-and-illnesses-in-2014.htm

Bureau of Labor Statistics (2018). Back injuries prominent in work-related musculoskeletal disorder cases in 2016. *The Economics Daily*. https://www.bls.gov/opub/ted/2018/back-injuries-prominent-in-work-related-musculoskeletal-disorder-cases-in-2016.htm

Burton, C. C. (2014). Diagnosing and managing carpal tunnel syndrome in primary care. *The British Journal of General Practice, 64*, 262–263.

Byeon, J., Kim, J., Jeong, H., Sim, Y., Kim, D., Choi, J., & Kim, G. (2013). Degenerative changes of spine in helicopter pilots. *Annals of Rehabilitation Medicine, 37*, 706.

Byström, S., Hall, C., Welander, T., & Kilbom, Å. (1995). Clinical disorders and pressure-pain threshold of the forearm and hand among automotive assembly line workers. *Journal of Hand Surgery, 20*, 782–790.

Cardona, A., Thiese, M., Kapellusch, J., Merryweather, A., Wood, E., & Hegmann, K. (2019). Role of biomechanical factors in resolution of carpal tunnel syndrome among a population of workers. *Journal of Occupational and Environmental Medicine, 61*, 340–346.

Casazza, B. (2012). Diagnosis and treatment of acute low back pain. *American Family Physician, 85*, 343–350.

Chawla, J. (2018). *Low back pain and sciatica*. https://emedicine.medscape.com/article/1144130-overview

Chen, J.-C., Chan, W., Katz, J., Chang, W., & Christian, D. (2004). Occupational and personal factors associated with acquired lumbar spondylolisthesis of urban taxi drivers in. *Occupational and Environmental Medicine, 61*, 992–998.

Chikenji, T., Gingery, A., Zhao, C., Passe, S. M., Ozasa, Y., Larson, D., & Amadio, P. C. (2014). Transforming growth factor-beta (TGF-beta) expression is increased in the subsynovial connective tissues of patients with idiopathic carpal tunnel syndrome. *Journal of Orthopaedic Research : Official Publication of the Orthopaedic Research Society, 32*(1), 116–122. https://doi.org/10.1002/jor.22485

Christ, W., & Dupuis, H. (1966). Uber die Beanspruchung die Wirbelsaule unter dem Einfluss sinusforminger und stochastischer Schwingungen. *Internationale Zeitschrift für Angewandte Physiologie, Einschliesslich Arbeitsphysiologie, 22*, 258–278.

Clark, B. D., Al-Shatti, T. A., Barr, A. E., Amin, M., & Barbe, M. F. (2004). Performance of a high-repetition, high-force task induces carpal tunnel syndrome in rats. *Journal of Orthopaedic and Sports Physical Therapy, 34*(5), 244–253. https://doi.org/10.2519/jospt.2004.34.5.244

Clark, B. D., Barr, A. E., Safadi, F. F., Beitman, L., Al-Shatti, T., Amin, M., & Barbe, M. F. (2003). Median nerve trauma in a rat model of work-related musculoskeletal disorder. *Journal of Neurotrauma, 20*(7), 681–695. https://doi.org/10.1089/089771503322144590

Clarke, M. L. (1998). The histopathology of de Quervain's disease. *Journal of Hand Surgery, 23B*, 732–734.

Cohen, S. P. (2015). Epidemiology, diagnosis, and treatment of neck pain. *Mayo Clinic Proceedings, 90*(2), 284–299. https://doi.org/10.1016/j.mayocp.2014.09.008

Contreras, O., Rebolledo, D. L., Oyarzun, J. E., Olguin, H. C., & Brandan, E. (2016). Connective tissue cells expressing fibro/adipogenic progenitor markers increase under chronic damage: relevance in fibroblast-myofibroblast differentiation and skeletal muscle fibrosis. *Cell Tissue Res, 364*(3), 647–660. https://doi.org/10.1007/s00441-015-2343-0

Cote, J. N. (2014). Adaptations to neck/shoulder fatigue and injuries. *Advances in Experimental Medicine and Biology, 826*, 205–228. https://doi.org/10.1007/978-1-4939-1338-1_13

Cote, P., Cassidy, J. D., & Carroll, L. (1998). The Saskatchewan health and back pain survey. The prevalence of neck pain and related disability in Saskatchewan adults. *Spine, 23*. https://doi.org/10.1097/00007632-199808010-00015

Cunningham, L., & Kelsey, J. (1984). Epidemiology of musculoskeletal impairments and associated disability. *American Journal of Public Health, 74*, 574–579.

Cutts, S. (2007). Cubital tunnel syndrome. *Postgraduate Medical Journal, 83*(975), 28–31. https://doi.org/10.1136/pgmj.2006.047456

da Costa, B., & Vieira, E. (2010). Risk factors for work. *American Journal of Industrial Medicine, 53*, 285–323.

Dale, A. M., Harris-Adamson, C., Rempel, D., Gerr, F., Hegmann, K., Silverstein, B., & Merlino, L. (2013). Prevalence and incidence of carpal tunnel syndrome in US working populations: pooled analysis of six prospective studies. *Scandinavian Journal of Work, Environment & Health, 39*(5), 495.

Dennett, X., & Fry, H. J. (1988). Overuse syndrome: a muscle biopsy study. *Lancet, 1*(8591), 905–908.

Descatha, A., Dale, A. M., Franzblau, A., Coomes, J.,& Evanoff, B. (2010). Diagnostic strategies using physical examination are minimally useful in defining carpal tunnel syndrome in population-based research studies. *Occupational and Environmental Medicine, 67*, 133–135.

Descatha, A., Dale, A., Jaegers, L., Herquelot, E., & Evanoff, B. (2013). Self-reported physical exposure association with medial and lateral epicondylitis incidence in a large longitudinal study. *Occupational and Environmental Medicine, 70*, 670–673.

Descatha, A., Leclerc, A., Chastang, J.-F., & Roquelaure, Y. (2003). Medial epicondylitis in occupational settings: prevalence, incidence and associated risk factors. *Journal of occupational and environmental medicine/American College of Occupational and Environmental Medicine, 45*(9), 993–1001.

Devereux, J., Vlachonikolis, I., & Buckle, P. (2002). Epidemiological study to investigate potential interaction between physical and psychosocial factors at work that may increase the risk of symptoms of musculoskeletal disorder of the neck and upper limb. *Occupational and Environmental Medicine, 59*, 269–277.

Driscoll, M., & Blyum, L. (2011). The presence of physiological stress shielding in the degenerative cycle of musculoskeletal disorders. *Journal of Bodywork and Movement Therapies, 15*(3), 335–342. https://doi.org/10.1016/j.jbmt.2010.05.002

Duckworth, T., & Blundell, C. M. (2010). *Lecture notes: Orthopaedics and fractures* (4th ed.). Wiley. ISBN: 978-1-405-13329-6

Eisenstein, A., & Parry, C. (1987). The lumbar facet arthrosis syndrome. *Journal of Bone and Joint Surgery, 69B*, 3–7.

Elliott, M. B., Barr, A. E., Clark, B. D., Amin, M., Amin, S., & Barbe, M. F. (2009). High force reaching task induces widespread inflammation, increased spinal cord neurochemicals and neuropathic pain. *Neuroscience, 158*(2), 922–931. https://doi.org/10.1016/j.neuroscience.2008.10.050

Elliott, M. B., Barr, A. E., Clark, B. D., Wade, C. K., & Barbe, M. F. (2010). Performance of a repetitive task by aged rats leads to median neuropathy and spinal cord inflammation with associated sensorimotor declines. *Neuroscience, 170*(3), 929–941. https://doi.org/10.1016/j.neuroscience.2010.07.041

Enoka, R. M., & Duchateau, J. (2008). Muscle fatigue: What, why and how it influences muscle function. *Journal of Physiology, 586*(1), 11–23. https://doi.org/10.1113/jphysiol.2007.139477

Erselcan, T., Topalkara, K., Nacitarhan, V., Akyuz, A., & Dogan, D. (2001). Carpal tunnel syndrome leads to significant bone loss in metacarpal bones. *Journal of Bone and Mineral Metabolism, 19*, 317–320.

Ettema, A. M., Amadio, P. C., Zhao, C., Wold, L. E., & An, K. N. (2004). A histological and immunohistochemical study of the subsynovial connective tissue in idiopathic carpal tunnel syndrome. *The Journal of Bone and Joint Surgery. American, 86-A(7)*, 1458–1466.

Ettema, A. M., Zhao, C., An, K. N., & Amadio, P. C. (2006). Comparative anatomy of the subsynovial connective tissue in the carpal tunnel of the rat, rabbit, dog, baboon, and human. *Hand, 1*. https://doi.org/10.1007/s11552-006-9009-z

Fadel, M., Lancigu, R., Raimbeau, G., Roquelaure, Y., & Descatha, A. (2017). Occupational prognosis factors for ulnar nerve entrapment at the elbow: a systematic review. *Hand Surg Rehabil, 36*(4), 244–249. https://doi.org/10.1016/j.hansur.2017.03.004

Falkiner, S., & Myers, S. (2002). When exactly can carpal tunnel syndrome be considered work-related? *ANZ Journal of Surgery, 72*, 204–209.

Fan, Z., Silverstein, B., Bao, S., Bonauto, D., Howard, N., Spielholz, P. N. L., & Viikari-Juntura, E. (2009). Quantitative exposure-response relations between physical workload and prevalence of lateral epicondyitis in a working population. *American Journal of Industrial Medicine, 52*, 479–490.

Farfan, H. (1973). *Mechanical Disorders of the Low Back*. Philadelphia: Lea and Febiger.

Fatoye, F., Gebrye, T., & Odeyemi, I. (2019). Real-world incidence and prevalence of low back pain using routinely collected data. *Rheumatology International, 39*(4), 619–626. https://doi.org/10.1007/s00296-019-04273-0

Faucett, J., Blanc, P., & Yelin, E. (2000). The impact of carpal tunnel syndrome on work status: implications of job characteristics for staying on the job. *Journal of Occupational Rehabilitation, 10*, 55–69.

Fedorczyk, J. M., Barr, A. E., Rani, S., Gao, H. G., Amin, M., Amin, S., & Barbe, M. F. (2010). Exposure-dependent increases in IL-1beta, substance P, CTGF, and tendinosis in flexor digitorum tendons with upper extremity repetitive strain injury. *Journal of Orthopaedic Research : Official Publication of the Orthopaedic Research Society, 28*(3), 298–307. https://doi.org/10.1002/jor.20984

Festen-Schrier, V., & Amadio, P. C. (2018). The biomechanics of subsynovial connective tissue in health and its role in carpal tunnel syndrome. *Journal of Electromyography and Kinesiology : Official Journal of the International Society of Electrophysiological Kinesiology, 38*, 232–239. https://doi.org/10.1016/j.jelekin.2017.10.007

Fisher, P. W., Zhao, Y., Rico, M. C., Massicotte, V. S., Wade, C. K., Litvin, J., & Barbe, M. F. (2015). Increased CCN2, substance P and tissue fibrosis are associated with sensorimotor declines in a rat model of repetitive overuse injury. *Journal of Cell Communication and Signaling, 9*(1), 37–54. https://doi.org/10.1007/s12079-015-0263-0

Foley, M., Silverstein, B., & Polissar, N. (2007). The economic burden of carpal tunnel syndrome: long-term earnings of CTS claimants in Washington State. *American Journal of Industrial Medicine, 50*, 155–172.

Fourneir, D. E., Kiser, P. K., Shoemaker, J. K., Battié, M. C., & Séguin, C. A. (2020). Vascularization of the human intervertebral disc: A scoping review. *JOR Spine, 3*(4), e1123. https://doi.org/10.1002/jsp2.1123

Freivalds, A. (2004). *Biomechanics of the Upper Limbs: Mechanics, Modeling, and Musculoskeletal Injuries*. CRC Press.

Froom, P., Froom, J., Van Dyk, D., Caine, Y., Ribak, J., Margaliot, S., & Floman, Y. (1984). Lytic spondylolisthesis in helicopter pilots. *Aviation and Space Environmental Medicine, 55*, 556–557.

Frost, P., & Andersen, J. (1999). Shoulder impingement syndrome in relation to shoulder intensive work. *Occupational and Environmental Medicine, 56*, 494–498.

Fry, H. (1986). Overuse syndrome of the upper limb in musicians. *Medical Journal of Australia, 144*, 182–185.

Fukuda, H., Hamada, K., & Yamanaka, K. (1990). Pathology and pathogenesis of bursal-side rotator cuff tears viewed from en bloc histologic sections. *Clinical Orthopaedics and Related Research*, 254, 75–80.

Gallagher, S., & Heberger, J. (2015). The effects of operator position, pallet orientation, and palletizing condition on low back loads in manual bag palletizing operations. *International Journal of Industrial Ergonomics, 47*, 84–92.

Garcia, M. G., Laubli, T., & Martin, B. J. (2015). Long-term muscle fatigue after standing work. *Human Factors, 57*(7), 1162–1173. https://doi.org/10.1177/0018720815590293

Geoghegan, J., Clark, D., Bainbridge, L., Smith, C., & Hubbard, R. (2004). 2004 Risk factors in carpal tunnel syndrome. *Journal of Hand Surgery (British and European), 29b*, 315–320.

Gerdle, B., Hilgenfeldt, U., Larsson, B., Kristiansen, J., Sogaard, K., & Rosendal, L. (2008). Bradykinin and kallidin levels in the trapezius muscle in patients with work-related trapezius myalgia, in patients with whiplash associated pain, and in healthy controls—A microdialysis study of women. *Pain, 139*(3), 578–587. https://doi.org/10.1016/j.pain.2008.06.012

Gerdle, B., Kristiansen, J., Larsson, B., Saltin, B., Sogaard, K., & Sjogaard, G. (2014). Algogenic substances and metabolic status in work-related Trapezius Myalgia: a multivariate explorative study. *BMC Musculoskeletal Disorders, 15*, 357. https://doi.org/10.1186/1471-2474-15-357

Gerr, F., Marcus, M., Ensor, C., Kleinbaum, D., Cohen, S., Edwards, A., & Monteilh, C. (2002). A prospective study of computer users: I. Study design and incidence of musculoskeletal symptoms and disorders. *American Journal of Industrial Medicine, 41*(4), 221–235.

Ghasemi-Rad, M., Nosair, E., Vegh, A., Mohammadi, A., Akkad, A., Lesha, E., & Hasan, A. (2014). A handy review of carpal tunnel syndrome: From anatomy to diagnosis and treatment. *World Journal of Radiology, 6*, 284.

Global Burden of Disease 2017 Disease and Injury Incidence and Prevalence Collaborators (2018). Global, regional, and national incidence, prevalence, and years lived with disability for 354 diseases and injuries for 195 countries and territories, 1990-2017: A systematic analysis for the Global Burden of Disease Study 2017. *Lancet*, 392(10159), 1789–1858. https://doi.org/10.1016/S0140-6736(18)32279-7

Gold, J., Mohamed, F., Ali, S., & Barbe, M. (2014). Serum and MRI biomarkers in mobile device texting: A pilot study. *Human Factors, 56*, 864–872.

Gold, J. E., Hallman, D. M., Hellström, F., Björklund, M., Crenshaw, A. G., Djupsjobacka, M., Heiden, M., Mathiassen, S. E., Piligian, G., & Barbe, M. F. (2026). Systematic review of biochemical biomarkers for neck and upper-extremity musculoskeletal disorders. *Scandinavian Journal of Work, Environment & Health, 42*, 103–124.

Gumina, S., Candela, V., Passaretti, D., Venditto, T., Carbone, S., Arceri, V., & Giannicola, G. (2014). Intensity and distribution of shoulder pain in patients with different sized postero-superior rotator cuff tears. *Journal of Shoulder and Elbow Surgery, 23*, 807–813.

Gupta, A., & Mahalanabis, D. (2006). Study of hand function in a group of shoe factory workers engaged in repetitive work. *Journal of Occupational Rehabilitation, 16*, 675–684.

Hadrevi, J., Barbe, M. F., Ortenblad, N., Frandsen, U., Boyle, E., Lazar, S., & Sogaard, K. (2019). Calcium fluxes in work-related muscle disorder: Implications from a rat model. *BioMed Research International*, 5040818. https://doi.org/10.1155/2019/5040818

Hadrevi, J., Ghafouri, B., Larsson, B., Gerdle, B., & Hellström, F. (2013). Multivariate modeling of proteins related to trapezius myalgia, a comparative study of female cleaners with or without pain. *PLoS One, 8*(9), 73285. https://doi.org/10.1371/journal.pone.0073285

Hadrevi, J., Turkina, M. V., Carlsson, A., Gerdle, B., Larsson, B., Hellstrom, F., & Ghafouri, B. (2016). Myosin light chains and calcium regulating protein differences in chronic musculoskeletal neck and shoulder pain. *Journal of Integrated OMICS, 6*(1), 1–8.

Hales, T., & Bernard, B. (1996). Epidemiology of work-related musculoskeletal disorders. *Orthopedic Clinics of North America, 27*, 679–709.

Harris-Adamson, C., Eisen, E., Kapellusch, J., Garg, A., Hegmann, K., Thiese, M., & Silverstein, B. (2015). Biomechanical risk factors for carpal tunnel syndrome: A pooled study of 2474 workers. *Occupation. Occupational and Environmental Medicine, 72*, 33–41.

Hasvold, T., & Johnsen, R. (1993). Headache and neck or shoulder pain- frequent and disabling conditions in the general population. *Scandinavian Journal of Primary Health Care, 11*, 219–224.

Hilliard, B. A., Amin, M., Popoff, S. N., & Barbe, M. F. (2020). Force dependent effects of chronic overuse on fibrosis-related genes and proteins in skeletal muscles. *Connect Tissue Res, 1–17*. https://doi.org/10.1080/03008207.2020.1828379

Hirata, H., Tsujii, M., Yoshida, T., Imanaka-Yoshida, K., Morita, A., Okuyama, N., & Uchida, A. (2005). MMP-2 expression is associated with rapidly proliferative arteriosclerosis in the flexor tenosynovium and pain severity in carpal tunnel syndrome. *Journal of Pathology, 205*(4), 443–450. https://doi.org/10.1002/path.1709

Holtermann, A., Hansen, J. V., Burr, H., & Sogaard, K. (2010). Prognostic factors for long-term sickness absence among employees with neck-shoulder and low-back pain. *Scandinavian Journal of Work Environment and Health, 36*(1), 34–41.

Hoogendoorn, W., Poppel, M., Bongers, P., Koes, B., & Bouter, L. (1999). Physical load during work and leisure time as risk factors for back pain. *Scandinavian Journal Work Environment and Health, 25*, 387–403.

Hoy, D. B. (2012). A systematic review of the global prevalence of low back pain. *Arthritis and Rheumatism, 64*, 2028–2037.

Huisstede, B., Bierma-Zeinstra, S., Koes, B., & Verhaar, J. (2006). Incidence and prevalence of upper-extremity musculoskeletal disorders. A systematic appraisal of the literature. *BMC Musculoskeletal Disorders, 7*, 7.

Huysmans, M. A., Blatter, B. M., & Beek, A. J. (2012). Perceived muscular tension predicts future neck-shoulder and arm-wrist-hand symptoms. *Occupational and Environmental Medicine, 69*(4), 261–267. https://doi.org/10.1136/oemed-2011-100279

Jacobson, J. A., Chiavaras, M. M., Lawton, J. M., Downie, B., Yablon, C. M., & Lawton, J. (2014). Radial collateral ligament of the elbow: Sonographic characterization with cadaveric dissection correlation and magnetic resonance arthrography. *Journal of Ultrasound in Medicine, 33*(6), 1041–1048. https://doi.org/10.7863/ultra.33.6.1041. Wiley

Jain, N. X., Barr-Gillespie, A. E., Clark, B. D., Kietrys, D. M., Wade, C. K., Litvin, J., & Barbe, M. F. (2014). Bone loss from high repetitive high force loading is prevented by ibuprofen treatment. *Journal of Musculoskeletal & Neuronal Interactions, 14*(1), 78–94.

Jinrok, O., Zhao, C., Amadio, P., An, K., Zobitz, M., & Wold, L. (2004). Vascular pathologic changes in the flexor tenosynovium (subsynovial connective tissue) in idiopathic carpal tunnel syndrome. *Journal of Orthopaedic Research, 22*, 1310–1315.

Kakosy, T., Nemeth, L., Kiss, G., Laszloffy, M., & Kardos, K. (2006). Clinical features of the hand-arm vibration syndrome in miners. *Orvosi Hetilap, 147*(18), 833–839.

Kehl, L. J., Trempe, T. M., & Hargreaves, K. M. (2000). A new animal model for assessing mechanisms and management of muscle hyperalgesia. *Pain, 85*(3), 333–343.

Kelsey, J. L., & White, A. A., 3rd (1980). Epidemiology of low back pain. *Spine, 6*, 133–142.

Kerr, C., Sybert, D., & Albarracin, N. (1992). An analysis of the flexor synovium in idiopathic carpal tunnel syndrome: Report of 625 cases. *Journal of Hand Surgery, 17*, 1028–1030.

Kiel, J., & Kaiser, K. (2019). Golfers Elbow. [Updated 2021 Jul 25]. In *StatPearls [Internet]*. Treasure Island (FL): StatPearls Publishing. Available from: https://www.ncbi.nlm.nih.gov/books/NBK519000/

Kietrys, D. M., Barr, A. E., & Barbe, M. F. (2011). Exposure to repetitive tasks induces motor changes related to skill acquisition and inflammation in rats. *Journal of Motor Behavior, 43*(6):465–476.

Kisala, A., Pluskiewicz, W., & Adamczyk, P. (2019). Skeletal status in women with carpal tunnel syndrome—A 1-yr prospective study. *Journal of Clinical Densitometry, 22*, 305–310.

Klyne, D., Barbe, M., & Hodges, P. (2017). Systemic inflammatory profiles and their relationships with demographic, behavioural and clinical features in acute low back pain. *Brain, Behavior and Immunity, 60*, 84–92.

Klyne, D. M., & Hodges, P. W. (2020). Circulating adipokines in predicting the transition from acute to persistent low back pain. *Pain Medicine, 21*(11), 2975–2985.

Koes, B. W., van Tulder, M., Lin, C. W., Macedo, L. G., McAuley, J., & Maher, C. (2010). An updated overview of clinical guidelines for the management of non-specific low back pain in primary care. *European Spine Journal: Official Publication of the European Spine Society, the European Spinal Deformity Society, and the European Section of the Cervical Spine Research Society, 19*(12), 2075–2094. https://doi.org/10.1007/s00586-010-1502-y

Kraushaar, B., & Nirschl, R. (1999). Tendinosis of the elbow (tennis elbow): Clinical features and findings of histological, immunohistochemical, and electron microscopy studies. *Journal of Bone and Joint Surgery American, 81-A*, 259–278.

Kurrpa, K., Viikari-Juntura, E., Kuosma, E., Huuskonen, M., & Kivi, P. (1991). Incidence of tenosynovitis or peritendinitis and epicondylitis in a meat-processing factory. *Scandinavian Journal of Work, Environment, and Health, 17*, 32–37.

Kuslich, S., Ulstrom, C., & Michael, C. (1991). The tissue origin of low back pain and sciatica: A report of pain response to tissue stimulation during operations on the lumbar spine using local anesthesia. *Orthopaedic Clinics North America, 22*, 18.

Larsson, B., & Sogaard, K. (2007). Work related neck–shoulder pain: A review on magnitude, risk factors, biochemical characteristics, clinical picture and preventive interventions. *Best Practice & Research Clinical Rheumatology, 21*, 447–463.

Larsson, B., Sogaard, K., & Rosendal, L. (2007). Work related neck-shoulder pain: A review on magnitude, risk factors, biochemical characteristics, clinical picture and preventive interventions. *Best Practice and Research Clinical Rheumatology, 21*(3), 447–463.

Laws, J. (1998). The hazards of HAVS. *Occupational Health and Safety, 67*, 45–46.

Leal, L. G., Lopes, M. A., & Batista, M. L., Jr. (2018). Physical exercise-induced myokines and muscle-adipose tissue crosstalk: A review of current knowledge and the implications for health and metabolic diseases. *Frontiers in Physiology, 9*, 1307. https://doi.org/10.3389/fphys.2018.01307

Lee, I., Kim, Y., Kang, D., Kim, S., Kim, I., & Kim, E. (2019). Distribution of age, gender, and occupation among individuals with carpal tunnel syndrome based on the National Health Insurance data and National Employment Insurance data. *Annals of Occupational and Environmental Medicine, 31*, 31.

Luopajärvi, T., Kuorinka, I., Virolainen, M., & Holmberg, M. (1979). Prevalence of tenosynovitis and other injuries of the upper extremities in repetitive work. *Scandinavian Journal of Rehabilitation Medicine, 5*(Suppl. 3), 48–55.

Malchaire, J., Cock, N., & Vergracht, S. (2001). Review of the factors associated with musculoskeletal problems in epidemiological studies. *International Archives of Occupational and Environmental Health, 74*, 79–90.

Manchikanti, L. (2000). Epidemiology of low back pain. *Pain Physician, 3*, 167–192.

Manusov, E. (2012). Evaluation and diagnosis of low back pain. *Primary Care, 39*, 471–479.

Marras, W., Parakkat, J., Chany, A., Yang, G., Burr, D., & Lavender, S. (2006). Spine loading as a function of lift frequency, exposure duration, and work experience. *Clinical Biomechanics, 21*(4), 345–352.

Mayer, T., & Gatchel, R. (1988). *Functional restoration for spinal disorders: The sports medicine approach*. Lea & Febiger.

McCarron, R., Wimpee, M., Hudkins, P., & Laros, G. (1987). The inflammatory effect of nucleus pulposus. A possible element in the pathogenesis of low-back pain. *Spine, 12*, 760–764.

McCauliffe, J. (2010). Tendon disorders of the hand and wrist. *Journal of Hand Surgery, 35A*, 846–853.

McHardy, A., Pollard, H., & Luo, K. (2007). One-year follow-up study on golf injuries in Australian amateur golfers. *American Journal of Sports Medicine, 35*, 1354–1360.

Miller, T., & Reinus, W. (2010). Nerve entrapment syndromes of the elbow, forearm, and wrist. *American Journal of Roentgenology, 195*, 585–594.

Miranda, H., Punnett, L., Viikari-Juntura, E., Heliövaara, M., & Knekt, P. (2008). Physical work and chronic shoulder disorder: Results of a prospective population-based study. *Annals of Rheumatic Diseases, 67*, 218–223.

National Institute for Occupational Safety and Health (1997). *Musculoskeletal disorders and workplace factors*. National Institute for Occupational Safety and Health.

National Research Council – Institute of Medicine (2001). *Musculoskeletal disorders and the workplace: low back and upper extremities*. Washington: DC, National Academy Press.

Neer, C. (1983). Impingement lesions. *Clinical Orthopaedics, 173*, 70–77.

Novak, C. B., Lee, G. W., Mackinnon, S. E., & Lay, L. (1994). Provocative testing for cubital tunnel syndrome. *Journal of Hand Surgery, 19*(5), 817–820. https://doi.org/10.1016/0363-5023(94)90193-7

O'Driscoll, S. W., Horii, E., Carmichael, S. W., & Morrey, B. F. (1991). The cubital tunnel and ulnar neuropathy. *Journal of Bone and Joint Surgery British, 73*(4), 613–617. https://doi.org/10.1302/0301-620X.73B4.2071645

Ohlsson, K., Attewell, R. G., Johnsson, B., Ahlm, A., & Skerfving, S. (1994). An assessment of neck and upper extremity disorders by questionnaire and clinical examination. *Ergonomics, 37*, 891–897.

Ortenblad, N., Lunde, P. K., Levin, K., Andersen, J. L., & Pedersen, P. K. (2000). Enhanced sarcoplasmic reticulum Ca(2+) release following intermittent sprint training. *American Journal of Physiology-Regulatory, Integrative and Comparative Physiology, 279*(1), 152–160. https://doi.org/10.1152/ajpregu.2000.279.1.R152

Ortenblad, N., & Stephenson, D. G. (2003). A novel signaling pathway originating in mitochondria modulates rat skeletal muscle membrane excitability. *Journal of Physiology, 548*(Pt 1), 139–145. https://doi.org/10.1113/jphysiol.2002.036657

Palmer, K. (2011). Carpal tunnel syndrome: The role of occupational factors. *Best Practice and Research in Clinical Rheumatology, 25*, 15–29.

Palmer, K., Harris, E., & Coggon, D. (2007). Carpal tunnel syndrome and its relation to occupation: A systematic literature review. *Occupational Medicine (London), 57*, 57–66.

Parsons, S., Breen, A., Foster, N. E., Letley, L., Pincus, T., Vogel, S., & Underwood, M. (2007). Prevalence and comparative troublesomeness by age of musculoskeletal pain in different body locations. *Family Practice, 24*, 308–316.

Pavan, P. G., Stecco, A., Stern, R., & Stecco, C. (2014). Painful connections: Densification versus fibrosis of fascia. *Current Pain and Headache Reports, 18*(8), 441. https://doi.org/10.1007/s11916-014-0441-4

Pelmear, P. (2003). The clinical assessment of hand-arm vibration syndrome. *Journal Occupational Medicine (London), 53*, 337–341.

Periasamy, M., & Kalyanasundaram, A. (2007). SERCA pump isoforms: Their role in calcium transport and disease. *Muscle & Nerve, 35*(4), 430–442.

Picavet, H., & Schouten, J. (2003). Musculoskeletal pain in the Netherlands: Prevalence's, consequences and risk groups, the DMC(3)-study. *Pain, 102*, 167–178.

Pink, M., & Tibone, J. (2000). The painful shoulder in the swimming athlete. *Orthopaedic Clinics of North America, 31*, 247–261.

Pope, D., Croft, P., Pritchard, C., & Silman, A. (1997). Prevalence of shoulder pain in the community: The influence of case definition. *Annals of Rheumatic Diseases, 56*, 308–312.

Pribicevik, M. (2012). The epidemiology of shoulder pain: a narrative review of the literature. In P. Ghosh (Ed.), *Pain in Perspective* (pp. 147–186). IntechOpen.

Punnett, L. (2005). Estimating the global burden of low back pain attributable to combined occupational exposures. *American Journal of Industrial Medicine, 48*, 459–469.

Rossignol, M., Leclerc, A., Allaert, F. A., Rozenberg, S., Valat, J. P., Avouac, B., . . . Hilliquin, P. (2005). Primary osteoarthritis of hip, knee, and hand in relation to occupational exposure. *Occupational and Environmental Medicine, 62*(11), 772–777.

Roto, P., & Kivi, P. (1984). Prevalence of epicondylitis and tenosynovitis among meatcutters. *Scandinavian Journal of Work, Environment, and Health, 10*, 203–205.

Saito, R. Y., Yano, M. Y., Angelini, L. C., Matos, D., Guimaraes, A. V., & Angelini, L. C. (2018). Prevalence of cubital tunnel syndrome among dock workers. *Revista Brasileira de Medicina do Trabalho, 16*(3), 270–276. https://doi.org/10.5327/Z1679443520180265

Sbernardori, M., & Bandiera, P. (2007). Histopathology of the A1 pulley in adult trigger fingers. *Journal of Hand Surgery, 32B*, 556–559.

Schafers, M., Sorkin, L. S., & Sommer, C. (2003). Intramuscular injection of tumor necrosis factor-alpha induces muscle hyperalgesia in rats. *Pain, 104*(3), 579–588. https://doi.org/doi:S0304395903001155

Schechtman, H., & Bader, D. (1997). In vitro fatigue of human tendons. *Journal of Biomechanics*, 829–835.

Schrier, V., Vrieze, A., & Amadio, P. C. (2020). Subsynovial connective tissue development in the rabbit carpal tunnel. *Journal of Veterinary Medical Science, 6*(4), 1025–1033. https://doi.org/10.1002/vms3.281

Schuind, F., Ventura, M., & Pasteels, J. (1990). Idiopathic carpal tunnel syndrome: Histologic study of flexor tendon synovium. *The Journal of Hand Surgery, 15*, 497–503.

Schwarzer, A., Aprill, C., & Bogduk, N. (1995). The sacroiliac joint in chronic low back pain. *Spine, 20*, 31–37.

Seitz, A., McClure, P., Finucane, S., Boardman, N., & Michener, L. (2011). Mechanisms of rotator cuff tendinopathy: Intrinsic, extrinsic, or both? *Clinical Biomechanics, 26*, 1–12.

Shah, N. P., Miller, T. T., Stock, H., & Adler, R. S. (2012). Sonography of supraspinatus tendon abnormalities in the neutral versus Crass and modified Crass positions: A prospective study. *Journal of Ultrasound in Medicine, 31*(8), 1203–1208. https://doi.org/10.7863/jum.2012.31.8.1203.Wiley

Sharma, P., & Maffulli, N. (2005). Tendon injury and tendinopathy: Healing and repair. *Journal of Bone and Joint Surgery (American), 87*, 187–202.

Shen, S., & House, R. (2017). Hand-arm vibration syndrome: What family physicians should know. *Canadian Family Physician, 63*, 206–210.

Shepherd, J., & Screen, H. (2013). Fatigue loading of tendon. *International Journal of Experimental Pathology, 94*, 260–270.

Shiri, R., Viikari-Juntura, E., Varonen, H., & Heliövaara, M. (2006). Prevalence and determinants of lateral and medial epicondylitis: A population study. *American Journal of Epidemiology, 164*, 1065–1074.

Silverstein, B. A., Fan, Z. J., Bonauto, D. K., Bao, S., Smith, C. K., Howard, N., & Viikari-Juntura, E. (2010). The natural course of carpal tunnel syndrome in a working population. *Scandinavian Journal of Work, Environment & Health*, 384–393.

Simons, D. G., & Travell, J. G. (1981). Myofascial trigger points, a possible explanation. *Pain, 10*(1), 106–109. https://doi.org/10.1016/0304-3959(81)90053-1

Sjøgaard, G., Lundberg, U., & Kadefors, R. (2000). The role of muscle activity and mental load in the development of pain and degenerative processes at the muscle cell level during computer work. *European Journal of Applied Physiology, 83*, 99–105.

Smidt, N. & van der Windt, D. A. (2006). Tennis elbow in primary care. *British Medical Journal, 333*, 927.

So, B., Kim, H. J., Kim, J., & Song, W. (2014). Exercise-induced myokines in health and metabolic diseases. *Integrative Medicine Research, 3*(4), 172–179. https://doi.org/10.1016/j.imr.2014.09.007

Stapleton, M. (2006). Occupation and carpal tunnel syndrome. *ANZ Journal of Surgery, 76*, 494–496.

Stauber, W. T. (2004). Factors involved in strain-induced injury in skeletal muscles and outcomes of prolonged exposures. *Journal of Electromyography and Kinesiology : Official Journal of the International Society of Electrophysiological Kinesiology, 14*(1), 61–70. https://doi.org/10.1016/j.jelekin.2003.09.010

Stenlund, B., Goldie, I., & Hagberg, M. (1993). Shoulder tendinitis and its relation to heavy manual work and exposure to vibration. *Scandinavian Journal of Work and Environmental Health, 19*, 43–49.

Stephens, R., Fatemi, A., Stephens, R., & Fuchs, H. (2001). *Metal Fatigue in Engineering* (2nd ed.). John Wiley & Sons.

Sternbach, G. (1999). The carpal tunnel syndrome. *The Journal of Emergency Medicine, 17*, 519–523.

Sterud, T., & Tynes, T. (2013). Work-related psychosocial and mechanical risk factors for low back pain: A 3-year follow-up study of the general working population in Norway. *Occupational and Environmental Medicine, 70*, 296–302.

Stockstill, J. W., Harn, S. D., Strickland, D., & Hruska, R. (1993). Prevalence of upper extremity neuropathy in a clinical dentist population. *Journal of the American Dental Association, 124*, 67–72.

Sun, H., Andarawis-Puri, N., Li, Y., Fung, D., Lee, J., Wang, V., & Flatow, E. L. (2010). Cycle-dependent matric remodeling gene expression response in fatigue-loaded rat patellar tendons. *Journal of Orthopaedic Research, 28*, 1380–1386.

Tanaka, S., Petersen, M., & Cameron, L. (2001). Prevalence and risk factors of tendinitis and related disorders of the distal upper extremity among US workers: Comparison to carpal tunnel syndrome*†. *American Journal of Industrial Medicine, 39*(3), 328–335.

Thomas, S. J., Reuther, K .E., Tucker, J. J., Sarver, J. J., Yannascoli, S. M., Caro, A. C., Voleti, P. B., Rooney, S. I., Glaser, D. L., & Soslowsky, L. J. (2014). Biceps detachment decreases joint damage in a rotator cuff tear rat model. *Clinical Orthopaedics and Related Research, 472*, 2404–2412.

Thomsen, J., Mikkelsen, S., Andersen, J., Fallentin, N., Loft, I., Frost, P., & Overgaard, E. (2007). Risk factors for hand-wrist disorders in repetitive work. *Occupational and Environmental Medicine, 64*, 527–533.

Thornton, G., Schwab, T., & Oxland, T. R. (2007). Cyclic loading causes faster rupture and strain rate than static loading in medial collateral ligament at high stress. *Clinical Biomechanics, 22*, 932–940.

Treaster, D., & Burr, D. (2004). Gender differences in prevalence of upper extremity musculoskeletal disorders. *Ergonomics, 47*, 495–526.

Van der Windt, D., Thomas, E., & Pope, D. (2000). Occupational risk factors for shoulder pain: A systematic review. *Occupational and Environmental Medicine, 57*, 433–442.

van Kampen, D., Berg, T., Woude, H., Castelein, R., Scholtes, V., Terwee, C., & Willems, W. (2014). The diagnostic value of the combination of patient characteristics, history, and clinical shoulder tests for the diagnosis of rotator cuff tear. *Journal of Orthopaedic Surgery Research, 9*, 40.

van Rijn, R. M., Huisstede, B. M., Koes, B. W., & Burdorf, A. (2009). Associations between work-related factors and specific disorders at the elbow: A systematic literature review. *Rheumatology (Oxford), 48*(5), 528–536. https://doi.org/10.1093/rheumatology/kep013

Vaquero-Picado, A., Barco, R., & Antuña, S. (2017). Lateral epicondylitis of the elbow. *EFORT Open Reviews, 1*, 391–397.

Vernon-Roberts, B., & Pirie, C. (1977). Degenerative changes in the intervertebral discs of the lumbar spine and their sequelae. *Rheumatology Rehabilitation*, *16*, 13–21.

Viikari-Juntura, E., & Silverstein, B. (1999). Role of physical load factors in carpal tunnel syndrome. *Scandinavian Journal of Work, Environment & Health*, *25*, 163–185.

Visser, B., & van Dieen, J. H. (2006). Pathophysiology of upper extremity muscle disorders. *Journal of Electromyography and Kinesiology*, *16*(1), 1–16. https://doi.org/10.1016/j.jelekin.2005.06.005

Waddell, G. (1987). Volvo award in clinical sciences: A new clinical model for the treatment of low-back pain. *Spine*, *12*, 632–644.

Walsh, T., Delahunt, E., & McCarthy, P. (2011). Effects of taping on thumb alignment and force application during PA mobilisations. *Manual Therapy*, *16*, 264–269.

Wolf, J., Sturdivant, R., & Owens, B. (2009). Incidence of de Quervain's tenosynovitis in a young, active population. *Journal of Hand Surgery*, *34A*, 112–115.

Wolf, J. M., Mountcastle S., Burks, R., Sturdivant, R. X., & Owens, B. D. (2010). Epidemiology of lateral and medial epicondylitis in a military population. *Military Medicine*, *175*, 336–339.

Yang, C., Leitkam, S., & Cote, J. N. (2019). Effects of different fatigue locations on upper body kinematics and inter-joint coordination in a repetitive pointing task. *PLoS One*, *14*(12), 0227247. https://doi.org/10.1371/journal.pone.0227247

Yoshii, Y., Zhao, C., Henderson, J., Zhao, K. D., An, K. N., & Amadio, P. C. (2011). Velocity-dependent changes in the relative motion of the subsynovial connective tissue in the human carpal tunnel. *Journal of Orthopaedic Research*, *29*, 62–66.

Yoshii, Y., Zhao, C., Zhao, K. D., Zobitz, M. E., An, K. N., & Amadio, P. C. (2008). The effect of wrist position on the relative motion of tendon, nerve, and subsynovial connective tissue within the carpal tunnel in a human cadaver model. *Journal of Orthopaedic Research*, *26*, 1153–1158.

Zajac, A., Chalimoniuk, M., Maszczyk, A., Golas, A., & Lngfort, J. (2015). Central and Peripheral Fatigue During Resistance Exercise. A Critical Review. *Journal of Human Kinetics*, *49*, 159–169. https://doi.org/10.1515/hukin-2015-0118

Zhang, Y. C. (2016). Intervertebral disc cells produce interleukins found in patients with back pain. *American Journal of Physical Medicine & Rehabilitation/Association of Academic Physiatrists*, *95*(6), 407.

Zugel, M., Maganaris, C. N., Wilke, J., Jurkat-Rott, K., Klingler, W., Wearing, S. C., & Hodges, P. W. (2018). Fascial tissue research in sports medicine: From molecules to tissue adaptation, injury and diagnostics: Consensus statement. *British Journal of Sports Medicine*, *52*(23), 1497. https://doi.org/10.1136/bjsports-2018-099308

3

Structure and Function of the Musculoskeletal System

A Systems View of the Musculoskeletal System

The musculoskeletal system is composed of a variety of specialized forms of tissues, including skeletal muscles, tendons, bones, joints, ligaments, and associated connective tissues. It also includes the nerves and blood vessels that bring innervation and blood supply to these structures. These tissues work together as a system, with skeletal muscles contracting as a result of nervous impulses leading to movement through force exertion on tendons, which then pull on bones. Most muscles cross one or more joints (producing movement in the joints that they cross) before attaching to the articulating bones that form a joint. With muscle contraction, one articulating bone is drawn toward the other. One bone is typically held in its original position, because other muscles stabilize it or contract in the opposing direction, or because the structure of the bone or joint makes it less movable. Ligaments provide stability to these joints. In this chapter, we will discuss the basic structure and function of each of these tissues, except for the basic structure and function nerves, which will be discussed in Chapter 4. Repair properties of each of these tissues will be discussed in Chapter 11.

Connective Tissues: General Overview

Connective tissues are the most abundant tissues in the body. They envelop, protect, support, and separate structures as well as bind structures together. Connective tissues also act as a cushion between tissues, provide a pathway for nerves and blood vessels into and out of individual tissues, and more. Most connective tissues have a rich nerve supply and blood supply (except for cartilage which is aneural and avascular, and tendons which have a scanty blood supply). Special connective tissue types include cartilage, osseous (bone), and vascular (blood). The matrixes of these connective tissues differ, with some being fluid (blood), semifluid, gelatinous, fibrous (tendon), or calcified (bone). In cartilage, for example, the matrix is firm but pliable, while in bone, the matrix is considerably harder but not pliable.

General Connective Tissue Structure

Cells

Fibroblasts are common support cells in connective tissues. They are mesenchymal pluripotent cells with great heterogeneity in their subtypes. Fibroblasts are key producers of collagen and are heavily involved in the continuous slow turnover of a tissue's extracellular matrix. When exposed

Musculoskeletal Disorders: The Fatigue Failure Mechanism, First Edition. Sean Gallagher and Mary F. Barbe.

to mechanical or physiological stress, fibroblasts adapt to their environment and have the ability to respond to and send local signals (e.g., cytokines and growth factors) (Dick, Miao, & Limaiem, 2020). Fibroblasts can also transform their phenotype into several other cell types for wound healing and replacement of damaged tissue (Dick et al., 2020). Other types of cells within connective tissues include adipocytes, macrophages (phagocytic immune cells), and plasma cells (cells that give rise to antibodies for immune defense). There are also mast cells that produce histamine and serotonin (chemicals that dilate small blood vessels) and heparin (an anticoagulant).

Extracellular matrix

The extracellular matrix of connective tissues consists of ground substance and fibers and plays a critical role as a scaffold within which tissues organize. The ground substance is the component of the matrix located between the cells and the fibers. It is typically a semifluid gel medium that serves for the passage of molecules through connective tissues and for the exchange of metabolites with the circulatory system (Young & Heath, 2000). It contains a mixture of long unbranched polysaccharide chains and water stabilized by glycosaminoglycans (GAGs), proteoglycans, and glycoproteins. The glycoproteins include structural (fibrillin and fibronectin), nonfilamentous (laminin, entactin, and tenascin), and integrin proteins (cell adhesion molecules). The typical gel-like property of the extracellular matrix is imparted by the large volume of these globular complexes and their hydrophilic nature (their highly charged side chains attract large volumes of water and ions), which, when combined, produces the characteristic turgor of the ground substance. The mechanical properties of a tissue's particular ground substance depend on the reinforcing fibrous proteins (collagen subtypes or elastin) or minerals (bone) to which these aggregates and other components are bound.

A number of types of fibrous proteins can be found in the ground substance of connective tissue. Collagen type I is the primary collagen in the dermis of skin (Figure 3.2), tendons, ligaments, and bone. It is formed by tropocollagen triple chains into larger fibrils (Iannarone, Cruz, Hilliard, & Barbe, 2019) that are visible under light microscopy. In contrast, collagen type II is the main collagen of hyaline cartilage and consists of fine filaments that cannot be visualized under light microscopy. Collagen type III is the major component of the fine reticular network within the bone marrow. It is also the first type of collagen deposited into developing or repairing tendons and bones. Elastin is a fibrous protein typically present as discontinuous fibrils (Figure 3.2) or sheets and confers the properties of stretch and elastic recoil (Young & Heath, 2000).

General Subtypes: Structure and Function

In this section, we summarize the general features of connective tissues and their function (see Table 3.1).

Loose connective tissue

Loose connective tissues are the most abundant in the body. In this general type of connective tissue (often divided into adipose, areolar, and reticular), the fibers are loosely woven and there are many cells. It is located around nerves and blood vessels, among others, and is composed of thin and relatively few fibers (collagenous, elastic, and/or reticular) and cell types, all embedded in a semifluid ground substance (Figure 3.1a). There are large numbers of cells and cellular processes, including fibroblasts, often adipocytes, immune cells, blood vessel and lymph vasculature cells, and neuronal processes (nerves) (Figure 3.1b). Functionally, this tissue provides cushioning, support, elasticity, and immune functions.

Table 3.1 General Features of Connective Tissues

Characteristic	Description
General types	• Loose (adipose, areolar, reticular); dense (e.g., tendon, cartilage, and bone); fascia (e.g., epimysium)
Cells	• Main cell types: Fibroblasts, adipocytes, resident macrophages, plasma cells
Extracellular matrix (ECM)	• Main composition: Polysaccharides, water, glycosaminoglycans (GAGs), proteoglycans, glycoproteins
	• Additional components: Collagen I/III, elastin, depending on subtype
Function	• Envelops, separates tissues and cells, cushions, supports, immune function, and more

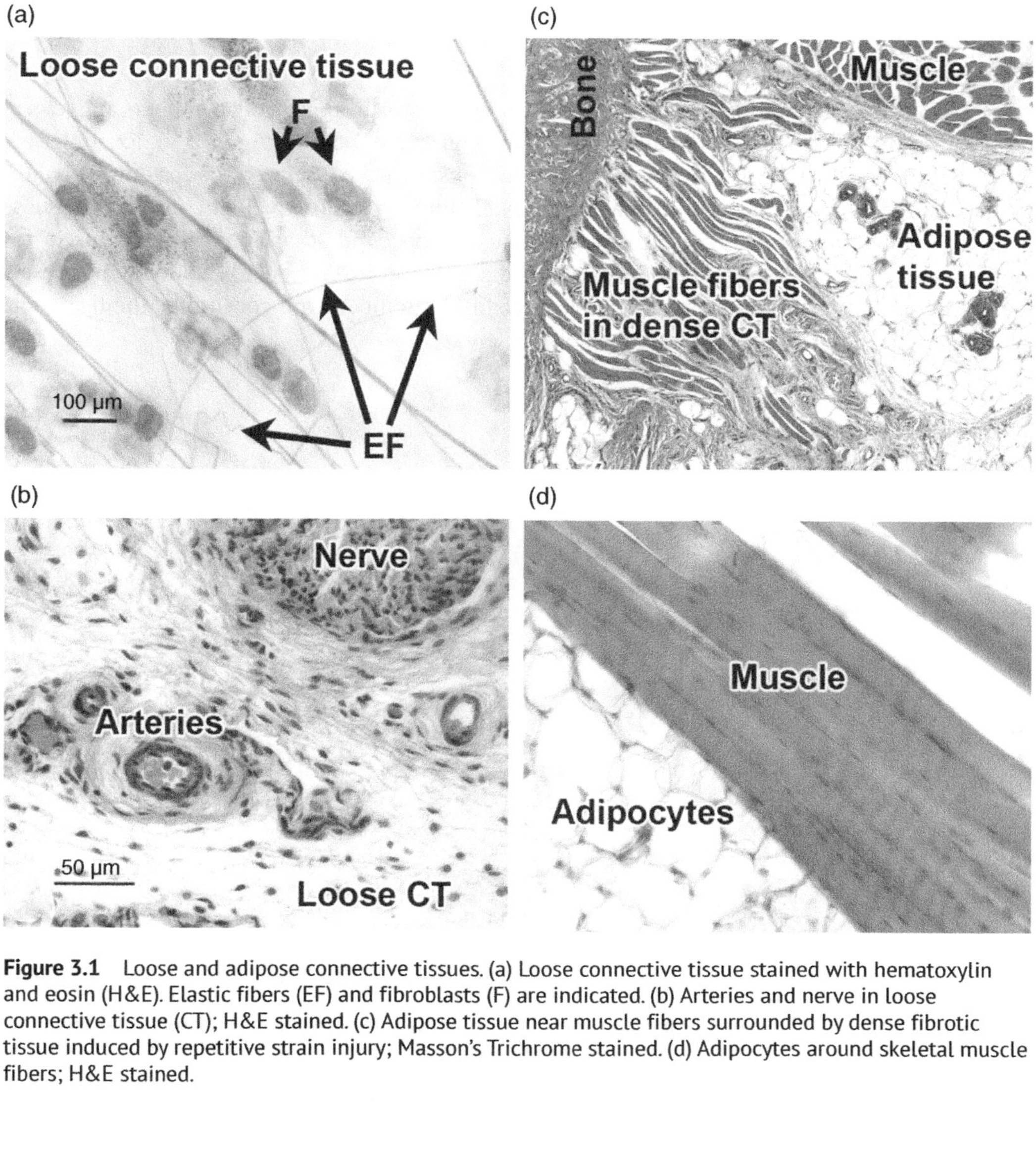

Figure 3.1 Loose and adipose connective tissues. (a) Loose connective tissue stained with hematoxylin and eosin (H&E). Elastic fibers (EF) and fibroblasts (F) are indicated. (b) Arteries and nerve in loose connective tissue (CT); H&E stained. (c) Adipose tissue near muscle fibers surrounded by dense fibrotic tissue induced by repetitive strain injury; Masson's Trichrome stained. (d) Adipocytes around skeletal muscle fibers; H&E stained.

Areolar tissue This type of loose connective tissue is the most widely distributed and is present in the dermis, around blood vessels, and nerves. It contains at one time or another, nearly all of the cell types normally found in connective tissue, including fibroblasts, macrophages, plasma cells, mast cells, adipocytes, and a few white blood cells. Its loose, randomly arranged fibers include collagen, elastic, or reticular. The ground substance is semifluid or gelatinous and contains primarily hyaluronic acid, chondroitin sulfate, dermatan sulfate, or keratan sulfate.

Adipose tissue Adipose tissue is primarily composed of adipocytes. It can be found in the subcutaneous layer of skin, the marrow of long bones, between muscles, and around nerves and joints (Figure 3.1c,d). It reduces heat loss through the skin and provides energy reserves, support, and protection.

Reticular tissue This type of loose connective tissue contains a fine network of collagen III fibers, often termed reticular fibers. It is present around blood vessels and muscle, within bone marrow, and in basement membranes.

Dense collagenous connective tissues

Dense connective tissues contain either regularly or irregularly arranged collagen fibers and fewer intercellular substance and cells than found in loose connective tissues (Figure 3.2). Examples of dense irregular connective tissues include the dermis of skin, deep fascia, the periosteum of bone, the perichondrium of cartilage, and organ capsules. Examples of dense regular connective tissues include tendons, ligaments, aponeuroses (thin flat tendon bands that connect one muscle to another or to bone), cartilage, and bone. Each is discussed in further detail separately in subsequent sections. Elastic tissue has a preponderance of elastic fibers and constitutes the ligament flava of vertebrae and arterial walls, among others.

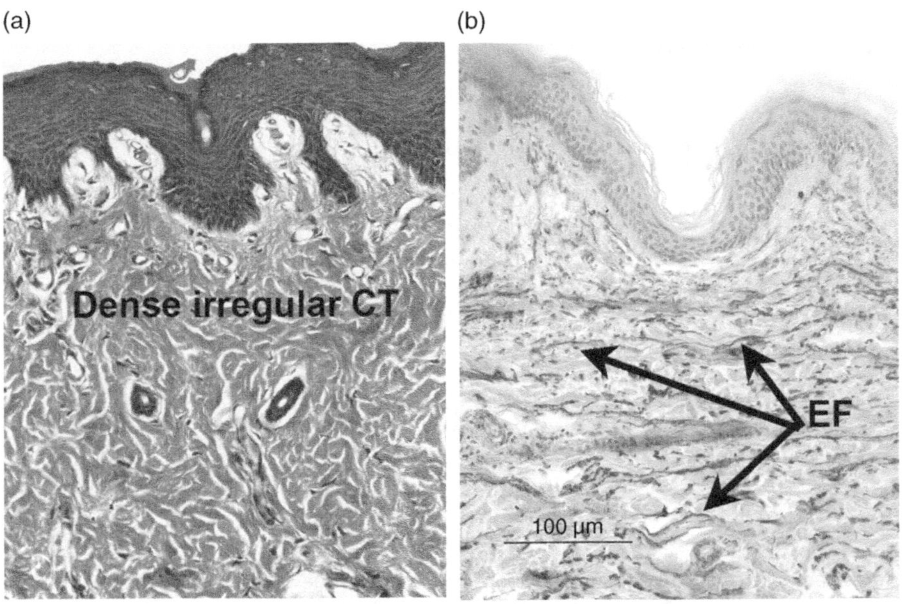

Figure 3.2 Dense irregular connective tissue in the dermis of the skin. (a) Masson's Trichrome staining detects the dense amount of collagen fibers. (b) Verhoeff Gieson Elastin Staining is used to detect elastic fibers (EFs). The black-stained EFs are surrounded by collagen fibers.

Fascia

Fascia is the term applied to the sheets or broad bands of fibrous connective tissue that (a) lies beneath the skin; (b) attaches, stabilizes, encloses, and separates muscle and tendons from each other; and (c) separates internal organs from each other. It is classified by layer (superficial, deep, visceral, or peritoneal fascia), function, or anatomical location. Superficial fascia is the subcutaneous layer of connective tissue that lies immediately deep to the skin. It serves as a storehouse of water and fat (which acts as insulation) and provides a pathway for nerves, vessels, and immune cells to travel between other tissues (Figure 3.1b). Deep fascia is a denser connective tissue that holds muscles and tendons together, fills spaces between tissues, and lines the body wall and extremities (e.g., the lower leg's crural fascia). Functionally, deep fascia allows free movement of muscles and tendons, carries blood vessels and nerves, and sometimes provides an attachment for muscle (e.g., the palmaris brevis muscle of the hand).

There are several extensions of deep fascia around and into individual muscles and tendons (Figure 3.3). The epimysium is the deep fascial dense connective tissue wrapping around the entire muscles. Invaginations of the epimysium into a muscle are termed perimysium (a type of irregular connective tissue) and endomysium (a type of reticular connective tissue). The epimysium, perimysium, and endomysium are all continuous with similar structures in tendons (epitenon, peritenon, and endotenon). Since tendons and aponeuroses (broad flat tendons) attach skeletal muscles to bones and other muscles, respectively, the continuity of these coverings allows skeletal muscles to produce movement.

Interstitial fascia or interstitium has been recently highlighted as a new term in the literature (Stecco & Caro, 2019; Stecco, Macchi, Porzionato, Duparc, & De Caro, 2011). By definition of its name, interstitial fascia is the located "between the cells." Anatomically, interstitial fascia is the highly vascularized and highly innervated superficial and deep fascial components mentioned earlier.

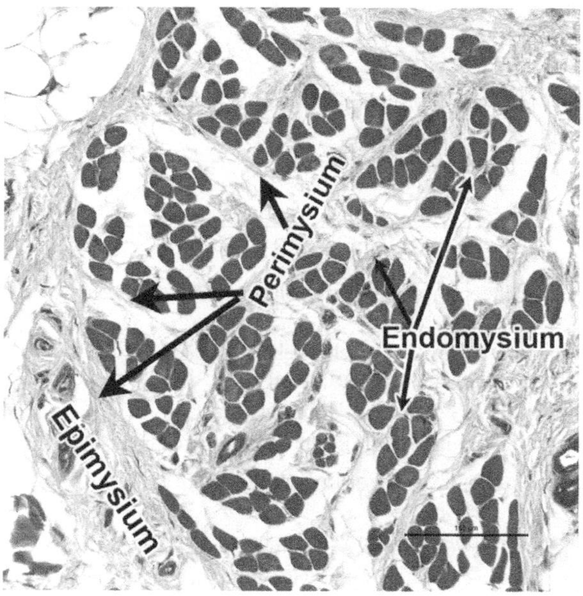

Figure 3.3 Extensions of deep fascia around and into individual muscle fibers. The epimysium (deep fascial fibrous connective tissue wrapping around entire muscle), perimysium (around individual fascicles), and endomysium (Endo; around individual muscle fibers/cells) are indicated.

Skeletal (Striated) Muscle

Muscle tissue consists of contractile cells that can be divided into skeletal (striated), cardiac, and smooth muscle subtypes. Skeletal muscle differs from the other two subtypes because it can be made to contract by conscious neural control, making it voluntary. Skeletal muscle tissue is composed of fused (i.e., multinuclear) specialized cells containing contractile proteins, connective tissue, blood vessels, and nerves (Table 3.2) (Gillies & Lieber, 2011). Muscle repair and adaptability is conferred by satellite and stem cells (both of which can replace damaged muscle cells) and neural innervation.

Skeletal Muscle Structure

Cells

Individual skeletal muscle fibers (also known as myofibers) are very long (up to 30 cm), cylindrical, typically arranged in parallel, and have diameters from 10 to 100 μm (Figures 3.4 and 3.5). They are multinucleated (more than one nucleus) as the result of the fusion of the mononucleated myoblasts that are muscle cell precursors. The nuclei are located just beneath the sarcolemma on the periphery of the sarcoplasm. The variation in muscle fiber diameters depends on many factors, such as age, gender, state of nutrition, physical training, or muscle damage. Physical training typically results in their enlargement of diameter and volume (hypertrophy), while their damage can lead to loss of cell volume and atrophy.

Muscle also contains satellite cells that are myogenic precursor cells (Mauro, 1961). Satellite cells are normally located beneath the basal lamina and adjacent to the sarcolemma of muscle fibers (Mauro, 1961; White & Esser, 1989). The satellite cells of young animals are referred to as myoblasts, are active, and initiate the process of muscle differentiation (Ishikawa, 1966; Snow, 1977). Yet, even in mature mammals in which satellite cells are typically quiescent, a muscle injury activates the satellite cells, driving them out of their quiescent state and initiating their proliferation

Table 3.2 Summary of Cells, Subtypes, Extracellular Matrix (ECM), and Function of Skeletal Muscle Under Normal Conditions

Characteristic	Description
Tissue type	• Contractile
Cells	• Main cell types: Individual muscle fibers (myofibers), myoblasts, satellite cells, bone marrow–derived stem cells • Additional cell types: Resident macrophages, endothelial cells associated with blood vessels throughout muscles, fibroblasts in sheaths, peripheral glial cells associated with nerve endings and neuromuscular junction
Subtypes	• Type I (slow-twitch/red), Type IIb (fast-twitch/white), Type IIa (intermediate), Type IIx
ECM	• Main composition: Collagen type I and glycoproteins in muscle proper, collagen IV in basement membrane • Additional components: Collagen III, collagen V, and elastin in fascial sheaths
Function	• Contraction and then movement of the endoskeleton to which the muscle is attached (bones and cartilage)

Based on Gillies, A. R., & Lieber, R. L. (2011). Structure and function of the skeletal muscle extracellular matrix. *Muscle Nerve 44*(3), 318–331. doi:10.1002/mus.22094.

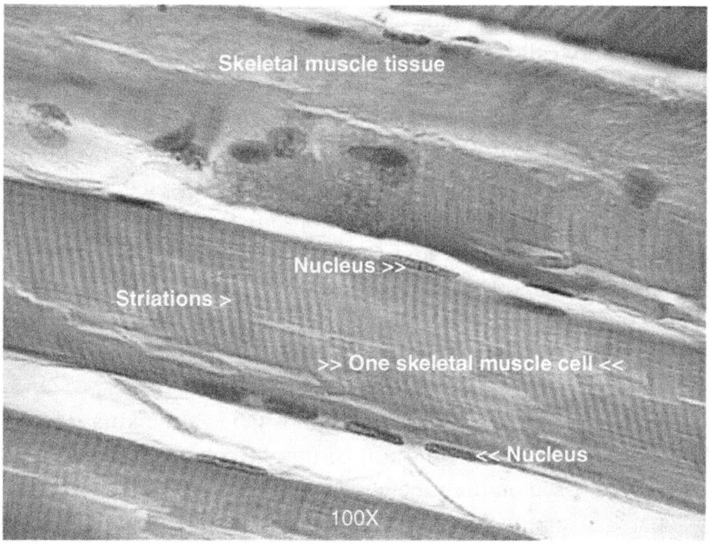

Figure 3.4 Single muscle cells (fiber) showing multinucleated nature and striations. From Tortora, G. J., & Derrickson, B. H. (Eds.), (2010). Muscle. In *Introduction to the human body*, 11th ed., Wiley.

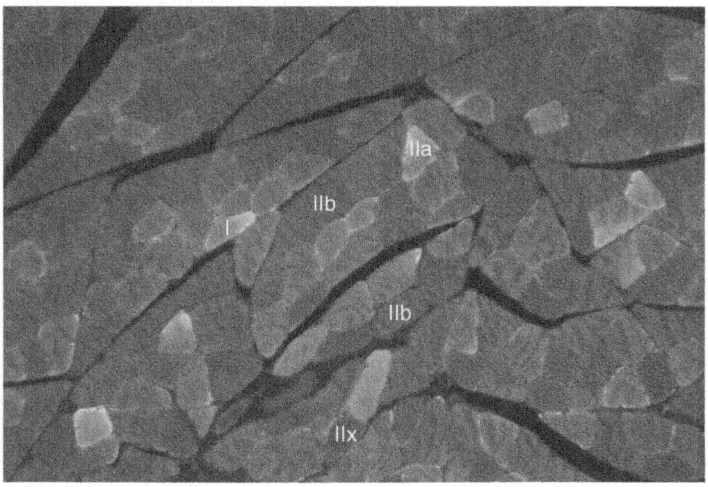

Figure 3.5 Distribution of different myosin heavy chains detected by immunofluorescence in a rat flexor digitorum muscle. This muscle is composed predominantly of type IIb (myosin heavy-chain type II) fast fibers. The banding seen is the myosin chains. A smaller number of fibers are type I, slow fibers. This muscle contains several intermediate fibers that stain for both types I and II myosin heavy chains. There are also some type IIx fibers that are unstained.

(Charge & Rudnicki, 2004). Thereafter, they undergo differentiation into myocytes and fuse either with each other or with existing myofibers for the repair of injured muscles (Charge & Rudnicki, 2004). A minor fraction of satellite cells regenerate themselves or self-renew and eventually return to a quiescent state (Collins et al., 2005). Bone marrow–derived stem cells that possess the ability to contribute to regeneration of injured skeletal muscle tissue have also been identified in human skeletal muscle (Stromberg et al., 2013). Thus, both satellite cells and bone marrow–derived stem cells play key roles in muscle growth and repair and are instrumental in the adaptation of muscle to various stimuli (Exeter & Connell, 2010). In pathological conditions and during muscle wound healing, inflammatory cells (neutrophils, macrophages, and lymphocytes) and myofibroblasts can be observed in muscle tissues (Barbe et al., 2021).

The connective tissue sheaths of muscles, described further below, contain fibroblasts, endothelial cells associated with blood vessels, nerve axons, and sometimes adipose cells and myofibroblasts. Muscles also contain resident macrophages that secrete various growth factors for the maintenance of the muscle fibers. The sites of neuromuscular junctions are the sites where nerve axons terminate on muscle fibers, and muscle spindles and Golgi tendon apparati are sensory receptors located within muscles and myotendinous junctions, respectively. These sites contain glial cells, the Schwann cells, and glial satellite cells, in additional to nerve axon terminals.

Metabolic subtypes

Muscle tissue obtains energy as adenosine triphosphate (ATP) and phosphocreatine kinase from both the aerobic metabolism of fatty acids and glucose and the anaerobic glycolysis. Skeletal muscle cells can be divided into three subtypes based on their metabolic and histochemical characteristics as well as their myosin heavy-chain subcomponents. Type I fibers, also known as slow-twitch fibers or "red" fibers, are small in size, contain many mitochondria and large amounts of myoglobin and cytochromes, and have high type I myosin heavy-chain content (Figure 3.5). Their glycolytic enzyme content is low. Myoglobin is an iron protein that binds O_2 and is the feature that makes these fibers appear dark red in color. Type I fibers obtain their energy primarily from aerobic oxidative phosphorylation of fatty acids. As a consequence, they are adapted for slow contractions over prolonged periods. Postural muscles of the back contain many type I fibers.

In contrast, type IIb, or fast-twitch fibers or "white" fibers, have an opposite metabolic profile. They are also large in size. They have abundant glycogen for the generation of APT via anaerobic metabolism, but fewer mitochondria and less myoglobin, giving them a pale whitish color. As a consequence, they depend on anaerobic glycolysis for energy and are adapted mainly for rapid contractions, although they undergo rapid physiological fatigue. These fibers are recruited during short-duration high-intensity activity, such as short sprints and maximum weight lifting.

Physiologically intermediate between slow and fast fibers are type IIa or intermediate fibers. They are also intermediate in size. They have many mitochondria and high myoglobin content and also contain a high amount of glycogen. Since they utilize both oxidative metabolism and anaerobic glycolysis, they are adapted for both rapid contracts and short bursts of energy. They are also intermediate in color and energy metabolism. There is high percentage of type IIa fibers in muscles used during sustained power activities, such as sprinting 400 m.

Experiments using myosin heavy-chain isoform immunostaining has also revealed an additional type of fiber, type IIx, that does not stain with antibodies against type I or II antibodies (and are thus unstained, as shown in Figure 3.5) (Pierobon-Bormioli, Sartore, Libera, Vitadello, & Schiaffino, 1981; Schiaffino, 2010). Interestingly, if nerves to slow and fast type fibers are exchanged experimentally, the fibers change their morphological and physiological features to conform to the innervating nerve.

Extracellular matrix

Collagen is the major structural protein in skeletal muscle extracellular matrix. It accounts for 1–10% of a muscle's dry weight (Dransfield, 1977; Schiaffino & Reggiani, 2011). Fibrillar types of collagen I and III predominate in the adult endomysium, perimysium, and epimysium (Listrat et al., 2000; Marvulli, Volpin, & Bressan, 1996). Type V collagen, another fibril-forming collagen, associates with types I and III and may form a core for type I collagen fibrils in the perimysium and endomysium (Fitch, Gross, Mayne, Johnson-Wint, & Linsenmayer, 1984). Elastin is also part of the fascial layers for the provision of structural elasticity. In contrast, the basement membranes of muscle fibers consist of a branched network structure of type IV collagen (Sanes, 1982). Many glycoproteins function as linker molecules between type IV collagen in the basement membrane and sarcolemma (Ervasti & Campbell, 1993). Interactions between these glycoproteins provide potential mechanisms for the transmission of lateral forces from myofibers (Grounds, Sorokin, & White, 2005).

Organization

Skeletal muscle is a hierarchically organized tissue that employs a bundling technique to develop its structure (Figure 3.6). Myofilaments are the chains of filamentous proteins located inside myofibrils. Groupings of myofibrils are bundled together into long cylindrically shaped muscle fibers (multinuclear muscle cells) by a plasma membrane that surrounds the cytoplasm (termed sarcolemma and sarcoplasm in muscles, respectively). Note, the sarcolemma is the plasma membrane of a striated muscle fiber; however, the sarcoplasmic reticulum, to be discussed shortly, is the smooth endoplasmic reticulum within muscle fibers. Next, the individual muscle fibers are bundled together into parallel bundles termed fascicles by a typically small amount of delicate connective tissue called the endomysium. The endomysium also occupies the space between individual muscle fibers (Figures 3.3 and 3.6). Most muscles are composed of multiple fascicles bundled together by a slightly denser collagenous connective tissue called the perimysium. These connective tissues contain cells (the most numerous being fibroblasts and macrophages), fibrous proteins (collagen and elastin), and ground substance in roughly equal parts. They are also flexible, well vascularized, innervated, and not very resistant to stress. Lastly, the entire muscle is surrounded by a dense external sheath of connective tissue called the epimysium (Figures 3.3 and 3.6). These various muscle-related connective tissue sheaths are linked together by thin septa of connective tissue that typically contain a small amount of collagen I and III and elastin. These connective tissue sheaths can undergo thickening as a consequence of increased collagen deposition in processes termed scarring or fibrosis, processes described further in Chapter 11.

Contractile proteins and the sarcomere

The arrangement of contractile proteins in skeletal muscle fibers gives rise to their light microscopic appearance of having cross-striations and thus the name "striated muscle" (Figures 3.4 and 3.6). These striations are alternating light and dark bands that are perpendicular to the long axes of muscle cells. The darker bands are called A bands and are visible due to their optical properties in polarized light (they are anisotropic); the lighter bands are called I bands (they are isotropic and do not alter their appearance in polarized light). Transmission electron microscopes reveal that each I band is bisected by a dark transverse line, termed the Z-disc (German, *Zwischenscheibe*, for "between the discs"). The repetitive functional subunit of the muscle fibers contractile apparatus is the *sarcomere* (Greek, *sarkos* + *mere*, part) and extends from Z disc to Z disc (Figure 3.7).

The sarcomere is filled with long cylindrical filamentous bundles termed myofibrils. Myofibrils have a diameter of 1–2 μm and run parallel to the long axis of the muscle fibers. Myofibrils consist of an end-to-end chain-like arrangement of sarcomeres that contain two types of myofilaments, thick and thin, that lie parallel to the long axis of the myofibril (Figure 3.6). These myofilaments are the contractile proteins of the myofibril. Each thin filament is composed of F-actin, tropomyosin, and troponin complexes. Troponin is a complex of three subunits: TnT that attaches to tropomyosin, TnC that binds calcium ions, and TnI that inhibits the actin–myosin interaction. Troponin

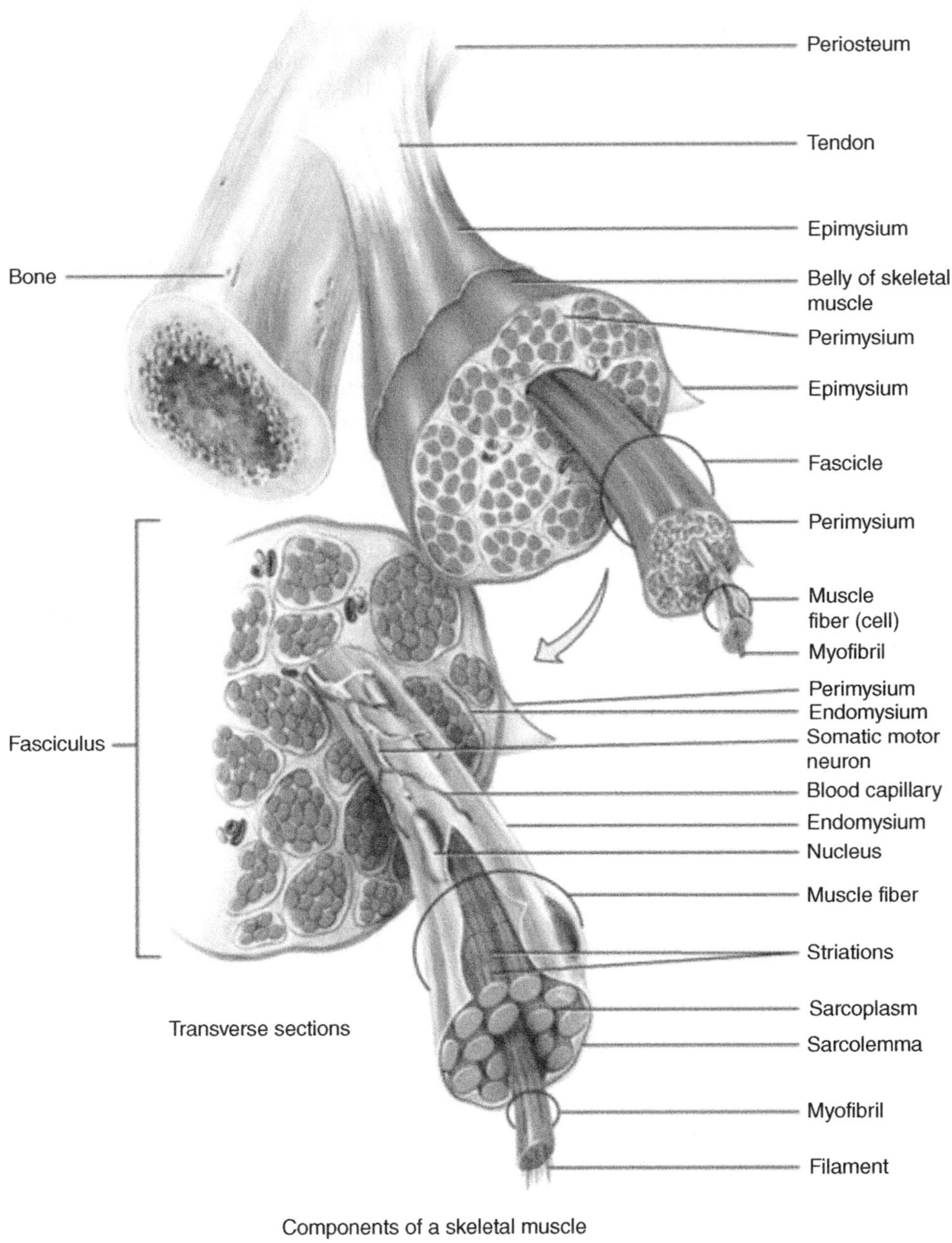

Figure 3.6 Structure of a skeletal muscle. Tortora, G. J., & Derrickson, B. H. (Eds.), (2010). Muscle. In *Introduction to the human body*, 11th ed., Wiley.

complexes are attached at regular intervals along each tropomyosin molecule. Each thick filament is composed of many myosin heavy-chain molecules bundled together along their rod-like tails, with their heads exposed and directed toward neighboring thin filaments. The thick myofilament bundles are held in place by myosin-binding proteins along the M line (German, *Mittelscheiber,*

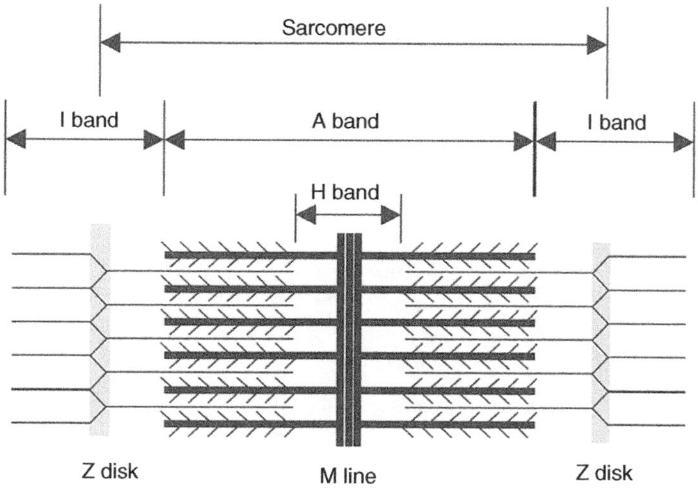

Figure 3.7 A simplified schematic of a sarcomere is shown. A sarcomere is composed of actin and myosin filaments that are organized into a characteristic pattern displaying A-, I-, M-, and Z-bands. Modified from Nayak, A. & Amrute-Nayak, M. (2020). SUMO system – A key regulator in sarcomere organization. *FEBS Journal, 287*, 2176–2190. https://doi.org/10.1111/febs.15263.

middle line). Small globular projections on one end of each heavy chain form the myosin heads that have ATP and actin-binding sites and the enzymatic capacity to hydrolyze ATP (Figure 3.10). Cross bridges are formed between the thin and thick filaments by the head of the myosin molecules plus a short part of its rod-like portion. These cross bridges are involved in the conversion of chemical energy to mechanical energy (Brunello et al., 2014). This structural biology generates the force necessary for the contraction of individual muscle fibers, which when bundled together into an entire muscle drive movement of the skeleton (via attachment of muscles and tendons to bones).

Sarcoplasmic reticulum and calcium storage and release

The sarcoplasmic reticulum of muscles is a membrane-bound structure that is similar to the smooth endoplasmic reticulum in other cells (a network of membranous tubules in the cytoplasm of eukaryotic cells that is in essence a transportation system). The sarcoplasmic reticulum is a key structure specialized in calcium ion (Ca^{2+}) storage (Figure 3.8). Depolarization of the sarcoplasmic reticulum membrane results in the release of Ca^{2+} ions. This release is initiated at the specialized neuromuscular junction (to be discussed shortly). For a uniform muscle contraction, the cell membrane of skeletal muscle fibers extends into and penetrates the center of the muscle fiber as a system of transverse (T) tubules that form a complex network encircling the A–I bands of each sarcomere. Adjacent to the opposite sides of each T-tubule are the expanded terminal cisternae of the sarcoplasmic reticulum. Two small cisternae of the sarcoplasmic reticulum and the T-tubule form a specialized complex known as a triad. It is this junction where a neurally mediated depolarization of the T-tubules is transmitted to the sarcoplasmic reticulum, stimulating a quick and widespread release of Ca^{2+}.

It is important to understand that muscle contraction depends on the availability of Ca^{2+} ions, while muscle relaxation occurs in the absence of Ca^{2+}. The sarcoplasmic reticulum (Figure 3.8) regulates Ca^{2+} flow necessary for rapid contraction and relaxation cycles. After depolarization of the sarcoplasmic reticulum, Ca^{2+} ions concentrated within cisterna are passively released into the

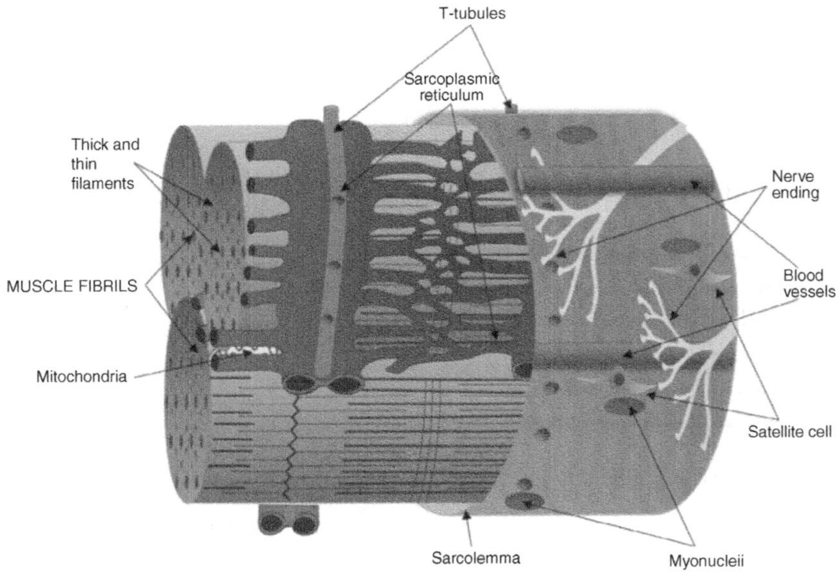

Figure 3.8 Diagram of the sarcoplasmic reticulum and T-tubule system of a mammalian skeletal muscle fiber. The sarcoplasmic reticulum enmeshes fibrils with transverse (T) tubules intersecting them. Invaginations of the T-tubules occur at the transition point of A and I bands in every sarcomere. The T-tubules are associated with terminal cisternae of the sarcoplasmic reticulum, forming triads. The cut surface of myofibrils also shows the thin and thick myofilaments. Satellite cells reside along the host muscle fiber, directly above the sarcolemma under the basal lamina of muscle and in proximity to the nuclei of muscle cells. Nerve endings and local capillaries extend along the length of the muscle fiber. The extracellular matrix, not shown here, successively encases each layer. Mukund, K. & Subramaniam, S. (2019). Skeletal muscle: A review of molecular structure and function, in health and disease. *Wiley Interdisciplinary Reviews: Systems Biology and Medicine, 12*, e1462./John Wiley & Sons/CC BY-4.0.

vicinity of the overlapping thick and thin filaments and bind to troponin. This allows bridging of the actin and myosin molecules. When the membrane depolarization ends, the sarcoplasmic reticulum actively transports the Ca^{2+} back into the cisternae, ending contractile activity.

Vascularization

Skeletal muscle is highly vascularized and can receive up to 80–85% of the heart's total cardiac output during heavy exercise (Figure 3.9) (Joyner & Casey, 2015). Muscle contraction requires a great deal of energy and, therefore, large amounts of nutrients and oxygen. Moreover, waste products (e.g., lactic acid) produced during the muscle's energy production reactions need to be eliminated. For this purpose, large blood vessels and nerves enter the epimysium and divide into branches that spread throughout the muscle in the perimysium and endomysium. Numerous capillaries run longitudinally through the endomysium as an "endomyseal capillary bed." There are frequent transverse anastomoses between these capillaries, resulting in a fine elongated capillary network that surrounds each muscle fiber.

Function of Skeletal Muscle Components

Proper function of skeletal muscle also requires careful coordination between muscle fibers and their proteins with connective tissues, blood vessels, and nerves. Overall, muscles, using their ability to contract, transmit their forces through tendons onto the endoskeleton (bones and cartilage), which allows the movement of the skeleton.

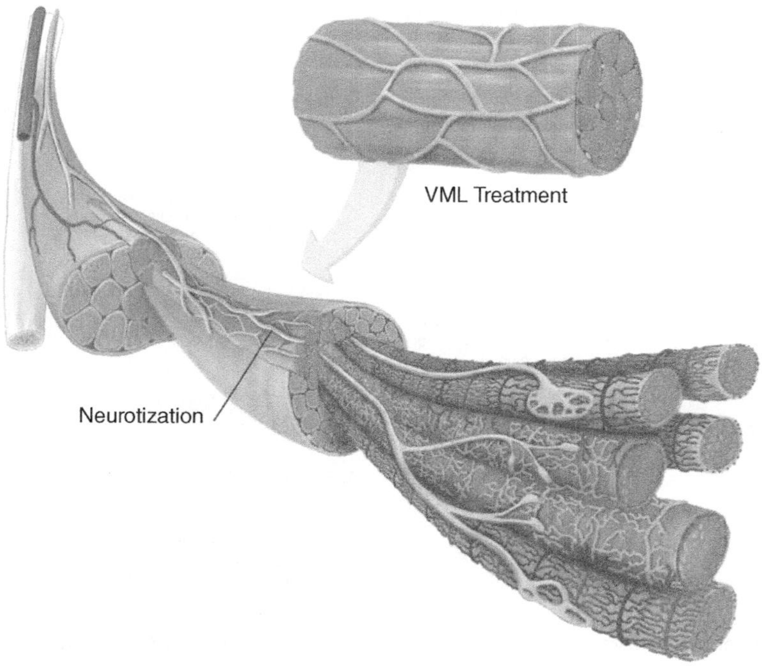

Figure 3.9 Vascular anatomy within skeletal muscle. (a) Highly organized vasculature with dense capillary networks run parallel to myofibers forming microvascular units optimized for nutrient transfer. Inset: Capillaries are embedded within myofiber sarcolemma, where mitochondria congregate at the contact site between capillary and myofiber. From: Gilbert-Honick, J. & Grayson, W. (2020). Vascularized and innervated skeletal muscle tissue engineering. *Advanced Healthcare Materials 9(1):* e1900626. Wiley.

Myosin filament sliding

The contraction of muscle tissues provides motion, maintenance of posture, and heat production. The mechanisms of contraction of sarcomeres are key to muscle function. The thin and thick filaments only partially overlap in resting sarcomeres (Figure 3.7). However, during contraction, the amount of overlap between these filaments increases due to sliding of the filaments past one another (Figure 3.10), which causes shortening of the sarcomere. This contraction is induced by an action potential produced at the myoneural synapse (the juncture of a somatic motor axon and a muscle fiber). At the sarcomere level, during contraction, a small subset of myosin heads align with available actin-binding sites. As the bound myosin heads move the actin, they provide for alignment of new actin–myosin cross bridges. The old bridges detach only after the myosin binds a new ATP molecule. This action resets the myosin head and prepares it for another contraction cycle. If no ATP is available, the actin–myosin complex become stable, which accounts for the extreme muscle rigidity associated with death (rigor mortis). A single muscle contraction is the result of hundreds of bridge-forming and bridge-breaking cycles. The contraction activity that leads to a complete overlap between thin and thick filaments continues until Ca^{2+} ions are removed, and the troponin–tropomyosin complex again covers the myosin-binding site.

Neuromuscular junction and muscle contraction

Skeletal muscle is considered as a voluntary muscle because it can be made to contract by conscious controls. In order for a skeletal muscle fiber to contact, it must first be stimulated by an impulse (an action potential) from a motor nerve cell. The neurons that stimulate muscles to

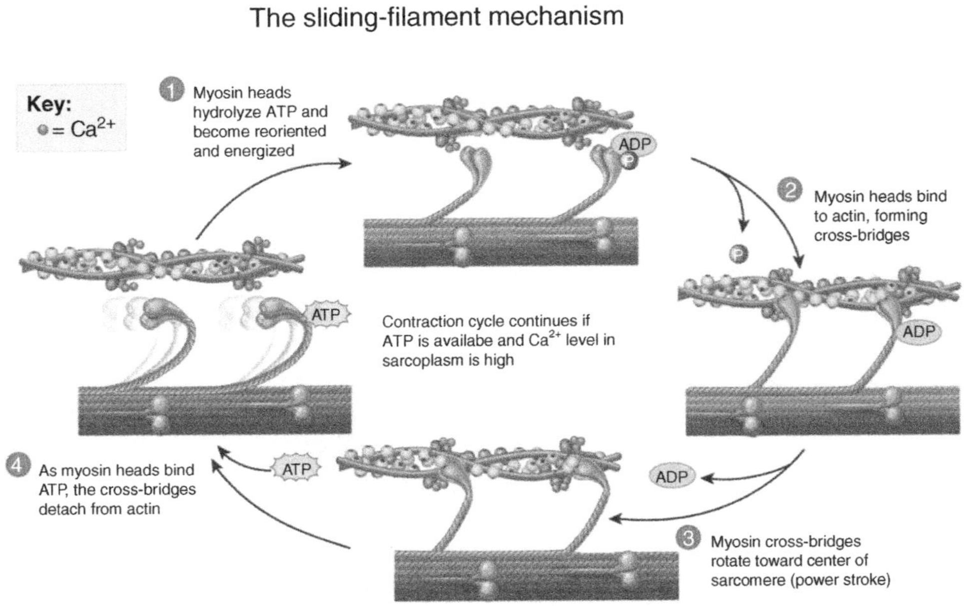

Figure 3.10 The sliding-filament mechanism. Tortora, G. J., & Derrickson, B. H. (Eds.), (2010). Muscle. In *Introduction to the human body*, 11th ed., Wiley.

contract are somatic (of the body) motor neurons and have cell bodies that originate in the spinal cord or brainstem and have nerve processes (axons) that extend into the periphery to muscles (see Chapter 4). In skeletal muscle, myelinated somatic motor nerves branch into the perimysium and divide into several terminal smaller branches that innervate the muscle fibers. At the site of innervation, the axon loses its myelin sheath and forms a dilated terminal situated within a trough on the muscle cell surface, the neuromuscular junction (also known as a motor end plate) (Figure 3.11). Within this axon terminal are numerous synaptic vesicles containing the neurotransmitter acetylcholine. When a somatic neuron fires and the action potential reaches the motor end plate, acetylcholine is released into a synaptic cleft (a space between the axonal terminal and the muscle). The synaptic cleft is a highly folded region of the sarcolemma that allows for more surface area. There are numerous mitochondria, ribosomes, and glycogen granules at this site. When acetylcholine binds to its receptor, Na^+ channels open and membrane depolarization results. Excess acetylcholine in the synaptic cleft is hydrolyzed by the enzyme cholinesterase to avoid prolonged contact of the neurotransmitter with its receptors. The depolarization is then propagated deep into the myofiber by the previously discussed transverse tubule system. At each triad (a T-tubule and two cisterna), the depolarization signal is passed to the sarcolemma reticulum. This results in a release of Ca^{2+} and initiation of the muscle cells's contraction cycle. When the depolarization ceases, the Ca^{2+} is actively transported back into the cisterna for storage, and the muscle cell relaxes.

Extracellular matrix/fascia

As previously mentioned and depicted (Figures 3.3 and 3.6), individual muscle fibers are bound together by a complex system of collagenous supporting tissue that link individual myofibers into a fascicle in order to form a single functional mass (Gillies & Lieber, 2011). The size of the

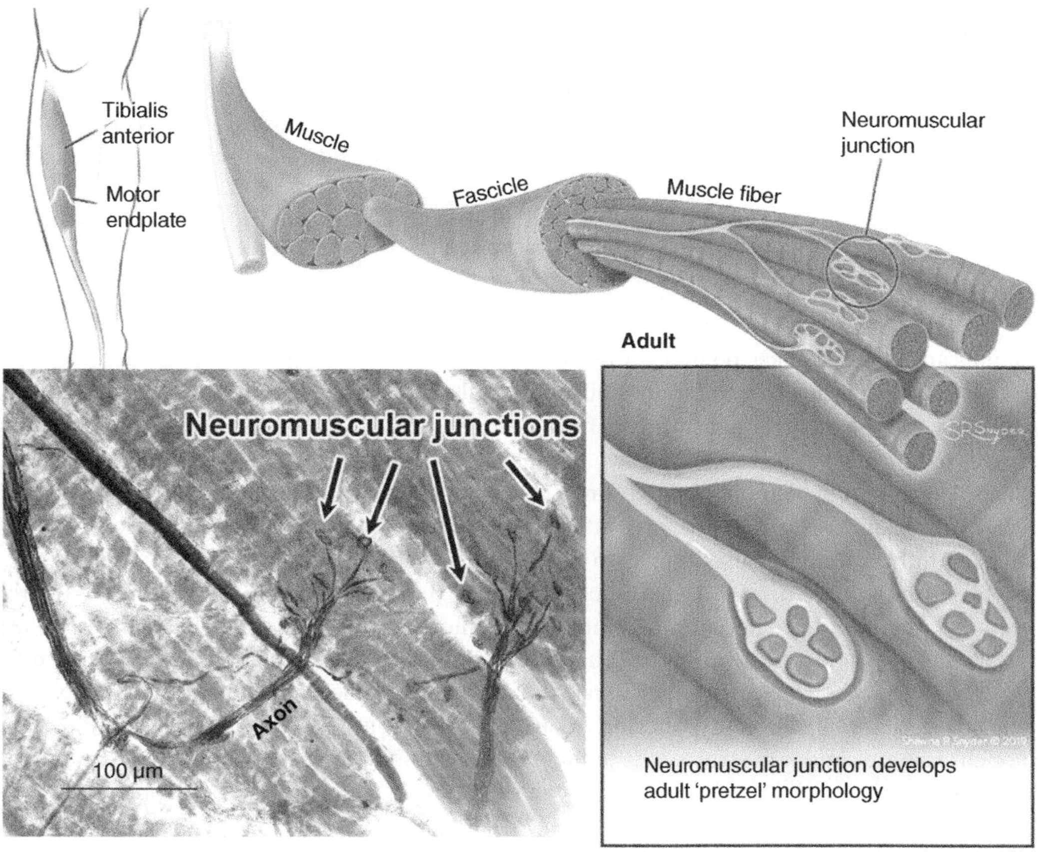

Figure 3.11 The neuromuscular junction. Adult skeletal muscle is highly organized with one neuronal branch innervating each myofiber at the neuromuscular junction, which exhibits a mature, pretzel morphology with direct overlap between the presynaptic nerve terminal bouton and the postsynaptic acetylcholine receptor clusters. Gilbert-Honick, J. & Grayson, W. (2020). Vascularized and innervated skeletal muscle tissue engineering. *Advanced Healthcare Materials* 9(1): e1900626. Wiley.

fasciculi reflects the function of a muscle. Muscles responsible for fine controlled movements, like those of the hand, have small fasciculi and a relatively greater proportion of perimysial supporting tissue. Larger muscles responsible for gross movements have large fascicles and relatively little perimysial tissue. Muscle fibers are also anchored by these fascial connective tissues. The external lamina transmits the contractile forces developed by the internal contractile proteins. The connective tissue framework becomes continuous with those of tendons, as well as bone or skin when muscles are directly attached to these latter structures. The extracellular matrix also serves as a biological reservoir of muscle stem cells. In both injured and diseased states, the extracellular matrix adapts dramatically, a property that has clinical manifestations for muscle function.

Muscle as an endocrine system

Skeletal muscle is also an endocrine system and serves as a major site of insulin-stimulated glucose disposal and homeostasis (Mukund & Subramaniam, 2019). It secretes a variety of cytokines and peptides, termed "myokines," including interleukin (IL)-8, IL-18, IL-15, insulin like growth factor

1 (IGF1), and fibroblast growth factor 21 (FGF21). These factors are regulated by muscle contractile activity and exercise. These myokines exert autocrine (self), paracrine (related only to the local vicinity of the organ producing the factor), and endocrine (systemic signaling) effects in a context-dependent manner that enables muscles to maintain metabolic homeostasis during health and exercise, and responses during chronic metabolic conditions and disorders. This will be discussed further in Chapters 11 and 15.

Tendon

Tendons are a type of dense regular connective tissue since they are arranged in a highly organized pattern with a clear predominance of collagen fibers over ground substance and cell numbers. They can also be thought of as a fibrous cord or band of variable length that anchor muscles to bone. Many muscles have two tendons at both their proximal and distal ends (such as the biceps muscle of the upper extremity), although some muscles attach directly to bone without a tendon (such as the proximal attachments of deep flexor and extensor muscles on the radius and ulna). Tendons may unit with muscles at the end of a muscle, or it may run along the side of the muscle or within its center for long or short distances, receiving muscle fibers along its lateral border. The point of union with a muscle is called a myotendinous junction (Kannus, 2000). Although tendons are characterized by their great tensile strength (Benjamin & Ralphs, 1998), they have dynamic characteristics that belie their appearance and respond to exercise or immobilization by altering their tensile strength (Woo & Buckwalter, 1988). Aponeuroses are similar in structure to tendons, although they are thinner sheet-like structures and connect one muscle to another muscle or to bone. The overall characteristics of tendons are summarized in Table 3.3.

Tendon Structure

Cells

A variety of distinctive cell types occur within tendons. Tenocytes are transformed from tenoblasts (immature tenocytes), which are rounded cells with large, ovoid nuclei (Borynsenko &

Table 3.3 Summary of Cells, Extracellular Matrix (ECM), Subregions, and Function Of Tendons Under Normal Conditions

Characteristic	Description
Tissue type	• Dense regular connective tissue
Cells	• Main cell types: Tenocytes, tenoblasts, tendon stem/progenitor cells (TSPC) • Additional cell types: Chondrocytes or synovial cells in tendon subregions, peripheral glial cells associated with nerve endings, fibroblasts in sheaths, endothelial cells associated with blood vessels in sheaths
ECM	• Main composition: 65–80% collagen I, water, proteoglycans, glycoproteins, elastin, mucin
Subregions	• Myotendinous junction, tendon midbody, enthesis
Function	• Transfer of tensile forces created by muscles onto bone; absorbs sudden shocks to limit muscle damage

Beringer, 1989). Tenocytes are flat tapered cells that appear spindle-shaped in longitudinal tissue sections and stellate (with long extensions) in cross sections. Tenocytes, a common synonym for differentiated fibroblast-like cells that lie within rows within the tendon proper, comprise about 95% of the cellular elements of a tendon. They lie sparingly in longitudinal rows between collagen fibrils (Figure 3.12) (Butler, Grood, Noyes, & Zernicke, 1978) and are aligned in parallel with the primary direction of force on the tendon. Tenocytes synthesize collagen and most other compounds of a tendon's extracellular matrix (Evans & Barbenel, 1975; Kjaer, 2004). Tendons also contain low numbers of stem/progenitor cells (tendon stem/progenitor cells, which are also regarded as tendon-derived stem cells). These cells show typical stem cell characteristics of self-renewal capacity (Li, Wu, & Liu, 2021). In tendon fascial sheaths, there are also different subpopulations of fibroblasts with different roles in matrix synthesis and cell migration during wound healing (Jozsa & Kannus, 1997). The remaining 5–10% of cells in a tendon includes chondrocytes (located at entheses, where the tendon attaches to bone, Figure 3.12c), endothelial cells associated with blood vessels, and peripheral glial cells associated with nerve processes. In pathological

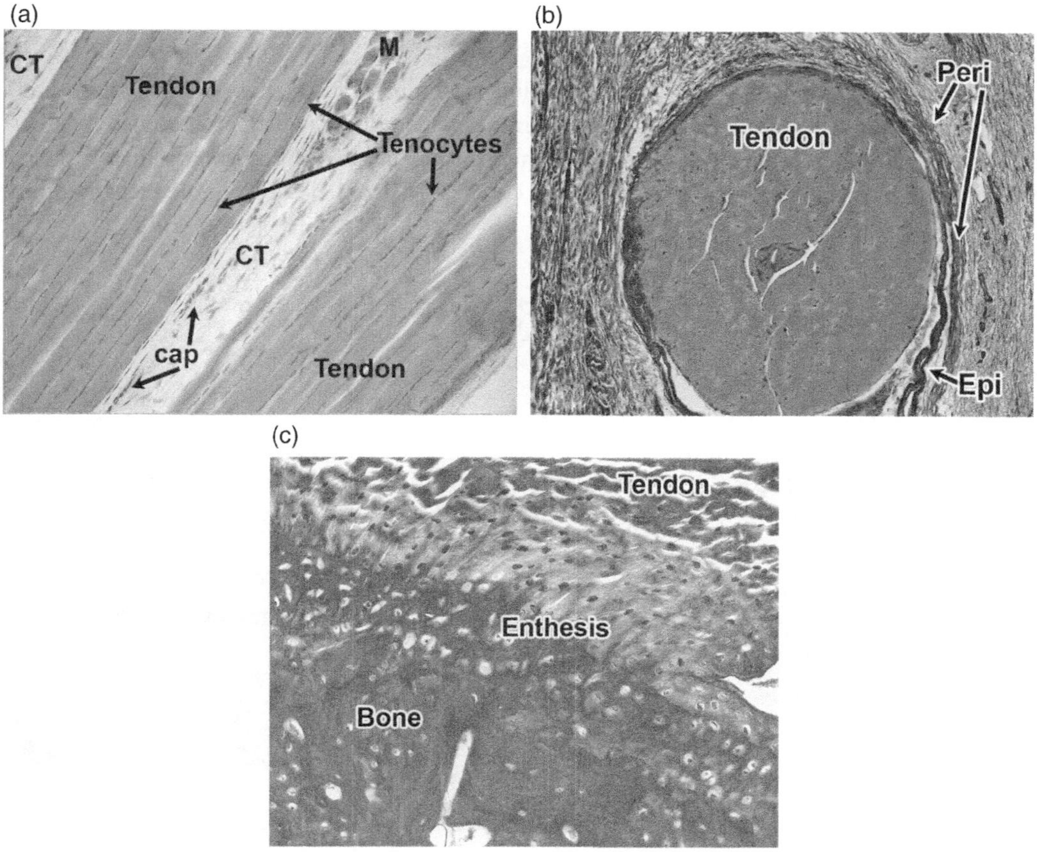

Figure 3.12 Tendon images. (a) Longitudinal tendon section, with examples of tenocytes (tendon fibroblast like cells) indicated. CT = loose connective tissue; cap = capillary; M = muscle fibers/cells. Hematoxylin and eosin (H&E) staining. (b) Cross-section through a small tendon in the palm. It lacks individual fascicles, so just the outer epitenon (epi) and peritenon (peri) layers are visible. Masson's Trichrome staining. (c) The tendon–bone intersection called an enthesis. Masson's Trichrome staining.

conditions and during wound healing, inflammatory cells (neutrophils, macrophages, and lymphocytes) and myofibroblasts can be observed in tendon tissues (Barbe et al., 2021; Fedorczyk et al., 2010; Jozsa & Kannus, 1997; Kietrys, Barr, & Barbe, 2011).

Extracellular matrix

The dry mass of a tendon accounts for about 30% of the total tendon mass, with water making up the remainder (Sharma & Maffulli, 2005). This dry mass portion is 65–80% collagen, 0.2% proteoglycans and inorganic substances, 1–2% elastin, and 4.5% other proteins (O'Brien, 1997). The most abundant type of collagen in tendons is collagen I (95%), with the remaining being collagen III and IV. In immature and healing tendons, collagen III is the initial collagen deposited by tenocytes (and occurs in a disorganized manner) and is subsequently replaced by collagen I. The direction of the collagen fibers is aligned linearly with the stresses exerted on the tendon. Several extracellular proteins cross-link and act as structural scaffolds for the larger collagen I interdigitating fibrils. These include decorin, fibromodulin, laminin 2, and tenascin C. The inorganic components (calcium and magnesium) are involved in growth, development, and normal metabolism of tendon tissue (Kannus, 2000). There is also an interstitial matrix (Figure 3.13) that contains ground substance, such as mucin (Ali et al., 2015).

Organization

Like muscle, tendons exhibit a hierarchical bundling structure (Figure 3.13). At the smallest level, collagen molecules (tropocollagen) are bundled into collagen fibrils, which are bundled together into interdigitating collagen fibrils. These are then further bundled into primary fiber bundles (subfascicles) by an endotenon connective tissue layer. The subfascicles are bundled together into

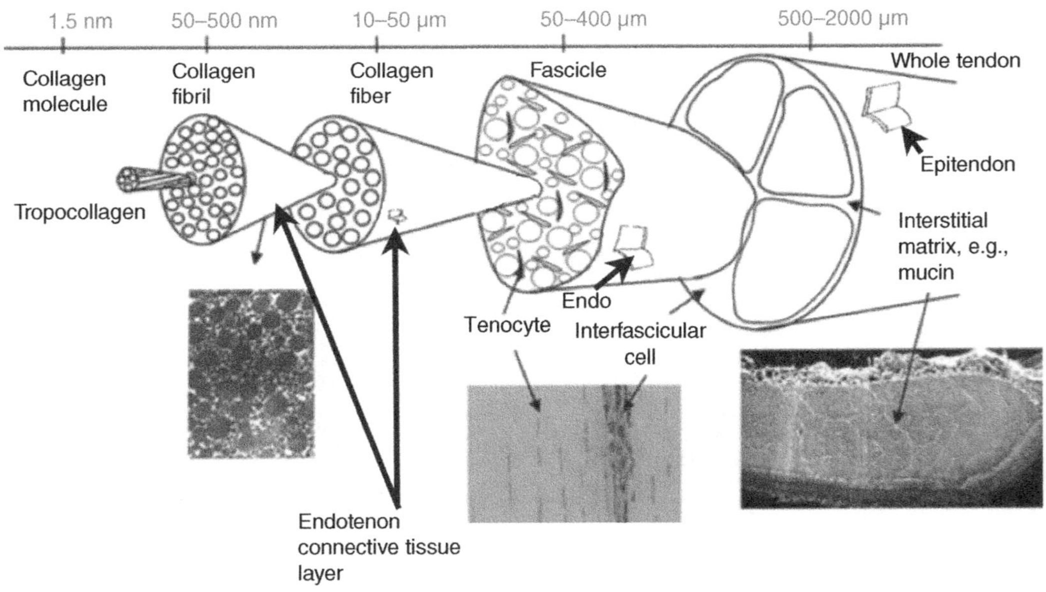

Figure 3.13 Schematic depicting the hierarchical structure of tendon, with inset images: Transverse sections show fibril and fascicle packing. The longitudinal histological section (hematoxylin and eosin) shows the tendon cell populations. Modified from: Screen, H. R., Berk, D. E., Kadler, K. E., Ramirez, F., & Young, M. F. (2015). Tendon functional extracellular matrix. *Journal of Orthopaedic Research*, *33*(6), 793–799, First published: 30 January 2015, doi: 10.1002/jor.22818. Wiley.

a larger fascicle that is also surrounded by endotenon. At the fascicle level, a characteristic "crimp" pattern can be seen histologically. Several fascicles are then bundled together to form the whole tendon, all of which are surrounded by an outer denser epitenon wrapping (Figures 3.12 and 3.13). This nested structure allows the bundles to slide independently from one another. As mentioned above, there are several components to the extracellular matrix of tendons that are hierarchically arranged and cross-linked together. This highly ordered structure provides strength, durability, high tensile strength, and stability during force transmission.

At the macroscopic level, tendons are not homogeneous structures. They can be broadly divided into three regions along their axis. There is a muscle–tendon junction (the myotendinous junction), a tendon midbody, and a tendon–bone junction (the enthesis) locates where tendons attach to bone. The myotendinous junction and enthesis have distinct structural, cellular, and molecular characteristics compared to the midbody of a tendon. The myotendinous junction displays a "zipper" like morphology, where skeletal muscle fibers and tendon collagen fibrils interdigitate. At this same point, the cytoskeletal network and basement membrane of muscle fiber bundles directly attach to the collagen fibrils of tendons. Regarding entheses (Figure 3.12c), some are primarily fibrous and noncartilaginous, although most tendon–bone attachments employ fibrocartilagenous entheses. The latter consist of four zones of connective tissue, listed in order from the tendon to the bone: (a) fibrous tissue originating from tendon (the aligned collagen fibrils surrounding fibroblasts resemble the tendon midbody), (b) uncalcified fibrocartilage, (c) calcified fibrocartilage, and (d) subchondral bone. This gradual change in structure reduces mechanical stress levels between the tensile tendon and the brittle bone.

Some tendons are also enclosed by tube-like synovial sheaths, for example, at the wrist and ankle. These sheaths are made up of two layers, both lined by flattened synovial cells of mesenchymal origin. The inner visceral layer is attached to the surface of the tendon, while the outer parietal layer is adjacent to neighboring structures. The space between these layers contains a viscous fluid similar in composition to the synovial fluid of synovial joints. This liquid is composed of water, proteins, hyaluroanate, and other glycosaminoglycans. This synovial secretion acts as a lubricant permitting easy sliding movements of a tendon within its sheath. Tendinitis or tenosynovitis is an inflammation of this tendon sheath and are painful conditions that can follow trauma, excessive strain, or excessive exercise (see Chapters 2 and 11).

Tendons have a very rich neural network and are often innervated from the muscles with which they are associated or from local nerves. There are many nerve endings at the sites of myotendinous junctions and bone–tendon junctions, including Golgi tendon organs and free nerve endings (which are typically pain fibers), as discussed further in Chapter 4. With regard to vascularization, the interior of healthy tendons is fairly devoid of blood vessels, with most of the blood vessels localized to the tendon sheaths.

Function of Tendon Components

Transfer of forces

The myotendinous junctions and entheses described earlier facilitate force transfer between these structures. For example, the myotendinous junctions allow tendons to absorb sudden shocks in order to limit muscular damage (Selvanetti, Cipolla, & Puddu, 1997), and the entheses transfer muscle tensile forces across tendons and onto bone, enabling joint flexion. For this purpose, the collagen fibers of tendons are continuous with those in the endomysium and perimysium connective tissue layers in muscles, as well as with the periosteum of bones. However, tendons fibrils do not run continuously from muscle to bone. Instead, stress is transferred through a hydrated proteoglycan-rich gel matrix in which the fibers of this fiber-reinforced composite are contained (Ker, 2002; Shepherd & Screen, 2013).

Mechanotransduction in tenocytes

Tenocytes are stellate in shape when examined in longitudinal sections, with elongated protrusions in all directions. These protrusions contact tenocytes within the same and adjacent rows, thus forming an intricate tendon network. There are gap junctions at these contact points. Gap junction proteins, such as, connexin 43, are expressed at these sites and are thought to regulate the transfer of proteins between tenocytes via mechanisms that are still unclear. Yet, these gap junctions are considered essential mediators of the mechanotransduction function of tenocytes (mechanotransduction is defined as a cell's response to mechanical cues by biochemical signals). Similar to other mechanosensitive cells, mechanotransductive responses are involved in tenoctye homeostasis, healing, and degeneration. Tenocyte homeostasis is regulated by the production of degradative enzymes (e.g., matrix metalloproteinases [MMPs]) and extracellular proteins (e.g., collagen). Altered mechanical loading promotes changes in mechanosensitive proteins, including integrins and the tenocyte transcription factor, scleraxis, which is important for tenogenesis. Altered mechanical loading also leads to increased production of transforming growth factor beta 1 (TGFbeta-1). TGFbeta-1 is a key regulator of differentiation, proliferation, and extracellular matrix production for most cell types, including tenocytes. The production of several other proteins is altered by mechanical loading, including the cytokine IL-1, cyclooxygenase 2 (COX2), platelet-derived growth factor (PDGF), and CCN2/CTGF (cell communication network factor 2, formally known as connective tissue growth factor). In this manner, altered mechanical loading can lead to catabolism (via a degradative environment) or anabolism (increased tenocyte biomechanical properties via altered production in the mix of extracellular matrix proteins).

Cartilage

Cartilage is unique in all of the body tissues in that it is typically avascular, aneural, and alymphatic (Tortora & Derrickson, 2010). Because of these properties, injuries and damage to cartilage can be difficult to detect until they are quite severe, and difficult from which to heal. The general features of cartilage are summarized in Table 3.4.

Structure

Cells

Chondrocytes are the prevalent cells of cartilage, with the number per matrix ratio differing with cartilage type. Chondrocytes arise from chondroblasts, which are proliferating cells that originate from mesenchymal cells after exposure to the transcription factor SOX9 [sex determining region Y (SRY)-box 9]. Chondroblasts produce type II collagen, aggrecan, proteoglycans, and glycosaminoglycans, and therefore, the cartilaginous matrix. They become embedded in individual lacunae within the matrix that they produce (Figure 3.15); once embedded, they become chondrocytes. Chondrocytes then maintain the cartilage matrix throughout life, although the numbers of chondrocytes reduce with age. Joint trauma, inflammation, and stress fractures that extend into the cartilage can lead to chondrocyte damage and severe structural damage of the cartilage (Xiong & O'Brien, 2012).

Table 3.4 Summary of Cells, Extracellular Matrix (ECM), Subtypes, and Function of Cartilage and its Subtypes Under Normal Conditions

Characteristic	Description
Tissue type	• Dense pliable connective tissue
Cells	• Main cell types: Chondrocytes, chondroblasts • Additional cell types: Mesenchymal stem cells (low in number)
ECM	• Hyaline cartilage: Collagen II (15–20%), water (60–80%), GAGs (e.g., hyaluronic acid) • Fibrocartilage: High collagen content, lower water content than hyaline • Elastic cartilage: High elastin fiber content
Subtypes	• Hyaline (and its subtype, articular cartilage), fibrocartilage, elastic
Function	• Hyaline: Protection of bony surfaces, especially at points of movement • Fibrocartilage: Strength and rigidity, joint support and fusion • Elastic cartilage: Resilience and pliability

Extracellular matrix

In general, the extracellular material of each type of cartilage is firm but pliable. Cartilage consists of a dense network of collagen fibers (the type dependent on the subtype of cartilage) and sometimes elastic fibers, each embedded in chondroitin sulfate (a jelly-like substance). The collagen fibers add great strength to cartilage, while the ability of cartilage to assume its original shape after deformation is due to the chondroitin sulfate. The three primary types of cartilage, namely hyaline (articular) cartilage, fibrocartilage, and elastic cartilage, can be distinguished from each other by the type of fibers within the matrix.

Organization

While the cell types are similar in each type of cartilage, the organization of cells and collagen/elastin fibrils differ extensively between types. The characteristics of each are described in detail next.

Hyaline Cartilage

Structure

Hyaline cartilage is the most abundant type of cartilage (Figure 3.14). It is located at the ends of long bones (where it is called articular cartilage; Figure 3.14a,b), epiphyseal growth plates (Figure. 3.14c,d), ribs (where it is called costal cartilage), and in parts of the larynx, trachea, bronchi, and bronchial tubes. During growth, chondrocytes and hyaline cartilage are also present within the epiphyseal plate, becoming hypertrophic and releasing factors necessary for osteoblast, osteoclast, and endothelial cell invasion needed for bone lengthening (Figure 3.14c,d). Hyaline cartilage contains numerous chondrocytes responsible for manufacturing, secretion, organization, and maintenance of the organic components of the extracellular matrix (Nordin & Frankel, 2012). The ground substance is homogeneous and amorphous and is composed of fine collagen type II fibrils embedded in a concentrated solution of proteoglycans. Specifically, the collagen content of hyaline cartilage ranges from 15 to 20% of the wet weight. The matrix of hyaline cartilage contains three types of glycosaminoglycans (hyaluronic acid, chondroitin sulfate, and keratin sulfate). The

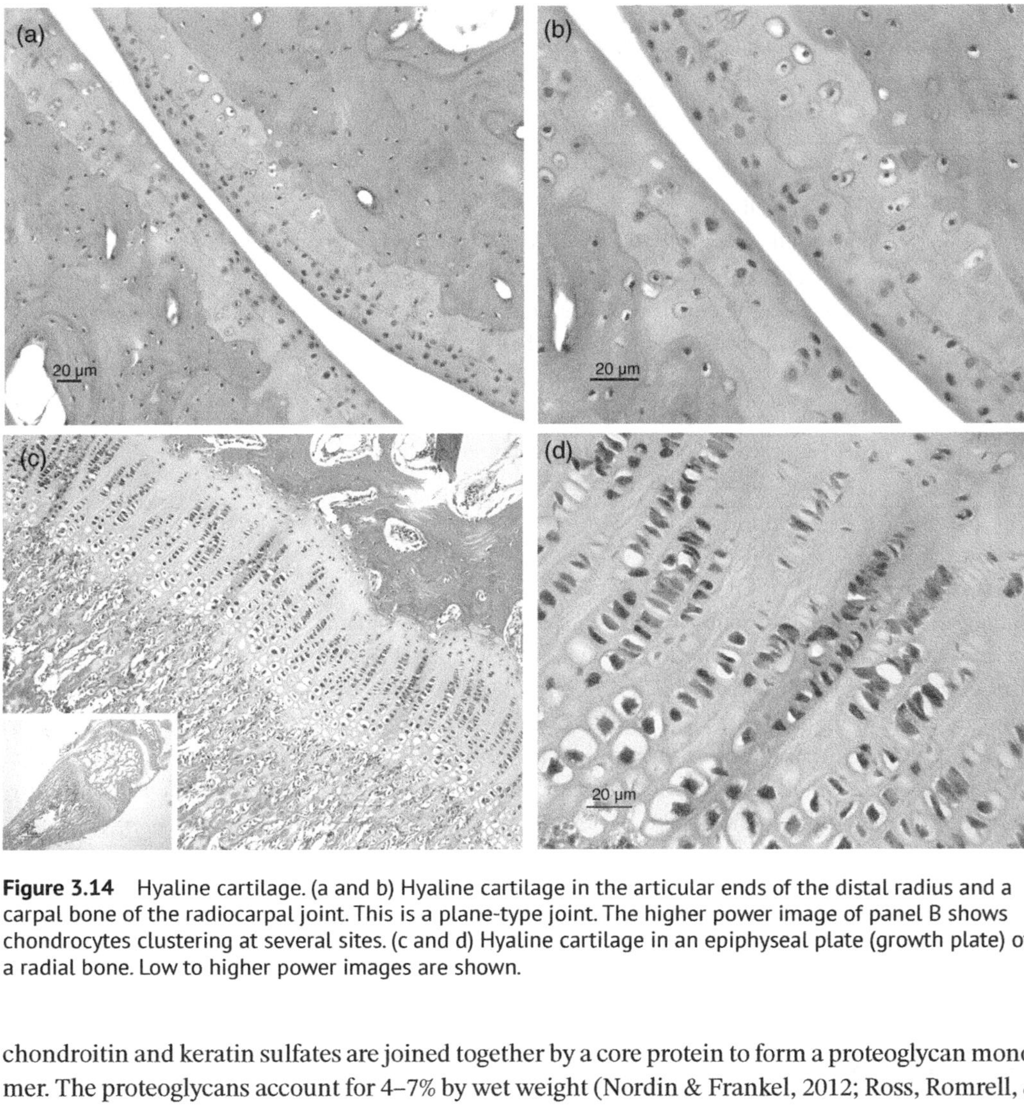

Figure 3.14 Hyaline cartilage. (a and b) Hyaline cartilage in the articular ends of the distal radius and a carpal bone of the radiocarpal joint. This is a plane-type joint. The higher power image of panel B shows chondrocytes clustering at several sites. (c and d) Hyaline cartilage in an epiphyseal plate (growth plate) of a radial bone. Low to higher power images are shown.

chondroitin and keratin sulfates are joined together by a core protein to form a proteoglycan monomer. The proteoglycans account for 4–7% by wet weight (Nordin & Frankel, 2012; Ross, Romrell, & Kaye, 1995). About 80 proteoglycans are associated with each hyaluronic acid molecule in large aggregates reinforced by linking-type proteins. These aggregates are bound to the thin collagen fibrils by electrostatic interactions and cross-linking glycoproteins. The remainder of the matrix is composed of water (60–78%), inorganic salts, and small amounts of link proteins, glycoproteins, and lipids. Some of the water is loosely bound, allowing diffusion of small metabolites to the chondrocytes, which is key in this typically avascular tissue.

Articular cartilage is a type of hyaline cartilage located in freely moving joints (Figure 3.14a,b) in which the joint is encased by an articular capsule and the bones connect with each other in a fluid-filled cavity known as the synovial cavity. Articular cartilage is organized into zones termed superficial, middle, deep, and a calcified zone (deepest). The most superficial zone is in contact with the synovial fluid that contains nutrients that diffuse into the cartilage. This zone protects the deeper layers from shear stresses and constitutes 10–20% of the thickness of articular cartilage. The chondrocytes in this upper zone are relatively high in number and flattened in shape, and the collagen fibers are tightly packed and are aligned in parallel to the articular surface. This combined structure resists the sheer, tensile, and compressive forces imposed by articulation and aids the protection and maintenance of the deeper structures. The middle zone represents 40–60% of the total cartilage volume. In this zone, the chondrocytes are spherical in shape and low in density and the collagen is obliquely organized (to help resist compressive forces). The deep zone of articular cartilage zone represents around 30% of the total cartilage volume. The collagen fibrils in this zone are arranged perpendicular to the articular surface and are large in diameter. The chondrocytes are arranged in columns (Figure 3.14a,b) that are in parallel to the collagen fibers and perpendicular to the joint line. As a consequence, this zone provides the greatest resistance to compressive forces. The deepest zone is the calcified cartilage layer (and is separated from the deep zone by a histological stain detectable "tide mark"). Like the deep zone, the collagen fibrils are arranged perpendicular to the articular surface. Unlike the other zone, calcification is present and the cell population is scare and hypertrophic. Its main purpose is to anchor collagen fibrils to the underlying subchondral bone.

Function

The large amounts of hyaluronic acid and other components in hyaline cartilage help retain water in the extracellular matrix. As a consequence, this type of cartilage provides resilience and pliability and is well adapted to serve in a weight-bearing joint, especially at points of movement. Hyaline cartilage also reduces friction and protects bony surfaces.

Fibrocartilage

Structure

Fibrocartilage is located at the intervertebral discs between the vertebrae (Figure 3.15), pubic symphysis, and in the menisci of knees. Fibrocartilage is distinct from hyaline cartilage in composition and structure. Fibrocartilage has a higher dry weight of collagen and less water, making it tougher and less resilient than articular cartilage. Its collagen fibers are thick (and therefore visible) and densely deposited in the tissue. In fact, the collagen fibers are so tightly packed that there is little evidence of an extracellular matrix. The chondrocytes are scattered among the many bundles of collagenous fibers.

Function

The structure of fibrocartilage combines both strength and rigidity; therefore, it is key to the support and fusion of joints in which it is present. Fibrocartilage is an anisotropic material that exhibits different strength capacities depending on the direction of loading (Murphy, Black, & Hastings, 2016). For example, it has been shown that fibrocartilage is strong during tension occurring in parallel to the orientation of the collagen fibers, but weaker during shear loading (Mansour, 2009).

Elastic Cartilage

Structure

The ligamentum flava joining the laminae of vertebrae is a type of elastic cartilage. Elastic cartilage is also present in the epiglottis, external ear, and auditory tubes. It is distinguished from other types of cartilage by the presence of elastic fibers in the matrix, in addition to the normal components of hyaline cartilage. As shown in Figure 3.16, a thread-like network of elastic fibers surrounds chondrocytes in this type of cartilage.

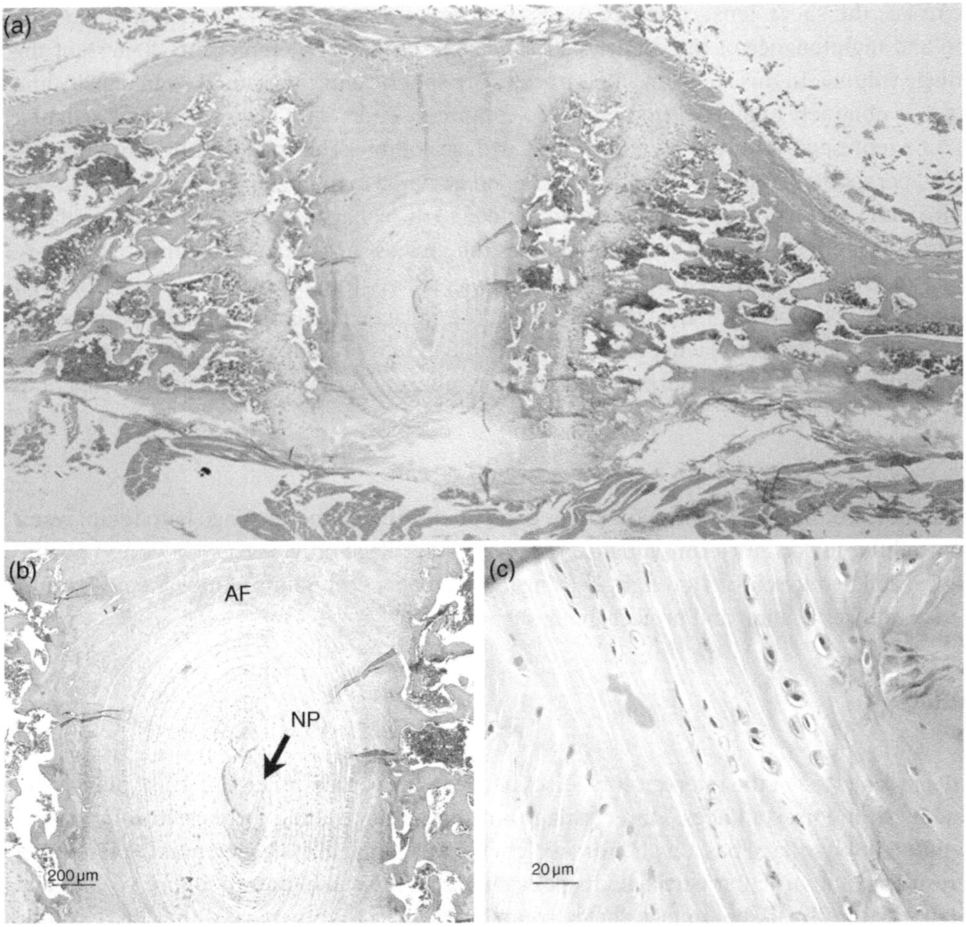

Figure 3.15 Fibrocartilage in the intervertebral discs between the vertebrae. (a) Low power image showing the disc between two rat lumbar level vertebrae. (b) Mid-power image showing fibrocartilage encircling the nucleus pulposus (the gelatinous interior of intervertebral discs) located in the middle of the disc. (c) High power image showing the presence of chondrocytes within thick collagen fibers in the fibrocartilage.

Function

The elastic materials in this type of cartilage give it elastic properties in addition to the resilience and pliability of its other hyaline cartilage components. Related to musculoskeletal tissue function, the elastic fibers in the ligamentum flava of the vertebra aid in the rebound of vertebrae from a flexed position to an upright position. Thus, elastic cartilage gives support and maintains the shape of its inclusionary structure. Unlike hyaline cartilage, the matrix of elastic cartilage does not calcify.

Bone

Bone is a complex and dynamic tissue that continuously undergoes renewal and repair throughout life to fulfill its functions. It bears the weight of the body and provides the framework (i.e., helps the body maintain its shape). The anchoring of muscles to bone also permits mechanical

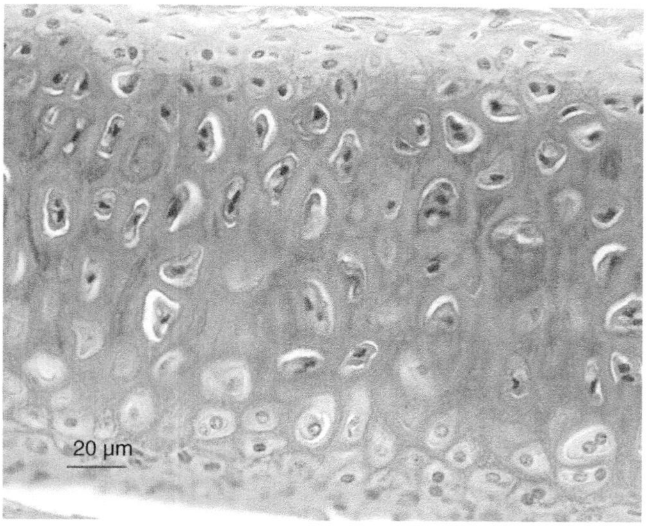

Figure 3.16 Elastic cartilage.

Table 3.5 Summary of Cells, Extracellular Matrix (ECM), Subtypes, and Function of Bone Under Normal Conditions

Characteristic	Description
Tissue type	• Dense mineralized connective tissue
Cells	• Main cell types: Osteoblasts, bone lining cells, osteocytes, osteoclasts, bone marrow–derived mesenchymal stem cells • Additional cell types: Hematopoietic cells in marrow spaces
ECM	• Collagen type I (~70%), 25% water, inorganic minerals (e.g., calcium, phosphorus)
Subtypes	• Cortical bone (compact bone), trabecular (cancellous/spongy bone)
Function	• Strength, stability, lever at points of attachment, storage of minerals/lipids/nutrients, blood cell formation

movement and locomotion by providing levers for the muscles (Clarke, 2008). Bone is composed of several cell types and a predominantly collagenous extracellular matrix (the osteoid) that becomes mineralized by the deposition of calcium hydroxyapatite. Bone also hosts hematopoietic cells and provides the environment for hematopoiesis within marrow spaces (which is also the storage site of iron) (Yang, 2010). Its general characteristics are summarized in Table 3.5.

Bone Structure

Cells

The cells in bone include osteoblasts, bone lining cells, osteocytes, and osteoclasts (Figure 3.17). They also contain nervous tissue, epithelial cells, and various types of hematopoietic cells. During bone growth and remodeling, there is a delicate balance between osteoblast and osteoclast function. This balance is orchestrated by osteocyte signaling, which dictates the outcome of loading on bone.

Osteoblasts—the producers of bone matrix Osteoblasts are derived from pluripotent mesenchymal stem cells of the osteochondroprogenitor lineage that have the potential to proliferate and

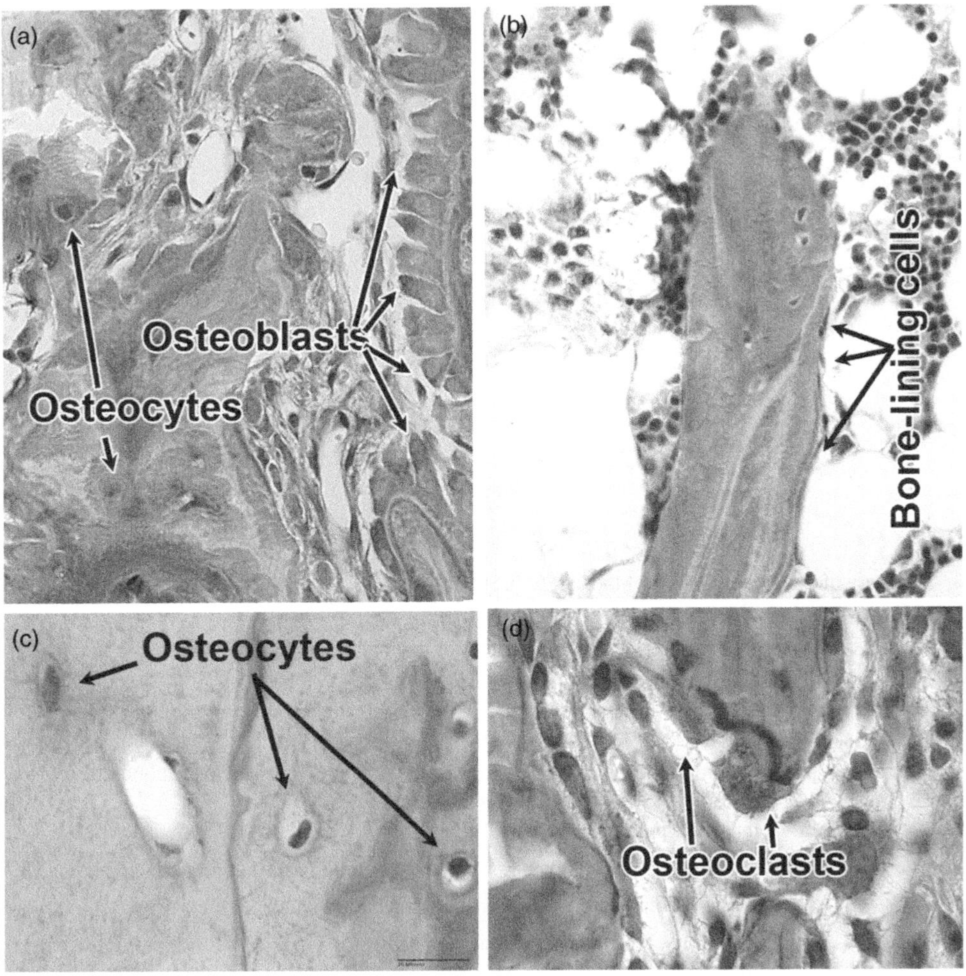

Figure 3.17 Bone cells. (a) Osteoblasts on the surface of trabeculae (larger cuboidal cells) and osteocytes that are embedded within the trabecular bone are depicted. (b) Bone lining cells are flat cells located on the surface of trabeculae. (c) A high power image of osteocytes, this time embedded within cortical bone. (d) Osteoclasts on the surface of trabecular bone.

differentiate into several connective tissue cell types depending on the stimulus within the local microenvironment. Given the appropriate stimuli, osteoprogenitor cells will first give rise to preosteoblasts and then osteoblasts (Caplan, 1991; Friedenstein, Chailakhyan, & Gerasimov, 1987; Owen, 1988; Pittenger et al., 1999; Yamaguchi et al., 1991). Osteoblasts are cuboidal mononucleated cells normally found at the bone surface (Figure 3.17a). They are responsible for the synthesis of the organic components of the bone matrix (the osteoid) and mediate its mineralization. Osteoblasts also produce a variety of other noncollagenous proteins, including osteocalcin (which is often used as a serum marker of bone formation). Osteoblasts are an important source of receptor-activated nuclear factor kappa B ligand (RANKL) that stimulates the differentiation and activation of osteoclasts (Boyce & Xing, 2007). Once osteoblasts become trapped and encased within the mineralized matrix, they are called osteocytes (Figure 3.17a,c).

Bone lining cells—effector cells on standby Bone lining cells originate from the same lineage as osteoblasts. They are mononucleated, flattened cells found lining surfaces in areas where there is no active bone formation (Figure 3.17b). They are believed to be a source of already committed osteogenic cells, known as dormant osteoblasts. They can be reactivated to the secreting form with the proper stimulus and under conditions that warrant active bone formation such as during mechanical stimulation, remodeling, and fracture repair (Miller, de Saint-Georges, Bowman, & Jee, 1989).

Osteocytes–the mechanotransducers and maintainers of bone Osteocytes are mature bone cells that live within the substance of bone and comprise 90–95% of all bone cells (Bonewald, 2007). Osteocytes are embedded in spaces (lacunae) in the interior of bone and are connected to adjacent cells by long cytoplasmic processes radiating from the cell body that lie within channels (canaliculi) throughout the mineralized matrix of bone (Figure 3.17) (Hirose et al., 2007; Lian & Stein, 2008). The processes of adjacent osteocytes make contact via gap junctions as well as with the osteoblasts and bone lining cells, maintaining the vitality of osteocytes by passing nutrients and metabolites between blood vessels and distant osteocytes (Jiang, Siller-Jackson, & Burra, 2007).

Osteocytes are believed to be the bone-sensing cells involved in mechanotransduction and thus the key regulators of bone remodeling. The gap junctions mentioned earlier aid in this function. Also, the osteocyte cell membrane is surrounded by interstitial fluid and extracellular matrix in which microtubules are embedded in order to transmit extracellular matrix mechanical changes to the osteocyte's actin filaments (Bakker et al., 2009). Osteocytes also communicate with surrounding cells via the release of biochemical factors and signaling molecules, such as bone morphogenetic proteins (BMPs), prostaglandin E2 (PGE2), and nitric oxide (NO) (Klein-Nulend, Bacabac, & Bakker, 2012).

Osteocytes are also actively involved in maintaining the bony matrix. They express osteoblast stimulating factor-1 after mechanical or muscular loading (Klein-Nulend & Bonewald, 2008). Osteocytes send inhibitory signals to osteoclasts to prevent bone loss during normal loading (Nakashima et al., 2011). Local damage (microcracks) of the osteoid matrix can compromise the osteocyte environment, disrupting the fluid flow, consequently reducing nutrients and oxygen supply to the embedded cells and creating oxidative stress (Al-Dujaili et al., 2011).

Osteoclasts–reallocate and remodel bone Osteoclasts differentiate after the fusion of bone marrow-derived mononuclear precursor cells of the monocyte–macrophage lineage in a process termed osteoclastogenesis. Osteoclasts are large multinucleated cells with a ruffled bottom in contact with the bone matrix (Figure 3.17d). They work in concert with osteoblasts in the constant turnover and remodeling of bone. They do this via their ability to secrete hydrochloric acid and other degradative enzymes, which, once activated, dissolve the bone matrix, creating a resorption pit underneath the cell. Osteoclasts are regulated by parathyroid hormone, calcitonin (from the thyroid gland), and pro-inflammatory cytokines (Boyce & Xing, 2007; Brabnikova Maresova, Pavelka, & Stepan, 2013; Nakashima & Takayanagi, 2011). As mentioned earlier, osteoclast activation is also mediated by the binding of osteoblast or osteocyte produced RANKL (a protein that plays an essential role in the recruitment, differentiation, activation, and survival of osteoclasts) (Burgess et al., 1999). Estrogen has a dual effect: Its presence increases bone formation and reduces bone resorption by enhancing osteoblast proliferation and function (Ernst, Heath, & Rodan, 1989; Majeska, Ryaby, & Einhorn, 1994); it also reduces bone turnover by reducing osteoclast activity (Hofbauer et al., 1999).

Extracellular matrix

Bone is a material constructed of a flexible collagenous matrix that is intermingled with rigid mineral crystals. Thus, bone is harder and less pliable than tendons or cartilage. The extracellular matrix of bone is produced by osteoblasts and consists of inorganic and organic components. For example, osteoid is defined as the unmineralized, organic portion of the bone matrix that forms prior to the maturation of bone tissue; it is composed primarily of collagen type I. In both unmineralized and mineralized bone, the organic component of bone (40% of bone's dry weight) include collagen type I fibers (90% of the organic matrix and ~97% of the collagenous proteins) and a number of noncollagenous proteins, such as osteocalcin and bone sialoprotein, which may orchestrate mineralization (Hu, Peel, Ho, Sandor, & Clokie, 2009; Robey et al., 1993). The inorganic component of bone represents about 60% of the dry weight of bone matrix and is composed mainly of abundant calcium and phosphorus, as well as smaller amounts of bicarbonate, citrate, magnesium, potassium, and sodium. Calcium forms hydroxyapatite crystals with phosphorus, although it is also present in an amorphous form (Junqueira & Carneiro, 2005; Khurana, 2009). Calcium hydroxyapatite crystals are arranged parallel to collagen fibers. This orientation maximizes the collagen's resistance to tensile (stretch) forces and calcium hydroxyapatite's resistance to compressive forces (Gartner & Hiatt, 2007; Sela, Amir, Schwartz, & Weinberg, 1987). In life, bones also have a large amount of water (~25% of the total bone weight) (Ailavajhala, Oswald, Rajapakse, & Pleshko, 2019; Ailavajhala, Querido, Rajapakse, & Pleshko, 2020).

Organization

According to their anatomical shape, bones are classified into four general categories: long, short, flat, and irregular bones. We will focus here on long bones. Long bones have two extremities (epiphyses), a cylindrical tube in the middle (diaphysis, also known as shaft of the bone), and a transitional zone between them (metaphyses) (Figure 3.18). The epiphysis is the expanded end of the bone that is covered by articular cartilage. The metaphysis is the junctional region between the epiphysis and the diaphysis and includes the growth plate (physis). The diaphysis is the shaft of long bones and is located in the region between metaphyses. The growth plate is a zone of endochondral ossification (cartilage-to-bone conversion) that mediates growth in bone length in an actively growing cartilage-to-bone region (Yang, 2010).

Bone tissue can also be classified by texture, matrix arrangement, maturity, or developmental origin (Yang, 2010). There are two main subtypes of bone: cortical and trabecular bone. Both types are chemically identical, but differ in terms of their structure, arrangement, and cell density. Approximately 80% of bone is cortical bone, with the remainder as trabecular bone (Carter & Hayes, 1977).

Trabecular bone (also known as cancellous or spongy bone) has numerous cavities (Figure 3.18). It is found mainly at the ends of many long bones and in areas like the ears and nose (Cooper, Milgram, & Robinson, 1966). Individual trabeculae are extensively connected and are oriented along the lines of mechanical stress on the bone in question. Trabecular bone is more metabolically active than cortical bone because of its much larger surface area for remodeling.

Cortical bone is dense in texture with few or no cavities, although it does contain pores for blood vessels, for example (Figures 3.18 and 3.19). Cortical bone is typically seen as the hard outer shell that surrounds trabecular bone or the centrally located marrow cavity. It is surrounded externally and internally by a periosteum and endosteum, respectively (Yang, 2010). Cortical bone is organized into Haversian systems or osteons (Figure 3.19), in which the lamellae are concentrically organized around a vascular canal, the Haversian canal. The blood supply of cortical bone enters from the periosteum via Volkmann canals, which also connect Haversian canals with each other (Brooks, 1963).

Lamellar bone is mature bone in which collagen fibers are arranged in parallel. It is located in both trabecular bone and cortical bone, the latter concentrically organized around a vascular canal.

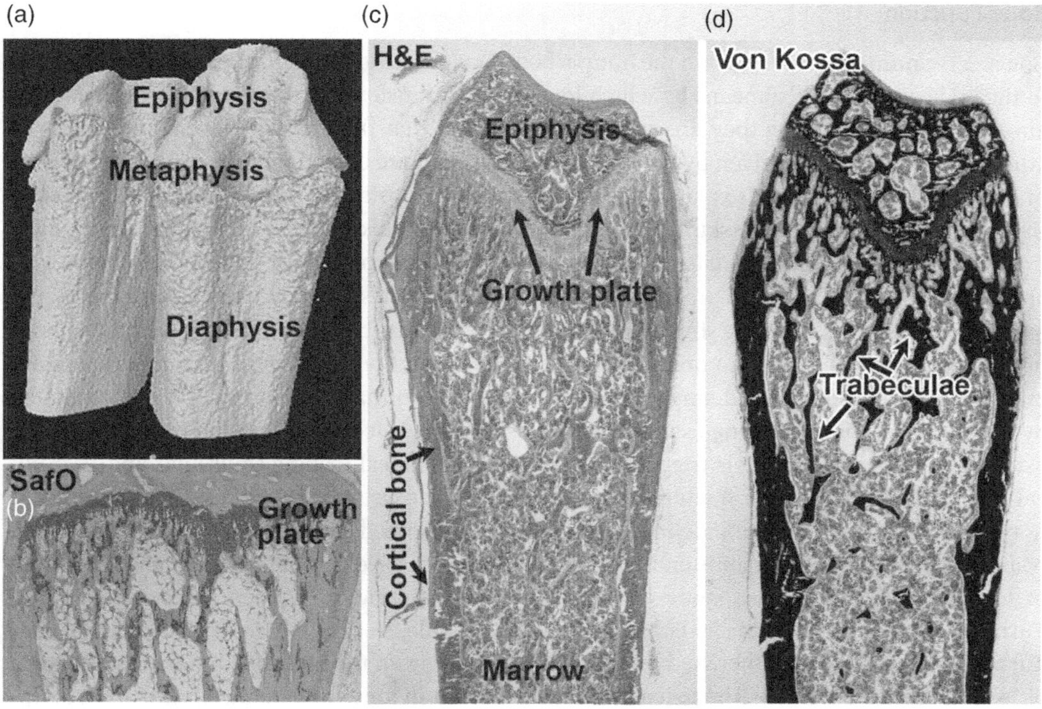

Figure 3.18 The organization of long bones. (a) Three-dimensional micro computed tomographic image of a rat's radius and ulna bones at the level of the wrist. (b) Staining a section of the radius with safranin O (Saf O) shows the location of cartilage in the epiphyseal plate (growth plate) and trabecular bone). (c) Hematoxylin and eosin staining showing the location of the growth plate proximal to the epiphysis, trabecular bone within the bone marrow region, and denser cortical bone on the outer edge of the bone. (d) Von Kossa staining of calcified trabecular and cortical bone.

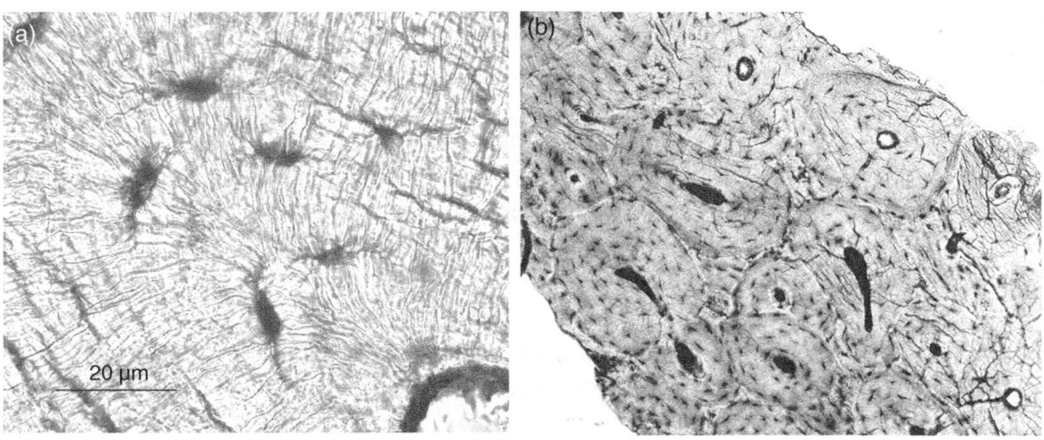

Figure 3.19 Osteons in cortical bone. (a) The osteocytes canaliculi are visible in the osteon. (b) Complete osteons (complete circles) and partial osteons left from past remodeling events are shown.

Bone Function

Bones serve numerous functions in the human body. Bones provide strength and structural stability to the body and provide a means by which loads can be transferred from one part of the body to another. Biomechanically, they are critical structures in that they provide levers and points of attachment for tendons (driven by muscle contraction) that are essential in permitting movement of the human body. Bones also play an important structural protective role for important organs of the body (most notably as the skull around the brain and the rib cage around the heart and lungs).

However, there is much more to bone than its structural and protective roles. Bones themselves are living dynamic organs and are quite complex in nature. These organs are constantly changing and remodeling to adapt to the stresses imposed them. This attribute permits both restorative and/or adaptive repair and helps to prevent fracture development when damage accumulation is not excessively rapid. Bone remodeling and maintenance is a normal, homeostatic process mediated by chondrocytes, bone-forming osteoblasts, bone-resorbing osteoclasts, and the mechanosensing osteocytes. Bone remodeling is triggered by growth, mechanical loading (muscular and/or cyclical), injuries (microcracks or fractures), and various local or systemic cytokines, chemokines, and hormones. During active remodeling, bone matrix is resorbed and replaced where needed in response to the loading demands on the bone. Many studies have demonstrated an anabolic effect of loading on bones in case studies or animal models (Schriefer, Warden, Saxon, Robling, & Turner, 2005; Srinivasan et al., 2003; Warden, Fuchs, Castillo, Nelson, & Turner, 2007; Zhang, Sun, Turner, & Yokota, 2007). Other studies show that depending on the intensity, frequency, and form of loading, persistent intense bone loading can also result in long-term damage, excessive resorption, and detrimental changes to the cartilage and bone [reviewed in (Barbe & Popoff, 2020)]. This topic will be explored further in Chapter 11.

Bone is also the site of a number of hematopoietic cells and blood cell formation—all essential to the body's nutrition and protection against infection and damaged tissue. Bones are a major site for the storage of minerals, especially calcium and phosphorus. Lastly, bone plays a critical role in storing nutrients and lipids that serve as an energy reserve for the body.

Ligament

Ligaments are structures that hold bones together at joints (Figure 3.20). They are made up of dense regularly arranged connective tissues with a predominance of collagenous fibers arranged into bundles, and a small number of fibroblastic-like or synoviocyte-like cells. Ligaments can be either extrinsic ligaments located outside a synovial joint or strategic reinforcing thickenings of a joint capsule (intrinsic ligaments). These features are summarized in Table 3.6.

Ligament Structure

Ligaments have similarities yet differences from tendons in important respects. Ligaments have a similar hierarchical organization of collagen structures as tendons, although the collagen fibers tend to be more loosely packed in ligaments (the collagen fibrils are slightly less in volume fraction and organization than tendon). However, ligaments have a higher percentage of proteoglycan matrix than tendons. Another significant difference in structure between ligaments and tendons is the amount of elastin found in ligaments. Elastin comprises less than 4% of the dry weight of tendons; in contrast, typical ligaments exhibit 4–9% elastin as dry weight, while some highly

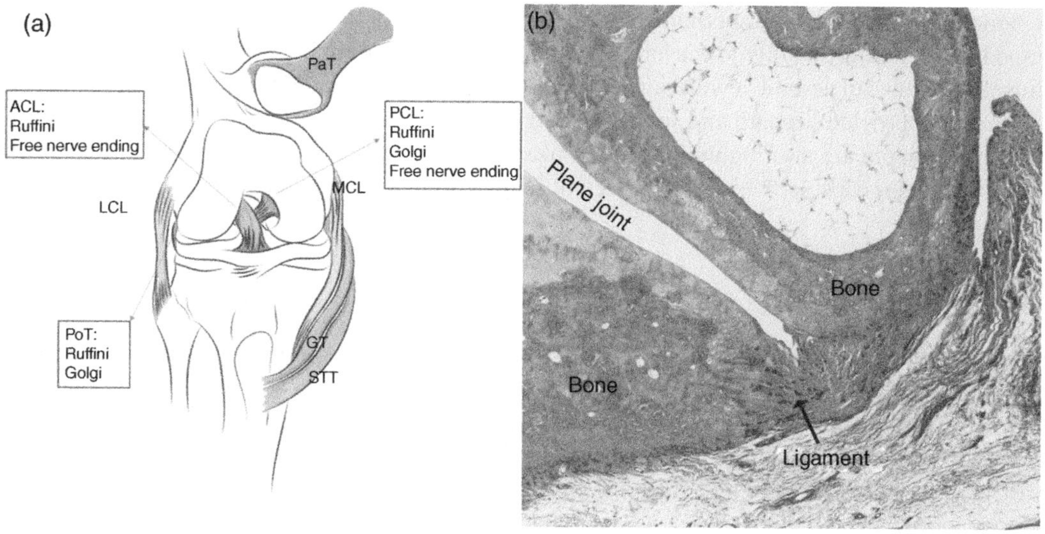

Figure 3.20 Ligaments. (a) A diagram showing the ligament of the knee: lateral collateral ligament (LCL), medial collateral ligament (MCL), anterior and posterior cruciate ligaments (ACL and PCL), and several other tendons. Sensory receptors present in the ligaments are listed and include free nerve endings (pain endings), Ruffini endings (pressure receptors), and Golgi tendon organs (tension receptors). From Cabuk, H., & Kuşku Çabuk, F. (2016). Mechanoreceptors of the ligaments and tendons around the knee. *Clinical Anatomy, 29*,(6),789–795. doi: 10.1002/ca.22743. (b) An image of a ligament joining carpal bones.

Table 3.6 Summary of Cells, Extracellular Matrix (ECM), Subtypes, and Function of Ligaments Under Normal Conditions

Characteristic	Description
Tissue type	• Dense regular connective tissues
Cells	• Fibroblastic synoviocyte-like type cells
ECM	• Collagen, proteoglycans, elastin (varies from 4 to 70% of dry weight dependent on ligament)
Subtypes	• Typical (4–9% elastin) to highly extensible (up to 70% extensible)
Function	• Support and strength to joints

extensible ligaments have over 70% elastin as dry weight. The elastin network in the ligament resides along and between the collagen fibers (Zitnay & Weiss, 2018).

Ligament Function

The function of ligaments is to provide support and structure to the joints (while providing some flexibility in joint motion). They also prevent excessive motion and provide feedback on positional information of the joints through sensory endings in the ligaments. Ligaments serve to join two or more bones together; both at rest and during the normal range of motion of the joint in question. Ligaments limit the range of motion through passive stabilization and guiding joints through their normal range of motion under tensile load. Thus, ligaments function to transfer forces from bone to bone in a particular joint, both at rest and during movement, and help to guide motion while providing structural stability to the joint. The range of motion of different joints can vary widely; thus, ligaments can assume a wide variety of shapes and sizes. Ligaments are pliant and flexible, but they also provide strength and support to the joint resulting from forces that may be applied.

Joint ligaments are also highly innervated near the site of attaching tendons and in the outer layer of the joint capsule. This innervation will be discussed further in Chapter 4.

Joints

Bones are too rigid to bend without damage. Fortunately, there are multiple bones throughout the body joined together by joints (the articulation or union between two or more bones or parts of bones). This segmentation of the skeleton allows for movement and segmental growth. As is the case with all aspects of the musculoskeletal system, the structure of a joint, specifically the manner in which the joints are held together, determines its function. Although there are many ways to classify joints, the simplest is a functional classification of little to no movement (synarthroses, syndesmoses, and synchondroses) versus freely movable (diarthroses) (Table 3.7).

Structure of Synarthroses

Synarthroses are bound together by either fibrous (symphyses and syndesmoses) or cartilaginous tissue (synchondroses). Symphyses are joints joined by fibrocartilage, in which the two opposing surfaces are covered by hyaline cartilage (thus, symphyses are also considered cartilaginous joints). The strength of the fibrocartilage allows for only a little movement but much stability, while the hyaline cartilage on the articulating surfaces allows for shock absorption. The pubic symphyses and intervertebral joints are examples of symphyses (Figure 3.15). The adjoining bones of fibrous syndesmoses are bound together by a thin sheet of fibrous tissue, either a ligament or a fibrous membrane. Since the fibrous tissue is flexible, these joints allow partial movement. The amount of movement allowed depends on the length of the fibers uniting the bones. Examples of syndesmoses are the suture joints of the skull and the union of the radius and ulna in the forearm by an

Table 3.7 Classifications of Joints

Classification type	Subtype	Description
Functional	• Little to no movement (synarthroses)	• Fibrous (symphyses and syndesmoses) • Cartilaginous (synchondroses)
	• Freely movable	• Diarthroses (all synovial joints)
Arthrokinematics	• Plane	• *Function:* Gliding, spinning, or a combination
	• Hinge • Saddle • Condyloid • Ball-and-socket • Pivot joints	• *Function:* Movement in one plane, usually sagittal, about one axis of rotation • *Function:* Biaxial (motion about two primary axes in two planes) or triaxial movement • *Function:* Biaxial movement • *Function:* Movement in all three axes • *Function:* Movement in one plane (uniaxial)

interosseous membrane. Synchrondroses are joints joined together by cartilage and permit slight bending in early life. A key example is the joining of the epiphysis of a long bone with the metaphysis by a cartilaginous growth plate (the physis) (Figure 3.14). This is a temporary synchondrosis since the growth plate eventually ossifies in the mature adult.

Structure of Diathroses (Synovial Joints)

Diarthroses are designed for movement and include all synovial joints. These are the most common types of joints and are defined as two or more bones whose ends are covered by hyaline cartilage, united by a fibrous tissue capsule that encloses the joint, and separated by a joint cavity. The cavity is filled with synovial fluid produced by a synovial membrane (a vascular connective tissue) lining the interior of the fibrous capsule. The synovial membrane cells produce and secrete synovial fluid, a lubricant that provides a smooth, nearly frictionless, gliding motion of opposing joint surfaces. The synovial fluid also nourishes the articular (hyaline) cartilage covering the bones. This type of joint allows the most movement, although lower stability. As a consequence, extrinsic and intrinsic ligaments usually reinforce synovial joints. Some synovial joints also have other distinguishing features such as menisci, labrums, or fibrocartilage articular discs that allow for shock absorption and/or additional stability. Nearly all of the joints of the upper and lower limbs are synovial.

Function of Joints

Arthrokinematics describes the movements occurring between the joint surfaces, such as rolling, spinning, and gliding of joint surfaces. As such, joints can be divided into plane, hinge, saddle, condyloid, ball-and-socket, and pivot joints. Plane joints are characterized by opposing bony surfaces that are flat or nearly so. The arthrokinematics of a plane joint includes gliding and spinning or a combination thereof. Gliding refers to a translation of one surface with respect to another, whereas spinning refers to a clockwise or counterclockwise rotation of one surface with respect to another. Depending on the precise curvature of the surfaces of a plane joint, their orientation, and their constraints by soft-tissue structures, the osteokinematics of plane joint movement ranges from uniaxial to triaxial. Examples of plane joints include the acromioclavicular joint, which is triaxial, and the vertebral zygopophyseal (facet) joints, which are uniaxial. Hinge joints are constrained to movement in one plane, usually sagittal, about one axis of rotation, usually mediolateral. The elbow joint is one example of a hinge joint. Saddle (sellar) joints are characterized by opposing surfaces that are concave and convex, but along opposite planes so that they are contoured to fit together. The osteokinematics of saddle joints are inconsistently described as either biaxial (motion about two primary axes in two planes) or triaxial. This inconsistency can be explained by the fact that the majority of motion typically occurs in two planes (usually flexion-extension and abduction-adduction), while there is a small amount of internal-external rotation. The carpometacarpal joint of the thumb is an example of a saddle joint in which flexion-adduction-internal rotation combine to produce the action of opposition. Condyloid joints are composed a one nearly spherical convex surface opposing a shallow, nearly flat concave surface. These joints are considered biaxial owing to the predominance of movement about two axes and in two planes. The arthrokinematics during movement of condyloid joints are described by the "concave–convex rule," which specifies that to maintain congruence of joint surfaces during bone movement, the convex condyloid component must roll in the direction of bony movement and glide in the opposite direction with respect to the concave component. Examples of condyloid joints include (a) the metacarpophalangeal joints of the fingers; (b) the knee joint, in which the distal femoral condyles articulate with the shallow, concave tibial plateaus; and (c) the atlanto-occipital joint between the occipital condyles and the atlas. Ball and socket joints are distinguished by one bone with an ovoid or spherical convex surface that moves within a relatively deep concave surface. Ball and socket joints allow movement about all three axes and in all three planes of motion, flexion-extension, abduction-adduction, and internal-external rotation. The coxofemoral (hip) and glenohumeral (shoulder) joints are examples of ball and socket joints. Lastly, pivot joints are characterized by one bone with a rounded process that moves within a sleeve or ring formed by the opposing bone. They permit rotation about a single axis and are, therefore, uniaxial joints. Examples include the proximal radioulnar and atlantoaxial joints.

Summary

This chapter discussed the main non-neural tissue types that comprise the musculoskeletal system. Tables 3.1–3.5 summarize each tissue type in detail under normal uninjured conditions, Table 3.7 summarizes joints by their main function versus arthrokinematics, while Table 3.8 provides a general summary overview. Differences in these tissues characteristics after injury are discussed in Chapter 11, and their interaction with the nervous system is discussed in Chapter 4.

Table 3.8 Summary of Non-Neural Tissues of the Musculoskeletal System

Tissue	Description	Main functions
Loose connective tissues • Adipose • Areolar • Reticular	Fibers are loosely woven with many cells, all embedded in a semifluid ground substance.	Provides cushioning, support, elasticity, and immune functions
Dense connective tissues -Irregular • Dermis of skin • Deep fascia • Periosteum • Perichondrium - Regular • Tendon • Cartilage • Bone	Characterized by regularly or irregularly arranged collagen fibers, and low intercellular substance. Primary cells are fibroblasts or fibroblast like cells in dense irregular connective tissues. Primary cells in tendons are tenocytes, chondrocytes in cartilage, and a number of cells including osteoblast and osteoclasts in bone.	• Tendon: Transfer of tensile forces created by muscles onto bone; absorbs sudden shocks to limit muscle damage. • Cartilage: Hyaline: Protection of bony surfaces, especially at points of movement; Fibrocartilage: Strength and rigidity, joint support and fusion; Elastic cartilage: Resilience and pliability • Bone: Strength, stability; lever at points of attachment; storage of minerals, lipids and nutrients; blood cell formation
Skeletal muscle	Contains contractile cells (myocytes) arranged in multinucleated striated long fibers (myofibers).	Contraction and then movement of the endoskeleton to which the muscle is attached
Ligaments	Dense regularly connective tissue with many collagenous fibers arranged into bundles; small number of fibroblastic-like cells	Support and strength to joints

Bibliography

Ailavajhala, R., Oswald, J., Rajapakse, C. S., & Pleshko, N. (2019). Environmentally-controlled near infrared spectroscopic imaging of bone water. *Scientific Reports*, *9*(1), 10199. https://doi.org/10.1038/s41598-019-45897-3

Ailavajhala, R., Querido, W., Rajapakse, C. S., & Pleshko, N. (2020). Near infrared spectroscopic assessment of loosely and tightly bound cortical bone water. *Analyst*, *145*(10), 3713–3724. https://doi.org/10.1039/c9an02491c

Al-Dujaili, S. A., Lau, E., Al-Dujaili, H., Tsang, K., Guenther, A., & You, L. (2011). Apoptotic osteocytes regulate osteoclast precursor recruitment and differentiation in vitro. *Journal of Cellular Biochemistry*, *112*(9), 2412–2423. https://doi.org/10.1002/jcb.23164

Ali, S., Cunningham, R., Amin, M., Popoff, S. N., Mohamed, F., & Barbe, M. F. (2015). The extensor carpi ulnaris pseudolesion: Evaluation with microCT, histology, and MRI. *Skeletal Radiol*, *44*(12), 1735–1743. https://doi.org/10.1007/s00256-015-2224-3

Bakker, A. D., Silva, V. C., Krishnan, R., Bacabac, R. G., Blaauboer, M. E., Lin, Y. C., . . . Klein-Nulend, J. (2009). Tumor necrosis factor alpha and interleukin-1beta modulate calcium and nitric oxide signaling in mechanically stimulated osteocytes. *Arthritis Rheum*, *60*(11), 3336–3345. https://doi.org/10.1002/art.24920

Barbe, M. F., Harris, M. Y., Cruz, G. E., Amin, M., Billett, N. M., Dorotan, J. T., . . . Bove, G. M. (2021). Key indicators of repetitive overuse-induced neuromuscular inflammation and fibrosis are prevented by manual therapy in a rat model. *BMC Musculoskelet Disord*, *22*(1), 417. https://doi.org/10.1186/s12891-021-04270-0

Barbe, M. F., & Popoff, S. N. (2020). Occupational activities: Factors that tip the balance from bone accrual to bone loss. *Exercise and Sport Sciences Reviews*, *48*(2), 59–66. https://doi.org/10.1249/JES.0000000000000217

Benjamin, M., & Ralphs, J. R. (1998). Fibrocartilage in tendons and ligaments--an adaptation to compressive load. *Journal of Anatomy*, *193*(Pt 4), 481–494. Retrieved from http://www.ncbi.nlm.nih.gov/pubmed/10029181

Bonewald, L. F. (2007). Osteocytes as dynamic multifunctional cells. *Annals of the New York Academy of Sciences*, *1116*, 281–290. https://doi.org/10.1196/annals.1402.018

Borynsenko, M., & Beringer, T. (1989). *Functional histology* (pp. 105–112). Boston: Little, Brown.

Boyce, B. F., & Xing, L. (2007). Biology of RANK, RANKL, and osteoprotegerin. *Arthritis Research and Therapy*, *9*(Suppl 1), S1. https://doi.org/10.1186/ar2165

Brabnikova Maresova, K., Pavelka, K., & Stepan, J. J. (2013). Acute effects of glucocorticoids on serum markers of osteoclasts, osteoblasts, and osteocytes. *Calcified Tissue International*, *92*(4), 354–361. https://doi.org/10.1007/s00223-012-9684-4

Brooks, M. (1963). Blood supply of long bones. *British Medical Journal*, *2*(5364), 1064–1065.

Brunello, E., Caremani, M., Melli, L., Linari, M., Fernandez-Martinez, M., Narayanan, T., . . . Reconditi, M. (2014). The contributions of filaments and cross-bridges to sarcomere compliance in skeletal muscle. *Journal of Physiology*, *592*(17), 3881–3899. https://doi.org/10.1113/jphysiol.2014.276196

Burgess, T. L., Qian, Y., Kaufman, S., Ring, B. D., Van, G., Capparelli, C., . . . Lacey, D. L. (1999). The ligand for osteoprotegerin (OPGL) directly activates mature osteoclasts. *Journal of Cell Biology*, *145*(3), 527–538. Retrieved from http://www.ncbi.nlm.nih.gov/pubmed/10225954

Butler, D. L., Grood, E. S., Noyes, F. R., & Zernicke, R. F. (1978). Biomechanics of ligaments and tendons. *Exercise and Sport Sciences Reviews*, *6*, 125–181. Retrieved from http://www.ncbi.nlm.nih.gov/pubmed/394967

Cabuk, H., & Kuşku Çabuk, F. (2016). Mechanoreceptors of the ligaments and tendons around the knee. *Clinical Anatomy, 29*(6), 789–795. https://doi.org/10.1002/ca.22743

Caplan, A. I. (1991). Mesenchymal stem cells. *Journal of Orthopaedic Research, 9*(5), 641–650. https://doi.org/10.1002/jor.1100090504

Carter, D. R., & Hayes, W. C. (1977). The compressive behavior of bone as a two-phase porous structure. *Journal of Bone Joint Surgery, A, 59*, 954–962.

Charge, S. B., & Rudnicki, M. A. (2004). Cellular and molecular regulation of muscle regeneration. *Physiological Reviews, 84*(1), 209–238. https://doi.org/10.1152/physrev.00019.2003

Chow, J. W., Wilson, A. J., Chambers, T. J., & Fox, S. W. (1998). Mechanical loading stimulates bone formation by reactivation of bone lining cells in 13-week-old rats. *Journal of Bone and Mineral Research, 13*(11), 1760–1767. https://doi.org/10.1359/jbmr.1998.13.11.1760

Clarke, B. (2008). Normal bone anatomy and physiology. *Clinical Journal of the American Society of Nephrology, 3*(Suppl 3), S131–S139. https://doi.org/10.2215/CJN.04151206

Collins, C. A., Olsen, I., Zammit, P. S., Heslop, L., Petrie, A., Partridge, T. A., & Morgan, J. E. (2005). Stem cell function, self-renewal, and behavioral heterogeneity of cells from the adult muscle satellite cell niche. *Cell, 122*(2), 289–301. https://doi.org/10.1016/j.cell.2005.05.010

Cooper, R. R., Milgram, J. W., & Robinson, R. A. (1966). Morphology of the osteon. An electron microscopic study. *The Journal of Bone and Joint Surgery, 48*(7), 1239–1271. Retrieved from http://www.ncbi.nlm.nih.gov/pubmed/5921783

Deng, Z. L., Sharff, K. A., Tang, N., Song, W. X., Luo, J., Luo, X., . . . He, T. C. (2008). Regulation of osteogenic differentiation during skeletal development. *Frontiers in Bioscience, 13*, 2001–2021. Retrieved from http://www.ncbi.nlm.nih.gov/pubmed/17981687

Dick, M. K., Miao, J. H., & Limaiem, F. (2020). *Histology, Fibroblast*. Treasure Island, FL: StatPearls.

Dransfield, E. (1977). Intramuscular composition and texture of beef muscles. *Journal of the Science of Food and Agriculture, 28*(9), 833–842. https://doi.org/10.1002/jsfa.2740280910

Ernst, M., Heath, J. K., & Rodan, G. A. (1989). Estradiol effects on proliferation, messenger ribonucleic acid for collagen and insulin-like growth factor-I, and parathyroid hormone-stimulated adenylate cyclase activity in osteoblastic cells from calvariae and long bones. *Endocrinology, 125*(2), 825–833. Retrieved from http://www.ncbi.nlm.nih.gov/pubmed/2752978

Ervasti, J. M., & Campbell, K. P. (1993). A role for the dystrophin-glycoprotein complex as a transmembrane linker between laminin and actin. *Journal of Cell Biology, 122*(4), 809–823. Retrieved from http://www.ncbi.nlm.nih.gov/pubmed/8349731

Evans, J. H., & Barbenel, J. C. (1975). Structural and mechanical properties of tendon related to function. *Equine Veterinary Journal, 7*(1), 1–8. Retrieved from http://www.ncbi.nlm.nih.gov/pubmed/1116491

Exeter, D., & Connell, D. A. (2010). Skeletal muscle: Functional anatomy and pathophysiology. *Semin Musculoskelet Radiol, 14*(2), 97–105. https://doi.org/10.1055/s-0030-1253154

Fedorczyk, J. M., Barr, A. E., Rani, S., Gao, H. G., Amin, M., Amin, S., . . . Barbe, M. F. (2010). Exposure-dependent increases in IL-1beta, substance P, CTGF, and tendinosis in flexor digitorum tendons with upper extremity repetitive strain injury. *Journal of Orthopaedic Research, 28*(3), 298–307. https://doi.org/10.1002/jor.20984

Fitch, J. M., Gross, J., Mayne, R., Johnson-Wint, B., & Linsenmayer, T. F. (1984). Organization of collagen types I and V in the embryonic chicken cornea: monoclonal antibody studies. *Proceedings of the National Academy of Sciences of the United States of America, 81*(9), 2791–2795. Retrieved from http://www.ncbi.nlm.nih.gov/pubmed/6326145

Friedenstein, A. J., Chailakhyan, R. K., & Gerasimov, U. V. (1987). Bone marrow osteogenic stem cells: in vitro cultivation and transplantation in diffusion chambers. *Cell Tissue Kinet, 20*(3), 263–272. Retrieved from http://www.ncbi.nlm.nih.gov/pubmed/3690622

Gartner, L. P., & Hiatt, J. L. (2007). *Color textbook of histology* (3rd ed.). Saunders,Inc.

Gilbert-Honick, J., & Grayson, W. (2020). Vascularized and innervated skeletal muscle tissue engineering. *Advanced Healthcare Materials, 9*(1), e1900626.

Gillies, A. R., & Lieber, R. L. (2011). Structure and function of the skeletal muscle extracellular matrix. *Muscle Nerve, 44*(3), 318–331. https://doi.org/10.1002/mus.22094

Grounds, M. D., Sorokin, L., & White, J. (2005). Strength at the extracellular matrix-muscle interface. *Scandinavian Journal of Medicine and Science in Sports, 15*(6), 381–391. https://doi.org/10.1111/j.1600-0838.2005.00467.x

Hirose, S., Li, M., Kojima, T., de Freitas, P. H., Ubaidus, S., Oda, K., . . . Amizuka, N. (2007). A histological assessment on the distribution of the osteocytic lacunar canalicular system using silver staining. *Journal of Bone and Mineral Metabolism, 25*(6), 374–382. https://doi.org/10.1007/s00774-007-0764-x

Hofbauer, L. C., Khosla, S., Dunstan, C. R., Lacey, D. L., Spelsberg, T. C., & Riggs, B. L. (1999). Estrogen stimulates gene expression and protein production of osteoprotegerin in human osteoblastic cells. *Endocrinology, 140*(9), 4367–4370. Retrieved from http://www.ncbi.nlm.nih.gov/pubmed/10465311

Hu, Z. M., Peel, S. A., Ho, S. K., Sandor, G. K., & Clokie, C. M. (2009). Induction of bone matrix protein expression by native bone matrix proteins in C2C12 culture. *Biomedical and Environmental Sciences, 22*(2), 164–169. https://doi.org/10.1016/S0895-3988(09)60041-6

Iannarone, V. J., Cruz, G. E., Hilliard, B. A., & Barbe, M. F. (2019). The answer depends on the question: Optimal conditions for western blot characterization of muscle collagen type 1 depends on desired isoform. *Journal of Biological Methods, 6*(3), e117. https://doi.org/10.14440/jbm.2019.289

Ishikawa, H. (1966). Electron microscopic observations of satellite cells with special reference to the development of mammalian skeletal muscles. *Zeitschrift für Anatomie und Entwicklungsgeschichte, 125*(1), 43–63. Retrieved from http://www.ncbi.nlm.nih.gov/pubmed/5973580

Jiang, J. X., Siller-Jackson, A. J., & Burra, S. (2007). Roles of gap junctions and hemichannels in bone cell functions and in signal transmission of mechanical stress. *Frontiers in Bioscience, 12*, 1450–1462. Retrieved from http://www.ncbi.nlm.nih.gov/pubmed/17127393

Joyner, M. J., & Casey, D. P. (2015). Regulation of increased blood flow (hyperemia) to muscles during exercise: A hierarchy of competing physiological needs. *Physiological Reviews, 95*(2), 549–601. https://doi.org/10.1152/physrev.00035.2013

Jozsa, L., & Kannus, P. (1997). Histopathological findings in spontaneous tendon ruptures. *Scandinavian Journal of Medicine and Science in Sports, 7*(2), 113–118. Retrieved from http://www.ncbi.nlm.nih.gov/pubmed/9211612

Junqueira, L. C., & Carneiro, J. (2005). *Basic histology text and atlas* (11th ed.). McGraw-Hill.

Kannus, P. (2000). Structure of the tendon connective tissue. *Scandinavian Journal of Medicine and Science in Sports, 10*(6), 312–320. Retrieved from http://www.ncbi.nlm.nih.gov/pubmed/11085557

Ker, R. F. (2002). The implications of the adaptable fatigue quality of tendons for their construction, repair and function. *Comparative Biochemistry and Physiology Part A: Molecular and Integrative Physiology, 133*(4), 987–1000. https://doi.org/10.1016/s1095-6433(02)00171-x

Khurana, J. S. (Ed.) (2009). *Bone pathology* (2nd ed.). Humana Press.

Kietrys, D. M., Barr, A. E., & Barbe, M. F. (2011). Exposure to repetitive tasks induces motor changes related to skill acquisition and inflammation in rats. *Journal of Motor Behavior, 43*(6), 465–476. https://doi.org/10.1080/00222895.2011.627897

Kjaer, M. (2004). Role of extracellular matrix in adaptation of tendon and skeletal muscle to mechanical loading. *Physiological Reviews, 84*(2), 649–698. https://doi.org/10.1152/physrev.00031.2003

Klein-Nulend, J., Bacabac, R. G., & Bakker, A. D. (2012). Mechanical loading and how it affects bone cells: the role of the osteocyte cytoskeleton in maintaining our skeleton. *Eur Cell Mater, 24,* 278–291. Retrieved from http://www.ncbi.nlm.nih.gov/pubmed/23007912

Klein-Nulend, J., & Bonewald, L. F. (2008). The osteocyte. In J. P. Bilezikian, L. G. Raisz, & T. J. Martin (Eds.), *Principles of bone biology* (3rd ed., pp. 153–174). Academic Press, ISBN 9780123738844, doi: https://doi.org/10.1016/B978-0-12-373884-4.00028-8

Kusters, Y. H., & Barrett, E. J. (2016). Liraglutide prevents microvascular insulin resistance and preserves muscle capillary density in high-fat diet-fed rats. *American Journal of Physiology-Endocrinology and Metabolism, 311*(3), E640-8. https://doi.org/10.1152/ajpendo.00205.2016

Li, Y., Wu, T., & Liu, S. (2021). Identification and distinction of tenocytes and tendon-derived stem cells. *Frontiers in Cell and Developmental Biology, 9,* 629515.

Lian, J. B., & Stein, G. S. (2008). Osteoblast biology. In D. Feldman, D. A. Nelson, & C. J. R. R. Marcus (Eds.), *Osteoporosis* (3rd ed.). Elseivier Inc.

Listrat, A., Lethias, C., Hocquette, J. F., Renand, G., Menissier, F., Geay, Y., & Picard, B. (2000). Age-related changes and location of types I, III, XII and XIV collagen during development of skeletal muscles from genetically different animals. *The Histochemical Journal, 32*(6), 349–356. Retrieved from http://www.ncbi.nlm.nih.gov/pubmed/10943849

Lynch, M. P., Stein, J. L., Stein, G. S., & Lian, J. B. (1995). The influence of type I collagen on the development and maintenance of the osteoblast phenotype in primary and passaged rat calvarial osteoblasts: Modification of expression of genes supporting cell growth, adhesion, and extracellular matrix mineralization. *Experimental Cell Research, 216*(1), 35–45. https://doi.org/10.1006/excr.1995.1005

Majeska, R. J., Ryaby, J. T., & Einhorn, T. A. (1994). Direct modulation of osteoblastic activity with estrogen. *The Journal of Bone and Joint Surgery, 76*(5), 713–721. Retrieved from http://www.ncbi.nlm.nih.gov/pubmed/8175820

Malaval, L., Modrowski, D., Gupta, A. K., & Aubin, J. E. (1994). Cellular expression of bone-related proteins during in vitro osteogenesis in rat bone marrow stromal cell cultures. *Journal of Cellular Physiology, 158*(3), 555–572. https://doi.org/10.1002/jcp.1041580322

Mansour, J. M. (2009). Biomechanics of cartilage. In C. Hughes (Ed.), *Kinesiology: The mechanics and pathomechanics of human movement* (2nd ed., pp. 66–79). Baltimore: Lippincott Williams & Wilkins.

Marvulli, D., Volpin, D., & Bressan, G. M. (1996). Spatial and temporal changes of type VI collagen expression during mouse development. *Developmental dynamics: An official Publication of the American Association of Anatomists, 206*(4), 447–454. https://doi.org/10.1002/(SICI)1097-0177(199608)206:4<447::AID-AJA10>3.0.CO;2-U

Mauro, A. (1961). Satellite cell of skeletal muscle fibers. *Journal of Biophysical and Biochemical cytology, 9,* 493–495. Retrieved from http://www.ncbi.nlm.nih.gov/pubmed/13768451

Miller, S. C., de Saint-Georges, L., Bowman, B. M., & Jee, W. S. (1989). Bone lining cells: Structure and function. *Scanning Microsc, 3*(3), 953–960. discussion 960-951. Retrieved from http://www.ncbi.nlm.nih.gov/pubmed/2694361

Mukund, K., & Subramaniam, S. (2019). Skeletal muscle: A review of molecular structure and function, in health and disease. *Wiley Interdisciplinary Reviews: Systems Biology and Medicine, 12,* e1462. Wiley

Murphy, W. L., Black, J., & Hastings, G. W. (2016). *Handbook of biomaterial properties* (2nd ed.). New York: Springer.

Nakashima, T., Hayashi, M., Fukunaga, T., Kurata, K., Oh-Hora, M., Feng, J. Q., . . . Takayanagi, H. (2011). Evidence for osteocyte regulation of bone homeostasis through RANKL expression. *Nature Medicine, 17*(10), 1231–1234. https://doi.org/10.1038/nm.2452

Nakashima, T., & Takayanagi, H. (2011). New regulation mechanisms of osteoclast differentiation. *Annals of the New York Academy of Sciences, 1240*, E13–E18. https://doi.org/10.1111/j.1749-6632.2011.06373.x

Nayak, A., & Amrute-Nayak, M. (2020). SUMO system – A key regulator in sarcomere organization. *FEBS Journal, 287*, 2176–2190. https://doi.org/10.1111/febs.15263

Nordin, M., & Frankel, V. H. (2012). *Basic biomechanics of the musculoskeletal system* (4th ed.). Philadelphia: Wolters Kluwer Health/Lippincott Williams & Wilkins.

O'Brien, M. (1997). Structure and metabolism of tendons. *Scandinavian Journal of Medicine and Science in Sports, 7*(2), 55–61. https://doi.org/10.1111/j.1600-0838.1997.tb00119.x

Owen, M. (1988). Marrow stromal stem cells. *Journal of Cell Science. Supplement, 10*, 63–76. Retrieved from http://www.ncbi.nlm.nih.gov/pubmed/3077943

Pierobon-Bormioli, S., Sartore, S., Libera, L. D., Vitadello, M., & Schiaffino, S. (1981). "Fast" isomyosins and fiber types in mammalian skeletal muscle. *Journal of Histochemistry and Cytochemistry, 29*(10), 1179–1188. https://doi.org/10.1177/29.10.7028858

Pittenger, M. F., Mackay, A. M., Beck, S. C., Jaiswal, R. K., Douglas, R., Mosca, J. D., . . . Marshak, D. R. (1999). Multilineage potential of adult human mesenchymal stem cells. *Science, 284*(5411), 143–147. Retrieved from http://www.ncbi.nlm.nih.gov/pubmed/10102814

Robey, P. G., Fedarko, N. S., Hefferan, T. E., Bianco, P., Vetter, U. K., Grzesik, W., et al. (1993). Structure and molecular regulation of bone matrix proteins. *Journal of Bone and Mineral Research: The Official Journal of the American Society for Bone and Mineral Research, 8*(Suppl 2), S483–S487. https://doi.org/10.1002/jbmr.5650081310

Ross, M. H., Romrell, L. J., & Kaye, G. I. (1995). *Histology: A text and atlas* (3rd ed.). Baltimore: Williams & Wilkins.

Sanes, J. R. (1982). Laminin, fibronectin, and collagen in synaptic and extrasynaptic portions of muscle fiber basement membrane. *Journal of Cell Biology, 93*(2), 442–451. Retrieved from http://www.ncbi.nlm.nih.gov/pubmed/7047538

Schiaffino, S. (2010). Fibre types in skeletal muscle: A personal account. *Acta Physiologica (Oxf), 199*(4), 451–463. https://doi.org/10.1111/j.1748-1716.2010.02130.x

Schiaffino, S., & Reggiani, C. (2011). Fiber types in mammalian skeletal muscles. *Physiological Reviews, 91*(4), 1447–1531. https://doi.org/10.1152/physrev.00031.2010

Schriefer, J. L., Warden, S. J., Saxon, L. K., Robling, A. G., & Turner, C. H. (2005). Cellular accommodation and the response of bone to mechanical loading. *Journal of Biomechanics, 38*(9), 1838–1845. https://doi.org/10.1016/j.jbiomech.2004.08.017

Screen, H. R., Berk, D. E., Kadler, K. E., Ramirez, F., & Young, M. F. (2015). Tendon functional extracellular matrix. *Journal of Orthopaedic Research, 33*(6), 793–799. https://doi.org/10.1002/jor.22818. Wiley

Sela, J., Amir, D., Schwartz, Z., & Weinberg, H. (1987). Ultrastructural tissue morphometry of the distribution of extracellular matrix vesicles in remodeling rat tibial bone six days after injury. *Acta Anat (Basel), 128*(4), 295–300. Retrieved from http://www.ncbi.nlm.nih.gov/pubmed/3037839

Selvanetti, A., Cipolla, M., & Puddu, G. (1997). Overuse tendon injuries: Basic science and classification. *Operative Techniques in Sports Medicine, 5*(3), 110–117. https://doi.org/10.1016/S1060-1872(97)80031-7

Sharma, P., & Maffulli, N. (2005). Tendon injury and tendinopathy: Healing and repair. *The Journal of Bone & Joint Surgery, 87*(1), 187–202. https://doi.org/10.2106/JBJS.D.01850

Shepherd, J. H., & Screen, H. R. (2013). Fatigue loading of tendon. *International Journal of Experimental Pathology, 94*(4), 260–270. https://doi.org/10.1111/iep.12037

Snow, M. H. (1977). The effects of aging on satellite cells in skeletal muscles of mice and rats. *Cell and Tissue Research, 185*(3), 399–408. Retrieved from http://www.ncbi.nlm.nih.gov/pubmed/597854

Sommer, B., Bickel, M., Hofstetter, W., & Wetterwald, A. (1996). Expression of matrix proteins during the development of mineralized tissues. *Bone, 19*(4), 371–380. Retrieved from http://www.ncbi.nlm.nih.gov/pubmed/8894143

Srinivasan, S., Agans, S. C., King, K. A., Moy, N. Y., Poliachik, S. L., & Gross, T. S. (2003). Enabling bone formation in the aged skeleton via rest-inserted mechanical loading. *Bone, 33*(6), 946–955. Retrieved from http://www.ncbi.nlm.nih.gov/pubmed/14678854

Stecco, C., & Caro, R. (2019). 2019 Ejtm special on muscle fascia. *European Journal of Translational Myology, 29*(1), 8060. https://doi.org/10.4081/ejtm.2019.8060

Stecco, C., Macchi, V., Porzionato, A., Duparc, F., & De Caro, R. (2011). The fascia: The forgotten structure. *Italian Journal of Anatomy and Embryology, 116*(3), 127–138. Retrieved from https://www.ncbi.nlm.nih.gov/pubmed/22852442

Stromberg, A., Jansson, M., Fischer, H., Rullman, E., Hagglund, H., & Gustafsson, T. (2013). Bone marrow derived cells in adult skeletal muscle tissue in humans. *Skelet Muscle, 3*(1), 12. https://doi.org/10.1186/2044-5040-3-12

Taichman, R. S. (2005). Blood and bone: two tissues whose fates are intertwined to create the hematopoietic stem-cell niche. *Blood, 105*(7), 2631–2639. https://doi.org/10.1182/blood-2004-06-2480

Tortora, G. J., & Derrickson, B. H. (Eds.) (2010). Muscle. In *Introduction to the human body* (11th ed.). Wiley.

Tu, X., Rhee, Y., Condon, K. W., Bivi, N., Allen, M. R., Dwyer, D., . . . Bellido, T. (2012). Sost downregulation and local Wnt signaling are required for the osteogenic response to mechanical loading. *Bone, 50*(1), 209–217. https://doi.org/10.1016/j.bone.2011.10.025

Warden, S. J., Fuchs, R. K., Castillo, A. B., Nelson, I. R., & Turner, C. H. (2007). Exercise when young provides lifelong benefits to bone structure and strength. *Journal of Bone and Mineral Research, 22*(2), 251–259. https://doi.org/10.1359/jbmr.061107

White, T. P., & Esser, K. A. (1989). Satellite cell and growth factor involvement in skeletal muscle growth. *Medicine and Science in Sports and Exercise, 21*(5 Suppl), S158–S163. Retrieved from http://www.ncbi.nlm.nih.gov/pubmed/2691828

Wijenayaka, A. R., Kogawa, M., Lim, H. P., Bonewald, L. F., Findlay, D. M., & Atkins, G. J. (2011). Sclerostin stimulates osteocyte support of osteoclast activity by a RANKL-dependent pathway. *PLoS One, 6*(10), e25900. https://doi.org/10.1371/journal.pone.0025900

Woo, S. L., & Buckwalter, J. A. (1988). AAOS/NIH/ORS workshop. Injury and repair of the musculoskeletal soft tissues. Savannah, Georgia, June 18–20, 1987. *Journal of Orthopaedic Research: Official Publication of the Orthopaedic Research Society, 6*(6), 907–931. https://doi.org/10.1002/jor.1100060615

Xiong, J., & O'Brien, C. A. (2012). Osteocyte RANKL: New insights into the control of bone remodeling. *Journal of Bone and Mineral Research, 27*(3), 499–505. https://doi.org/10.1002/jbmr.1547

Yamaguchi, A., Katagiri, T., Ikeda, T., Wozney, J. M., Rosen, V., Wang, E. A., . . . Yoshiki, S. (1991). Recombinant human bone morphogenetic protein-2 stimulates osteoblastic maturation and inhibits myogenic differentiation in vitro. *Journal of Cell Biology, 113*(3), 681–687. Retrieved from http://www.ncbi.nlm.nih.gov/pubmed/1849907

Yang, Y. J. (2010). Histology of the bone. http://www.emedicine.com/orthoped.htm.

Young, B., & Heath, J. W. (2000). In B. Young & J. W. Heath (Eds.), *Wheater's functional histology*. Philadelphia: Churchill Livingstone, in imprint of Harcourt Publishers Limited.

Zhang, P., Sun, Q., Turner, C. H., & Yokota, H. (2007). Knee loading accelerates bone healing in mice. *Journal of Bone and Mineral Research, 22*(12), 1979–1987. https://doi.org/10.1359/jbmr.070803

Zitnay, J. L., & Weiss, J. A. (2018). Load transfer, damage, and failure in ligaments and tendons. *Journal of Orthopaedic Research, 36*(12), 3093–3104. https://doi.org/10.1002/jor.24134

4

Structure and Function of the Nervous System and Its Relation to Pain

Overview

We first provide a systems overview of the nervous system, briefly defining central, peripheral, and automatic nervous systems. We then introduce basic structures of the nervous system (neurons and glia) followed by the structure and function of the nerve system. We follow this by describing interactions of peripheral and then central nervous systems that interact with the musculoskeletal system and then describe pain, pain exacerbation, and pain persistence (which occurs after peripheral and/or central sensitization mechanisms) since pain symptoms are the key characteristics of tissue injury and fatigue failure.

A Systems View of the Nervous System

The central nervous system (CNS) comprises the brain and spinal cord, while the peripheral nervous system (PNS) comprises everything outside of the dura mater (the outermost membrane enveloping the CNS). Although specific components of these systems are spatially separated and are categorized differently, each system communicates with the other. Peripheral nerves convey neural messages from sensory organs, receptors, and endings in afferent (sensory) nerves towards the CNS. Within the CNS, this afferent information is integrated and efferent and other responses are generated. The CNS sends efferent signals toward the periphery through peripheral nerves to targets in the body. If muscles receive efferent electrophysiological signals that result in muscle contractions, these signals are considered as motor signals (Figure 4.1). If the efferent signals are received by glands, organs, or other nonmuscular targets, they are considered as effector signals since they produce an effect in the end organs, such as the release of neurotransmitters or hormones.

Somatic is defined as "of, related to, or effecting, the body" (Merriam-Webster, 2021). Therefore, the somatic nervous system includes peripheral nerves that receive and convey both conscious and unconscious afferent information from the head, neck, body wall, and extremities to the CNS, where the sensory information is processed and interpreted. The somatic nervous system also comprises CNS structures that plan and execute efferent motor information for the main purpose of voluntary motor control, and the peripheral nerves that carry this efferent information to striated muscles in the head, neck, body wall, and extremities.

Musculoskeletal Disorders: The Fatigue Failure Mechanism, First Edition. Sean Gallagher and Mary F. Barbe.

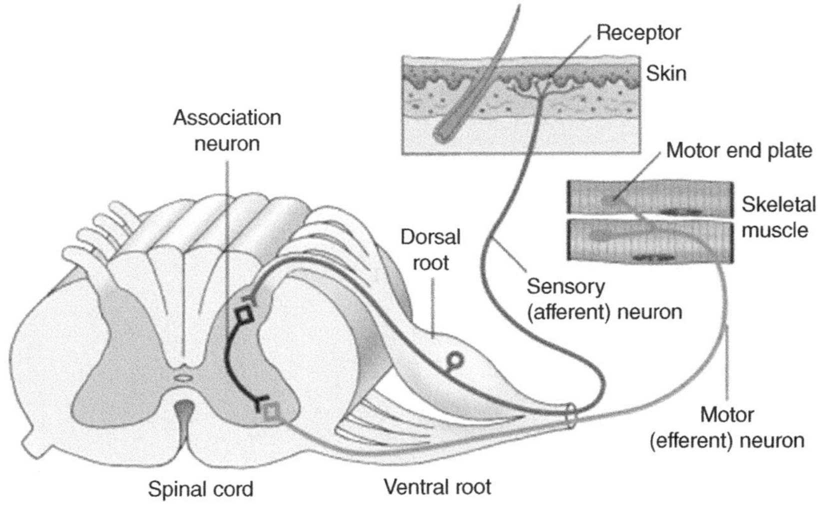

Figure 4.1 Sensory (afferent) nerves send signals from peripheral sensory terminals or receptors in distal targets (e.g., skin) through dorsal roots to the CNS (spinal cord or brain). Nerve axons that transmit commands from the CNS to end organs, including muscles, are considered efferents. If these efferent axons innervate muscles, they are considered a motor. Pakurar, A. S., & Bigbee, J. W. (2004). *Digital histology, an interactive CD atlas*. Figure 8.2. Wiley. ISBN 0-471-64982-1.

The autonomic nervous system also comprises neural structures of the PNS and CNS that regulate involuntary bodily functions, such as heart rate, blood pressure, pupil dilation, body temperature, sweating, digestion, gastrointestinal motility, and bladder function. A variety of brain, brainstem, and spinal cord structures are involved in these autonomic motor regulatory functions. Peripheral nerves convey autonomic motor efferent signals to smooth muscles in arteries and skin, cardiac muscle, glands, and organs. The autonomic nervous system can be further divided into sympathetic and parasympathetic nervous systems. The sympathetic nervous system is often called the "fight or flight system," since it is responsible for regulating the body's rapid involuntary response to dangerous or stressful situations. Activation of the sympathetic nervous system results in the release of hormones that can enhance brain alertness, accelerate heart rate, widen bronchial passages and quicken breathing (to raise fresh oxygen levels to the brain), increase the release of glucose for quick energy, decrease motility in the large intestines, increase peristalsis in the esophagus, and induce pupillary dilation, piloerection (goosebumps), and perspiration (sweating). Sympathetic activation causes vasoconstriction of arteries and veins to increase resistance and decrease distal blood flow. The parasympathetic system is the "rest and restoration system" since it counters with a homeostatic return of blood pressure, breathing rate, hormone release, and digestion to normal levels.

Functions of the sympathetic nervous system are pertinent to musculoskeletal disorders since disturbances in this system are related to symptoms of complex regional pain syndrome type I. This term encompasses reflex sympathetic dystrophy and causalgia. Complex regional pain syndrome is a painful condition that can be caused by irritative injuries of the peripheral nerves. It is characterized by symptoms of severe burning pain, glossy skin, swelling, redness, and sweating. Many patients with complex regional pain syndrome are workers with compensation claims (Lazaro, 2017). Pathological responses in the sympathetic nervous autonomic system also contribute to the hand-arm vibration syndrome (HAVS), as mentioned in Chapter 2.

An Introduction to Cellular Components of the Nervous System

Neurons

Neurons are specialized cells that have unique and diverse morphological features that allow them to transmit specific signals to and from tissues or other neurons. All neurons, despite their some shape differences, share some similar structures (Table 4.1; Figure 4.2). The neuronal cell body is the portion of the cell surrounding the nucleus that contains the majority of the cell's organelles. It is the metabolic and genetic center of this cell type. Dendrites extend from the cell body and are highly branched processes that are specialized for receiving incoming information. The cell body and dendrites are the primary receptive portions of a neuron. An axon is the long projection of a neuron that is specialized for carrying a neuron's electrical signal (the action potential). A single axon typically arises from each neuron, although branching along the axon (termed collateral branches) may occur. Axons typically terminate as multiple small branches that can be focused to quite broad on the end target (termed the axonal arborization). It is within these axon terminals that the axonal action potential is converted into a chemical signal via the release of a neurotransmitter that is then received by the target cell, which may be a muscle, another neuron, organ, and more.

Table 4.1 Basic Arrangements of Neuronal Cell Bodies and Their Processes

System	Groups of cell bodies	Bundle of processes
Central nervous system (CNS)	Nucleus or cortex (gray matter)	Tracts/pathways in white matter
Peripheral nervous system (PNS)	Ganglia	Nerve

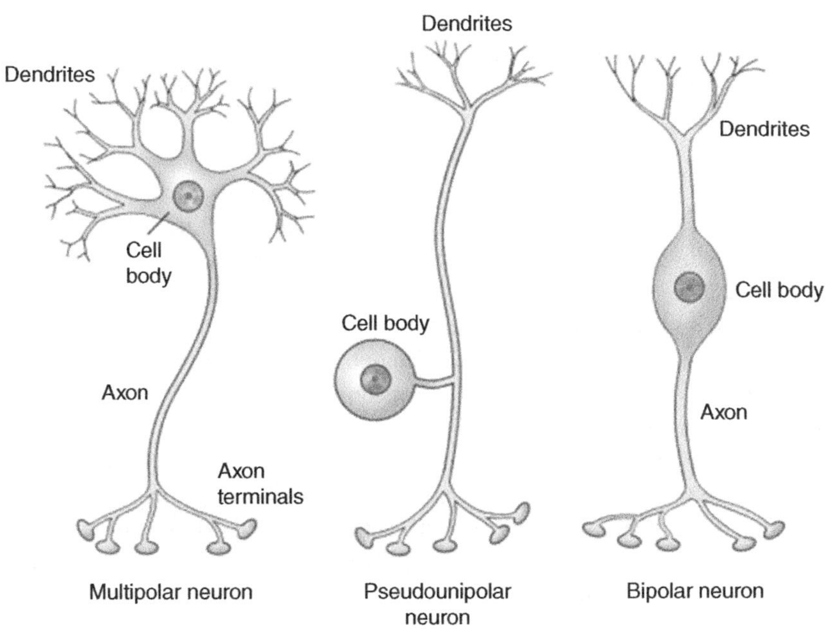

Figure 4.2 Types of neurons based on shape. Pakurar, A. S., & Bigbee, J. W. (2004). *Digital histology, an interactive CD atlas*. Figure 8.2. Wiley. ISBN 0-471-64982-1.

Table 4.2 Examples of Neurotransmitters and Neuropeptides

Excitatory	• Promote the generation of an action potential	• Acetylcholine, adrenaline, catecholamines (e.g., substance P), dopamine, glutamate, histamine, and norepinephrine (also known as noradrenaline)
Inhibitory	• Suppress the generation of an action potential	• Dopamine, GABA (gamma-aminobutyric acid), glycine, and serotonin (5-hydroxytryptamine, 5-HT)

Note. Dopamine effects can either be excitatory or inhibitory, with effects based on the type of receptor to which it is binding.

Neurons synthesize neurotransmitter substances or their precursors in their cell bodies. Neurotransmitters are chemical substances that are transported along the axon and then released at their terminal endings. These chemicals diffuse across narrow intercellular spaces (synaptic clefts) before binding to specific receptors incorporated into the membrane of the muscle cell, postsynaptic neuron, gland, or other end-organ structure. There are many types of neurotransmitters. Some neurotransmitters are excitatory and promote the generation of an action potential in a postsynaptic neuron, including glutamate, norepinephrine, and substance P (Table 4.2 provides a number of examples). Others are inhibitory neurotransmitters and suppress the generation of an action potential, including gamma-aminobutyric acid (GABA) and serotonin. Neurons are also metabolically very active and expend much energy maintaining ionic gradients across their plasma membranes, as will be discussed later in section "Structure and Function of the Peripheral Nervous System."

Neurons also contain cytoskeletal components that are arranged in parallel bundles throughout the neuronal cell body, under the cell membrane, and along the length of axons and dendrites. Intermediate filaments are one type of cytoskeletal component that provides structural support. Microtubules are another type of cytoskeletal component that is critically involved in the axonal transport of several neurotransmitter substances, enzymes, membrane subcomponents, and other cellular constituents. Changes after damage to various neural structures, including these cytoskeletal components, will be discussed further in Chapter 6.

Glial Cells

Neuroglial cells (typically called glial cells) are an important part of the neural microenvironment and are comprised mostly of Schwann cells and satellite cells in peripheral neural structures, and microglia, oligodendrocytes, and astrocytes in the CNS. Glial cells are critical for maintaining extracellular fluid homeostasis and providing metabolic support to neurons. Both Schwann cells in the PNS and oligodendrocytes in the CNS synthesize and maintain the insulating myelin sheaths that surround axons (Figure 4.3; Table 4.3). Satellite cells are found in dorsal root ganglia and surround the cell bodies of sensory neurons. Microglial cells are a specialized population of macrophages located within the CNS that have immune and phagocytic functions, such as the ability to phagocytose infected, damaged or dying neurons, and injured brain and spinal cord tissues. Astrocytes make up the majority of CNS glial cells, provide lactate to neighboring neurons for fuel (either from glucose taken up from the blood or by metabolizing glycogen), and are involved in maintaining the blood–brain barrier. Both astrocytes and satellite cells stabilize the extracellular fluid in which they reside by removing potassium ions and neurotransmitters from synaptic clefts and recycling them so that they can be used again for synaptic transmission.

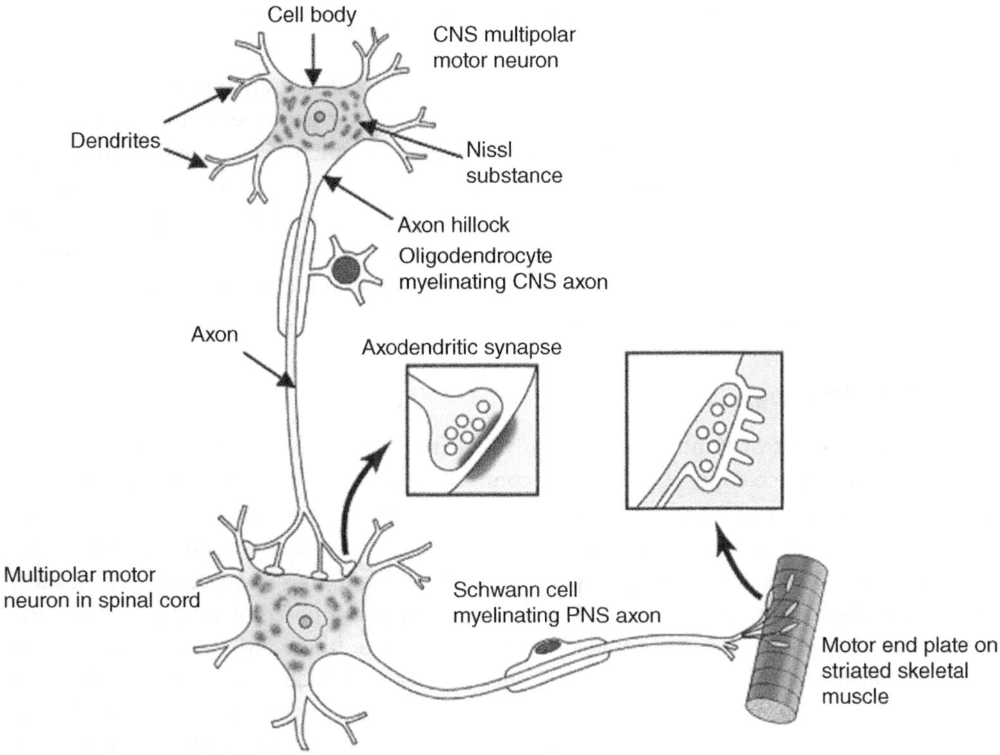

Figure 4.3 Typical multipolar neurons with glial cells that myelinate depicted: oligodendroctyes (myelinate central nervous system axons) and Schwann cells (myelinated peripheral nerve system axons). CNS (central nervous system), PNS (peripheral nervous system). Leichnetz, G. R. (2006). *Digital neuroanatomy. Figure 1.10b.* Wiley. ISBN: 0-470-04000-9.

Table 4.3 Main Types of Neuroglia and Their Properties

Neuroglia	Location	Function
Oligodendrocytes	CNS, mainly in white matter	In white matter of the CNS, they form myelin sheaths. In gray matter of the CNS, they surround neurons.
Schwann cells	Peripheral nervous system only	Myelinate axons and surround unmyelinated axons in the PNS. Function as phagocytes during axonal degeneration.
Protoplasmic astrocytes	CNS, gray matter	Support and isolate neurons; sequester Na^+ ions; metabolize extracellular neurotransmitters; repair damage to the CNS by forming glial scar tissue; surround unmyelinated axons.
Fibrous astrocytes	CNS, white matter	Same as protoplasmic astrocytes
Microglia	CNS	Phagocytize damaged nerve tissue in the CNS

Structure and Function of the Peripheral Nervous System

The PNS consists of spinal nerves arising from the spinal cord as well as cranial nerves arising from the brain. Spinal nerves typically contain both sensory and motor axons, and are organized on either side of the vertebral column, one pair for each vertebral segment. Dorsal and ventral nerve roots connect the spinal cord to the spinal nerves, with dorsal roots typically carrying afferent input and ventral roots typically carrying motor output (Figure 4.1). Peripheral ganglia are groups of afferent and/or efferent nerve cell bodies that are located outside of the CNS. Dorsal root ganglia are bundles of sensory neuron cell bodies located at each segmental level of the spinal column from cervical level 1 through coccygeal levels.

Peripheral Nerve Histology

Peripheral nerves consist of bundles of axons divided into fascicles (one or more fascicles per nerve) surrounded by three concentric layers of connective tissues, namely the epineurium, perineurium, and endoneurium (Figure 4.4). As described in Chapter 3 for muscles and tendons, the outer "epi" layer, termed the epineurium in nerves, is the outermost layer of dense irregular connective tissue and is composed of collagen and elastin fibrils. Groupings of nerve fibers (fascicles) are bundled together by the perineurium. The perineurium is composed of multiple concentric layers of flattened epithelial-like cells embedded in a connective tissue layer of collagenous and elastin fibrils arranged in circumferential, longitudinal, and oblique orientations (Rosso & Guck, 2019; Ushiki & Ide, 1990). The innermost connective tissue layer of a nerve is the endoneurium. It surrounds the axons and is composed of collagen types I, II, and IV fibrils, the latter in close association with the Schwann cell's basal lamina (Ushiki, Hayashi, & Ide, 1990).

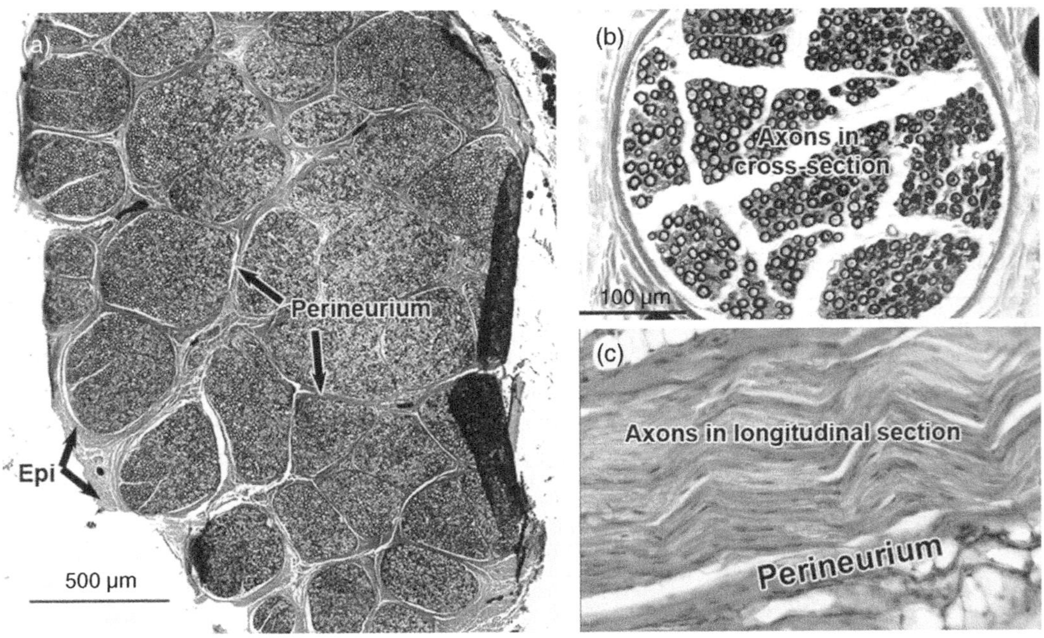

Figure 4.4 Peripheral nerve histological sections. (a) A cross-section of a large nerve with epineurium (Epi) and perineurium is shown. (b) A smaller nerve, with clear axonal profiles shown in the cross-section. (c) Longitudinal section of a small peripheral nerve with perineurium shown.

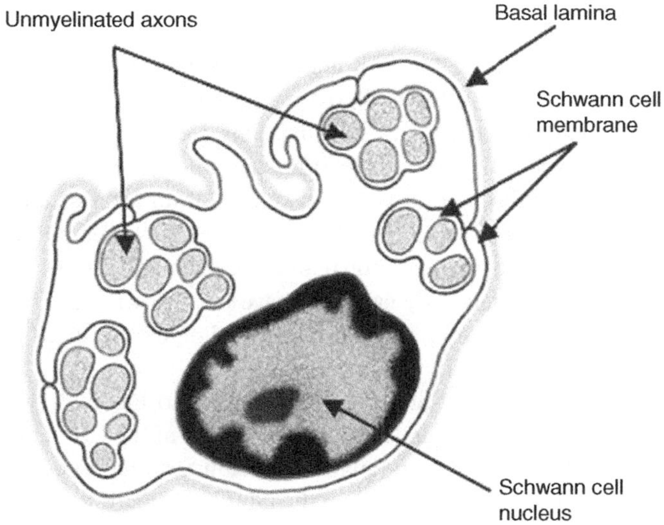

Figure 4.5 Schwann cells around unmyelinated peripheral nerve axons. Leichnetz, G. R. (2006). *Digital neuroanatomy.* Figure 1.10b. Wiley. ISBN-10 0-470-04000-9.

The axons with a nerve contain a mix of somatic motor, autonomic motor, and sensory axons, depending on the nerve in question. The axons have an undulated course longitudinally through peripheral nerves. Individual axons are surrounded by either myelinating or non-myelinating Schwann cells that provide nutritional and metabolic support to the axons (Figures 4.3 and 4.5). Although typically not described in histological texts, the Schwann cell's basal lamina comprises another extracellular matrix encasement of nerve axons and is composed of collagen type IV, fibronectin, laminin, and heparin sulfate proteoglycans (Ushiki et al., 1990). Large diameter axons are enveloped by multiple wrappings of concentric layers of Schwann cells that form a myelin sheath that surrounds these larger axons. Medium-sized axons are less myelinated, while smaller-sized axons are simply enveloped by the cytoplasm of a Schwann cell and are thus called unmyelinated (Figure 4.5). Between Schwann cells, there are short intervals of axons regions that are not covered by a myelin sheath. These intervals are known as the Nodes of Ranvier and are important for saltatory conduction of the axon's action potential. The rate of conduction of an axon's action potential is proportional to the amount of myelin so that larger axons show faster conduction than smaller unmyelinated axons.

Other tissues and cell types in peripheral nerves include blood vessels, as well as macrophages and fibroblasts. Transperineurial blood vessels link epineurial and endoneurial vascular plexuses and pierce the innermost layers of the perineurium (Myers, Kalichman, Reisner, & Powell, 1986; Myers, Murakami, & Powell, 1986). Resident noninflammatory macrophages are present within nerve bundles and contribute to maintenance functions. Infiltrating macrophages and mast cells can also be present, typically transiently, when needed for clean-up and repair after axonal injury. There are also fibroblasts within and surrounding nerve bundles (termed intraneural and extraneural fibroblasts, respectively) that can contribute to increases in the deposition of collagen within and around nerves in instances of fibrotic nerve encapsulation and resultant pathology (Clark, Al-Shatti, Barr, Amin, & Barbe, 2004; Clark et al., 2003). Fibrotic nerve encapsulation can be one cause of carpal tunnel symptoms, as discussed previously in Chapter 2 and will be discussed further in Chapter 11.

Synapses, Including Neuromuscular Junctions

Synapses are highly specialized intercellular junctions that link neurons together into nervous system pathways. Their basic components are defined in Table 4.4. Intercellular synaptic junctions also link neurons and their effector cells, such as in neuromuscular junctions. Neurotransmitters diffuse across synaptic clefts before binding to specific receptors incorporated into the membrane of the postsynaptic structure. Classically, neuron-to-neuron synapses consist of an axon of one neuron synapsing on the dendrites of another neuron (an axodendritic synapse). However, many axons synapse on other axons (an axo-axonic synapse) or directly on neuronal cell bodies. Dendrites can synapse on other dendrites, and cell body-to-cell body synapses have been described. The response in the post-synaptic structure can be excitatory or inhibitory depending on the specific neurotransmitter(s) released and the specific functional nature of the synapse.

Neuromuscular junctions are also termed motor endplates (Figure 4.3; See also Figure 3.11). These junctions are a specialized synapse between large alpha motor neurons from the CNS and the sarcolemma of a muscle fiber. At each of these motor end plates, the axon terminal loses its myelin sheath and divides into clusters of small swollen terminals on the muscle fiber surface. The motor endplate occupies a recess on the skeletal muscle's cell surface and is covered by an extension of the cytoplasm of the last Schwann cell surrounding the axon. The endoneurium investing the nerve becomes continuous with the delicate collagenous investing endomysium of the muscle fiber. The postsynaptic membrane of the neuromuscular junction is deeply folded into parallel secondary synaptic clefts. The presynaptic terminal of a somatic (skeletal) motor unit contains numerous synaptic vesicles that contain the neurotransmitter acetylcholine. When a nerve impulse arrives at the tip of the axon terminal, acetylcholine is released into the synaptic cleft that binds to specific receptors on the muscle membranes for acetylcholine (nicotinic receptors). This causes ion channels to open and the flow of sodium ions into the muscle cell that then initiates a sequence of steps that cumulates in a muscle contraction, as described earlier in Chapter 3 (section "Sarcoplasmic Reticulum and Calcium Storage and Release").

Basic Nerve Physiology

Most neurons have a negative resting membrane potential, meaning that when the cell is not sending or receiving any signals, the inside of the cell is negatively charged. A change in the membrane

Table 4.4 Structure of a Synapse

Component	Description
Presynaptic component	• Distal end of axon branches, each branch terminating in swelling or button, is called the terminal bouton. • Bouton contains synaptic vesicles/granules that contain neurotransmitters and numerous mitochondria.
Synaptic gap/cleft	• Separation (20–30 nm) between pre-and post-synaptic cells
Postsynaptic component	• Formed by the membrane of the postsynaptic neuron or muscle cell and contains receptors for neurotransmitters.
Bouton en passant	• Small swellings along the length of axons that allow a single axon to contact many cells.

Modified from Pakurar, A. S., & Bigbee, J. W. (2004). *Digital histology, an interactive CD atlas*. Figure 8.2. Wiley. ISBN 0-471-64982-1.

potential towards a more positive potential is called depolarization, which, if of great enough magnitude, leads to the opening of voltage-gated ion channels (such as Na^+ channels) and further neuronal depolarization in the form of an action potential. Ion pumps and ion channels are critical for maintaining the resting membrane potential, as well as for re-establishing the membrane potential after cell depolarization occurs. Alternately, some signals hyperpolarize the membrane, which makes it more difficult for the membrane potential to depolarize enough to reach the threshold potential.

Sensory nerves are activated at their terminal endings by external stimuli, such as touch, heat, or pH changes or chemicals in the extracellular fluids. This input is integrated at the axon terminus into a membrane potential that is called a receptor potential (Figure 4.6a). Receptor potentials vary in amplitude depending on the intensity of the stimulus (a higher stimulus opens more ion channels and for longer durations). Receptor potentials can summate over time (temporally) and/or spatially (Figure 4.6b). Spatial summation occurs when multiple presynaptic neurons together release enough neurotransmitters to create a cumulative amplitude-graded postsynaptic receptor potential in the postsynaptic neuron. Temporal summation is the product of a single neuron sending repeated action potential to the nerve terminal causing a cumulative response on the second-order neuron. However, only when a neuron's cell's membrane reaches a specific threshold, do voltage-gated channels open to stimulate an action potential.

The action potential is the conductive potential of an axon (Figures 4.6a and 4.7). The action potential differs significantly from the receptor potential just discussed in that there is no graded

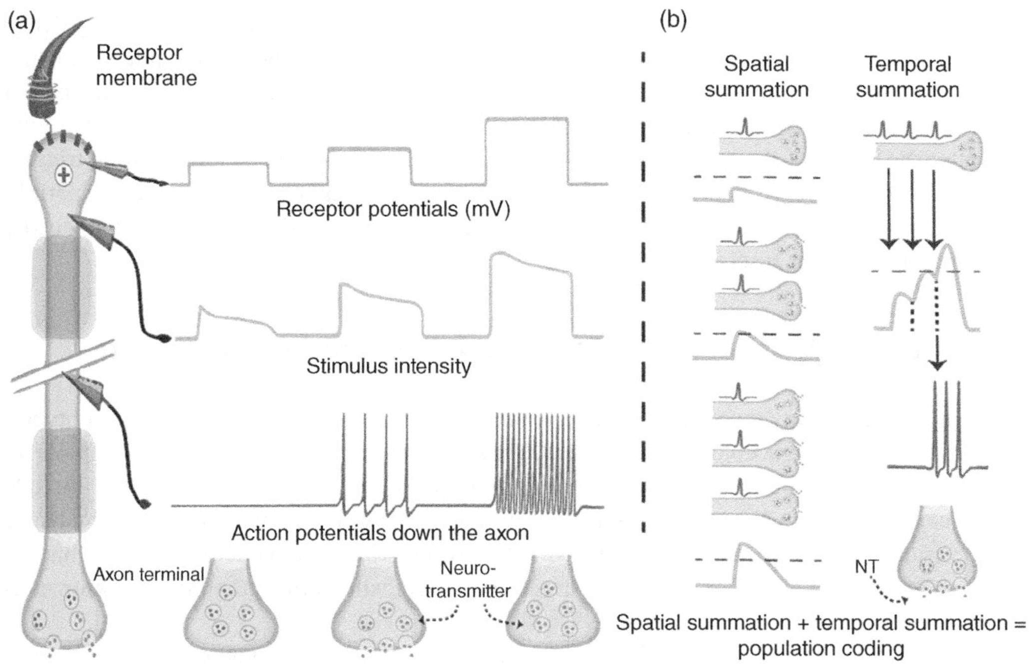

Figure 4.6 (a) Stimulus-induced amplitude-graded receptor potentials at receptors of the primary sensory neuron. Frequency-dependent response at the nerve terminals causes the selective release of neurotransmitters. The greater the receptor potential, the higher the frequency of action potentials generated. (b) A depiction of spatial and temporal summation. Chapman, K. B., Yousef, T. A., Foster, A., Stanton-Hicks M.D., & van Helmond, N. (2020). Mechanisms for the clinical utility of low-frequency stimulation in neuromodulation of the dorsal root ganglion. *Neuromodulation*, *24*(4), 738–745. https://doi.org/10.1111/ner.13323. Wiley.

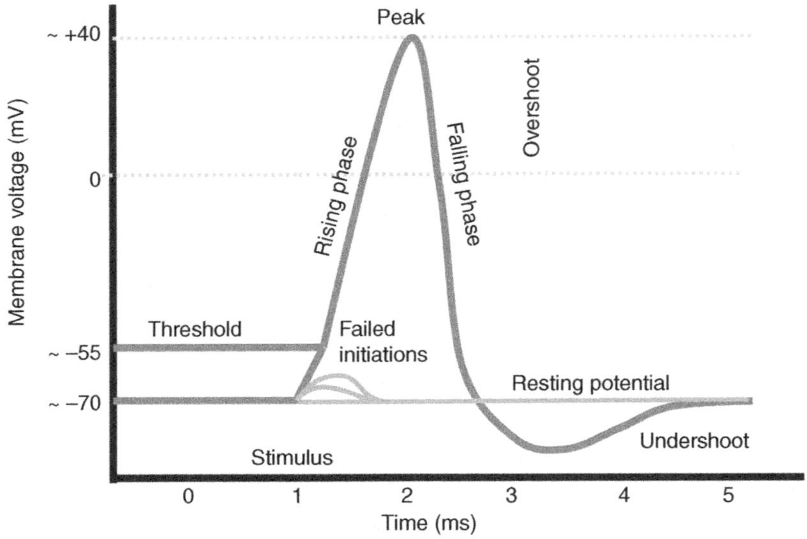

Figure 4.7 A schematic view of an idealized action potential that illustrates its various phases as the action potential passes a point (the threshold) on a cell's membrane. Action potential/Wikipedia/GNU Free Documentation License.

response or summation. An action potential is the activation of an all-or-none electrical signal. Physiologically, and action potential is a rapid swing in the polarity of the voltage from negative to positive and back. As shown in Figure 4.7, it has a rising phase, a falling phase, an undershoot, and then a return to its resting potential. The action potential does not dwell in one spot, instead, it travels along the axon from the site of activation to its terminal end, without degrading the signal (no matter the length of the axon). The depolarization associated with an action potential triggers the release of neurotransmitters from central synaptic terminals (Figure. 4.6a). For sensory peripheral nerves, these central terminals are located in the spinal cord or the brain stem (for sensory spinal or cranial nerves, respectively).

Interactions of Peripheral Nerves with the Musculoskeletal System

Although there are many types of sensory receptors, they can be divided into two main subtypes: exteroceptors and interoceptors (Table 4.5). Primary exteroceptive sensory systems relate to vision, audition, olfaction, taste, and somatosensation. Somatosensory exteroceptors include (a) mechanoreceptors in skin that respond to deformation, movement, and tension on the tissue and (b) various types of nociceptors that respond to noxious stimuli; and chemoreceptors that are sensitive to acids and increased histamine. Nociceptors are pain endings that are also known as free nerve endings or C fibers.

Interoception is the process by which an organism senses, interprets, integrates, and regulates interoceptive signals. Interoreceptors sense the internal condition and include: (a) mechanoreceptors in muscles, joint capsules, tendons, and ligaments that respond to deformation, movement, and tension on the tissue; (b) nociceptors that respond to noxious stimuli and that are often free nerve endings; (c) chemoreceptors like acid sensory endings in muscles that respond to increases in lactic acid after exercise, for example; and (d) proprioceptors (Latin, *prioprius*, one's own) located in musculoskeletal tissues that respond to internal forces and positions.

Table 4.5 Comparison of Exteroreceptors Versus Interoreceptors

Exteroreceptors	• Special Sensory: Vision, audition, olfaction, taste • Somatosensation: Mechanoreceptors in the skin that respond to deformation, movement, and tension; nociceptors in the skin; chemoreceptors in skin
Interoreceptors	• Mechanoreceptors in muscles, joint capsules, tendons, and ligaments that respond to deformation, movement, and tension. • Nociceptors that respond to noxious stimuli and that are often free nerve endings. • Chemoreceptors like acid sensory endings in muscles (e.g., that respond to lactic acid). • Proprioceptors in musculoskeletal tissues that respond to internal forces and positions.

Innervation of Skin

In skin, polymodal nociceptors respond to high intensity mechanical, mechanical heat–cold, or itch, with the perceived sensation reported by the subject, begin burning, dull, aching or freezing pain, or itch. Unimodal nociceptors include mechanical receptors that respond to high-intensity mechanical stimuli to induce burning, dull or aching pain sensations. There are also noxious heat receptors that respond to high-intensity heat, and chemical receptors that respond to several substances in the extracellular fluids, including bradykinin, serotonin, and prostaglandin. The perceived sensation reported by the patient after stimulation of either noxious heat or chemical nociceptors is burning pain. Similar nociceptors can be found in muscles, joints, and viscera.

Innervation of Deep Fascia

Since fascia can be a source of pain (fascitis) and perhaps non-specific low back pain as well as other non-specific pain, the identification of nociceptive fibers in fascial tissue has attracted recent interest (Mense & Hoheisel, 2016). For example, thoracolumbar fascia has been shown to contain many presumably nociceptive fibers, including small free nerve endings that stained positive for calcitonin gene-related peptide (CGRP), Substance P and transient receptor potential vanilloid 1 (TRPV1; a transmembrane ion channel that can be opened by tissue acidosis (a pH below 5.9), noxious high temperatures (above 42 °C), and capsaicin (Mense & Hoheisel, 2016). The density of these presumably nociceptive fibers increases in upper and lower layers of the inflamed thoracolumbar fascia, compared to non-inflamed, further supportive of their nociceptor roles. Ruffini endings and Pacinian corpuscles have also been found in the human thoracolumbar fascia (Yahia, Rhalmi, Newman, & Isler, 1992) and deep fascia of the limbs (as free nerve endings). Ruffini endings are known to detect tissue stretch, deformation, and warmth, while Pacinian corpuscles detect transient tissue pressure and high-frequency vibration (Molnar & Gair, 2021). Such innervation by proprioceptors may allow deep fascial layers to participate in peripheral motor control (e.g., postural control), since it is a tissue that can transmit the tension generated by muscles to distant body segments (Stecco et al., 2008).

Innervation of Muscles

Muscles receive alpha and gamma motor neuron innervation. They also contain a number of sensory endings, including muscle spindles (mechanoreceptors), free nerve endings, and chemical receptors.

Muscle spindles (sensory muscle receptor)

Muscle fibers can be divided into striated extrafusal and intrafusal fiber types. The extrafusal muscle fibers are the ones described above and in Chapter 3 that contract after innervation and activation of a neuromuscular junction (the motor endplate) by large alpha motor neuronal axons. However, there are also smaller intrafusal muscle fibers that are part of an encapsulated sensory muscle receptor known as the muscle spindle (Figure 4.8).

Muscle spindles consist of highly modified muscle fibers (i.e., the striated intrafusal muscle fibers) that are aligned in parallel with and surrounded by the extrafusal skeletal muscle fibers. The muscle spindles are the proprioceptors of skeletal muscles (Figure 4.8). They consist of capsules that contain the intrafusal fibers (nuclear bag and nuclear chain fibers). The sensory axons from

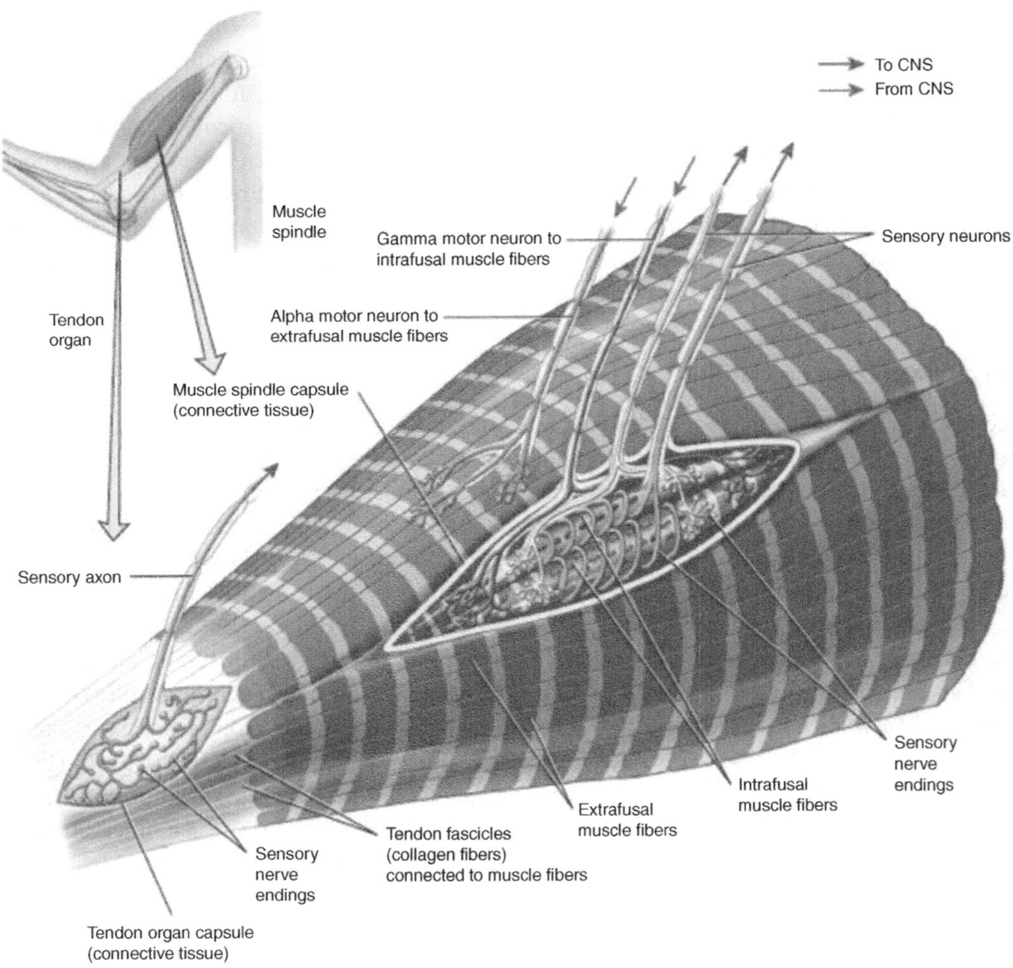

Figure 4.8 Innervation of muscles and tendons. Depiction of an alpha motor neuron to extrafusal muscle fibers (which innervate neuromuscular junctions), gamma motor neurons to intrafusal muscle fibers (also known as muscle spindles), sensory neurons from the muscle spindles that project sensory information to the central nervous system. A sensory nerve ending, the Golgi tendon organ, in the tendon is also shown. Tortora, G. J. & Derrickson, B. H. (Eds.). (2010). Chapter 16, Sensory, motor, and integrative systems. *Introduction to human body* (11th ed.). Wiley.

the nuclear bag fibers are type Ia afferents (also termed annulospiral endings), while the sensory axons from the nuclear chain fibers are type Ia and II (also termed flower spray endings). Each project sensory information from this muscle receptor into the dorsal horn of the spinal cord. The intrafusal muscle fibers are innervated by gamma motor neurons (whose cell bodies are located within the ventral horns of the spinal cord) that are also termed fusimotor neurons. The explicit assignment of gamma motor neurons is to control the tension of intrafusal muscle fibers so that they are ready and able to respond to any extrafusal muscle stretch. This is possible because there are two types of gamma motor neurons that relate to the fast (dynamic) and slow (static) muscle stretches (Rohrle, Yavuz, Klotz, Negro, & Heidlauf, 2019). Both static and dynamic type gamma motor neurons innervate the nuclear bag fibers, while only static type gamma motor neurons innervate the nuclear chain fibers; each work together to modify the sensitivity of the muscle spindle. The gamma motor neurons receive input from several descending motor pathways (corticospinal and reticulospinal tracts), which co-activate both the gamma and alpha motor neurons. In addition, there are beta motor neurons that provide both intra- and extrafusal muscle innervation (Rohrle et al., 2019). Similar to gamma motor neurons, the beta motor neurons have two distinct types that control either dynamic or static sensitivity of intrafusal and innervate extrafusal fibers. In this selected skeletal innervation organization, the dynamic beta motor neurons innervate nuclear bag intrafusal and slow contracting type extrafusal muscle fibers, while the static ones innervate the longest of the intrafusal muscle fibers (which are the nuclear chain fibers) and fast contracting extrafusal muscle fibers. In combination, these components detect changes in the length of the surrounding extrafusal muscle and the rate of that change. The muscle spindle also helps regulate the amount of effort required to perform movements with variable amounts of muscular force.

Other muscle innervation, e.g., nociceptors and chemoreceptors

Sensory nociceptors in muscles are responsible for painful sensations after muscle damage. These nerve endings are often identified by the expression of substance P and calcitonin gene-related peptide neuropeptides that are synthesized in the cell bodies of sensory neurons (i.e., in their cell bodies that are located in dorsal root ganglia). These neuropeptides are released as extracellular vesicles from the peripheral terminals of axons within the muscles. Substance P and calcitonin gene-related peptides show increased release in response to inflammatory responses in muscle tissues. Muscles are also sensitive to pH changes, particularly acidic changes because a decrease in pH also increases the activity of nociceptors (as a result of muscle acidosis). Knockout mouse experiments have revealed that the allodynia is due to acid-sensing ion channels in the muscles, specifically the Acid Sensing Ion Channel 1a (*ASIC3*) (Gregory, Gautam, Benson, & Sluka, 2018; Sluka, Winter, & Wemmie, 2009). Macrophage activation also plays a critical role. Activation of macrophages due to acidosis is accompanied by increases in several pro-inflammatory cytokines. The increase in inflammatory cytokines within muscle further activates the nociceptors, enhancing symptoms of pain. Irrespective of the cause, increases in muscle nociceptor or chemoreceptor activity produce a painful response observed as increased withdrawal of limbs on probing (indicative of increased sensitivity of nociceptors). This response is due to stimulation of a sensory-spinal cord-motor withdrawal reflex, as described further in section "Spinal Sensory-Motor Reflex Circuits." Increases in muscle pain are also termed muscle hyperalgesia or myalgia.

Both substance P and calcitonin gene-related peptides are commonly associated with blood vessels in the richly innervated extrafusal muscle. There is also sympathetic adrenergic innervation of the blood vessels within muscles that appear to regulate blood flow.

Innervation of Tendons

Like muscles, tendons also contain sensory nerves, including Golgi tendon organs, Ruffini endings, Pacinian corpuscles, free nerve endings (which are typically pain fibers), and sympathetic adrenergic innervation of their blood vessels (that are primarily located in the tendon sheaths). Golgi tendon organs are sensory endings located at the junction of the muscle and its tendon. They are specialized in detecting changes in tension within tendons during muscle stretch and contractions; they are also sensitive to the velocity of tension development (Figures 4.8 and 4.9). Their role is to inhibit motor activity if the tension becomes excessive and to help regulate the amount of effort required to perform movements with variable amounts of force.

Innervation of Bone

Hilton's Law, postulated in 1863 by John Hilton, states that the nerves that supply muscles and skin also supply the underlying joint. Since then, several studies have determined that both sensory and autonomic nerve fibers innervate mineralized bone, the bone marrow, and the periosteum. Myelinated and unmyelinated nerve terminals reside within a bone, closely associated with the vasculature, and in close proximity to osteoblasts, osteoclasts, and bone marrow adipocytes. Much of the anatomical information about the innervation of bone comes from the pain literature, since skeletal pathologies like fracture, osteoarthritis, osteoporosis, and bone metastases, are associated with bone pain. Nerve sprouting in bone and periosteum is responsible for bone pain.

Bone innervation is highly dynamic and has also been demonstrated to be important for bone acquisition and homeostasis. Both sensory and sympathetic innervation increases dramatically

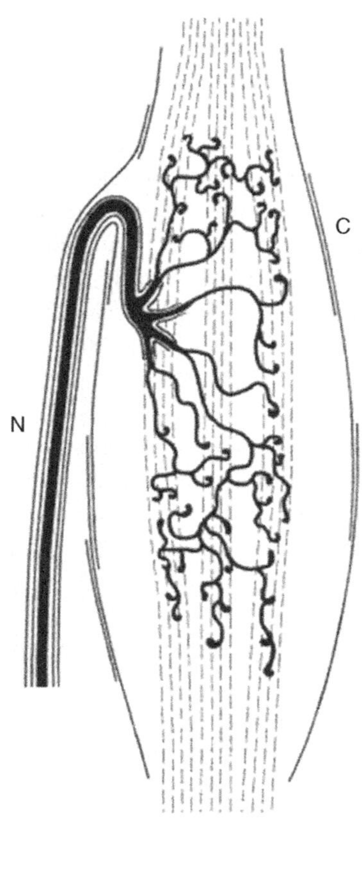

Figure 4.9 A Golgi tendon organ. The vertical dashed lines represent the collagen fibrils of the tendon. C = Capsule, N = nerve. Blumer, R., Lukas, J. R., Wasicky, R., & Mayr, R. (2000). Presence and morphological variability of Golgi tendon organs in the distal portion of sheep extraocular muscle. *The Anatomical Record 258*, 359–368./John Wiley & Sons.

during fracture healing and cancer metastases. Surgical or chemical denervation (with capsaicin, which destroys TRPV1 expressing sensory neurons mentioned earlier with muscle innervation) reduces bone acquisition and fracture healing. The role of bone innervation beyond pain has been investigated using antibodies against nerve growth factor (NGF) and its receptor, TrkA. Inhibition of NGF/TrkA signaling reduces the pain from fracture but does not delay the healing process.

Additionally, despite the classical role of sensory neurons to transmit afferent signals to the CNS, many also secrete neuropeptides that have an effect on a target tissue. Anatomical evidence points toward a role of these in response to mechanical loading, especially after a fracture. Substance P, calcitonin gene-related peptide (CGRP), and vasoactive intestinal peptide (VIP) expressing sensory fibers, as well as neuropeptide Y and glutamate expressing nerve endings are present in the periosteum, bone marrow, and on the trabecular bone of the metaphysis. This dense network of nerve fibers exhibits mechanosensory and site-specific sprouting after a fracture. Both CGRP and substance P expressing nerve endings sprout within callus sites during the healing process in sites of maximal bone loading and bone formation. For example, the bony callus on the highly loaded concave side of an angulated fracture has more CGRP and substance P nerve sprouting, compared to the less-loaded convex side. Neuropeptide Y positive fibers also increase during the early inflammatory phase in the bone-forming concave side, as well as during the later remodeling phase in the convex side. The latter occurs in parallel with bone resorption and thinning of the callus. In contrast, complete denervation delays fracture healing.

Innervation of Ligaments and Other Joint Structures

Joint ligaments and the periosteum associated with the adjoining bones are highly innervated with nociceptors near the site of attaching tendons where they merge with the outer layer of the joint capsule. Although poorly vascularized, the outer layer of joint capsules is highly innervated by a variety of somatic sensory fibers mediating sensations of pain, proprioception, pressure, and vibration. Thus, any swelling from disease or trauma stimulates nociceptors (pain endings) in joint structures gives rise to the sensation of pain in or near a joint. Ligaments also contain proprioceptors, such as Golgi tendon organ-like receptors (tension receptors), Ruffini endings (detect tissue stretch or deformation), and Pacinian corpuscles (pressure receptors) that signal tension and pressure changes (Molnar & Gair, 2021; Stecco et al., 2010). The joint capsule also contains Ruffini-type endings and Pacinian corpuscles (small, elongated Pacinian corpuscles). These receptors respond to the bending of joints (proprioception), as do some of the free nerve endings in the joint capsule. These types of joint capsule receptors play a protective function against the extremes of hyperextension and hyperflexion. Thus, part of the role of ligaments and joint capsules is in the sensation of pain or pressure within or near a joint.

In contrast, the inner layer of the joint capsule is the synovial membrane. It is highly vascularized but poorly innervated. The articular cartilage also lacks innervation. Thus the synovial membrane and the articular cartilage are insensitive to pain.

Central Nervous System Components that Interact with the Musculoskeletal System

The functional divisions of the nervous system include the somatosensory, motor control, autonomic, visual, auditory, vestibular, reticular, limbic, and higher cortical systems. There are a number of functional divisions of the CNS that interact with the musculoskeletal system. Systems that are key to sensory perception, responses to pain, and motor control are summarized in Table 4.6.

Table 4.6 Main Functional Divisions of the CNS that Interact with the Musculoskeletal System

System	Description	Subdivisions and basic functions
Somatosensory system	Sensory stimulation from the musculoskeletal system of the head, neck, body wall, and extremities is received and processed by the somatosensory system. This system also provides feedback that influences the motor, attention, and other systems of the CNS.	• **Peripheral sensory receptors and nerve terminals** • **Reflex circuits** in spinal cord • Dorsal-column medial lemniscal pathway: carries fine touch, joint sensation, 2-point discrimination, and vibratory input for conscious detection. • **Anterolateral System** (Ascending pain pathways): carries signals concerning nociception (pain, crude touch) and skin temperature for conscious and unconscious perception. • **Spinocerebellar pathways**: carries sensory input to the cerebellum for unconscious processing (for balance and fine coordination purposes)
Motor system in control of movement	A complex and hierarchical neuromuscular system consisting of a number of brain regions involved in the control of movement that is superimposed on motor neurons and reflex circuits in the spinal cord gray matter. Spinal cord neurons and circuitry implement the contraction of muscles and movement.	• Corticospinal and corticobulbar tracts: responsible for voluntary motor activity. • Basal Ganglia: control of voluntary motor movement, procedural learning, cognition. • Cerebellum: involuntary control of coordination and timing of movement, balance, equilibrium, and muscle tone. • Spinal cord: contains **motor neurons and reflex circuits** that are directly linked with the musculoskeletal system.
Reticular system	Interconnected circuits of neurons in the tegmentum of the brain stem, lateral hypothalamus, and thalamus.	• **Pain modulation, both excitatory and inhibitory** • Arousal and level of consciousness • Sleep
Limbic system	Involved in memory and memory processing, feeding behaviors, olfaction, "fight-or-flight" responses, aggression, expression of emotions, autonomic nervous system control, various aspects of sexual responses, and pain modulation (enhancement, persistence, or dampening).	• Hippocampal formation: memory and memory processing. • **Limbic lobe (mesocortex): involved in pain modulation**, feeding, olfactory, emotional, sexual responses • Neocortex. involved in pain processing and modulation

Subdivisions to be discussed in this chapter are bolded.

Spinal Sensory-Motor Reflex Circuits

First, we have to define regions of the spinal cord that are dedicated to sensory and motor functions. The spinal cord is divided into gray matter, which is the location of unmyelinated neuronal cell bodies, and white matter, which is the location of myelinated axons that are part of ascending and descending pathways (Figure 4.10). The gray matter is further divided into ventral and dorsal horns. The ventral horns of the spinal cord contain neuronal cell bodies that receive descending

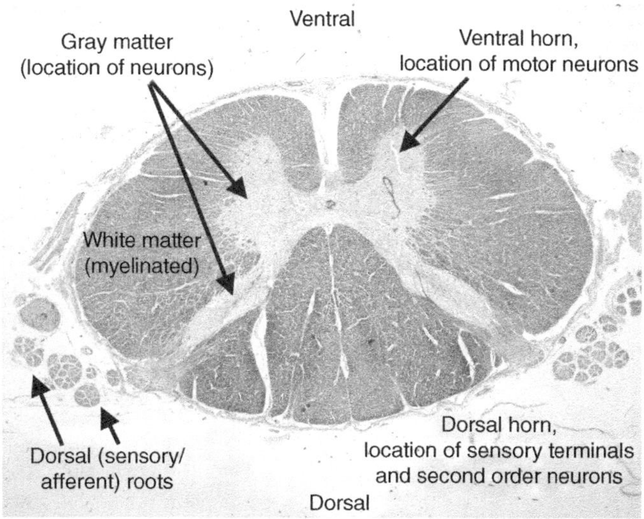

Figure 4.10 A spinal cord cut cross-sectionally. Figure generated by Barbe.

motor information from the motor cortex, and that then send efferent axons out into the periphery to innervate muscles (also known as motor efferent neurons). In contrast, the dorsal horns of the spinal cord contain neuronal cell bodies that receive incoming information from peripheral sensory axons, and that then send axons to the brainstem and brain for the processing of this sensory information (also known as the location of sensory terminals from the periphery and the location of secondary order neurons that project to the brain, Table 4.6; Figure 4.11).

The incoming sensory and outgoing motor neurons are part of simple reflex circuits of sensory and motor neurons (Figure 4.1) that provide rapid, stereotypical reactions to help maintain end-organ homeostasis. These are involuntary reflex circuits that are stimulated in response to sensory input into a structure that results in stereotyped motor output. The basics of a reflex circuit include: (a) a sensory neuron is activated by a sensory receptor in the end organ; (b) the sensory axons carry an afferent signal from the end organ or skin into the spinal cord where it synapses on a multipolar motor neuron; and (c) the motor neuron's axon then carries an efferent motor signal to skeletal muscle to initiate a contraction.

There are several simple reflex circuits in the spinal cord, including the myotatic reflex, Golgi tendon organ reflex, and nociceptive-specific reflexes. The myotatic reflex is an involuntary, ipsilateral muscle stretch reflex, occurring due to proprioceptive input. This reflex is stimulated by a brisk tap to the muscle's tendon. Tapping the tendon delivers a quick stretch to the whole muscle and the muscle spindles embedded in parallel to the extrafusal muscle fibers. The primary afferent endings of the muscle spindle receptor are stimulated by the quick stretch. These Ia afferents then depolarized and that signal is transmitted by axonal action potentials to the spinal cord, before directly synapsing on alpha motor neurons located in the ventral horn of the spinal cord. The alpha motor neurons depolarize, action potentials are propagated back to neuromuscular junctures located in the same muscle, acetylcholine is released that binds to the muscle receptors, and the muscle fibers contract. Thus, this is a monosynaptic reflex (sensory afferents synapse on motor effects to create muscle contraction). Other names for this simple myotatic reflex are the phasic stretch reflex and muscle stretch reflex.

Golgi tendon organ reflexes are another type of proprioceptive reflex. Tendon tension is registered by the Golgi tendon organs. This stretch information is propagated to the spinal cord by type 1B afferents that then innervated interneurons that inhibit (rather than excite) the alpha motor

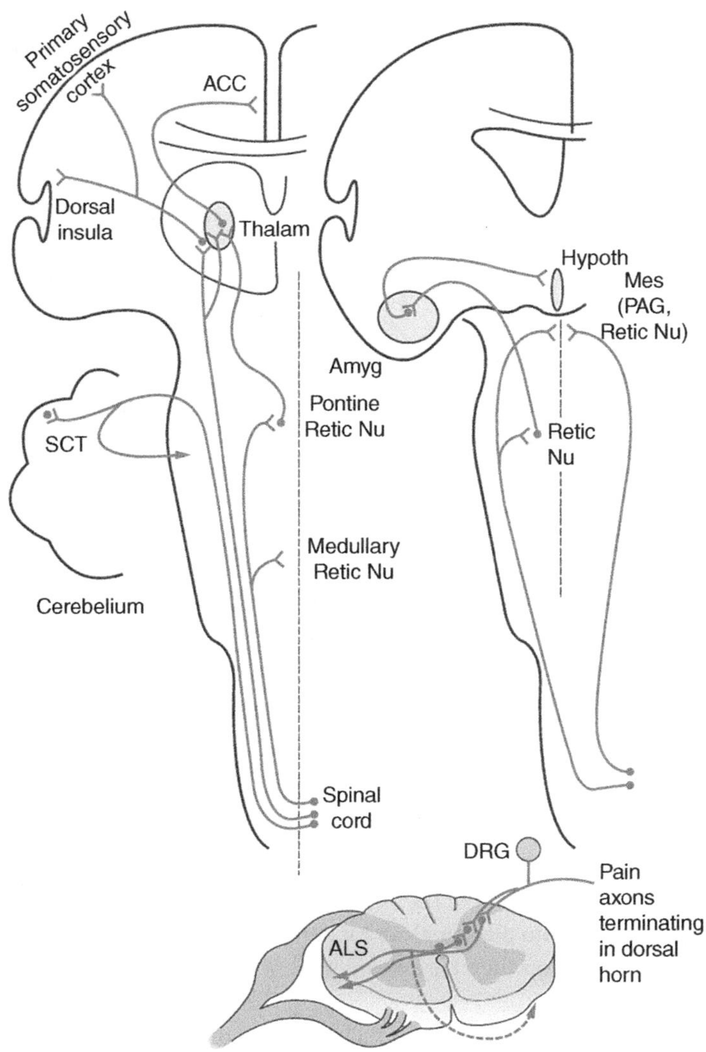

Figure 4.11 Diagram of the spinocerebellar tract and anterolateral system (ALS), a system of ascending pathways and structures involved in processing pain. Dorsal horn projection neurons receiving input from nociceptors project to the cerebellum via the spinocerebellar tract (SCT) as well as through a variety of subcortical and cortical nuclei and centers involved in the transmission of pain. These include several limbic cortices, including the amygdala (Amyg), anterior cingulate cortex (ACC), and dorsal insular cortex (Dorsal Insula). They also project to several brainstem reticular nuclei (Retic Nu), the hypothalamus (Hypoth), paraaqueductal gray (PAG), and the thalamus (Thalam). Relay thalamic nuclei project to the primary somatosensory cortex area. Other abbreviations include dorsal root ganglion (DRG). Modified from Rubertone, J. A., & Barbe, M. F. (2005). Wound healing and pain. In S. L. Michlovitz & T. P. Nolan (Eds.), *Modalities for therapeutic intervention* (4th ed., pp 15–40). PA: F. A. Davis.

neuron of the same muscle, resulting in an autogenic inhibition of the muscle so that the tension ceases. Synergistic muscles may also be inhibited. The role of this reflex is to adjust muscle activity, in concert with muscle spindle and descending supraspinal motor control input, with the purpose of preventing muscles from exerting enough force to prevent muscles from exerting enough force to tear the tendon. Unfortunately, this protective mechanism can fail if force buildup is very rapid, which may lead to tendon rupture.

Nociceptive-specific neurons that are located in the ventral horns of the spinal cord, also known as the motor horns, are primarily involved in reflexive motor responses to pain (e.g., withdrawal reflexes to pain). The same simple reflexes are stimulated as described above.

Ascending Pathways of Pain Transmission

Pain impulses are carried from the spinal cord to the brain in pathways located together in the anterolateral region of the spinal cord, thereby explaining the name of the pathway—the anterolateral system (Table 4.6; Figure 4.11). This system is a composite bundle of pathways that begin in the spinal cord and that terminate in the thalamus, a variety of brain stem regions (e.g., nuclei of the reticular formation and mesencephalon, also known as the midbrain), or thalamus-limbic regions (e.g., the hypothalamus). Specific subcomponents are named for their origin and termination and include the spinothalamic, spinoreticular, spinomesencephalic, and spinohypothalamic-limbic pathways (Boadas-Vaello et al., 2016; Bourne, Machado, & Nagel, 2014).

The spinothalamic tract is the primary ascending pain pathway and is the most studied of the known pain pathways (Bourne et al., 2014). The subcomponent of the anterolateral system carries not only pain and temperature sensibilities to the brain, but also crude tactile and pressure modalities from mechanoreceptors with large receptive fields (which means that there is lower specificity as to the peripheral location of these stimuli, once processed by the brain). There are three sets of neurons in this multi-synaptic pathway. First, axons of peripheral nociceptors (thought of as primary sensory neurons) synapse on nociceptive-specific neurons located in the dorsal horns of the spinal cord. These spinal cord sensory neurons are second-order sensory neurons. Most of their axons decussate (cross from one side to the other) in the spinal cord before ascending contralaterally (i.e., on the opposite side of the spinal cord) in the anterolateral region of the spinal cord's white matter. Their axons synapse on relay nuclei in the thalamus that project directly to the primary somatosensory cortex responsible for the perception of the precise type, location, and perception of noxious and non-noxious impulses. For example, this pathway, namely the spinothalamic pathway, provides information on pain quality (e.g., burning, sharp, dull).

The spinoreticular tract consists of the second-order nociceptor neurons that project to reticular formation nuclei scattered throughout the brainstem. A number of these reticular nuclei then send axonal projections directly or indirectly to limbic cortices that contribute to the emotional (affective) components of pain (e.g., increased stress). Spinomesencephalic axons project to the periaqueductal gray in the midbrain. Nuclei in the periaqueductal gray (as well as reticular formation nuclei) are involved in the modulation of pain, including enhancement, and other non-discriminative affective components of pain (Garland, 2012). Spinohypothalamic axons project from the spinal cord to the hypothalamus, the center of supraspinal autonomic control. These projections affect neuroendocrine and cardiovascular outputs in response to pain (e.g., nausea and increased heart rate, respectively) (Bourne et al., 2014). Although the spinocerebellar pathway depicted in Figure 4.11 is not an actual component of the anterolateral system, the cerebellar projections of these dorsal horn neurons aid in proprioception and the postural adjustments needed during reflexive responses to painful stimuli. Thus, the polysynaptic nature of the ascending circuitry from nociceptor neurons in the spinal cord allows for not only specific pain perception and location but also the emotional context of pain, enhancement of pain signals, neuroendocrine and cardiovascular outputs in response to pain.

Descending Modulatory Pathways of Pain Transmission

Descending axons from the periaqueductal gray nuclei and other reticular nuclei in the midbrain and medulla contribute to pain modulation. Their axons terminate in the dorsal horns of the spinal cord and release inhibitory neurotransmitters, such as serotonin and encephalin. This release of inhibitory neurotransmitters leads to an inhibition of the firing of primary sensory fibers or second-order projection neurons that are conveying nociceptive (pain) information. Thus, these descending pain pathways are primarily inhibitory in nature (Lau & Vaughan, 2014).

Pain

Pain is defined as the unpleasant sensory and emotional experience associated with, or resembling that associated with, actual or potential tissue damage (Pain, 2018). It is a personal experience that is influenced by a person's learned concepts and expectations of pain. It is also affected by biological, psychological, and social factors, as one can postulate from the complicated nature of the just described ascending and descending pain pathways.

Types of Pain

There are many types of pain, as shown in Table 4.7. This table shows many of the terms used to describe pain by clinicians, and clinical and basic science researchers. For example, acute pain is typically defined as pain of rapid or sudden onset. It is described as being sharp and localized and serves to warn the organism of impending tissue damage. This type of pain has also been termed nociceptor pain since nociception is the physiological sensory process of encoding and signaling of noxious stimuli to the central nervous system after activation of nociceptor endings (Woller, Eddinger, Corr, & Yaksh, 2017).

However, alterations in peripheral or central pain pathways elicited by inflammation, tissue or nerve damage, and more, can alter one's perception of stimuli. Various types of altered pain perceptions to stimuli include allodynia (a painful response to a normally nonpainful stimulus, such as light touch) and hyperalgesia (a heightened painful response to a noxious stimulus). Pain occurring as a result of inflammatory responses (e.g., inflammatory cytokine release from injured tissues or tissues affected by inflammatory disorders and diseases) can induce hypersensitivity to both painful and nonpainful stimuli. Such inflammatory pain may improve as the inflammation resolves (Jain et al., 2014; Taneja, Della Pasqua, & Danhof, 2017; Xin et al., 2017), although a chronic inflammatory condition can become associated with perpetuated pain symptoms even with remission of inflammatory signs due to negative neuroplastic changes in the dorsal root ganglia, spinal cord, and brain (Woller et al., 2017). Such hypersensitivity as a consequence of peripheral or central nervous system changes is discussed further below in the peripheral and central sensitization sections. There are also several types of stimulus-independent pain, such as spontaneous pain (the presence of pain symptoms despite a lack of stimuli).

Pain symptoms are considered persistent or chronic when they persist despite no obvious sign of nonneural tissue injury. Persistent or chronic pain after tissue or nerve injury, chemotherapy, or in association with metabolic disorders (such as diabetes and viral infections), cancer, or arthritis can be the result of chronic neuroinflammation, dysfunction, or pathological changes in nociceptor signaling or other aspects of the maladaptive neuroplasticity in the peripheral or central nervous

Table 4.7 Pain Terminology (Pain, 2018)

Pain term	Description
Acute pain	• Pain of rapid or sudden onset; described as sharp and localized.
Allodynia/ hypersensitivity	• Pain due to a stimulus that does not normally provoke pain, e.g., light touch, stroking of the skin, light pressure or pinch, movement of a joint, moderate cold or warmth. A lowered threshold.
Causalgia	• A syndrome of sustained burning pain, allodynia, and hyperpathia after a traumatic nerve lesion, often combined with vasomotor and sudomotor dysfunction and later trophic changes.
Central sensitization	• Increased responsiveness of nociceptive neurons in the CNS to their normal or subthreshold afferent input.
Dysesthesia	• An unpleasant abnormal sensation, whether spontaneous or evoked (as compared to paresthesias, which should not be unpleasant although the sensation could be borderline).
Hyperalgesia	• Heightened pain from a stimulus that normally provokes pain (reflects pain on a suprathreshold stimulation).
Hyperesthesia	• Increased sensitivity to stimulation, excluding the special senses. May refer to various modes of cutaneous sensitivity including touch and thermal sensation without pain, as well as to pain.
Hyperpathia	• A painful syndrome characterized by an abnormally painful reaction to a stimulus, especially a repetitive stimulus and an increased threshold. A raised threshold and increased response.
Inflammatory pain	• Pain occurring from inflammation, e.g., inflammatory cytokine and mediator release from injured tissues.
Neuralgia	• Pain in the distribution of a nerve or nerves.
Neuritis	• Inflammation in a nerve or nerves; a term used when nerve inflammation is thought to be present.
Neuropathic pain	• Pain caused by a lesion or disease of the somatosensory nervous system (peripheral or central). A clinical description that requires a demonstrable lesion or diagnosed disease.
Neuropathy	• Disturbance of function or pathology in a nerve (mono-neuropathy, mononeuropathy multiplex, or polyneuropathy).
Nociception	• The neural process of encoding noxious stimuli. Can be autonomic (e.g., elevated blood pressure) or behavioral (motor withdrawal reflex or a nocifensive behavior).
Nociceptive neuron	• A central or peripheral neuron of the somatosensory nervous system that is capable of encoding noxious stimuli.
Nociceptive pain	• Pain that arising from actual or threatened damage to non-neural tissue and due to activation of nociceptors (in contrast with neuropathic pain).
Peripheral sensitization	• Increased responses to painful or a normally subthreshold stimulus by primary afferents in the periphery.
Persistent or chronic pain	• Pain of long duration with a slower, gradual onset; described as dull, diffuse, and poorly localized
Recurrent pain	• Recurring or episodic; pain that accompanies a re-injury; may be a painful episode associated with a disease process, e.g., rheumatoid arthritis
Spontaneous pain	• The presence of pain symptoms despite a lack of stimuli.

systems. For example, neuropathic pain is a form of persistent pain that has been re-defined by the International Association for the Study of Pain (IASP) as pain caused by a lesion or disease of the peripheral or central somatosensory nervous system (Kosek et al., 2016). Whatever the term used, most agree that persistent and neuropathic pain conditions are linked to physiological attributes other than the normal neuronal transmission of sensory inputs.

Neuroplasticity and Pain

The term *neuroplasticity,* a phenomenon that occurs in both the peripheral and central nervous systems, is broadly defined as the altered functioning of the nervous system in response to different environmental conditions. Maladaptive plasticity underlies the pathophysiologic states involved in chronic pain conditions. When nociceptive pathways are suddenly activated by stimuli that are normally not painful (allodynia), when symptoms of pain are heightened or exaggerated in response to the inducing stimulus (hyperalgesia), or when pain symptoms are present in the absence of any stimulus (spontaneous pain), sensitization has occurred.

Peripheral sensitization

Peripheral sensitization is defined as altered nociceptor function with a reduced threshold of activation and enhanced responsiveness (Spiegel et al., 2017). This results from both direct and indirect mechanisms, such as (a) increased numbers of immune cells that secrete proinflammatory cytokines; (b) an increase in mediators in an extracellular "inflammatory soup" that maintains enhanced activation of the afferent terminals; (c) alterations or dysregulation of the expression of ion channels in the peripheral afferent terminals; (d) increased spontaneous or ectopic activity in the neuron; and (e) even alterations in surrounding cells that maintain the enhanced activity (Gold & Gebhart, 2010; Latremoliere & Woolf, 2009; Spiegel et al., 2017; St John Smith, 2017; Voscopoulos & Lema, 2010; Woller et al., 2017; Yan et al., 2017).

With regard to the "inflammatory soup," a variety of chemical mediators are released from injured cells and infiltrating immune cells into the extracellular matrix/fluid in the local injured site that then sensitize the peripheral end terminals of the nociceptors. Proinflammatory cytokines and neuropeptides released from activated pain terminals and sometimes macrophages (e.g., CGRP and substance P, nerve growth factor, norepinephrine, capsaicin, histamine, serotonin, and prostaglandin E_2) are among the chemical mediators that can lower the threshold of nociceptors (Gold & Gebhart, 2010; Voscopoulos & Lema, 2010; Yan et al., 2017). Other mediators including proteases, additional growth factors, chemokines, and damage-associated molecular patterns (DAMPs) continue to be identified (Kiguchi, Kobayashi, Saika, Matsuzaki, & Kishioka, 2017; Lacagnina, Watkins, & Grace, 2017; Yan et al., 2017). These latter mediators have a variety of cellular origins. Cellular sources of inflammatory cytokines include damaged tissue cells, damaged axons and cells within the nerve (Schwann cells, intraneural fibroblasts, satellite glial cells), and infiltrating immune cells (mast cells, neutrophils, lymphocytes, and macrophages) (Al-Shatti, Barr, Safadi, Amin, & Barbe, 2005; Kiguchi et al., 2017). Sensory afferent terminals express receptors for nearly every component of the inflammatory soup so that such exposure decreases the stimulation threshold, which increases their responsiveness (Woller et al., 2017; Yan et al., 2017). Under conditions of inflammation and peripheral sensitization, even non-nociceptive mechanoreceptors may elicit enhanced responses to pressure and movement, and high-threshold nociceptors respond to less intense stimuli, all of which increase pain sensations to various types of stimuli.

Such maladaptive neuroplasticity may be the common mechanism of pain associated with inflammatory diagnoses (i.e., diagnoses that end in "itis") (Woller et al., 2017). There are studies showing increased levels of tumor necrosis factor-alpha at the mid-axonal level and tissue inflammation around an axon increased firing activity of a nociceptor axon (termed ectopic discharge). For example, as a result of peripheral sensitization, presynaptic changes of the afferent neurons increase the release of neurotransmitters from their central terminals within the spinal cord dorsal horns. According to several investigators, this afferent barrage of excitatory transmitters into the dorsal horn is the presynaptic component of central sensitization.

Central sensitization

The phenomenon of central sensitization is defined as adaptations within the CNS to external or internal stimuli that are characterized by (a) abnormal pain responses such as hyperalgesia or allodynia; (b) diverse biochemical and cellular adjustments including altered neurotransmitter, receptor, or ion channel expression; and/or (c) changes in the structure and functional properties of neurons (Woolf, 2011). Changes in the synaptic network involving the nociceptor neurons are signs of persistent CNS changes that lead to sensitization (Woolf, 2010). Two distinct forms of central sensitization have been described: activity-dependent and transcription-dependent (Latremoliere & Woolf, 2009; Woolf, 2011). The activity-dependent form is a rapid central response induced by afferent nociceptor input that produces short-lasting synaptic changes, in turn enhancing synaptic transmission in the spinal cord (Latremoliere & Woolf, 2009; Woolf, 2007). Such changes may be an immediate response to activity-induced excitatory facilitation and diminished inhibition (Kuner, 2010). The transcription-dependent form refers to a slow induction of central changes in synaptic transmission distinguished by prolonged effects in which neuroplasticity may outlast the initial input or require low-threshold peripheral drive (Kuner, 2010; Latremoliere & Woolf, 2009).

Other proposed mechanisms of central sensitization and persistent pain are changes in calcium permeability, receptor overexpression, and synapse location (Lacagnina et al., 2017; Meacham, Shepherd, Mohapatra, & Haroutounian, 2017) as well as disrupted circuitry and neurotransmitter imbalances in the ascending and descending modulatory pain pathways (Meacham et al., 2017). Cortical and subcortical maladaptive plasticity has also been proposed to underlie central sensitization (Meacham et al., 2017). Altered synaptic spine density, or axonal degeneration or regeneration and aberrant connectivity, along with changes in glial function affect nociceptive molecular signaling, and in turn contribute to the persistence of pain (Kuner, 2010).

Summary

Details of this chapter are summarized in Table 4.8. In each tissue, there exist sensory receptors that translate a tissue's state into neural signals. This information is carried back along afferent fibers to the central nervous system. Key to this point and important to subsequent chapters, is that the sensation of pain is a critical learning tool by which sentient beings, such as humans, learn to avoid tissue damage and injury. For example, muscle spindle and Golgi tendon sensory receptors aid in the avoidance of tissue damage by signaling the amount of tissue tension and stretch. Their simple neural sensory-in and motor-out spinal cord circuits then signal muscle relaxation as needed to avoid tissue damage. Sensory free nerve endings also signal pending tissue damage and stimulate avoidance strategies (both perceived and reflexive).

Table 4.8 Summary

- The CNS comprises the brain and spinal cord, while the PNS comprises neural structures outside of the dura mater.
- Neurons are specialized cells that are able to conduct signals to and from tissues and other neurons.
- Glial cells are supportive cells to neurons. They provide myelination, metabolic support, and maintain homeostasis of a neuron's extracellular fluid.
- Some glial cells can also become phagocytic to clean up neural tissue damage.
- Most musculoskeletal tissues are innervated by nerves, including muscles, tendons, bone, ligament, and other joint structures. Only muscles receive motor innervation.
- There are many types of pain as well as many types of potential responses (perception of type and location, emotional responses, neuroendocrine responses, and cardiovascular responses, to name a few).

Bibliography

Al-Shatti, T., Barr, A. E., Safadi, F. F., Amin, M., & Barbe, M. F. (2005). Increase in inflammatory cytokines in median nerves in a rat model of repetitive motion injury. *Journal of Neuroimmunology, 167*(1–2), 13–22. https://doi.org/10.1016/j.jneuroim.2005.06.013

Blumer, R., Lukas, J. R., Wasicky, R., & Mayr, R. (2000). Presence and morphological variability of Golgi tendon organs in the distal portion of sheep extraocular muscle. *The Anatomical Record, 258*, 359–368. Wiley

Boadas-Vaello, P., Castany, S., Homs, J., Alvarez-Perez, B., Deulofeu, M., & Verdu, E. (2016). Neuroplasticity of ascending and descending pathways after somatosensory system injury: Reviewing knowledge to identify neuropathic pain therapeutic targets. *Spinal Cord, 54*(5), 330–340. https://doi.org/10.1038/sc.2015.225

Bourne, S., Machado, A. G., & Nagel, S. J. (2014). Basic anatomy and physiology of pain pathways. *Neurosurgery Clinics of North America, 25*(4), 629–638. https://doi.org/10.1016/j.nec.2014.06.001

Chapman, K. B., Yousef, T. A., Foster, A., Stanton-Hicks, M. D., & van Helmond, N. (2020). Mechanisms for the clinical utility of low-frequency stimulation in neuromodulation of the dorsal root ganglion. *Neuromodulation., 24*(4), 738–745. https://doi.org/10.1111/ner.13323. Wiley

Clark, B. D., Al-Shatti, T. A., Barr, A. E., Amin, M., & Barbe, M. F. (2004). Performance of a high-repetition, high-force task induces carpal tunnel syndrome in rats. *Journal of Orthopaedic & Sports Physical Therapy, 34*(5), 244–253. https://doi.org/10.2519/jospt.2004.34.5.244

Clark, B. D., Barr, A. E., Safadi, F. F., Beitman, L., Al-Shatti, T., Amin, M., . . . Barbe, M. F. (2003). Median nerve trauma in a rat model of work-related musculoskeletal disorder. *Journal of Neurotrauma, 20*(7), 681–695. https://doi.org/10.1089/089771503322144590

Garland, E. L. (2012). Pain processing in the human nervous system: A selective review of nociceptive and biobehavioral pathways. *Primary Care, 39*(3), 561–571. https://doi.org/10.1016/j.pop.2012.06.013

Gold, M. S., & Gebhart, G. F. (2010). Nociceptor sensitization in pain pathogenesis. *Nature Medicine, 16*(11), 1248–1257. https://doi.org/10.1038/nm.2235

Gregory, N. S., Gautam, M., Benson, C. J., & Sluka, K. A. (2018). Acid sensing ion channel 1a (ASIC1a) mediates activity-induced pain by modulation of heteromeric ASIC channel kinetics. *Neuroscience, 386*, 166–174. https://doi.org/10.1016/j.neuroscience.2018.06.033

Jain, N. X., Barr-Gillespie, A. E., Clark, B. D., Kietrys, D. M., Wade, C. K., Litvin, J., . . . Barbe, M. F. (2014). Bone loss from high repetitive high force loading is prevented by ibuprofen treatment. *Journal of Musculoskeletal and Neuronal Interactions, 14*(1), 78–94. Retrieved from https://www.ncbi.nlm.nih.gov/pubmed/24583543

Kiguchi, N., Kobayashi, D., Saika, F., Matsuzaki, S., & Kishioka, S. (2017). Pharmacological regulation of neuropathic pain driven by inflammatory macrophages. *International Journal of Molecular Sciences, 18*(11). https://doi.org/10.3390/ijms18112296

Kosek, E., Cohen, M., Baron, R., Gebhart, G. F., Mico, J. A., Rice, A. S., . . . Sluka, A. K. (2016). Do we need a third mechanistic descriptor for chronic pain states? *Pain, 157*(7), 1382–1386. https://doi.org/10.1097/j.pain.0000000000000507

Kuner, R. (2010). Central mechanisms of pathological pain. *Nature Medicine, 16*(11), 1258–1266. https://doi.org/10.1038/nm.2231

Lacagnina, M. J., Watkins, L. R., & Grace, P. M. (2017). Toll-like receptors and their role in persistent pain. *Pharmacology & Therapeutics, 184*, 145–158. https://doi.org/10.1016/j.pharmthera.2017.10.006

Latremoliere, A., & Woolf, C. J. (2009). Central sensitization: A generator of pain hypersensitivity by central neural plasticity. *The Journal of Pain, 10*(9), 895–926. https://doi.org/10.1016/j.jpain.2009.06.012

Lau, B. K., & Vaughan, C. W. (2014). Descending modulation of pain: The GABA disinhibition hypothesis of analgesia. *Current Opinion in Neurobiology, 29*, 159–164. https://doi.org/10.1016/j.conb.2014.07.010

Lazaro, R. P. (2017). Complex regional pain syndrome: Medical and legal ramifications of clinical variability and experience and perspective of a practicing clinician. *Journal of Pain Research, 10*, 9–14. https://doi.org/10.2147/JPR.S119308

Leichnetz, G. R. (2006). *Digital neuroanatomy. Figure 1.10b*. Wiley. ISBN: 0-470-04000-9

Meacham, K., Shepherd, A., Mohapatra, D. P., & Haroutounian, S. (2017). Neuropathic pain: Central vs peripheral mechanisms. *Current Pain and Headache Reports, 21*(6), 28. https://doi.org/10.1007/s11916-017-0629-5

Mense, S., & Hoheisel, U. (2016). Evidence for the existence of nociceptors in rat thoracolumbar fascia. *Journal of Bodywork and Movement Therapies, 20*(3), 623–628. https://doi.org/10.1016/j.jbmt.2016.01.006

Merriam-Webster. (2021). Merriam-Webster Dictionary. Retrieved from https://www.merriam-webster.com/dictionary/somatic

Molnar, C., & Gair, J. (2015). *Concepts of Biology* [1st Canadian Edition]. BCcampus. Retrieved from https://opentextbc.ca/biology/.

Myers, R. R., Kalichman, M. W., Reisner, L. S., & Powell, H. C. (1986). Neurotoxicity of local anesthetics: Altered perineurial permeability, edema, and nerve fiber injury. *Anesthesiology, 64*(1), 29–35. Retrieved from https://www.ncbi.nlm.nih.gov/pubmed/3942334

Myers, R. R., Murakami, H., & Powell, H. C. (1986). Reduced nerve blood flow in edematous neuropathies: A biomechanical mechanism. *Microvascular Research, 32*(2), 145–151. https://doi.org/10.1016/0026-2862(86)90050-6

IASP. (2018). Terminology. Retrieved from https://www.iasp-pain.org/resources/terminology/

Pakurar, A. S., & Bigbee, J. W. (2004). *Digital histology, an interactive CD atlas. Figure 8.2*. Wiley. ISBN: 0-471-64982-1

Rohrle, O., Yavuz, U. S., Klotz, T., Negro, F., & Heidlauf, T. (2019). Multiscale modeling of the neuromuscular system: Coupling neurophysiology and skeletal muscle mechanics. *Wiley Interdisciplinary Reviews: Systems Biology and Medicine, 11*(6), e1457. https://doi.org/10.1002/wsbm.1457

Rosso, G., & Guck, J. (2019). Mechanical changes of peripheral nerve tissue microenvironment and their structural basis during development. *APL Bioengineering, 3*(3), 036107. https://doi.org/10.1063/1.5108867

Rubertone, J. A., & Barbe, M. F. (2005). Wound healing and pain. In S. L. Michlovitz & T. P. Nolan (Eds.), *Modalities for therapeutic intervention* (4th ed., pp. 15–40). PA: F. A. Davis.

Sluka, K. A., Winter, O. C., & Wemmie, J. A. (2009). Acid-sensing ion channels: A new target for pain and CNS diseases. *Current Opinion in Drug Discovery & Development, 12*(5), 693–704. Retrieved from https://www.ncbi.nlm.nih.gov/pubmed/19736627

Spiegel, D. R., Pattison, A., Lyons, A., Ansari, U., McCroskey, A. L., Luehrs, E., . . . Le, S. (2017). The role and treatment implications of peripheral and central processing of pain, pruritus, and nausea in heightened somatic awareness: A review. *Innovations in Clinical Neuroscience, 14*(5–6), 11–20. Retrieved from https://www.ncbi.nlm.nih.gov/pubmed/28979822

St John Smith, E. (2017). Advances in understanding nociception and neuropathic pain. *Journal of Neurology, 265*, 231–238. https://doi.org/10.1007/s00415-017-8641-6

Stecco, C., Macchi, V., Lancerotto, L., Tiengo, C., Porzionato, A., & De Caro, R. (2010). Comparison of transverse carpal ligament and flexor retinaculum terminology for the wrist. *Journal of Hand Surgery (American volume), 35*(5), 746–753. https://doi.org/10.1016/j.jhsa.2010.01.031

Stecco, C., Porzionato, A., Lancerotto, L., Stecco, A., Macchi, V., Day, J. A., & De Caro, R. (2008). Histological study of the deep fasciae of the limbs. *Journal of Bodywork and Movement Therapies, 12*(3), 225–230. https://doi.org/10.1016/j.jbmt.2008.04.041

Taneja, A., Della Pasqua, O., & Danhof, M. (2017). Challenges in translational drug research in neuropathic and inflammatory pain: The prerequisites for a new paradigm. *European Journal of Clinical Pharmacology, 73*(10), 1219–1236. https://doi.org/10.1007/s00228-017-2301-8

Tortora, G. J., & Derrickson, B. H. (2010). *Introduction to the human body* (11th ed.). Wiley.

Ushiki, T., Hayashi, S., & Ide, C. (1990). The filamentous meshwork in the Schwann cell basement membrane as revealed by transmission and scanning electron microscopy. *Archives of Histology and Cytology, 53*(5), 523–530. https://doi.org/10.1679/aohc.53.523

Ushiki, T., & Ide, C. (1990). Three-dimensional organization of the collagen fibrils in the rat sciatic nerve as revealed by transmission- and scanning electron microscopy. *Cell and Tissue Research, 260*(1), 175–184. https://doi.org/10.1007/BF00297503

Voscopoulos, C., & Lema, M. (2010). When does acute pain become chronic? *British Journal of Anaesthesia, 105*(Suppl 1), i69–i85. https://doi.org/10.1093/bja/aeq323

Woller, S. A., Eddinger, K. A., Corr, M., & Yaksh, T. L. (2017). An overview of pathways encoding nociception. *Clinical and Experimental Rheumatology, 35 Suppl 107*(5), 40–46. Retrieved from https://www.ncbi.nlm.nih.gov/pubmed/28967373

Woolf, C. J. (2007). Central sensitization: Uncovering the relation between pain and plasticity. *Anesthesiology, 106*(4), 864–867. https://doi.org/10.1097/01.anes.0000264769.87038.55

Woolf, C. J. (2010). What is this thing called pain? *Journal of Clinical Investigation, 120*(11), 3742–3744. https://doi.org/10.1172/JCI45178

Woolf, C. J. (2011). Central sensitization: Implications for the diagnosis and treatment of pain. *Pain, 152*(3 Suppl), S2–S15. https://doi.org/10.1016/j.pain.2010.09.030

Xin, D. L., Hadrevi, J., Elliott, M. E., Amin, M., Harris, M. Y., Barr-Gillespie, A. E., & Barbe, M. F. (2017). Effectiveness of conservative interventions for sickness and pain behaviors induced by a high repetition high force upper extremity task. *BMC Neuroscience, 18*(1), 36. https://doi.org/10.1186/s12868-017-0354-3

Yahia, L., Rhalmi, S., Newman, N., & Isler, M. (1992). Sensory innervation of human thoracolumbar fascia. An immunohistochemical study. *Acta Orthopaedica Scandinavica, 63*(2), 195–197. https://doi.org/10.3109/17453679209154822

Yan, Y. Y., Li, C. Y., Zhou, L., Ao, L. Y., Fang, W. R., & Li, Y. M. (2017). Research progress of mechanisms and drug therapy for neuropathic pain. *Life Sciences, 190*, 68–77. https://doi.org/10.1016/j.lfs.2017.09.033

5

Fundamental Biomechanics Concepts

Introduction

Consider a worker whose job is to palletize bags of cement that weigh 225 N (~50 pounds) coming off a conveyor belt. He performs 6 lifts/min (from conveyor to pallet), throughout his entire 8-hr work shift, 5 days a week. Or consider a starting major league baseball pitcher who is called upon to throw dozens of 150 km/hr fastballs as part of his job every few days. It would seem obvious that the performance of these tasks would result in repetitive stress to specific regions of the musculoskeletal system and would increase the risk of injury on individual joints bearing the brunt of these activities. In fact, we know workers who perform manual materials handling tasks experience significant stress (particularly in the low back region) and are at increased risk of low back disorders (e.g., NIOSH, 1997). We also know that major league pitchers have a much higher than average prevalence of shoulder and elbow injuries, with shoulder injuries accounting for 31% of injuries and elbow injuries accounting for another 26% of major league pitcher injuries (Posner, Cameron, Wolf, Belmont, & Owens, 2011). The same trends hold true for pitchers at the high-school and minor league ranks (Lesniak et al., 2013; Lin, Wong, & Kazam, 2018). But what is the mechanism through which repetitively applied stresses results in damage to musculoskeletal tissues? And how should we go about ascertaining the risk of musculoskeletal injury for these individuals?

An important first step in assessing the risk of stressful tasks is to use the science of *biomechanics* to calculate the loads imposed on susceptible joints. Biomechanics has been defined as "The study of mechanical laws relating to the movement or structure of living organisms" (Concise Oxford English Dictionary, 2011). Biomechanics is an interdisciplinary science, drawing from fields such as engineering, physiology, and materials science to better understand the mechanical processes present in dynamic biological systems. As the name implies, a major emphasis in biomechanics is the application of classical (Newtonian) mechanics to understand the reaction of various bodily structures to the application of physical loads. The goal is to enhance our knowledge of the loads placed on biological materials, and the reactions of these materials to such loads.

Note that the examples in the preceding introduction involve activities that are repetitive in nature. A major focus of this book is to understand how repetitive loading of the musculoskeletal system leads to the development of tissue damage as the result of a fatigue failure process. However, before we can address this issue in detail, certain fundamental mechanical and biomechanical principles need to be understood. The purpose of this chapter is to cover the fundamentals of biomechanics that are important to the understanding of how musculoskeletal tissues are stressed, and their reactions to this stress. A comprehensive treatment of biomechanical methods is beyond the scope of the current book, and other sources can be sought to provide additional detail should the reader so desire (e.g., Chaffin, Andersson, & Martin, 2006; Nordin and Frankel, 2012; Özkaya, Leger, Goldsheyder, & Nordin, 2017). However, it is important to understand certain fundamental concepts to understand the mechanisms leading to damage of musculoskeletal tissues.

In this chapter, we will introduce basic biomechanical modeling concepts along with examples of how these principles can be applied to evaluate the effects of external loads placed on the system, and musculoskeletal tissue responses to these loads. The idea is to gain an understanding of how the loads that our musculoskeletal system experiences every day can lead to the development of musculoskeletal disorders. An understanding of the biomechanical loading experienced by the body is an important first step in this process.

The interest in examining the human body as a mechanical system has a long history and includes the work of such luminaries as Aristotle (384–322 B.C.), Leonardo da Vinci (1452–1519), Galileo Galilei (1564–1642), Giovanni Alfonso Borelli (1608–1679) and Sir Isaac Newton (1642–1726) (Kroemer, 1988). Aristotle, for example, wrote a book entitled "De Motu Animalium" (On the Movement of Animals), which described animal bodies as mechanical systems, including descriptions of how muscles worked. Aristotle also subjected muscles to geometric analysis for the first time. Leonardo da Vinci (1452–1519), often credited as the originator of biomechanics, performed in-depth anatomical studies of cadavers using mechanical principles, and studied the actions of the muscles by tracing their lines of action (between muscle origins and insertions) and also investigated joint function. Galileo analyzed the function and strength of bone, while Borelli estimated the position of the human center of mass (Innocenti, 2018).

While all of these contributions have been essential to the development of biomechanics, clearly the most important of these (and one of the truly monumental achievements in the history of science) was the discovery of three basic laws that govern the application of forces and the resultant motion of objects by Sir Isaac Newton (1643–1727). These laws, compiled in the *Principia Mathematica* (Newton, 1687), provide the basis for assessing loads experienced by materials (including musculoskeletal tissues). Basic knowledge of these laws is important for understanding the process by which musculoskeletal tissues incur injury. We will begin by examining these laws and understanding their importance.

Newton's Laws

Newton's First Law

Newton's first law states that an object at rest will stay at rest, or an object in motion will remain in motion (in a straight line and having constant velocity), as long as the net forces exerted on this object are zero. The first law is represented by the following equation:

$$\Sigma F = 0 \tag{5.1}$$

This equation sets the condition for the states in which there is either *no motion* or *no change in motion* of an object. The preceding equation assumes the presence of an *inertial reference system*, that is, a frame of reference in which a body (with zero net force acting upon it) is experiencing a total absence of acceleration. Establishing the "no change in motion" state implies directly that if there *is* a change of motion of an object, acceleration must be present.

Newton's Second Law

Newton's second law defines force as a function of the mass of an object interacting with the acceleration experienced by that object. For linear motion, this relationship is given by

$$F = ma \tag{5.2}$$

where F signifies the applied force, m represents the mass of the object, and a is the linear acceleration of the object to which force has been applied. Mass is assumed to be constant in this formulation. If multiple forces are brought to bear on the object, then F can be represented as the vector sum of the forces applied. If the object has no acceleration, the object state reverts to the first law.

When an angular acceleration is experienced by an object, Newton's second law is described by the following equation:

$$M = I\alpha \tag{5.3}$$

where M represents the resultant moment of force acting on the object, I represents the mass moment of inertia of the object, and α is the angular acceleration experienced by the object.

In these formulations of the second law, as the material properties m or I increase in magnitude, they will exhibit increased resistance to changes in motion (Özkaya et al., 2017). The second law makes clear that if an object is experiencing a change in motion, that object must be experiencing an application of force.

Newton's Third Law

Newton's third law states that every time a force is imposed on an object, that object must exert a force equal in magnitude and opposite in direction to the imposed force. That is, when an object has a force imposed on it, the following relationship will apply:

$$F_{A\rightarrow B} = -F_{B\rightarrow A} \tag{5.4}$$

This law reveals that force application is never a one-sided affair. Forces applied to an object must instead be thought of as a force *interaction* between the objects, and once an object exerts a force on another object, the reaction force will instantaneously mirror the forces placed upon it (Figure 5.1). Neither force can exist without the presence of its pair. Thus, if your hand presses down on the top of a table, the table will instantaneously generate an equal and opposite force pressing up on your hand.

A key aspect of these third law "partner" forces is that they *must* act on different objects. Since both are forces, each will be equivalent to their own particular mass times their respective acceleration. This means that even though the forces acting on the two objects are equal, if the objects have different masses, the accelerations experienced by the two objects will be proportionally different.

In order to utilize Newton's laws for biomechanical analyses, we need to introduce certain concepts used in evaluating forces and their effects on objects. These quantities include *scalars, vectors,* and *moments.*

Scalars

A scalar quantity is one that is completely specified by its magnitude. Such quantities require only a number and the appropriate units of measurement for complete specification. Examples of scalars relevant to biomechanical analyses may include such quantities as mass, length, time, density, volume, and energy.

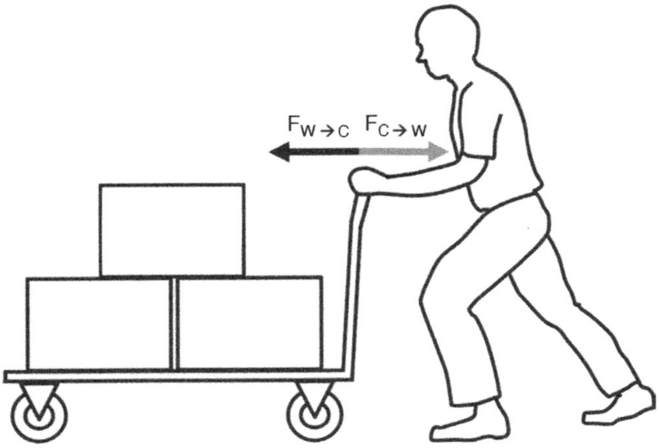

Figure 5.1 An example of Newton's third law of motion. The worker pushes on the cart with a given force ($F_{W\rightarrow C}$). The cart will simultaneously exert a force precisely mirroring the force exerted on it by the worker ($F_{C\rightarrow W}$). This reaction force will always be equal in magnitude and opposite in direction. The two forces must always be equal, but the accelerations experienced by the objects will differ in proportion to their respective masses.

Vectors

A vector is a quantity that contains two pieces of information: a magnitude and a direction. Forces are represented by vectors as they contain both a magnitude (i.e., the amount of the force applied), and a direction in which that force is applied. Vectors are typically represented by a one-headed arrow. For example, in the case of a figure (such as a free-body diagram) demonstrating a force being applied to an object, the base of the arrow will be affixed to point of the force application, and the arrow will indicate the direction in which the force is being applied. The length of the arrow is scaled to represent the magnitude of the forces, with shorter arrows representing smaller force magnitudes and longer arrows representing larger forces. Figure 5.2 provides an example of a force vector, wherein a 5.1 kg box lying on a surface is being acted upon by the gravitational force of the Earth (9.8 m/s^2), resulting in a 50 N downward force.

Moments

In physics, a *moment* represents the tendency of an object to rotate in a certain direction, which is a function of two variables: the magnitude of the applied force and the perpendicular distance between the applied force line of action and the axis of rotation of the object. An example is

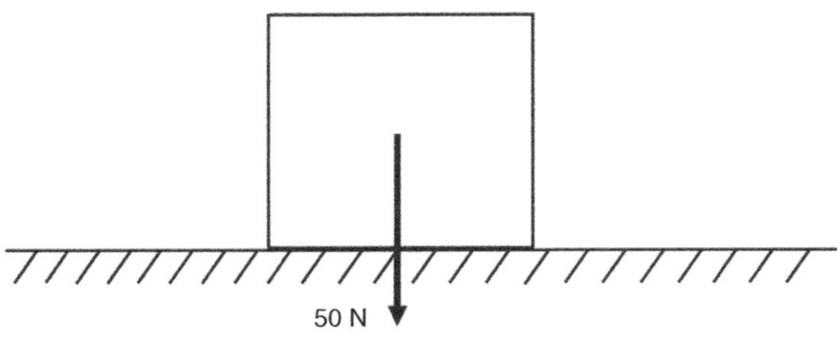

Figure 5.2 A 50 N downward force vector created by gravitational acceleration (9.81 m/s^2) acting on an object having a 5.1 kg mass.

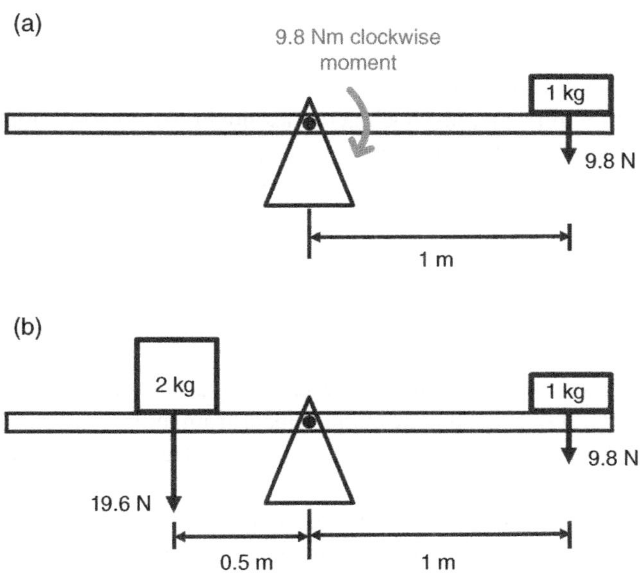

Figure 5.3 Moment example: (a) a 1 kg (9.8 N) load placed 1 m to the right of the balance pivot point creates a 9.8 Nm clockwise moment. (b) a 2 kg (19.6 N) load used to bring the scale back into balance must be placed at half the distance to create an equivalent (counterbalancing) moment.

provided in Figure 5.3. In Figure 5.3a, a balance is shown on which a 1 kg load is placed 1 m away from the pivot point. This 1 kg load, acted upon by the gravitational pull of the Earth, creates a 9.8 N downward force. This force acts with a 1-m lever arm (or distance) from the pivot to create a 9.8 Newton-meter (Nm) moment creating a tendency for the balance rotate in a clockwise direction.

If we had a 2 kg mass (creating a 19.6 N force—double that of the previous load) and wanted to bring the balance back to level, we could place it on the opposite side of the balance but to achieve an equivalent moment on the left, we would have need to halve the distance from the pivot point to achieve a 9.8 Nm counterclockwise moment to bring the balance back to level. Obviously, the smaller the lever arm of the counterbalancing object, the greater the mass (and ultimately force) will have to be to achieve system balance. As will be seen shortly, this concept is critically important in understanding the large forces experienced by musculoskeletal tissues during physical activity.

The terms "moment" and "torque" are similar concepts but there is an important distinction between the two terms. A torque is a particular type of moment that is the result of *a force couple*. A force couple is the result of two equal and opposite noncollinear forces acting on a body. Thus, all torques are moments, but not all moments are torques. For example, if you were using a wrench to tighten a bolt, we would say that your hand force (acting at a distance from the bolt) exerts a moment about the bolt, but that the jaws of the wrench create a force couple (i.e., a torque) on the head of the bolt.

Moments are critically important in biomechanical analyses, as will be seen shortly. The body regularly experiences external moments (for example, a load lifted in the hands) that must be counteracted by the development of moments internal to the body (using muscle force). As will be illustrated in the next section, muscles often operate on very small lever arms, thus requiring the generation of substantial forces when external loads are applied to the body. This, in turn, leads to large stresses on musculoskeletal tissues (often applied repetitively), which can be consequential to the health of the affected tissues.

Biomechanical Modeling

Fortunately, we can take advantage of Newton's laws to model the effects of forces imposed on the musculoskeletal system due to various stressful activities. Such activities might include (but are not limited to) work in occupational settings or participating in athletic activities. As we will see, these models can be very useful in helping to understand the impact of loadings that place mechanical stress on tissues.

The musculoskeletal system in humans is complex and highly dynamic, the nature of which makes precise understanding of the effects of loading on system components challenging. From a mechanical standpoint, the fact that musculoskeletal tissues are viscoelastic tissues means that these materials will respond differently to the same magnitude of loading depending on the rate at which the loading is applied. If a tendon is loaded at a low strain rate it will absorb mechanical energy more readily but will be less effective at transferring mechanical loads from muscle to bone. If the strain rate is high, the tendon will become stiffer, have a higher ultimate strength, and will be more effective at transmitting loads.

In addition to the changeable response of tissues to the rate of mechanical loading, there are a number of related physiological events occurring simultaneously. Nutrients and oxygen must be supplied to musculoskeletal tissues during physical activity, and delivery of these essential resources can be inhibited due to factors such as blood flow occlusion caused by muscle contraction, leading to physiological fatigue (Broxterman et al., 2015). Furthermore, musculoskeletal tissues are load sensitive and will remodel themselves according to the stresses applied (or not applied) to them. A limited number of high-stress exertions can lead to adaptive tissue strengthening, while a lack of stress can lead to atrophy. Damaged tissues can be repaired; however, the ability to do so is highly variable and dependent on factors such as the characteristics of the tissue itself, and the age and gender of the individual, as discussed in detail in Chapter 12. In fact, there is so much going on in this system that permits us the ability to move, it can seem daunting to comprehend the myriad of factors that might lead to dysfunction of the system.

In the face of such complexity, it can be helpful to simplify the system to allow for a reasonable estimation of the effects of loading experienced by the human body. One common simplifying assumption used by biomechanists is to model the musculoskeletal system as a system of rigid links connected by pin joints. Though neither of these assumptions is accurate, their use allows us analysis procedures that can provide insight into the effects of loading on the musculoskeletal system. A commonly employed simplification is to assess biomechanical demands using a *static* biomechanical model, even though tasks may be dynamic in nature. This simplification avoids the additional complexity associated with dynamic biomechanical analysis; however, it will result in estimates that may significantly underestimate the forces and moments acting on musculoskeletal tissues. The following sections will examine some basic tenets of biomechanical models of the musculoskeletal system and will provide examples of static and dynamic biomechanical modeling approaches.

Static Biomechanical Modeling

The simplest method of assessing the biomechanical impact of loading on the musculoskeletal system is using static biomechanical models. This method of assessing is applicable in situations where a person is simply holding a load (say a 5-kg dumbbell), or if it can be assumed to be moving the load in a constant velocity (i.e., with negligible acceleration). In a static biomechanical analysis, it is assumed that the system is in *static equilibrium*, meaning that the sum of all external forces and moments acting on the system is zero. It also assumes that all the bodies in the system are made of non-deformable *rigid bodies*. In reality, all materials deform to some extent when loaded, however, sometimes the deformation is so small that the assumption of no deformation is reasonable.

To achieve a state of static equilibrium, two conditions must be present. First, the system in question must be in *translational equilibrium*. This means that the net force (a summation of all force vectors) acting on the system must equal zero. If this condition is true, then the linear acceleration of the system must be zero as well. The second condition needed to achieve static equilibrium is that the system must also be in *rotational equilibrium*. A body is in rotational equilibrium if the vector sum of all moments applied to the system is also equal to zero. Thus, in accordance with Newton's first law of motion, static equilibrium requires both of the following equations to be satisfied:

$$\sum F = 0 \text{ and } \sum M = 0 \tag{5.5}$$

That is, the condition of static equilibrium stipulates that the sum of the forces acting on the system must equal zero, and the sum of the moments acting on the system must also equal zero.

In performing a biomechanical analysis involving the human body, there are two categories of force that will influence the stress experienced by musculoskeletal tissues. These are *external forces* and *internal forces*. External forces include the effects of gravity on body segments and other loads experienced by the body, such as those resulting from activities such as manual handling of objects, operation of vibrating hand tools, or other loads. However, in terms of understanding the development of injury in musculoskeletal tissues, it is the *internal forces* borne by musculoskeletal tissues that are of particular interest, as these will provide us an understanding of the stresses and strains experienced by tissues putting them at risk of injury. However, it is critical to understand the enormous influence of external loads on consequent internal force requirements.

As an example of static biomechanical analysis, let's assume that we have a person holding a dumbbell that weighs 5 kg (approximately 11 pounds), as shown in Figure 5.4. The upper arm link in this example is perpendicular and the forearm-hand link parallel to the floor. The distance from

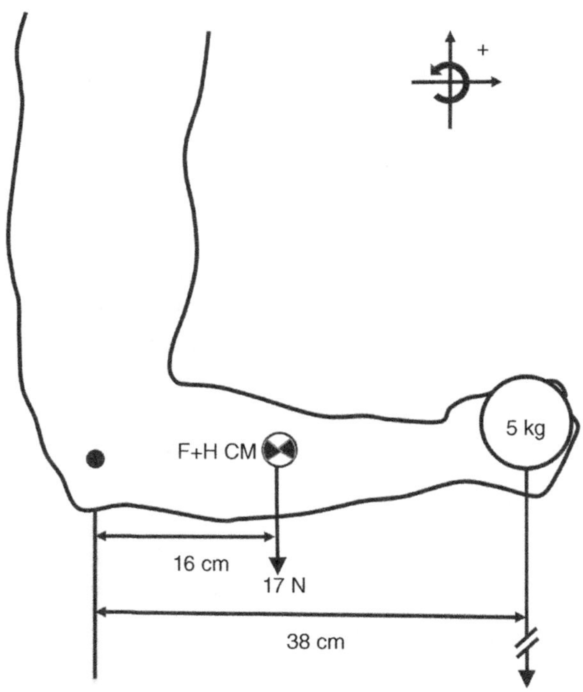

Figure 5.4 Free body diagram of weight-holding example. Note sign convention (F + H CM = Forearm/hand center of mass; ● = Elbow joint center).

the elbow to the load is 38 cm. In addition to the weight of the dumbbell, we must also consider the weight of the forearm and hand, which will also contribute a moment about the elbow. We will assume the sum of this weight acts at the *center of mass* of the forearm and hand. The center of mass is an imaginary point that represents the distribution of mass of an object and is considered the point at which the entire mass of the object is acting. In the current example, we will assume the mass of the forearm-hand link is 1.73 kg and the weight 17.0 N, and the distance from the elbow joint to the center of mass of the forearm-hand link is 16 cm. We will initially solve for the external forces acting on the body and then determine the internal forces that must be developed by muscle to maintain static equilibrium of the system.

If we first consider the load of the dumbbell itself, we can take the mass of this load and multiply it by the acceleration applied to the mass due to gravity (approximately 9.8 m/s^2). This results in the weight of the load (a force) being 49 N:

$$\text{Weight}\left(\text{N}\right) = 5\,\text{kg} * 9.8\,\text{m}/\text{s}^2 = 49\,\text{N} \tag{5.6}$$

Since the distance from the elbow is 38 cm (or 0.38 m), and the force of gravity acts in a downward direction, just the load itself will result in an 18.62 Newton-meter (Nm) clockwise moment (clockwise being negative):

$$\text{Load moment} = -49\,\text{N} * 0.38\,\text{m} = -18.62\,\text{Nm} \tag{5.7}$$

However, there is another mass that must also be accounted for in calculating the moment about the elbow joint, the mass of the forearm-hand segment, which weighs 17 N when considering the acceleration due to gravity (1.73 kg $*$ 9.8 m/s^2). The force associated with this segment will be assumed to act at the segment's center of mass, which we estimate to be 16 cm from the elbow joint:

$$\text{F\&H moment} = -17\,\text{N} * 0.16\,\text{m} = -2.72\,\text{Nm} \tag{5.8}$$

This moment is also clockwise and must be added to the moment associated with the 5 kg load to obtain the total (counterclockwise) moment about the elbow:

$$M_E = -18.62\,\text{Nm} + \left(-2.72\,\text{Nm}\right) = -21.34\,\text{Nm} \tag{5.9}$$

The total forces in this example also need to be obtained:

$$\text{Force}\left(\text{load} + \text{F\&H}\right) = -49.0\,\text{N} + \left(-17\,\text{N}\right) = -66\,\text{N} \tag{5.10}$$

Equations 5.9 and 5.10 provide us with all the necessary information regarding the external forces acting on the load and the forearm-hand segment. However, it should be apparent that currently the system is not in equilibrium (i.e., forces and moments acting on the joint do not equal zero). There must be an equal and opposite moment acting about the elbow joint to counteract the moments of the load and the forearm-hand segment, and there must also be an equal and opposite force at the elbow joint to counteract the downward forces of the load and forearm-hand to achieve static equilibrium.

To calculate the reactive force at the elbow joint, we can use the following equation:

$$F_{load} + F_{F\&H} + RF_E = 0 \tag{5.11}$$

Here, F_{load} is the force due to the load (N), $F_{F\&H}$ is the force due to the weight of the forearm and hand (N), and RF_E is the reaction force at the elbow. Solving we get:

$$-49\,\text{N} + \left(-17\,\text{N}\right) + RF_E = 0 \tag{5.12}$$

RF_E must equal 66 N.

For the reactive moment at the elbow, we can use the following equation:

$$M_{load} + M_{F\&H} + RM_E = 0 \tag{5.13}$$

Here, M_{load} is the moment due to the weight of the load times its distance from the elbow (Nm), $M_{F\&H}$ is the moment due to the weight of the forearm and hand taken at its center of mass (Nm) times its distance from the elbow (Nm), and RM_E is the reactive moment at the elbow. We can plug in the moments we have calculated previously:

$$-18.62\,\text{Nm} + (-2.72\,\text{Nm}) + RM_E = 0 \tag{5.14}$$

Thus, the reactive moment about the elbow must be +21.34 Nm.

Thus, to maintain static equilibrium, there must exist a counterclockwise moment of 21.34 Nm acting about the elbow and an upward force of 66 N to counter the downward forces of the load and forearm-hand link. Figure 5.5 provides the counterbalancing forces and moments at the elbow joint:

The question then becomes, "What is the mechanism by which the restorative (i.e., counterclockwise) moment is generated?" To answer this question, we must look to the forces generated *inside* the body, usually the result of contracting muscle. To simplify this analysis, we will assume that there is only one elbow flexor muscle attached to bone by a single tendon (this assumption is often referred to as using a "single equivalent muscle"). In this simplified analysis, we will also assume that the force generated by the muscle is perpendicular to the floor and that the "elbow flexor" tendon is attached to the forearm bones with a lever arm of 5 cm (0.05 m). Because this lever arm is small with respect to those of the load and the forearm-hand center of mass, the muscle forces produced will have to be considerably larger to create an equivalent and opposite counteracting moment. The following equation provides the relationship needed to determine the required muscle force:

$$d * F_m = 21.34\,\text{Nm} \tag{5.15}$$

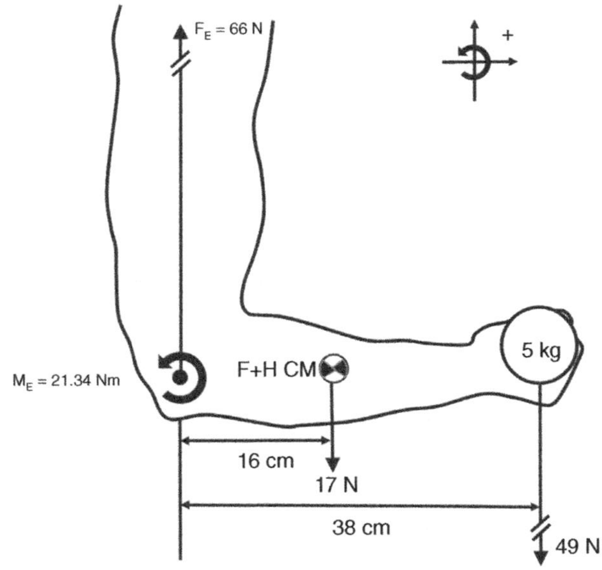

Figure 5.5 Reactive moment and reactive forces acting at the elbow.

where d represents the muscle moment arm and F_m is the muscle force. Dividing the counterclockwise moment by the muscle moment arm gives:

$$F_m = \frac{21.34\,\text{Nm}}{0.05\,\text{m}} = 426.8\,\text{N} \tag{5.16}$$

This result shows that simply holding a 5 kg mass in the hand requires a muscle force of 426.8 N (nearly 100 pounds of force) to maintain static equilibrium. Note the reaction force at the elbow must now be modified due to the introduction of the muscle force and becomes negative due to the positive muscle force:

$$F_{load} + F_{F\&H} + F_m + RF_E = 0 \tag{5.17}$$

Or

$$-49\,\text{N} + \left(-17\,\text{N}\right) + 426.8\,\text{N} + RF_E = 0 \tag{5.18}$$

Giving a reaction force at the elbow (RF_E) of −360.8 N (Figure 5.6).

Many books on biomechanics note the large muscle forces required to maintain the static equilibrium of a load in the hands and leave it there. Certainly, the large muscle forces associated with holding a modest load are interesting of their own accord. However, if we want to go further and understand the effects of such a load on the potential for injury development in musculoskeletal tissues, the earlier result is not the end of the story. It is incumbent on us to go a step further so that

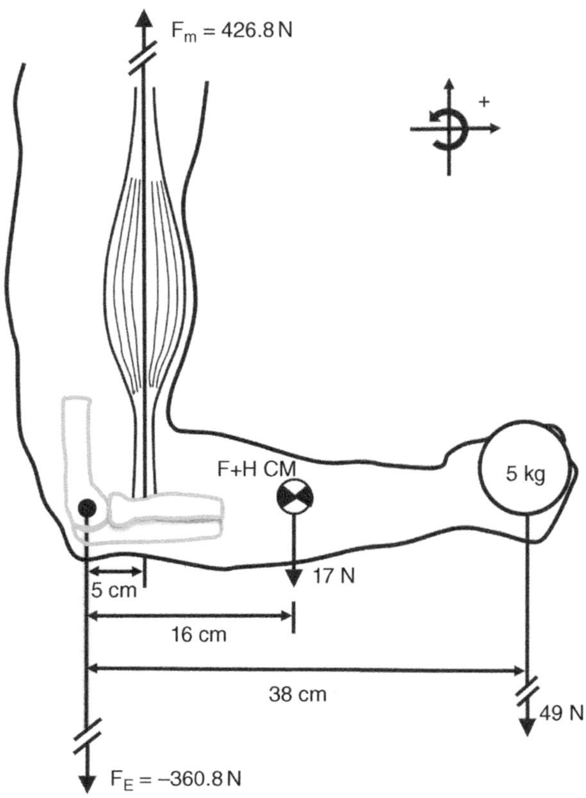

Figure 5.6 Biomechanical analysis including internal (muscle) forces. The muscle must generate 426.8 N of force to counterclockwise moments due to the load and weight of the forearm and hand. Note reaction force at the elbow (F_E) has turned negative in response to large muscle forces (−360.8 N).

we can understand the consequences of exposure to such forces (and the stresses and strains experienced by musculoskeletal tissues), particularly when such stresses are experienced repeatedly.

Whenever a force is applied to a tissue, the tissue is compelled to either deform or accelerate (typically the former). When deformation of an object (such as a tendon) occurs, an internal resistance to deformation is created within the material. This internal resistance is known as *stress* and (in accordance with Newton's laws) must be equal in magnitude and opposite in direction to the applied force. The stress is distributed over the cross-sectional area of the material in question and is expressed in units of force per cross-sectional unit area. When examining the development of damage to musculoskeletal tissues (for example, tendons), we want to understand the *stress* and the resultant *strain* (deformation) experienced by these tissues. It should be noted that we must abandon our assumption of rigid body mechanics (as in the preceding example) when we start examining what is happening at the tissue level (Litsky and Spector, 1994).

For this calculation, we need to take the force being transmitted by the tendon to the bone (in this case 426.8 N) and divide by the cross-sectional area of the tendon to determine the stress experienced by this tissue. If we assume an elbow flexor tendon cross-sectional area of 25 mm^2 (Walton, Li, Pennings, Agur, & Elmaraghy, 2015), we can estimate a stress of 17,072,000 Pascal (Pa), or 17.1 megapascal (MPa) on the tendon:

$$Stress = \frac{F(\text{Newtons})}{A(\text{square meters})} = \frac{426.8\,\text{N}}{0.000{,}025\,\text{m}^2} = 17{,}072{,}000\,\text{Pa} = 17.1\,\text{MPa} \tag{5.19}$$

This increase in stress will necessarily lead to a commensurate increase in deformation (or strain) on tissues making up the tendon. The amount of damage that might accrue in the tendon will be a function of the number of times such a load is experienced, the amount of time the exertion is sustained, and exposure to other loads that might be experienced in combination with the current one. Data from cyclic loading of tendons *ex vivo* (Schechtman and Bader, 1997) suggest that the average tendon loaded at this level of stress if loaded repetitively would last over 300,000 cycles.

Now suppose we were to increase the load in the hand to 15 kg in our biomechanical example. If one follows the calculations outlined earlier (using identical assumptions), the muscle force required to maintain equilibrium would be 1,172 N, roughly equivalent to 263 pounds of force. The stress on the tendon would now equal 46.9 MPa (nearly triple the previous stress) and the collagen fibers making up the tendon would be placed under much greater tensile strain. The increase in strain will lead to an elevated risk of damage to the tendon, particularly if such a strain is experienced repeatedly. At this level of stress, an average tendon would last approximately 5,000 cycles when loaded repetitively, according to results of *ex vivo* tests (Schechtman and Bader, 1997). If the load in the hand was 25 kg, the required muscle force to maintain static equilibrium would be 1,916 N (431 pounds), and the estimated cycles to failure would be approximately 100 cycles.

Table 5.1 summarizes the data from the calculations provided earlier. The use of traditional static biomechanical analysis techniques demonstrates that increasing hand loads result in increasingly greater reactive elbow moments, and, due to the third-class lever arrangement of the system, the muscle forces required to hold the load are large (equivalent to 100–430 pounds of muscle force). However, if we are interested in the development of damage to musculoskeletal structures (in this case the tendon), we must go further to estimate the stress in the tendon and the number of cycles it would take to initiate the process of fatigue failure at each stress level. As can be seen, while the biomechanical parameters and stress increase linearly with increased hand load, estimated cycles to failure exhibit an exponential decline.

Table 5.1 Estimates of Biomechanical Parameters (Elbow Moment, Required Muscle Force), Resultant Tendon Stress, and Estimated Cycles to Failure Associated with Hand Loads of 5, 15, and 25 kg as Discussed in the Text

Hand load (kg)	Elbow moment (Nm)	Required muscle force (N)	Tendon stress (MPa)	Estimated cycles to failure
5	21.3	427	17.1	310,000
15	58.6	1,172	46.9	5,000
25	95.8	1,916	76.6	100

Dynamic Biomechanical Modeling

The previous example employed a static two-dimensional biomechanical analysis as an introductory illustration of biomechanics principles. As mentioned earlier, a fundamental assumption of this analysis technique is that the system is not experiencing any acceleration. While there are certainly examples of tasks that can be fairly modeled using static analysis methods (such as holding a suitcase at one's side or tasks involving minimal acceleration), human activities usually involve dynamic motion, and such motion may involve considerable acceleration. Such dynamic activities can result in substantial increases in stress on musculoskeletal tissues that can significantly impact their *fatigue life* (cycles to failure). To analyze dynamic tasks, we must consider both the *kinematics* and *kinetics* of motion. Kinematics is simply the study of motion without consideration of the forces responsible for that motion. Kinetics, on the other hand, is the study of the forces that cause motion, in accordance with Newton's laws.

Motion is generally divided into two types: translational (linear) and angular (rotational). Each of these types of motion has its own specific equations to quantify both the kinematics and kinetics of motion. In the case of translational (linear) motion, a three-axis Cartesian coordinate system is traditionally used to assess measures of displacement, velocity, and acceleration. The three-dimensional displacement vector of an object can be calculated by

$$s = (x_f - x_i)i + (y_f - y_i)j + (z_f - z_i)k \tag{5.20}$$

where s is the three-dimensional displacement, x_f and x_i represent the final and initial positions in the x-direction, and i represents a unit vector in the x-direction. Similarly, y_f and y_i represent the final and initial positions in the y-direction, and j represents a unit vector in the y-direction, and z_f and z_i represent the final and initial positions in the z-direction, with k representing a unit vector in the z-direction.

If one desires to obtain the instantaneous velocity of an object, the change in the displacement of the object with respect to time would be calculated. This relationship, defined by the term instantaneous velocity, is represented by the following equation:

$$v = ds/dt \tag{5.21}$$

The average velocity is represented by the following equation:

$$\bar{v} = \Delta s/\Delta t \tag{5.22}$$

which has units of meters per second (m/s). Instantaneous and average linear acceleration is defined as the change in velocity with respect to time, which are represented by the following equations:

$$a = dv/dt \tag{5.23}$$

$$\bar{a} = \Delta v / \Delta t \tag{5.24}$$

When dealing with angular motion, it is common to use polar rather than Cartesian coordinates. As can be seen, the equations for kinematics of angular motion are analogous to the equations for rectilinear motion. For example, angular displacement is given by the following equation, which relates the radius (r) of a circle, the angle θ (in radians), and the arc length s:

$$s = r\theta \tag{5.25}$$

The angular velocity is the derivative of the angular position with respect to time and is the first derivative of the angular displacement. symbolized by the Greek letter omega (ω):

$$\omega = \frac{d\theta}{dt} = \dot{\theta} \tag{5.26}$$

The average angular velocity ($\bar{\omega}$) describes the change in angular position of a rotating object between two time points (t_1 and t_2) and is defined by the ratio of change in the angular position of the object over the time interval of interest:

$$\bar{\omega} = \frac{\theta_2 - \theta_1}{t_2 - t_1} \tag{5.27}$$

where θ_1 and θ_2 represent the angular positions of the rotating object at t_1 and t_2, respectively.

A change in the angular velocity of a rotating object over time is known *as angular acceleration*, which is derivative of angular velocity with respect to time. Angular acceleration is generally represented by the Greek letter alpha (α):

$$\alpha = \frac{d\omega}{dt} = \ddot{\theta} \tag{5.28}$$

The average angular acceleration represents the change in angular velocity over a given time period and is denoted by $\bar{\alpha}$:

$$\bar{\alpha} = \frac{\omega_2 - \omega_1}{t_2 - t_1} \tag{5.29}$$

When evaluating the kinetics associated with motion, the effects of force on the object in question must be considered. Two types of force act on a rotating object. The first is a tangential force, which is governed by the following equation:

$$F_t = mr\alpha \tag{5.30}$$

where m is the mass of the object, r represents the distance of the objects center of mass from the point of rotation of the object, and α is the angular acceleration of the rotating object.

A second force acting on the rotating object is called the *normal force*, which acts perpendicular to the axis of rotation:

$$F_n = mr\omega^2 \tag{5.31}$$

When evaluating the moments acting on a rotating object, there are several components that need to be considered. These include the moment associated with the weight of the body (such as a rotating body segment) acting at a distance from the center of rotation of an object (typically about a joint center), a moment imposed by a load held in the hand times the distance of that load from the joint center, and/or a component due to the mass of the body resisting any change in angular velocity known as the *mass moment of inertia*. The larger the mass moment of inertia, the more difficult it becomes to alter the angular acceleration of an object.

The mass moment of inertia of a body is the result of the sum of the masses (from the multitude of particles of which the object is composed) multiplied by the square of its distance from the axis of rotation. The volume and density of the object and its distribution of mass will have a considerable influence on the mass moment of inertia. For objects of a given mass, if the center of mass is close to the center of rotation, the resistance to rotation will be lower compared to that when the center of mass is farther away. The moment of inertia, considered at the center of mass of an object under angular acceleration (I_{cm}), is denoted by the following equation (Freivalds, 2004):

$$M = I_{cm}\alpha \tag{5.32}$$

indicating that the net torque is a function of the mass moment of inertia times the angular acceleration. This is simply Newton's second law applied to angular rotation.

Because the body's segments do not rotate about their center of mass but at joint centers, it is helpful to be able to calculate the net moment about joint centers. A method known as the parallel axis theorem is employed to allow the calculation of the net torque at the joint centers. The theorem states the following relationship exists with respect to the moment of inertia:

$$I = I_c + mr_c^2 \tag{5.33}$$

where I is the mass moment of inertia that exists about an axis parallel to one of the objects centroidal axes, I_c is the moment of inertia about that centroidal axis, m is the total mass of the object, and r_c is the shortest distance between these two axes. Figure 5.7 provides an example of the parallel axis theorem. In this example, a depiction of the forearm and hand are presented diagrammatically. The moment of inertia about the center of mass is 0.009 kg m^2. However, the forearm does not rotate about its center of mass, but about the elbow joint, represented by O in the figure. If the distance between O and the center of mass (CM) is 0.16 m and the mass of the forearm-hand link is 1.735 kg, the mass moment of inertia about the elbow joint (I_O) would be 0.053 kg m^2.

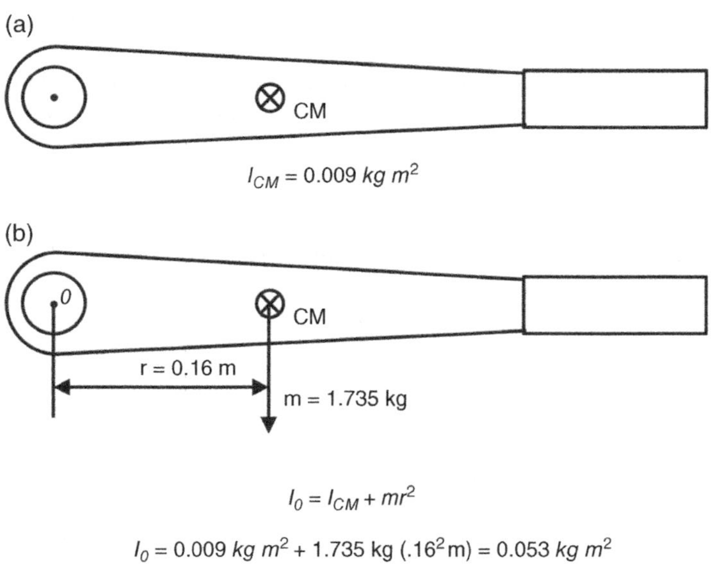

Figure 5.7 Example of the use of the parallel axis theorem. (a) The mass moment of inertia at the center of mass of the forearm-hand link (I_{CM}) is 0.009 kg m^2, (b) using the parallel axis theorem, the mass moment of inertia about the elbow joint (I_O) is 0.053 kg m^2.

The information provided earlier can be used as a basis for the development of dynamic biomechanical models to estimate the forces and moments associated with motions or tasks of interest to musculoskeletal researchers. As with the static analyses performed earlier, the dynamic model must include all relevant forces acting on the body segment in question. These include the inertial forces associated with segment motion, the forces associated with gravitational acceleration on the body segment and any additional external loads present. Anthropometry of the body segment being analyzed, including the distances from the joint center to locations of interest (center of mass of the segment and any external load handled), will be necessary. Typically, we will be solving for the muscle forces required to perform the tasks and the magnitude of the reaction force experienced by the joint bearing the brunt of the load.

To illustrate dynamic biomechanical analysis techniques, we will use the data from the prior static analysis and introduce dynamic motion to see how the moments about the elbow and the required muscle forces are affected by the introduction of motion.

Consider an individual who is lifting a 5 kg load involving rotation of the forearm-hand link about the elbow. Let's assume that at the time that the forearm and hand link is parallel with the ground (90° from the vertical (θ), the link has an instantaneous angular velocity of 6 rad/s and an instantaneous angular acceleration of 75 rad/s^2. As with the previous static example, we also assume that the weight of the forearm and hand link is 17 N, the lever arm from the elbow joint center to the single muscle equivalent tendon is 5 cm (a), the distance from the elbow to the center of mass of the forearm and hand link is 16 cm (b) and that the lever arm from the elbow joint to the 5 kg load is 38 cm (c). We will also assume that the mass moment of inertia of the of the forearm and hand (calculated at the elbow joint) is I_o = 0.053 kg m^2. We would like to ascertain the net torque produced about the elbow joint, the muscle force required to perform the task, and the magnitude of the reaction force acting on the elbow joint.

In order to get the net moment (M_0) (acting counterclockwise) about the elbow joint due to the rotational motion, we simply have to multiply the mass moment of inertia by the angular acceleration:

$$M_0 = I_o\alpha = \left(0.053\text{kg/m}^2\right)\left(75\text{rad/s}^2\right) = 3.975\,\text{Nm} \tag{5.34}$$

The net torque represents the rotational effects of all external forces acting on the forearm and hand link (Özkaya et al., 2017). In this example, there will be three external forces having rotational effects. These include the forces exerted by the elbow flexor tendon (transmitted muscle force), the weight of the forearm and hand link (acting at its center of mass), and the weight of the load being held by the hand, each having their own respective lever arms (as illustrated in Figure 5.8). Therefore, the magnitude of the net moment M_0 about the elbow joint due to the muscle force (F_m), the weight of the forearm and hand (W) and the load (L) would be:

$$M_0 = M_m - M_w - M_l \tag{5.35}$$

where M_m represents the moment created by the tendon, M_w represents the moment created by the weight of the forearm segment, and M_l represents the moment due to the hand load. The moments can be represented by their respective forces and lever arms:

$$M_0 = aF_m - bF_w\,sin\theta - cF_l\,sin\theta \tag{5.36}$$

We can then solve for the unknown muscle force by rearranging:

$$F_m = \frac{M_0 + bWsin\theta + cLsin\theta}{a} \tag{5.37}$$

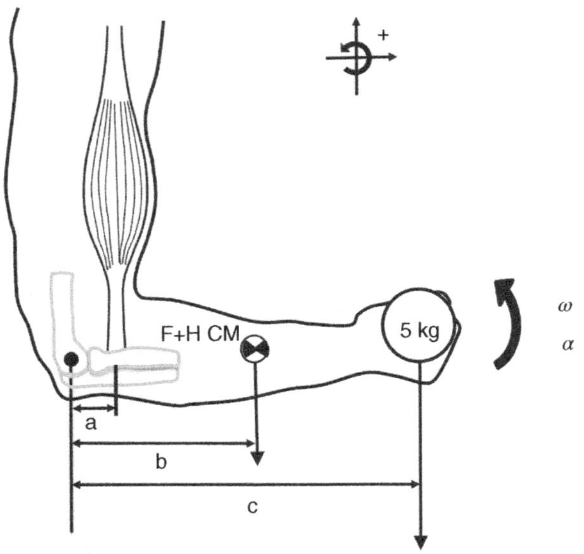

Figure 5.8 Dynamic biomechanical example.

Inputting the information provided, we can then obtain an estimate of the required muscle force for the dynamic lift:

$$F_m = \frac{3.975\,\text{Nm} + (0.16\,\text{m})(17\,\text{N})(\sin 90^\circ) + (0.38\,\text{m})(49\,\text{N})(\sin 90^\circ)}{0.05} = 506.3\,\text{N} \tag{5.38}$$

Comparing the required muscle forces associated with the current dynamic exertion to the earlier static analysis, it can be seen the dynamics associated with handling a 5 kg load increases the required muscle forces by approximately 19%. The dynamic task will increase the stress and strain experienced by tendons and decrease the number of cycles to failure associated with handling the 5 kg load compared to the static holding task. The greater the magnitude of the dynamic component, the greater this effect will be. However, it should also be noted that because the tissues of the musculoskeletal system are viscoelastic, they will become somewhat stiffer and stronger depending on the rate at which dynamic loads are applied.

Summary

The preceding examples illustrate the benefits of biomechanical analysis in developing an appreciation of the forces and moments that may be imposed on the musculoskeletal system during the performance of simple tasks. As indicated previously, this information can be used to assess the muscle forces required to perform these tasks. However, if one wants to use this information to get an appreciation of how these muscle forces or joint reaction forces might lead to the development of a musculoskeletal tissue injury, fatigue failure methods may be employed. This latter step is not often considered in the biomechanical literature but would seem quite useful in improving our understanding of the development of damage in tissues of the musculoskeletal system leading to MSDs.

Of course, we must recognize that there are several assumptions and limitations related to the biomechanical techniques provided earlier. For example, the earlier examples assume that the segments are rigid bodies and that joints are pin joints, neither of which is accurate. We have assumed in our examples that there is one single elbow flexor muscle responsible for the required muscle force as opposed to several (in reality). We have not included antagonistic muscle forces that will be clearly present (in this case forces from the elbow extensors), which would increase the forces required by the agonist muscle(s). The analyses here assume two-dimensional planar movement which is generally reasonable for these actions in the preceding examples, but we must recognize that human activities typically involve complex three-dimensional motion. Clearly, complex three-dimensional full-body dynamic biomechanical analyses require use of sophisticated computer-based models.

Despite these limitations, biomechanical modeling can provide us with useful information regarding the nature of forces and moments acting on body segments. Muscle forces will have an impact on musculoskeletal tissues. For example, when the biceps muscle generates a tensile force, it will create stress in the tendon leading to a strain (or deformation) of that tendon. The greater the muscle force (and stress), the greater the deformation. At the molecular level, the deformation is the result of forces internal to the tendon (and the particles that make up that tendon) pulling on particles above and below them and in line with the long axis of the tendon. If this action is performed repetitively, these internal molecular forces may weaken and eventually experience a breaking of the molecular bonds leading to damage initiation.

Different types of materials will have their own distinctive responses to the forces and moments experienced during life. Understanding how the materials that make up our musculoskeletal system respond to the loads imposed upon them is important in our understanding of the development of damage in musculoskeletal tissue. Chapter 6 will detail the material properties of these tissues and discusses implications with respect to the development of MSDs.

Bibliography

Broxterman, R., Craig, J., Smith, J., Wilcox, S., Jia, C., Warren, S., & Barstow, T. (2015). Influence of blood flow occlusion on the development of peripheral and central fatigue during small muscle mass handgrip exercise. *The Journal of Physiology*, *593*, 4043–4054.

Chaffin, D., Andersson, G., & Martin, B. (2006). *Occupational biomechanics*. New York: Wiley.

Concise Oxford English Dictionary (2011). *Biomechanics*. London: Oxford University Press.

Freivalds, A. (2004). *Biomechanics of the upper limbs: Mechanics, modeling, and musculoskeletal injuries*. Boca Raton: CRC Press.

Innocenti, B. (2018). Biomechanics: A fundamental tool with a long history (and even longer future!). *Muscles, Ligaments and Tendons Journal*, *7*, 491–492.

Kroemer, K. (1988). Chapter: 3. Biomechanical Models. In K. Kroemer, S. Snook, S. Meadows, & S. Deutsche (Eds.), *Ergonomic Models of Anthropometry, Human Biomechanics and Operator-Equipment Interfaces: Proceedings of a Workshop* (pp. 19–42). Washington, DC: National Research Council.

Lesniak, B., Baraga, M., Jose, J., Smith, M., Cunningham, S., & Kaplan, L. (2013). Glenohumeral findings on magnetic resonance imaging correlate with innings pitched in asymptomatic pitchers. *American Journal Sports Medicine*, *41*, 2022–2027.

Lin, D., Wong, T., & Kazam, J. (2018). Shoulder injuries in the overhead-throwing athlete: Epidemiology, mechanisms of injury, and imaging findings. *Radiology*, *286*, 370–387.

Litsky, A., & Spector, M. (1994). Biomaterials. In S. Simon (Ed.), *Orthopaedic Basic Science* (pp. 447–486). Chicago: American Orthopaedic Society for Sports Medicine.

Newton, I. (1687). *Philosophiae naturalis principia mathematica*. Londini: Jussu Societatis Regiæ ac Typis Josephi Streater; prostat apud plures Bibliopolas.

NIOSH (1997). *Musculoskeletal disorders and workplace factors*. Cincinnati, OH: National Institute for Occupational Safety and Health.

Nordin, M., & Frankel, V. (2012). *Basic biomechanics of the musculoskeletal system*. Baltimore: Lippincott, Williams & Wilkins.

Özkaya, N., Leger, D., Goldsheyder, D., & Nordin, M. (2017). *Fundamentals of biomechanics*. New York: Springer.

Posner, M., Cameron, K., Wolf, J., Belmont, P. J., & Owens, B. (2011). Epidemiology of major league baseball injuries. *American Journal of Sports Medicine*, *39*, 1676–1680.

Schechtman, H., & Bader, D. (1997). In vitro fatigue of human tendons. *Journal of Biomechanics*, *30*, 829–835.

Walton, C., Li, Z., Pennings, A., Agur, A., & Elmaraghy, A. (2015). A 3-dimensional anatomic study of the distal biceps tendon: Implications for surgical repair and reconstruction. *Orthopaedic Journal of Sports Medicine*, *3*, 6.

6

Material Properties of Musculoskeletal and Peripheral Nerve Tissues

Overview

During the process of evolution, the development of increasingly complex life-forms necessitated the innovation of systems to support the needs of more complex organisms (Kardon, 2011). The answer to this need was the development of a complex system of materials that would allow support of more complex organ systems, allow the body (organism) to maintain its shape, and permit the organism to move around freely. The system that would eventually develop would comprise several distinct types of materials, each with its own specific characteristics and roles.

Previous chapters have described the general structure and function of materials that make up the musculoskeletal system and the biomechanical forces and moments that may be experienced by musculoskeletal tissues. This chapter will focus on the responses of various musculoskeletal tissues to the application of physical loads. Specifically, we will discuss some important fundamentals of materials science, the mechanical characteristics of musculoskeletal tissues, and the way they respond to different types of loading. The material characteristics of musculoskeletal tissues, and how these materials respond to loads imposed upon them, are a critical aspect of how and why injuries develop in musculoskeletal tissues. We will briefly discuss principles of fatigue failure (i.e., cumulative damage development in materials to application of repeated stress) in this chapter; however, Chapter 7 will focus in detail on fatigue failure responses of tissues comprising the musculoskeletal system.

Fundamentals of Materials Science

Hooke's Law

A fundamental relationship useful in understanding the effect of forces on materials is Hooke's law. Hooke's law represents a simple proportionality between two quantities: the force required to displace an object and the degree to which that object is lengthened. The equation for Hooke's law is shown as follows:

$$F = kx$$

where the force (F) needed to extend or compress an elastic object by some distance x is proportional to the distance the object is stretched times a constant (k). Typically, this relationship is

Musculoskeletal Disorders: The Fatigue Failure Mechanism, First Edition. Sean Gallagher and Mary F. Barbe.

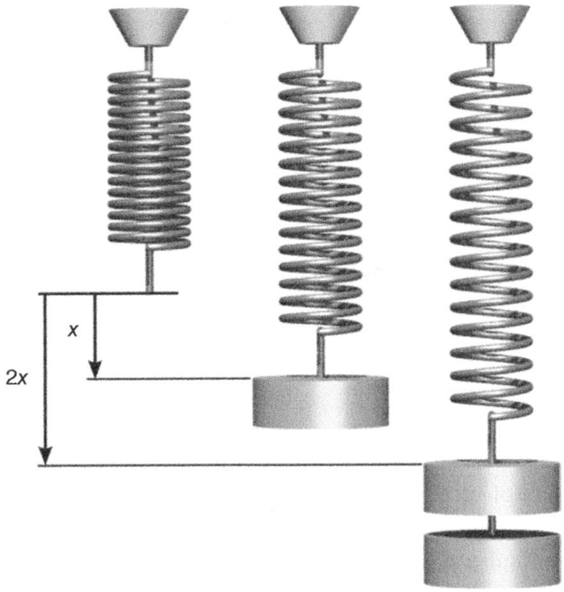

Figure 6.1 The displacement of the spring is proportional to the force applied to the spring according to Hooke's law. Svjo–own work, CC BY-SA 3.0, https://commons.wikimedia.org/w/index.php?curid=25398333, freely available.

demonstrated using a spring (specifically an "ideal" spring). The extension of the spring is proportional to the force applied, as illustrated in Figure 6.1. Hooke's law holds true as long as the material being extended remains well within its elastic limit. When the material stays below its elastic limit, it will typically return to its original length using a restorative force generated within the material.

Stress Versus Strain

Consider a force being applied to an elastic material, such as a rubber bungee cord. If the bungee cord is fixed on one end and a tensile force is applied to the other end, the cord will be deformed (stretched), and a restorative force will be generated inside the cord. If the tensile load is removed, this restorative force will allow the bungee cord to return to its original shape. In diagrams, this restorative force is usually depicted using an arrow representing a single vector. In reality, however, the restorative force will be distributed across the entire cross-sectional area of the cord. The distribution of this restorative force throughout the cross-sectional area of the bungee cord is known as *stress*, and a *stress field* will be present in the bungee cord. Stress is designated by the Greek letter σ and is simply the internal restorative force divided by the cross-sectional area of the bungee cord:

$$stress(\sigma) = \frac{F}{A}$$

where F is the restorative force and A represents the cross-sectional area of the material (in this case, the bungee cord). Since stress represents a force (whose unit is Newtons) over an area (whose unit is m^2), the unit for stress is given in N/m^2 and is named as "pascal (Pa)" in honor of Blaise Pascal, the French mathematician, physicist, and theologian. As a Newton represents less than 4 ounces of force and the area is a square meter, 1 Pascal is a very low level of stress. When dealing with stresses experienced by musculoskeletal tissues, the magnitude of stress experienced by these tissues can be in millions or billions of Pascals, denoted megapascals (MPa) and gigapascals (GPa), respectively.

Material stress can always be resolved into three fundamental types: *tension, compression,* and *shear.* Figure 6.2 provides graphical examples of the responses of a material to tensile, compressive, and shear forces. On the molecular level, stress represents internal forces exerted by adjacent particles acting upon one another. For example, if an individual were standing upright and holding two 10 kg loads in their hands with arms at their sides, particles of the bony structures of the arms would be pulling on particles above and below them by interatomic attractive forces (creating *tension*); furthermore, in the bony structures of the legs, each particle would be pushing down on particles underneath (creating *compression*). The sum of these individual intermolecular forces adds up to the total force being experienced by the material in question, and when normalized by the cross-sectional area, it represents the stress experienced by the material.

Material stress will, in turn, result in deformation (or *strain*) of the material, the nature of which is dictated by the nature of the stress involved. *Strain* is defined as the change in length (compared to its original length) caused by a stress, and is represented by the following equation:

$$\epsilon = \frac{l - l_0}{l_0}$$

where ϵ equals strain (a unitless measure often expressed as a percentage), l represents the deformed object length, and l_0 represents the original length. For example, if a 15-in. bungee cord were stretched 3 in., it would be said to experience a strain of 20%.

As illustrated in Figure 6.2, when an object is placed under tension, it will experience a lengthening deformation (strain) along the dimension under tension. When this occurs, there will also be secondary deformations in other dimensions. In tension, for example, the material will become

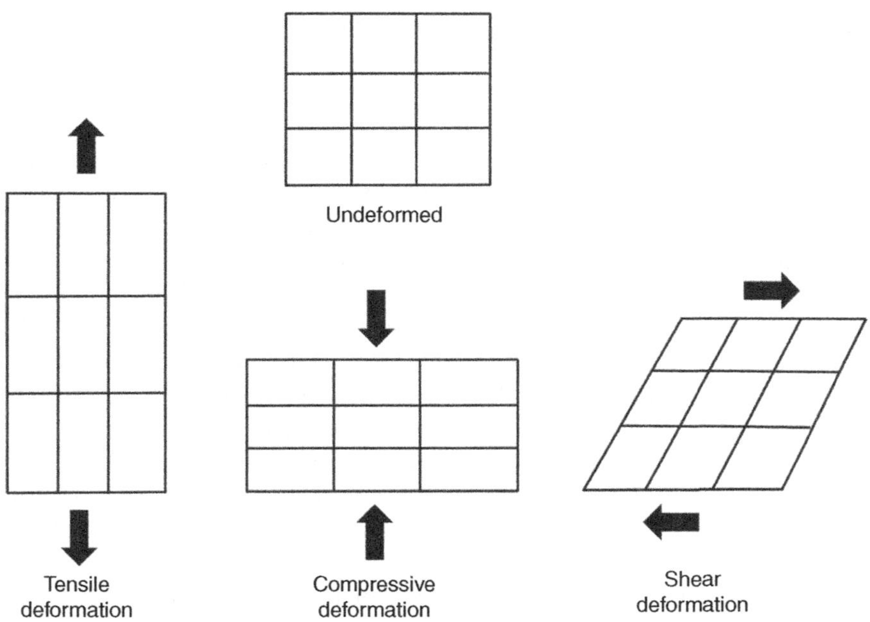

Figure 6.2 An undeformed object and the same object under tensile, compressive, and shear deformation. Adapted from Black, J. (1988). *Orthopaedic biomaterials in research and practice.* Churchill-Livingstone.

thinner as it increases in length. If the material experiences compressive loading, it will deform primarily by shrinking in height; however, the material will also experience a secondary increase in width. Shear loading results when forces act in opposite directions at different levels of the structure. For example, a force is pushing to the right at the top of a structure, while at the same time the bottom of the structure experiences a force pushing to the left. This will cause deformation of the object in two directions (opposite to one another).

Note that when a material such as a rubber bungee cord is placed in tension, the cross-sectional area will not be uniform across the length of the material. For example, the cross-sectional area may be smaller in the center. The restorative force acting over a decreased cross-sectional area will result in increased stress in the center of the bungee cord as opposed to regions further from the middle. The enhanced concentration of stress experienced in the central region makes it more likely that this site will be the first to incur material damage. That is, the molecular attractive forces in the center will be under the greatest strain in this region and would be most likely to experience damage, either in single or (more typically) in repetitive force applications.

The extent of deformation experienced by a material depends on a number of factors, including the nature and structure of the material being loaded, the nature of the load (magnitude, direction, and duration), and environmental factors (such as heat and humidity) (Ozkaya, Leger, Goldsheyder, & Nordin, 2017). Compressive and tensile loading are commonly referred to as either *axial loading* or *normal loading*, as they refer to loads where the force is exerted normal to a fixed axis. Shear loading differs from axial loading in that the loading direction is perpendicular to the normal axis. Shear stress causes parallel planes of a material to slide past one another. Shear stress is generally represented using the Greek letter *tau*:

$$\tau = \frac{F}{A}$$

where τ represents shear stress, F is the applied force, and A is the cross-sectional area over which the shear stress is applied. The unit for shear stress is Pascals (N/m^2).

Stress–Strain Curve and Young's Modulus

There are a wide variety of materials in the world, each of which has its own unique molecular makeup. Depending on this molecular structure, materials will exhibit different strain responses to the application of stress. The relationship between stress and strain for a material is often depicted on a *stress–strain curve*. Stress–strain curves provide a great deal of useful information regarding material properties. Figure 6.3 shows a typical stress–strain curve for a tendon subjected to a continuously increasing tensile stress. Several regions can be identified at which the material will exhibit different behaviors as stress and strain increase. At very low levels of stress and strain, tendons and ligaments exhibit a feature called the "toe" region, which is indicative of a relatively large increase in strain compared to the increase in stress in this region. This response is associated with straightening the wavy crimp of relaxed collagen fibers. Once this crimp is straightened out, the stress–strain curve will enter a linear region (up to point A), where the proportion of stress and strain remains equivalent. The relationship of stress and strain in this region is described by a measure known as the *modulus of elasticity*, or *Young's modulus*. The *modulus of elasticity* has the same units as stress and can be determined at any point along the linear portion of the curve and is represented by the following equation:

$$E = \frac{stress}{strain}$$

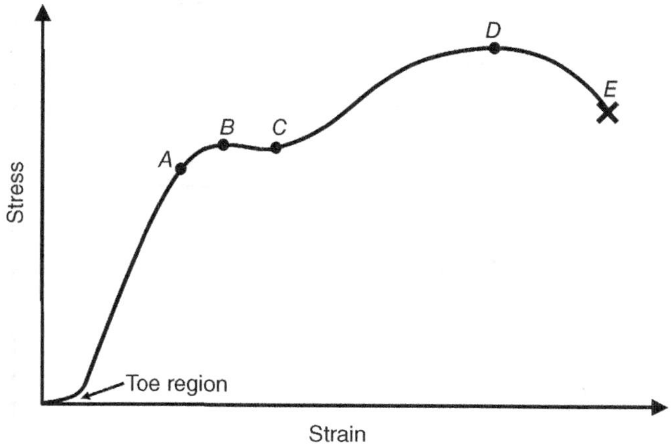

Figure 6.3 Material stress–strain curve. *A*=proportional limit, *B*=elastic limit, *C*=yield stress point, *D*=ultimate stress, *E*=rupture.

where *E* is the elastic (Young's) modulus, stress is the stress at any given point along the curve, and strain is the strain associated with that given point. The higher the modulus, the greater the stress it takes to generate a strain in a material.

Point A is known as the *proportional limit*. Beneath this limit, the material will exhibit elastic behavior in which the material will return to its original shape. The material will also maintain elastic behavior between the proportional limit (point A) and the elastic limit (point B) in Figure 6.3; however, the relationship between stress and strain will no longer be proportional (linear) in this range. Beyond point B, the material will begin to experience *plastic deformation*. Point C denotes the material's *yield point* (i.e., the amount of stress beyond which the material will no longer return to its original shape). The stress associated with the yield point is known as *yield stress*. After the yield point, there is a region where small increases in stress will again lead to large increases in material deformation, leading to point D, which represents the *ultimate stress* that can be borne by the material. Beyond this point, stress may decrease; however, the strain may continue to increase in a so-called "necking" process that may occur prior to failure. Finally, point E represents the point of final *material rupture* or *fracture*.

Material Deformation of Musculoskeletal Tissues

Viscoelastic Properties

All musculoskeletal and nerve tissues comprise materials that exhibit *viscoelastic* behavior. The term "viscoelastic" is derived from two terms: *viscosity* (a fluid property that measures resistance to "flow" under shear stress) and *elasticity* (a characteristic of solid materials to regain their original shape when deformed). Thus, musculoskeletal tissues possess both fluid and solid material characteristics. These characteristics have a tremendous bearing on the reaction of musculoskeletal tissues to loading, which differ significantly from engineering materials such as metals or plastics. The paragraphs that follow provide some of the important differences between viscoelastic materials and other types of materials in terms of their responses to applied stress.

One of the most important differences between typical engineering materials as opposed to viscoelastic materials is that viscoelastic materials exhibit different material characteristics depending on the rate at which they are loaded. Figure 6.4 demonstrates the strain response of cortical bone as a function of strain rate. As can be seen in this figure, faster strain rates require larger amounts of stress to achieve equivalent strains. Thus, stress–strain responses of viscoelastic

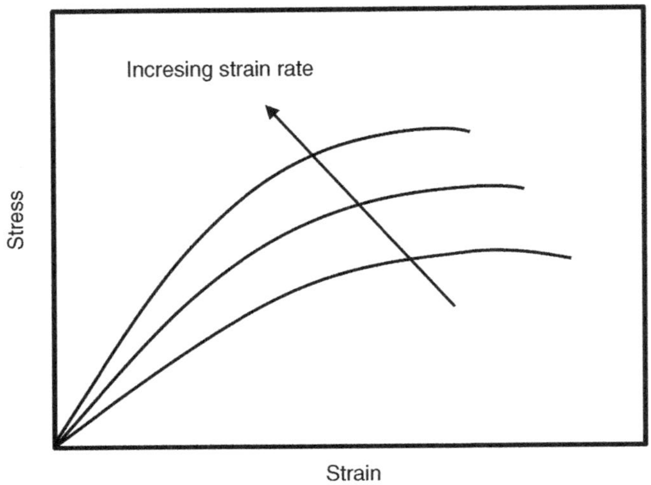

Figure 6.4 Relationship of stress and strain for a cortical bone at different strain rates. Increasing strain rate leads to a stiffer material and is associated with an increase in Elastic/Young's modulus. Adapted from Black, J. (1988). *Orthopaedic biomaterials in research and practice.* Churchill-Livingstone.

materials are time-dependent. Increased strain rate causes an increase in the *brittleness* of viscoelastic materials and an increase in *Young's modulus.*

For viscoelastic materials, the energy associated with a strain is partly stored in the material as potential energy, while some energy is dissipated as heat (regardless of whether the stresses experienced are high or low). [Note: See Table 6.1 for material characteristics definitions.]

Responses of Viscoelastic Materials to Static Loading Conditions

In addition to the changes in material characteristics associated with the load rate in viscoelastic materials, time-dependent changes occur during exposure to static loading conditions, leading to *creep responses* in the material. Experiments have been developed to assess the responses of these materials to various loading conditions. One such experiment, known as a creep and recovery test, is shown in Figure 6.5. When an instantaneous stress is applied to a perfectly elastic material (such as a rubber band), the strain response will be immediate and will remain constant until the stress is released, wherein the strain will immediately return to zero. The response of a viscoelastic material to the same stress regimen will be quite different. When the instantaneous stress is applied, the tissue will at first experience a small instantaneous strain but will subsequently experience strain in a gradual exponential manner. This is known as *creep strain* (see Figure 6.5). If the stress is immediately released, there will be a degree of instantaneous strain recovery (*elastic recovery*) followed by an exponential decrease in strain (*anelastic recovery*). If the material is a viscoelastic solid, recovery will be slow but complete. However, if the material is a viscoelastic fluid, it may never experience full recovery, resulting in permanent deformation.

The stress-relaxation procedure is used to examine the responses of a material to a stress that is instantaneously applied and then held at the same stress level indefinitely (Figure 6.6). In response to such a loading regimen, an elastic material will experience an immediate strain, and this strain will be maintained for as long as the stress is present. Viscoelastic materials will also experience a strain but will then undergo a period of stress relaxation, where the material will experience decreased stress. Viscoelastic solids will never decrease to a stress level of zero, while viscoelastic fluids will eventually achieve a zero-stress level.

Table 6.1 Definitions of Common Material Characteristics

Brittle	A brittle material is the opposite of a ductile material. Brittle materials will demonstrate a sudden failure without much plastic deformation. Not to be confused with weakness. Brittle materials can be very strong, such as diamonds.
Creep	The tendency of a solid material to move slowly or deform permanently under the influence of persistent mechanical stress.
Ductile	A material that will experience a large plastic deformation prior to failure.
Durability	The ability of a material to withstand wear or damage.
Elasticity	Resistance of a material to stress and its ability to regain its original form when deformed.
Flexibility	The ability of a material to deform under stress.
Heterogeneous	A material with dramatic variations in strength from one region to another.
Homogeneous	A material that does not vary from location to location in the material.
Isotropic versus Anisotropic	An *isotropic* material responds to stress in the same manner no matter the direction of loading. Most musculoskeletal tissues are *anisotropic,* meaning that they will vary in their stress response depending on the direction of loading.
Plasticity	The propensity of a solid material to undergo permanent deformation under load.
Recovery	With *elastic recovery*, there is a degree of instantaneous strain recovery after the release of a stress; *anelastic recovery* is an exponential decrease in strain after the release of a stress and usually occurs after the period of elastic recovery.
Resilience	The ability to absorb energy without experiencing permanent deformation. Resilience is measured by taking the area under the stress–strain diagram in the elastic region only.
Stiffness	The stiffness of a material as represented by the value of *Young's modulus*. The higher the modulus, the stiffer is the material and the more resistant to deformation it will be.
Toughness	A measure of the capacity of a material to withstand permanent deformation. This measure is represented by the area under the stress–strain diagram curve. The greater the area under the curve, the tougher the material is considered to be.
Viscosity	The resistance of a fluid to gradual deformation (flow) due to stress.
Yield strength	The stress at which a material will start to deform plastically.
Young's modulus	The modulus of elasticity; the relationship of stress and strain.

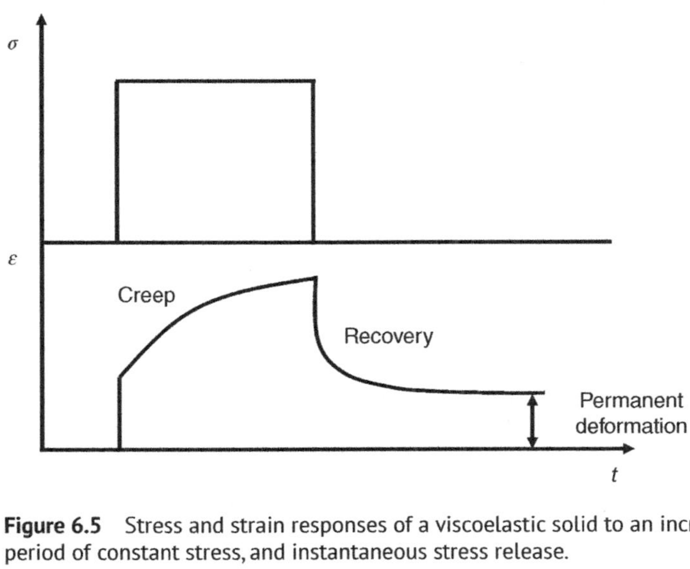

Figure 6.5 Stress and strain responses of a viscoelastic solid to an increase in instantaneous stress, a period of constant stress, and instantaneous stress release.

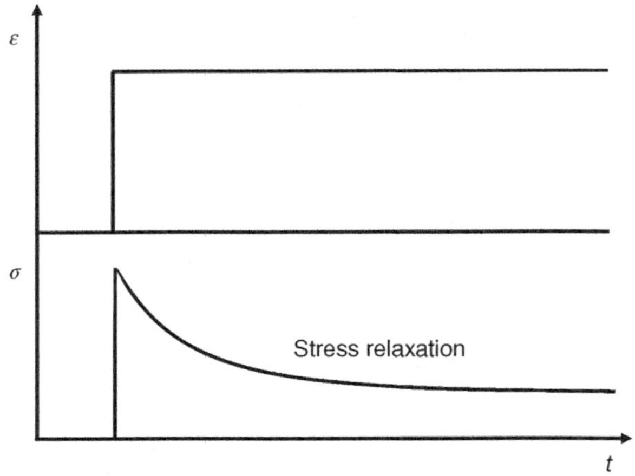

Figure 6.6 Stress-relaxation response of a viscoelastic solid subjected to a constant strain.

Hysteresis

Viscoelastic materials, even when stressed below their yield point, exhibit an elastic recovery curve that differs from the original stress–strain curve associated with its deformation (Figure 6.7). The area between the two curves represents energy that is dissipated, usually as heat. Such a response is not typically observed with elastic–plastic materials. The Morrow Energy Model (Morrow, 1964) is often used to assess the amount of energy dissipation and helps to estimate the number of cycles a viscoelastic material will last in repetitive loading.

The stress–strain relationship associated with cyclic loading and unloading of viscoelastic materials is considerably more complex than that observed under the static tests mentioned earlier. Figure 6.7 presents typical loading and unloading paths for cyclic loading of viscoelastic materials. While loading and unloading paths for elastic materials will follow the same slope, in viscoelastic materials loading and unloading curves associated with cyclic loading are markedly different. In

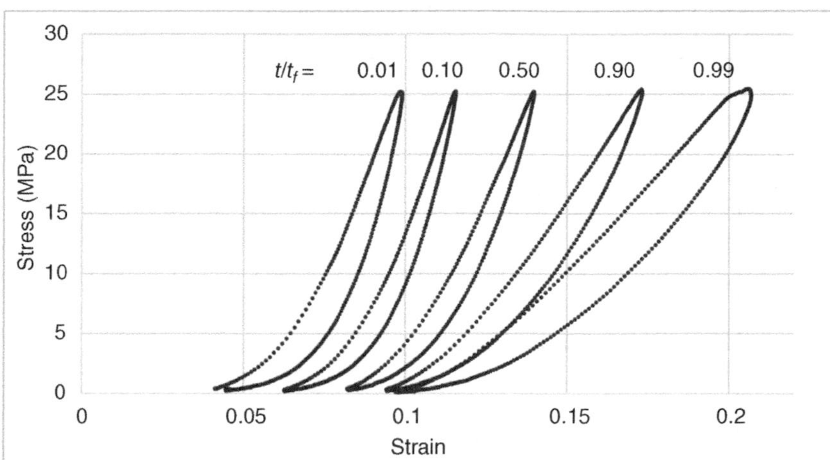

Figure 6.7 Hysteresis is evident in cyclic loading of a tendon at various percentages of fatigue life. The loading and unloading pathways for the viscoelastic material differ significantly. The area between the curves represents the inelastic work done (or energy dissipated) usually as heat. (*Note.* t/t_f represents the proportion of time with respect to the final time). Smith, N. (2019). *In vitro tensile fatigue of human flexor digitorum profundus and superficialis tendons* (Doctoral Dissertation). Auburn University.

elastic materials, the loading portion leads to the buildup of potential energy, which is fully recovered in the unloading phase. However, in viscoelastic materials, while there is still a buildup of potential energy in the material during loading, there will also be a certain amount of energy dissipated (in the form of heat) during the loading and unloading process. The loading and unloading curves for the viscoelastic materials form a loop, which is called the *hysteresis loop*. The area inside the hysteresis loop represents the work or energy dissipated (usually as heat) during the loading and unloading process.

General Characteristics of Deformation in Musculoskeletal Tissues

Many nonbiologic materials such as metals and ceramics exhibit elastic–plastic loading behavior, which means that these materials will respond instantaneously to the application (or release) of a load. Unlike these materials, biologic tissues are composite materials that exhibit a time-dependency in response to loading (Litsky & Spector, 1994). Composite materials exhibit some degree of flow or creep in response to an applied load. The viscous response of the musculoskeletal tissues to loading should not be surprising given the high percentage of fluids present in the composition of the human body (including musculoskeletal tissues). For example, muscle is estimated to be composed of approximately 80% water, and even bone comprises approximately 30% water (Mitchell, Hamilton, Steggerda, & Bean, 1945). In tendons and ligaments, the extracellular matrix is composed of about 55–70% water (Kaya, Karahan, & Yilmer, 2019).

When a load is released on a viscoelastic material, the recovery from deformation is also a time-dependent viscoelastic process. Some of the deformation experienced in loading will be recovered immediately upon release of the load. However, the subsequent recovery of the deformation will require an extended period of time, and some portion of the deformation may never be recovered (Litsky & Spector, 1994). The loss of energy to viscous flow experienced by viscoelastic materials at any stress level cannot be fully recovered and is dependent on factors such as stress level, duration of loading, and temperature.

Isotropy Versus Anisotropy

One characteristic of a so-called "ideal material" is that the material is completely homogeneous and will exhibit the same properties (e.g., strain) no matter the direction of the applied stress. This property is known as *isotropy*. Biologic structures, on the other hand, are composed of structural elements that help to achieve desired material properties for their particular purpose, which always require a greater capacity for strength in certain directions as opposed to others. Thus, biological tissues tend to exhibit large differences in material strength depending on the direction of applied loading. This property is known as *anisotropy*. Musculoskeletal tissues are *anisotropic* by nature. That is to say, their material strength will vary significantly depending on the direction in which they are loaded. This becomes evident when observing material characteristics such as Young's modulus and ultimate stress in different loading modalities. For example, bone is approximately twice as strong in axial compression compared to shear loading. This appears to be a function of the microarchitecture of trabecular bone, whose design favors resistance to compressive forces (Sanyal, Bayraktar, Kwon, & Keaveny, 2012).

An example of the anisotropy of musculoskeletal tissues is shown in Table 6.2 for the ultimate stresses of human femoral cortical bone exposed to longitudinal, transverse, and shear loading (Reilly & Burstein, 1975). As can be seen in this table, the ultimate stress for this type of bone is

Table 6.2 Anisotropic Loading Responses of the Human Femoral Cortical Bone

Loading direction	Ultimate strength (MPa)
Longitudinal compression	205 (17.3)
Longitudinal tension	135 (15.6)
Shear	65 (4.0)

Reilly, D., & Burstein, A. (1975). The elastic and ultimate properties of compact bone tissue. *Journal of Biomechanics*, 8, 393–405 and Keaveny, A., Morgan, E., & Yeh, O. (2003). *Bone mechanics*. McGraw-Hill.

strongest when loaded in longitudinal compression, followed by longitudinal tension and shear. As can be seen, the highest mean ultimate stress (205 MPa in longitudinal compression) is more than 3 times greater than the lowest mean ultimate stress (65 MPa in shear). While the anisotropic properties of bone are often used as examples of this property, it is important to recognize that anisotropic behavior is observed for all musculoskeletal tissues, including soft tissues such as tendons and ligaments. For many musculoskeletal materials, anisotropy appears to be the result of the manner in which collagen fibers are distributed and aligned in the tissue (Chanda & Callaway, 2018).

Material Properties of Musculoskeletal Components

Tendons/Ligaments

Tendons and ligaments are both fibrous connective tissues made primarily of bundles of collagen fibers. Their different functions (tendons connect muscle to bone and ligaments connect bone to bone) do lead to some differences in structure (notably increased elastin fibers in ligaments). However, their material structure and response to loading are generally quite similar. Thus, the material characteristics of both will be considered together in this section.

Strength

A tendon is an exceptionally strong structure when under tension, and it has been estimated that 1 cm^2 is capable of bearing a static load of over 1,000 kg (Elliott, 1965; Shadwick, 1990). This represents approximately 50% of the tensile strength of stainless steel (Robi, Jakob, Matevz, & Matjaz, 2013). The cross-sectional area and the content and quality of the collagen are the primary determinants of tendon and ligament strength. It has been estimated that tendons can withstand stresses of over 100 MPa. In fact, stresses of up to 110 MPa have been measured in the Achilles tendon *in vivo* (Komi, Fukashiro, & Jarvinen, 1992). The human extensor digitorum longus was found to average approximately 100 MPa in tests of ultimate stress (Schechtman & Bader, 1997). However, different tendons appear to vary in terms of ultimate stress, in part due to factors such as aging and function (Shepherd & Screen, 2013). For example, in tests of ultimate tensile stress in the human patellar tendon, younger donors (aged 29–50) exhibited an average ultimate stress of 64.6 (±15.0) MPa, while older donors (aged 64–93) showed an average ultimate stress of only 53.6 (±10.0) MPa (Johnson et al., 1994). The ultimate tensile strength of the tendon has been shown to correlate highly ($r^2 = 0.79$) with the elastic modulus derived from the stress–strain curve, with stiffer tendons exhibiting increased strength (Matson, Konow, Miller, Konow, & Roberts, 2012).

Not surprisingly, differences in structural aspects of ligaments versus tendons have an impact on their relative strength. The fact that collagen fibrils are less densely packed in ligaments, compared to tendons means that ligaments have less tensile strength per cross-sectional area. The less-dense collagen fiber makeup of ligaments leads to more space for ground substance between the collagen fascicles, a substance that does not provide much assistance in resisting tensile forces (Amis, 2004). As a result of these structural differences, ligaments exhibit decreased tensile strength for a given cross-sectional area than do the denser and better-organized tendons. In general, it has been found that the ultimate stress of a typical ligament is approximately 40 MPa (Amis, 2004), whereas the ultimate stress of tendons has been known to exceed 100 MPa (Schechtman & Bader, 1997).

Strain

When tendons or ligaments are not under strain, there is some slack built into the tissue in the form of a wavy crimp of the collagen fibers. When stress is first applied, the initial response is the straightening out of these crimped fibers. This straightening of the crimped fibers results in the "toe" region of the stress–strain curve in which there is a relatively large increase in strain compared to the increase in stress in this region. The strain associated with the toe region is typically in the range of 1–2%. With a further increase in stress, the stress–strain curve enters a linear region, which ranges from approximately 2–4% strain in tendons. In this region, tendons and ligaments demonstrate elastic behavior and when unloaded they will return to their original form. If strain exceeds 4%, microscopic failure of collagen fibrils will begin to appear and will become more prevalent as strain continues to increase. When the strain exceeds the 8–10% strain range, macroscopic failure will occur (Sharma & Maffulli, 2005). While many tendons and ligaments fail at approximately 10% strain, there are reports of tendons failing in the 15–20% range (Johnson et al., 1994). In rare cases, ligaments with very high amounts of elastin can be strained to 30% without failure, though approximately 10–15% is more common (Martin, Burr, Sharkey, & Fyhrie, 2015). Resilience (the fraction of energy returned in cyclic length changes) in mammalian tendons has been shown to be generally high, ranging from 86 to 97% (Matson et al., 2012).

A simple model of the increase in stiffness observed during uncrimping and gradually increasing stiffness of tendons and ligaments can be seen in Figure 6.8 (Hollister, 2021). As this model

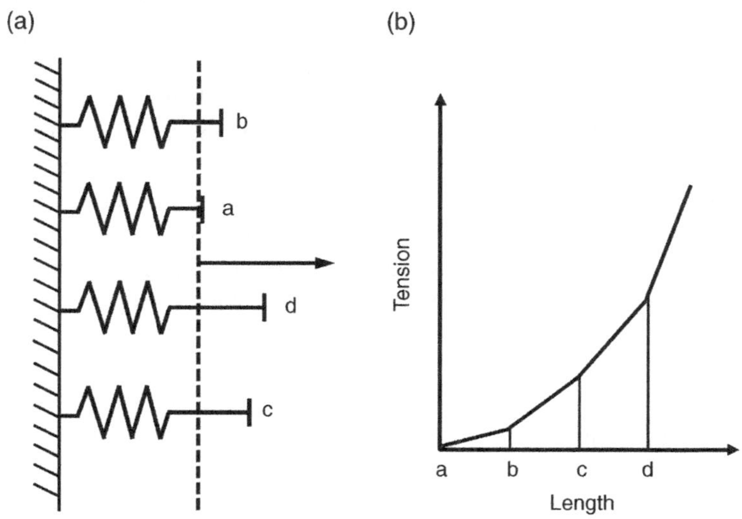

Figure 6.8 Model of the nonlinear stress–strain relationship in tendon and ligaments. (a) Model of individual collagen fibers engaging at different points as tendon/ligament experiences tensile stress, (b) summation of the effects of fibers engaging as tendon/ligament elongates. Redrawn from class notes: http://websites.umich.edu/~bme332/ch10ligten/bme332ligamenttendon.htm.

demonstrates, the stretching of the ligament causes individual collagen fibrils to straighten out and begin to take on the load. As more and more fibrils become engaged (each contributing a small amount of tensile force), the stiffness of the ligament will continue to increase. Once all fibers are engaged, continued increases in stress will cause fibers to endure increased strain, eventually leading to damage to individual fibers (a so-called microfailure). If stress increases further, additional fibers (especially those near the initial failure) will take on additional stress and may themselves fail. As these failures mount, eventually there will be a decreased stiffness response apparent in the stress–strain curve, and the material will start to fail, and may rupture. Studies have suggested that avulsion of the medial collateral ligament occurs at approximately 8% strain (Woo, Orlando, Camp, & Akeson, 1986).

Rupture strains in ligaments seem to be similar whether the rupture is due to cyclic loading or creep. In both cases, strain at rupture was in the range of 14–19% (Thornton, Schwab, & Oxland, 2007).

As mentioned previously, viscoelastic materials exhibit different responses based upon the rate at which they are loaded. This fact should be borne in mind as one considers the stress–strain curve discussed in the preceding section. If the material is loaded at a faster rate, it will exhibit increased stiffness. At slower rates of loading, the material will have a more viscous response, due to the water and proteoglycan constituents of the ligament. Thus, it can be said that the stress–strain curve can take different shapes even for the same tendon/ligament based on the rate of loading applied. Both ligaments and tendons also experience stress relaxation and creep. Results of studies on the viscoelastic properties of ligament show a nonlinear behavior in which the rate of creep is dependent upon stress level, and the rate of stress relaxation is dependent upon strain level (Provenzano, Lakes, Keenan, & Vanderby, 2001). Furthermore, relaxation has been found to be a faster process than creep in ligament, which is consistent with the previous experimental observations (Thornton, Oliynyk, Frank, & Shrive, 1997).

Elastic modulus

The elastic modulus of vertebrate tendons and ligaments has a wide range of values from 200–2,000 MPa, with an average of 1 GPa (Martin et al., 2015; Matson et al., 2012). Some of this variability may be due to real material property differences; however, some may also be due to differences in measurement techniques, including methods of determining the cross-sectional area of the tissue. Differences in sample storage and preparation may also impact obtained values for the elastic modulus. Recent advances in ultrasound have made it possible to measure the elastic modulus *in vivo* and track changes in the elastic modulus throughout an exercise intervention. For example, a study involving exercise in an older population has demonstrated a 69% increase in tendon elastic modulus with exercise (Reeves, Magnaris, & Narici, 2003). This would suggest that aged, exercised tendons may become stiffer and stronger and less susceptible to damage. It has also been suggested that changes in the elastic modulus with training may reduce susceptibility to fatigue damage (Buchanan & Marsh, 2001).

Anisotropy

Tendons and ligaments normally function in a uniaxial fashion; thus, there is generally little literature regarding the anisotropic features of these structures. However, even in normal joint function, there may be significant departures from pure uniaxial loading, including compression, shear, bending, and torsion, as well as complex combinations of these loading modes (Lynch, Johannessen, Wu, Jawa, & Elliott, 2003). In the few studies that have examined the transverse modulus, it has been found that the axially aligned modulus is on the order of two orders of magnitude greater than the transverse modulus of tendons (Quapp & Weiss, 1998). These results indicate that the elastic behavior of tendons is highly anisotropic and that off-axis loading of the tendon will encounter a material with a dramatically reduced stiffness and potentially more vulnerable to damage (Lynch et al., 2003).

Age

Researchers who have investigated the effects of aging on the mechanical properties of tendons and ligaments have reported varying findings. Maturation of tendon from youth to middle age is generally associated with an increase in elastic modulus and strength (Haut, Lancaster, & DeCamp, 1992; O'Brien, Reeves, Baltzopoulos, Jones, & Maganaris, 2010). Studies of human tendons tested *in vitro* have generally shown either a lack of change in the strength and elastic modulus of tendons due to age or a slight decline (Svensson, Heinemeier, Couppé, Kjaer, & Magnusson, 2016). These results are similar to those found in animal studies. Studies employing ultrasound to examine tendon deformation *in vivo* suggest either no change or a slight decline in modulus with aging (Carroll et al., 2008; Kubo, Kanehisa, Miyatani, Tachi, & Fukunaga, 2003; Stenroth, Peltonen, Cronin, Sipila, & Finni, 2012).

Effects of exercise

The effects of exercise on tendon/ligament mechanical properties have been studied by numerous authors (Svensson et al., 2016). Animal studies have reported findings indicating both no effect of exercise on mechanical properties of tendons (Legerlotz, Schjerling, Langberg, Bruggemann, & Niehoff, 2007; Viidik, 1969) or an increase in strength and stiffness (Woo et al., 1980; Woo, Gomez, Woo, & Akeson, 1982). In human studies, it has generally been found that tendon stiffness is greater in trained athletes (Couppe et al., 2008; Kubo, Kanehisa, Kawakami, & Fukunaga, 2000). Increase in strength appears to be more related to an increase in the size of the tendon, as opposed to an improvement in the mechanical quality of the tissue itself (Couppe et al., 2008). Ligaments experiencing beneficial exercise loading demonstrate an increase in mass, stiffness, and load to failure (West & Fu, 2005). As mentioned earlier, exercise in older adults led to an increase in the elastic modulus of tendons and a tendon that is less susceptible to damage (Reeves et al., 2003).

Effects of injury and repair

Healthy tendon comprises a matrix that is highly aligned in the direction of muscle loading (Sharma & Maffulli, 2005). However, injury to the tendon can result in significant and long-lasting detrimental effects on the tendon's mechanical properties. The mechanical strength of a damaged tendon is correlated with the phases of the damage and healing process (Gelberman, Goldberg, An, & Banes, 1987). In the initial inflammatory phase, the injured region is no longer filled with strong collagen fibers, but with clotted blood, fluid, and damaged tissues not capable of bearing a significant load. The tendon will begin to regain strength more quickly when fibroplasia begins along with the deposition of granulation tissue (Gelberman et al., 1987). During this process, collagen fibrils are laid down; however, in the initial absence of a mechanical stimulus, they are deposited in a random fashion and are lacking in strength. Over time, and with the guidance of controlled mechanical loading, the organization of the collagen architecture in the scar tissue repair will start to improve. Though improved, the scar tissue never achieves the organizational structure of the original tendon. As a result, the injured tendon rarely achieves the mechanical quality of the original tendon (Sharma & Maffulli, 2005).

Cartilage

There are three primary types of cartilage in the human body: hyaline (or articular) cartilage, fibrocartilage, and elastic cartilage, as discussed in Chapter 3. The material properties of hyaline cartilage and fibrocartilage will be considered separately. We will discuss their following characteristics: ultimate strength and stress–strain relationships.

Articular cartilage

Articular cartilage is a type of hyaline cartilage (as discussed in Chapter 3) that consists of a thin layer of low-friction soft tissue that overlies the joint surface, such as in diarthrodial joints (Lu & Mow, 2008). The main function of this material is to provide a smooth, lubricated surface allowing smooth joint motion and to facilitate the transmission of loads to the underlying bone. It offers several important biomechanical functions including wear resistance and shock absorption. While articular cartilage can and does experience damage due to fatigue, this material is one of the most resilient tissues of the human body in terms of its ability to withstand high cyclic loads (Sophia Fox, Bedi, & Rodeo, 2009).

Strength The structural strength of hyaline cartilage is primarily provided by type II collagen fibrils and proteoglycans (Nordin & Frankel, 2012). Type II collagen fibrils have high tensile strength and stiffness; however, they provide little in the way of compressive strength. A common method of testing the mechanical properties of articular cartilage is the indentation test. One of the benefits of this test is that mechanical properties of the cartilage can be measured while the cartilage is still attached to the bone (Lu & Mow, 2008).

The ultimate strength of both superficial and deep zones of the articular cartilage of human knees aged 8–91 years was performed in a study by Kempson (1982). In these tests, the cartilage was oriented according to the primary alignment of the collagen fibers and the ultimate tensile strength of the cartilage was recorded by a load cell using a strain rate of 5 mm/min. Results of this experiment (provided in Tables 6.3 and 6.4) demonstrated that the ultimate tensile strength increased in the teens and twenties but experienced a significant decline with advancing age (Kempson, 1982).

Strain Articular cartilage responds to stress in a nonlinear fashion, due to the large amount of water contained in the material (Lu & Mow, 2008). As a result, evaluation of the biomechanical behavior of articular cartilage usually involves dividing the response into two phases: (a) the interstitial fluid phase and (b) the porous-permeable solid phase. Examination of the tensile loading response of the material requires the use of low strain rates to avoid biphasic flow effects of the material (Nordin & Frankel, 2012). In a stress–strain curve for tensile strength, there are

Table 6.3 Tensile Fracture Stress (MPa) of Femoral Condyle Hyaline Cartilage in the Superficial and Deep (800 μm Beneath the Surface) Zones by Age in Males

	10–19	20–29	30–39	40–49	50–59	60–69	70–79	80–89	90–99
Sup	29 (20–38)	38 (32–50)	32 (21–36)	—	20 (15–26)	19 (17–23)	—	9 (7–11)	—
Deep	28 (27–29)	23 (14–32)	19 (13–29)	—	13 (12–18)	14 (9–17)	—	7 (3–9)	—

Based on Kempson, G. (1982). Relationship between the tensile properties of articular cartilage from the human knee and age. *Annals of the Rheumatic Diseases, 41*, 508–511.

Table 6.4 Tensile Fracture Stress (MPa) of Femoral Condyle Hyaline Cartilage Superficial and Deep (800 μm Beneath the Surface) Zones by Age in Females

	10–19	20–29	30–39	40–49	50–59	60–69	70–79	80–89	90–99
Sup	32 (27–37)	41 (36–44)	—	21 (12–28)	—	15 (13–20)	9 (7–11)	12 (8–16)	12 (9–16)
Deep	32 (29–47)	26 (21–28)	—	14 (12–19)	—	11 (5–15)	4 (1–10)	8 (5–10)	3 (1–4)

Based on Kempson, G. (1982). Relationship between the tensile properties of articular cartilage from the human knee and age. *Annals of the Rheumatic Diseases, 41*, 508–511.

three primary regions: the toe region, the linear region, and failure. The toe region is nonlinear with respect to stress and strain because this region represents the region where collagen fibers pull out from bone and realign (Nordin & Frankel, 2012). In the subsequent linear region, all the straightened and aligned fibers are being stretched (Figure 6.9). Failure occurs when these collagen fibers rupture (Figure 6.9). The ultimate strain experienced by bovine cartilage specimens was approximately 25% when loaded in a plane parallel to the preferred fiber orientation and 30% when loaded in a perpendicular fashion (Sasazaki, Shore, & Seedhom, 2006). Rupture of the articular surface led to rapid failure in subjacent layers with continued loading (Sasazaki et al., 2006).

Elastic modulus The elastic modulus of articular cartilage has been studied by several authors (Kempson, Muir, Pollard, &Tuke, 1973; Silver, Bradica, & Tria, 2001; Silver, Bradica, & Tria, 2002). Tensile stress–strain curves indicate that the superficial zone of articular cartilage has an elastic modulus of approximately 7.0 GPa parallel to the cleavage line and 2.2 GPa perpendicular to the cleavage line. The large elastic modulus in type II collagen fibers of healthy articular cartilage is comparable to that of type I collagen in tendons and indicates a large capacity for energy storage during load-bearing activities as walking (Silver et al., 2002). Elastic modulus of deeper layers has been found to exhibit decreased elastic moduli (4.91–5.64 GPa), which may indicate a lack of parallel orientation of the collagen fibrils in these regions (Silver et al., 2002).

Anisotropy Articular cartilage demonstrates an anisotropic response to tensile loading in the superficial layer (Kamalanathan & Broom, 1993; Kempson, 1979; Sasazaki et al., 2006). When one compares the ratio of tensile strength in the direction parallel to the original fiber orientation versus perpendicular loading, one finds that the ratio is approximately 1.6–2.0 in bovine specimens but is reported to be closer to 3.0 in human cartilage (Kempson, 1979). A notable finding in studies of the mechanical properties of articular cartilage is that the collagen meshwork would reorient according to the direction of loads applied. This reorientation of the collagen becomes more prominent at higher strains when loaded in the perpendicular direction (Kamalanathan & Broom, 1993; Sasazaki et al., 2006).

Age As shown in Tables 6.3 and 6.4, the ultimate strength of cartilage declines significantly after the age of 70. Aging also appears to decrease the deformation observed in articular cartilage; however, sex and physical training status do not appear to alter cartilage deformation significantly (Eckstein, Hudelmaier, & Putz, 2006). A study examining patellar cartilage thickness compared a younger cohort of men and women (aged 18–40 years) to an older cohort (50–75 years) (Hudelmaier et al., 2001). Results demonstrated no significant difference in the cartilage thickness in the younger versus older men; however, a significantly lower thickness (−12%) was observed in the

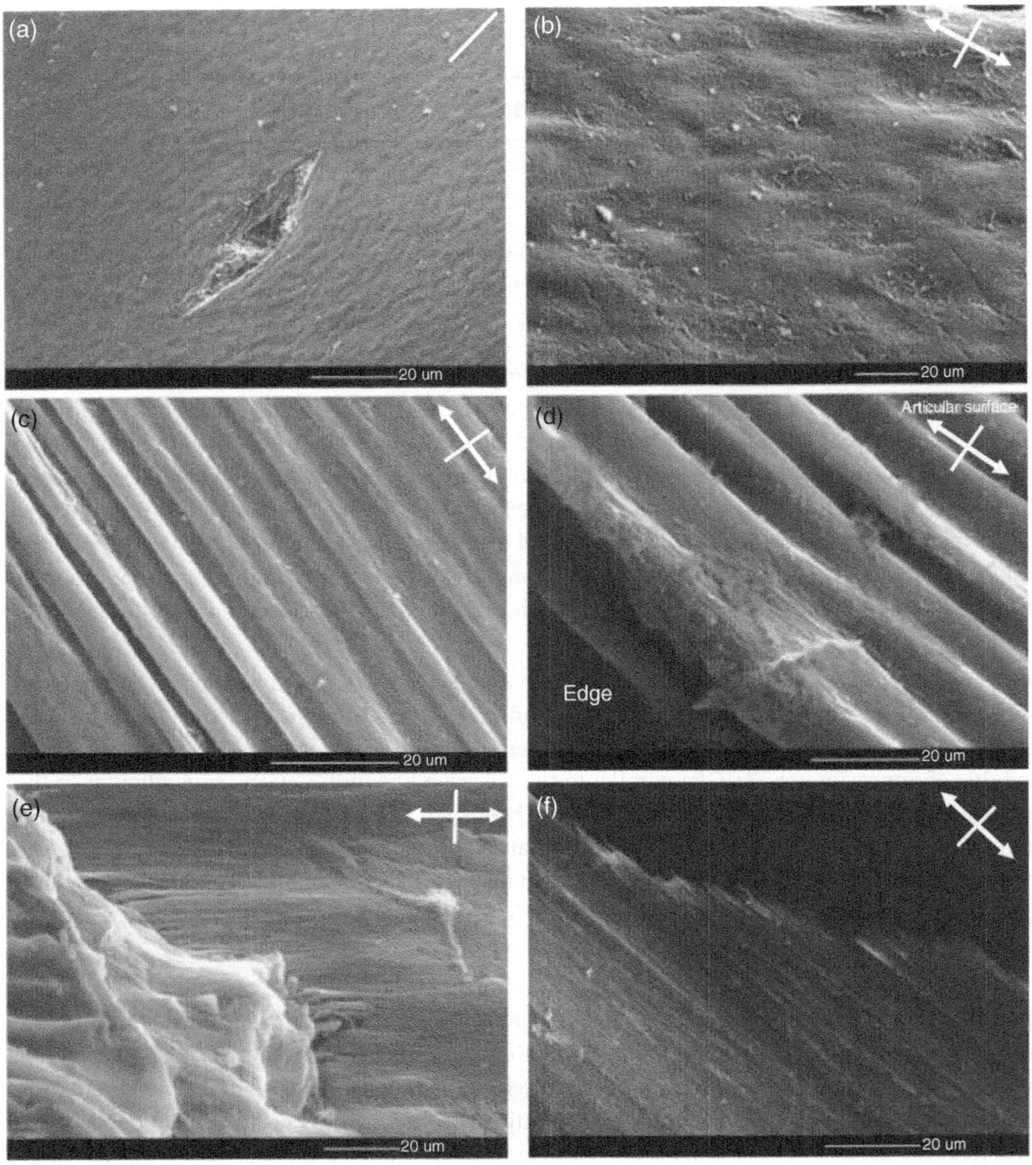

Figure 6.9 Scanning electron micrographs showing the mechanism of cartilage failure in the tensile mode in the perpendicular group. Double-headed arrow represents the direction of the applied strain. Strain was applied perpendicular to the split white line. (a) at 0% strain, the fibrillar meshwork within the articular surface was predominantly oriented in the direction of the split line. (b) As the strain increased, the ridges became evident on the articular surface. (c) At 15% strain, bundles of ridges (~3 microns in diameter) that were aligned parallel to the direction of the applied strain were evident. (d) At 25% strain, there were initial signs of rupture in the sheath-like material covering the ridges, which exposed the individual fibrils inside the ridges themselves. Much greater strain was required for fibrillar reorientation in the perpendicular group, compared to the parallel one. (e) At 30% strain, the articular surface ruptures. This rupture exposed the fibrils within the subjacent layer, which aligned parallel to the applied strain. (f) Finally, the rupture spread from the articular surface throughout the thickness of the articular cartilage and resulted in complete failure. Sasazaki, Y., Shore, R., & Seedhom, B. (2006). Deformation and failure of cartilage in the tensile mode. *Journal of Anatomy*, 208, 681–694.

older women as opposed to the younger group. On other joint surfaces of the knee, this study found age-related cartilage thinning of approximately 4% per decade in both men and women (Hudelmaier et al., 2001).

Effects of exercise In the past couple of decades, *in vivo* assessment of both the deformation of human articular cartilage during short-term exercise and long-term functional adaptations due to regular exercise has become possible through the use of *magnetic resonance imaging* (MRI) (Eckstein et al., 2006). Results of these studies have demonstrated that human cartilage shows little in the way of deformation during physiological loading and that the deformation experienced is regained in a relatively short period of time (Eckstein et al., 2006). Factors such as age, sex, and training activities appear to lead to a decrease in deformation; however, an absence of loading is associated with thinning of the articular cartilage (Eckstein et al., 2006). Cartilage that experiences intermittent compressive loads appears to result in increased proteoglycan synthesis (Parkkinen, Lammi, Helminen, & Tammi, 1992); however, increased loading does not appear to increase cartilage thickness in elite athletes (Carter, Wong, & Orr, 1991).

Effects of injury and repair Osteoarthritis is a degenerative disease of articular cartilage and is believed to be associated with an enzymatic cleavage of cartilage collagen and proteoglycans that may lead to damage development that significantly decreases the energy storage capacity of cartilage. The elastic modulus may be reduced by an order of magnitude in osteoarthritic cartilage, compared to healthy cartilage. The resulting loss of elastic energy storage in the cartilage may result in further degradation of the cartilage tissue (including fibrillation and fissure development). These degenerative changes may lead to further stress concentrations in the tissue, leading to accelerated wear with further exposure to repeated stress (Silver et al., 2001). If the injury extends to the subchondral bone, a spontaneous repair can occur; however, the reparative tissue (fibrocartilage) is substandard (less durable and lacking in smoothness) (Hayes, Brower, & John, 2001).

Fibrocartilage

As described in Chapter 2, fibrocartilage is typically found in regions where tendons and ligaments meet bone where it serves as a transitional material. Regions that employ fibrocartilage include the intervertebral disc, the menisci of knee joints, and the temporomandibular joint in the jaw. Fibrocartilage protects bony surfaces through its tough yet pliable tissue. Fibrocartilage is found in regions of the body typically subjected to compression. It has been postulated that fibrocartilaginous zones within chondral insertions may act to reduce fatigue failure in bones by providing a more gradual transition from soft tissue to hard bone (Schneider, 1956). Functionally, fibrocartilage interdigitates with the underlying bone and serves to increase the cross-sectional area of the interface between the two structures (Doschak & Zernicke, 2005). This serves to decrease stress concentrations when loads are experienced.

Strength The reported tensile mechanical strength of fibrocartilage is lower than that of articular cartilage. In general, the tensile strength of fibrocartilage (menisci and intervertebral discs) is reported to be approximately 10 MPa. The ultimate stress of fibrocartilage was examined in a study of the meniscus (Bullough, Munuera, Murphy, & Weinstein, 1970). In this study, the ultimate stress of the lateral meniscus was tested for three regions (i.e., anterior, central, and posterior) using the axis parallel to the fiber orientation. Results of these tests demonstrated ultimate stresses of 10.37 MPa for the anterior region, 6.31 MPa for the central region, and 6.87 MPa for the posterior location (Bullough et al., 1970). On the other hand, when ultimate stress was tested in a perpendicular axis to the alignment of the fibers, the ultimate stress found in the anterior, central, and posterior regions of the meniscus were found to be 0.80, 0.88, and 0.54 MPa, respectively, demonstrating anisotropic nature of the fibrocartilage.

Strain The strain of fibrocartilage at rupture (about 13%) is less than that of articular cartilage (about 25%) but greater than the average strain of tendon at failure (8–10%) (Yamada, 1970). In compression, the strength of fibrocartilage is similar to that of hyaline cartilage but exhibits less stiffness (Benjamin & Evans, 1990).

Elastic modulus The elastic modulus of fibrocartilage is about half that of articular cartilage (Arnoczky, Adams, Dehaven, Eyre, & Mow, 1988; Procter, Schmidt, Whipple, Kelly, & Mow, 1989). Table 6.5 provides information regarding the elastic modulus of both lateral and medial meniscus specimens by region (proximal, middle, and distal), with an overall average of 10.61 MPa. As can be seen from this table, the lateral meniscus demonstrates higher stiffness characteristics when compared to the medial meniscus. Furthermore, the middle zones of both menisci tended to show lower elastic moduli as compared to proximal and distal specimens. In general, distal specimens demonstrated increased stiffness compared to the proximal specimens.

Anisotropy Structures made of fibrocartilage (e.g., menisci and intervertebral discs) are composed primarily of type I collagen and, as demonstrated by the ultimate strength characteristics of fibrocartilage earlier, are anisotropic. Thus, mechanical properties will vary considerably based on the direction of testing relative to the collagen mesh and are the result of the interaction of the material constituents of the tissue. Fibrocartilage has two distinct phases: a solid phase that is due to the presence of collagen fibers, cells, proteoglycans, and proteins (and their orientation), and a fluid phase consisting of water and dissolved electrolytes (Gharpuray, 1998). The viscoelastic response observed is the result of fluid flow through the material and molecular relaxation of collagen and proteoglycans (Hayes & Bodine, 1978). The anisotropic behavior is primarily the result of the orientation of the collagen fiber inside the proteoglycan gel (Gharpuray, 1998).

Table 6.5 Elastic Modulus Values (MPa) for Fibrocartilage in Lateral and Medial Menisci

	Anterior	**Central**	**Posterior**	**Average**
Lateral				
• Proximal	10.00 (4.29)	14.17 (5.88)	14.62 (9.62)	12.93 (6.46)
• Middle	4.07 (1.86)	10.14 (4.65)	4.21 (1.26)	6.14 (2.62)
• Distal	13.01 (8.76)	13.24 (6.96)	21.24 (6.30)	15.83 (7.37)
Medial				
• Proximal	6.75 (5.15)	9.31 (7.46)	13.53 (8.44)	9.86 (6.96)
• Middle	3.59 (1.43)	5.60 (2.23)	2.03 (0.54)	3.74 (1.37)
• Distal	9.50 (6.35)	16.51 (9.00)	22.62 (7.18)	16.21 (7.47)

Values in parentheses represent the standard deviation.
Based on Bullough, P., Munuera, L., Murphy, J., & Weinstein, A. (1970). The strength of menisci of the knee as it relates to their fine structure. *Journal of Bone and Joint Surgery (British)*, 52, 564–567.

Aging Among the numerous effects of age are changes in the materials constituting the joints, including fibrocartilage. These changes can lead to decreases in joint mobility and may restrict an individual's ability to participate in a wide range of activities. One of the notable changes in fibrocartilage with age is a loss in water content, believed to stiffen joints of which fibrocartilage is a structural member and will result in decreased joint movement (Buckwalter, 1995; Levangie & Norkin, 2005). Avascularity often accompanies the development of degeneration, as seen in the central region of the menisci in the knee joint (Ghosh & Taylor, 1987) or the triangular cartilage disc of the wrist joint (Mikic, 1978). Other degenerative changes to fibrocartilage may also occur, including a loss of cellularity and increase in the proportion of type II collagen (Buckwalter, 1995). Disorganization of the extracellular matrix, affecting the biomechanical properties of fibrocartilage can also occur due to age or other influences (Arnoczky et al., 1988; Oda, Tanaka, & Tsuzuki, 1988).

Effects of exercise Studies indicate that the mechanical loading of fibrocartilage plays a major role in the physiologic, pathologic, and repair responses of this tissue (McNulty & Guilak, 2015). As with other tissues, the benefits of exercise require a certain amount of loading (physiologic loading), but not an excessive degree (pathologic loading). Physiologic loading of the meniscus, for example, leads to beneficial changes in the composition of fibrocartilage and can lead to decreased matrix degradation and increased anti-inflammatory cytokines. A modest amount of dynamic compression (~10% strain) leads to increased anabolic processes and decreased effects of the inflammatory cytokine IL-1, which can improve tissue repair response. Cyclic hydrostatic pressure and tensile strain on the meniscus can lead to an increased expression of anabolic genes and a decrease in catabolic and inflammatory responses. Pathological loading can include too little or too much strain. For example, immobilization can lead to negative impacts on meniscal structure and function, leading to decreased cell viability and an increase in the expression of proinflammatory cytokines. Too much loading (greater than 20% compressive strain) will lead to catabolic responses in the tissue and increased inflammation. Strains over this level will lead to cell death and a reduction in tissue metabolism (McNulty & Guilak, 2015).

Effects of injury and repair Fibrocartilage is an avascular structure, which makes it susceptible to degeneration. Degeneration of fibrocartilage may occur as the result of aging or in response to biomechanical loading or a combination of the two (Benjamin & Evans, 1990). Degeneration is apparent in fibrocartilage of knee joint and intervertebral discs (Benjamin & Evans, 1990). As the discs degenerate, fibrocartilage will proliferate into the inner annulus and nucleus pulposus, increasing the stiffness and reducing the elasticity of these latter tissues. This often follows the mineralization and bony invasion of the cartilage endplate (Oda et al., 1988). Mineralization and bone invasion will considerably reduce the pliability of the cartilage endplate.

Bone

Bones are a major constituent of the musculoskeletal system and are important in providing strength and structural stability to the body. The material properties of bone are dynamic and complex in nature and a bone experiences both short-term and long-term changes during its lifetime. Bone will adapt in the short term (to the extent possible) to the mechanical loads it experiences and will add bone mass to regions experiencing higher stress and will resorb bone in areas exposed to low stresses, per Wolff's law (Mow & Huiskes, 2005). Yet, there are also studies showing that increasing weight-bearing loads and muscle-loading exercise to excessive levels is associated with diminishing returns in bone mass and quality and can even lead to increased stress fractures

(Bourrin, Genty, Palle, Gharib, & Alexandre, 1994; Saunier & Chapurlat, 2018; Umemura, Ishiko, Yamauchi, Kurono, & Mashiko, 1997).

Strength

The ultimate strength of bone varies considerably according to the gender and age of the individual and the mineral content of the bone. Some of the factors known to influence bone material properties include collagen fiber orientation, degree of mineralization of the bone matrix, geometry, porosity, and presence of fatigue microdamage (Martin, 1993). In addition, as shown in Table 6.2, bone strength is highly influenced by the nature of the load experienced. For example, bone is strongest in compression, then in tension (66% of compressive strength), and is much weaker in shear (only 33% of compressive strength) (Reilly & Burstein, 1975). The age and sex of an individual also play a large role in bone strength. Figure 6.10 provides the compressive and tensile strengths of femoral cortical bone for males and females by age based on data by Havaldar and colleagues (Havaldar et al., 2014).

Strain

It can be challenging to measure the stress–strain relationship of whole bones due to the variation in material properties and the geometry of the whole bone. Usually, such tests are performed using 3- or 4-point bending tests in which the bone is supported at the end and subjected to point loads along its length to ascertain the tolerable bending and shear stresses (Sharir, Barak, & Shahar, 2008). More frequently, bone samples of uniform shape are obtained from whole bone and are used to estimate the bone material properties (Sharir et al., 2008). Yamada (1970) estimated the ultimate elongation strain on bone as between 1.41 and 1.59% (Yamada 1970).

Elastic modulus

Young's modulus can be estimated from such tests but must be considered only as estimates due to the complexities and lack of homogeneity of the bone material and geometry. Due to the variability of samples, testing methods, and anisotropy, a wide range of values for Young's modulus have been observed in bones. The axial modulus for cortical bone averages approximately 20 GPa, while the

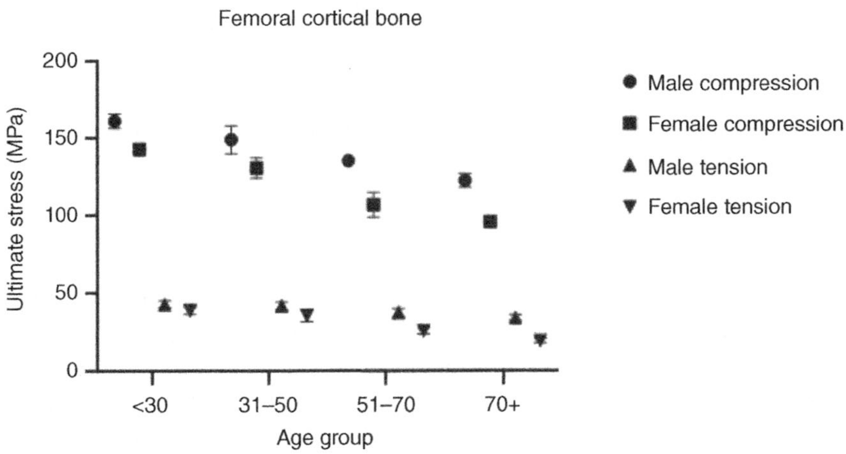

Figure 6.10 Ultimate stress values for femoral cortical bone samples from males and females by age group (Based on Havaldar, R., Pilli, S., & Putti, B. (2014). Insights into the effects of tensile and compressive loadings on human femur bone. *Advanced Biomedical Research, 3*, 101).

modulus for cortical bone in the transverse direction is only about 40–50% of this value (Sharir et al., 2008). The elastic modulus for trabecular bone has been found to be approximately 10% lower than that of cortical bone in the axial direction (Bayraktar et al., 2004). When loaded transversely, however, the modulus for trabecular bone is found to be slightly higher than for transversely loaded cortical bone. In addition, the modulus for cortical bone loaded transversely has been found to be approximately 40% lower than in axial tests (Turner, Rho, Takano, Tsui, & Pharr, 1999).

The modulus of bone is clearly a function of bone density (Helgason et al., 2008). Studies examining this relationship have been performed, and while all agree that there is a positive correlation between the two, there is immense variability between studies. This is undoubtedly due to several factors, including the complexities of experimental techniques to measure Young's modulus and variation of the geometry of the specimens. The relationship between density and stiffness also appears to depend to a degree on the location in the body (Helgason et al., 2008). Bone mineral content (a measure that combines bone density and size) has also been shown to be positively correlated with stiffness (Meyers, Chen, Lin, & Seki, 2008).

Anisotropy

Bones are constructed of two types of bone, cortical and trabecular (cancellous), which are made of similar materials, but which exhibit greatly different structural characteristics (as described in Chapter 3). Both types of bone exhibit anisotropic properties, with greater strength when loaded in compression than when loaded in tension or shear. Table 6.2 provides the results of tests of ultimate strength on human cortical bone in longitudinal compression and tension, and in shear loading (Keaveny, Morgan, & Yeh, 2003; Reilly & Burstein, 1975). These results demonstrate that the tensile strength of bone is approximately two-thirds of compression, and that shear strength is only about one-third of the compressive strength. The elastic modulus of bone also demonstrates anisotropy, for example, the elastic modulus of cortical bone is approximately 20 GPa, while the modulus in transverse loading is approximately half this value (Sharir et al., 2008). A structure model index (SMI) is widely used to measure the prevalence of plate- or rod-like structures in trabecular bone. This index exploits the change in surface curvature that occurs as a structure varies from spherical (SMI = 4; i.e., "rods") to cylindrical (SMI = 3) to planar (SMI = 0, "i.e., plates") (Hildebrand & Ruegsegger, 1997; Salmon, Ohlsson, Shefelbine, & Doube, 2015). The degree of anisotropy is decreased if the trabeculae structure changes from more rod-like to more plate-like (indicated by a decreased SMI) because the plate-like structure is thought to be stronger (Liu et al., 2010). Such a change, which typically occurs in response to loading in young adults (Massicotte et al., 2015), increases not just trabecular bone strength but also overall bone strength. An increase in the degree of anisotropy is indicative of disorganization in trabecular structure and distribution and an overall weaker bone that is less resistant to mechanical loading due to increased stiffness (Ding et al., 2003; Ding, Odgaard, & Hvid, 2003).

Age

Aging has been shown to significantly affect the stiffness of cortical bone. In a study examining the elastic modulus of cortical bone specimens aged 35–92 years using a 3-point bending test, it was determined that the elastic modulus decreased at a rate of 2.3% per decade (Zioupos & Currey, 1998). Aging is generally associated with the loss of bone "quality," which may be associated with factors such as architectural changes, changes in the compositional components, and events at the micromechanical level, such as accumulation of microdamage (Zioupos, 2001). This loss of bone "quality" includes increases in marrow area, thinning (cortical and trabecular), intracortical bone porosity, osteoclastic resorptive spaces, arterial spaces, and woven bone formation (Turner, 2007).

Effects of exercise

Exercise has an immense effect on the strength of bone and has an important role to play with respect to the maintenance of healthy bone, especially with respect to fractures, including osteoporotic fractures (Russo, 2009). A key reason for this is the critical influence of muscle force on the mechanical properties of bone (Russo, 2009). It is apparent that bone does not respond in an anabolic manner when subjected to static loads. Instead, it responds best to dynamic loads, which provides a maximal osteogenic mechanical stimulus. Such stimuli can consist of a limited number of high magnitude activities (Rubin & Lanyon, 1985); however, lower magnitude dynamic activities can also be used as long as the frequency is sufficiently high (Rubin et al., 2004).

Effects of injury and repair

Injury to bone is related to the mechanical loading experienced and the strength of the bone. For example, the strength of bone decreases with age as a result of bone loss, and fracture risk increases as a result. Data from prospective studies demonstrated that a decrease in standard deviation by one in bone mass can lead to a 50–100% increase in fracture risk of non-spinal bone (Melton et al., 1993). It is generally accepted that the repair and remodeling of bone is activated by damage development and/or mechanical load. Unlike most other tissues, bone is capable of returning to pre-injury strength (Russo, 2009). Bone appears to have unique plasticity in this regard, and one that appears to be present at all ages. Bone health and the bone healing process appear to be strongly correlated with forces generated by its attached muscles. Clearly, these structures are both anatomically and functionally linked, and it appears that muscle mass and strength are critical to both healing and the maintenance of bone health (Russo, 2009).

Skeletal Muscle

Muscle is capable of producing remarkable amounts of force and may be required to do so repeatedly. While this capability would seem important and beneficial for an individual, it is clear that the repetitive forces generated by the muscle are sufficient to lead to damage to the muscle itself as well as to tendons and other musculoskeletal structures (Proske & Morgan, 2001). Muscle also performs several other functions essential to the maintenance of bodily health. For example, skeletal muscle plays important roles in blood circulation (via the skeletal muscle pump), breathing, control of blood pressure, the body's thermal homeostasis, and endocrine function, to name a few. In addition, muscles also serve as a storehouse for amino acids used by the body in the synthesis of organ-specific proteins (Wolfe, 2006).

Strength

Relatively few studies have tested the material strength of skeletal muscle. In a study of mechanically tested native bone-muscle samples obtained from human femora, it was found that muscle fibers tested in line with parallel fiber orientation ($47.6\,N \pm 11.5$) yielded higher tensile strength than those with perpendicular fiber orientation ($14.8\,N \pm 4.1$), indicating a significant anisotropic response. The location of failure was generally observed to be in the central region of muscle fibers (Schleifenbaum et al., 2016).

A separate study examined mechanical responses of goat muscle to tensile loading (Kuthe, Uddanwadiker, & Ramteke, 2014). Five samples of goat skeletal muscle were performed at a load rate of 1 mm/min both in line with the fiber orientation and at a 45° angle with respect to the fiber orientation. Muscle was found to be considerably stiffer along the axis of fiber orientation and exhibited a tensile ultimate strength of 0.44 MPa (110 N maximum load), while at a 45° orientation to the fiber orientation, the ultimate strength was 0.23 MPa with a maximum load of 43 N. The displacement to failure was less in the longitudinal direction (15.3 mm) compared to the 45° off-axis orientation (17.8 mm) (Kuthe et al., 2014).

Takaza and colleagues reported a study on the passive mechanical properties of skeletal muscle using the longissimus dorsi muscle from the pig (Takaza, Moerman, Gindre, Lyons, & Simms, 2013). These authors performed a tensile test on passive muscle along the muscle fiber axis as well as 30°, 45°, 60°, and 90° to that axis. These authors found that the transverse (90°) condition showed a linear response and the highest stiffness; however, failure occurred at relatively small levels of stretch. In the axis of the muscle fibers, the strain was nonlinear in nature and much less stiff, and failure occurred at much higher levels of strain. At intermediate angles of pull, the muscle exhibited a systematic progression of stress response in line with the responses described earlier (Takaza et al., 2013).

Strain

The stress–strain characteristics of muscle vary significantly according to its contraction state. Passive (uncontracted) muscle exhibits a nonlinear stress–strain curve, as seen in Figure 6.11. As passive muscle starts being pulled from resting length, little resistance to stress is initially encountered. However, as individual muscle fibers continue to stretch some fibers will reach their passive stretch limit and resistance to stress starts to increase. As more and more muscle fibers reach their passive stretching limit, resistance to stress begins to increase exponentially and reaches a maximum strain at about 1.6 times the initial muscle length.

The contracting (tetanized) muscle exhibits a dramatically different curve. As seen in Figure 6.11, the starting length for the tetanized muscle is one-half of the resting length of the uncontracted muscle. The contracted muscle fibers exhibit an immediate and linear increase in strain in response to tension. This relationship continues until the muscle reaches the original resting length. At this length, the binding of actin and myosin filaments is optimized. A decrease in tension is subsequently observed with increasing length, indicating that the actin-myosin binding sites are now decreasing. However, after a period of time, the muscle's passive elements begin to kick in, and increasing length starts to demonstrate increasing tension development in the muscle, to a point where it exceeds the tension achieved with the actin-myosin binding sites were optimal.

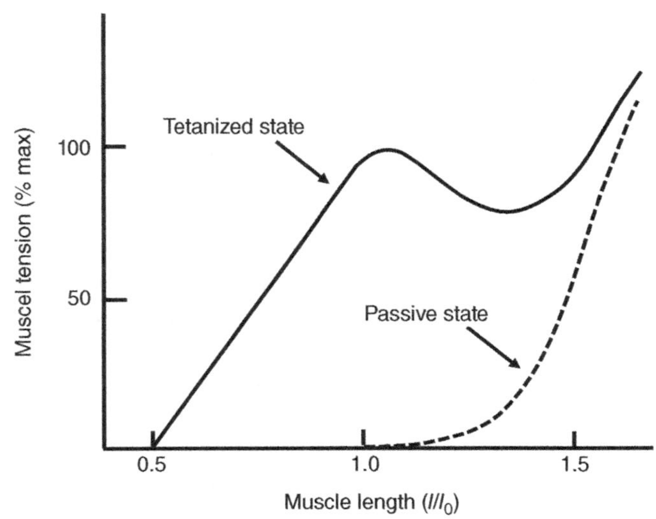

Figure 6.11 Muscle strain response in tetanized and passive states. Redrawn from Aubert, X., Roquet, M. L., & Van Der Elst, J. (1951). The tension-length diagram of the frog's sartorius muscle. *Archives internationales de physiologie, 59*, 239–241.

Elastic modulus

As mentioned previously, Young's modulus for tendons averages approximately 1 GPa. This modulus is somewhat higher than a softwood such as pine (0.6 GPa). The modulus for bone is approximately 20 GPa, similar to that seen in some hardwood trees (~15 GPa). In contrast, the modulus for a passive muscle under tension is approximately 10 kPa, which is slightly lower than that of rubber (20 kPa). These results indicate that bone is the stiffest and muscle the least stiff material of the connective tissues (Lieber, 2002).

Anisotropy

Studies of the mechanical and structural properties of skeletal muscle (such as anisotropy) are less prevalent than for most other materials. However, as might be expected with a material having a primarily unidirectional fiber structure, muscles demonstrate significant anisotropy when loaded in directions that are off-axis. A study examining the tensile loading of muscle from the goat was performed in which tests were either tested along the muscle length versus 45° off the main axis of the muscle. Results of this analysis demonstrated that greater stiffness was observed in the direction of the fibers compared to tensile loading at a 45° angle. In the longitudinal direction, the ultimate tensile strength exhibited was 0.44 MPa with a maximum load of 110 N, while in the direction 45° inclined to the muscle fibers, the ultimate tensile strength was 0.23 MPa with a maximum load of 43 N. This demonstrates that as fiber orientation changes within the muscle, the stiffness of the muscle tissue will change as well, demonstrating anisotropic mechanical behavior (Kuthe et al., 2014).

Age

The force output of muscle typically experiences a significant decline due to the aging process. On average, there is a 30% decrease in muscle strength and a 40% reduction in muscle mass from the second to seventh decades of life (Rogers & Evans, 1993). The loss of muscle mass is a significant factor in the reduction in force and reflects a loss of both Type I and (especially) Type II muscle fibers, along with a reduction in the size of remaining fibers. However, it has been clearly demonstrated that resistance training exercises can elicit moderate to strong effects in terms of increasing muscle force output in healthy older people (Liberman, Fortia, Beyer, & Bautmans, 2017). If the resistance training is of sufficient magnitude and duration, muscle hypertrophy can be achieved along with an increased rate of oxygen uptake, increases in capillary growth, and increased oxidative enzyme activity (Rogers & Evans, 1993). These adaptations may have beneficial effects on several age-related diseases (e.g., obesity, coronary artery disease, Type II diabetes, and osteoporosis) (Rogers & Evans, 1993).

Effects of exercise

The positive adaptations observed in muscles exposed to resistance training are well known (Nordin & Frankel, 2012). A recent review of the effects of resistance training in randomized control trials of older adults provides a good overview of typical adaptations observed and identifies factors that appear to maximize these effects (Borde, Hortobágyi, & Granacher, 2015). For example, all studies demonstrated significant strength improvements with resistance training, with large effects seen in one repetition maximum weightlifting for both the upper and lower extremities and moderate effects in maximum voluntary contractions (MVCs) in lower extremity studies. In this review, resistance training was found to result in small effects in muscle size; however, other studies have reported that resistance training results in significant muscular hypertrophy, with women experiencing a gain of about 80% of that experienced by males (similar to the percentage strength gains observed between sexes) (Brumitt & Cuddeford, 2015). Factors associated with increased strength gain include the training period (the more weeks of training the better), the training intensity (70–79% of the one-repetition max), and the total time under tension (6 s provided the maximal gain) (Borde et al., 2015).

In terms of rest, it was found that a rest period of 60 s between sets was associated with larger strength gains and that a rest period of 4 s between repetitions within a set was found to be optimal (Borde et al., 2015).

Lack of exercise (decreased use of muscle force) will, of course, lead to decreased strength and muscle atrophy (Gao, Arfat, Wang, & Goswami, 2018). Several conditions may result in disuse of muscle and wasting of muscle tissues, including diabetes (Bonaldo & Sandri, 2013), cancers (Stephens et al., 2010), cardiovascular disease (Gordon, Kelleher, & Kimball, 2013), muscular diseases and/or neurodegenerative disorders (Sandri, 2010; Verdijk et al., 2012), and conditions that lead to immobilization or bed rest. These conditions will lead to decreased muscle mass, strength, reduced muscle fiber cross-sectional area, changes in fiber type distribution, and changes in protein metabolism (decreased synthesis and increased degradation) (Gao et al., 2018).

Effects of injury and repair

Skeletal muscle continuously adapts to changes in its mechanical environment through modifications in gene expression and protein stability that affect its physiological function and mass. However, mechanical stresses commonly exceed the parameters that induce adaptations, producing instead acute injury. Damage to skeletal muscle is often the result of unaccustomed work or exercise, particularly exercise that involved repeated eccentric (i.e., muscle lengthening) contractions (Clarkson & Hubal, 2002). It should not be surprising that repeated eccentric exertions are associated with injury to muscle fibers, as this mode of contraction is known to result in the highest level of force development, compared to isometric or concentric muscle contractions (Nordin & Frankel, 2012). The latter two contraction modes can also lead to muscle injury although eccentric contractions have a much greater likelihood of doing so and in a shorter timeframe (Armstrong, 1984).

Healing time for exercise-induced muscle damage is dependent on the damage accrued during the exercise, which is, in turn, due to the force magnitude experienced by the muscle and the number of repetitions performed (Peake, Neubauer, Della Gatta, & Nosaka, 2017). The immediate post-exercise strength loss is a useful measure with which to estimate the duration of strength loss (Crameri et al., 2007; Malm et al., 2004). If the strength loss remains <20%, recovery will take (on average) 2 days. If the strength loss is 50%, muscle strength may not be fully recovered for more than a week (Jamurtas et al., 2005; Paulsen, Crameri, et al., 2010; Paulsen, Egner, et al. 2010).

Material Properties of Peripheral Nerves

Peripheral nerves are complex structures of axons, and their myelin sheaths are bundled together by several layers of connective tissue (see Chapter 4). Biomechanically, they have been described as cables that gain flexibility and elasticity at the expense of strength when small fibers are substituted for larger ones (Beel, Groswald, & Luttges, 1984). Peripheral nerves are tethered proximally to the spinal cord, at branch points and to the surrounding paraneural and myofascial tissues. As a consequence, they undergo mild to moderate tensile stress, shear or compression forces during limb and joint movement and locomotion, particularly at sites where nerves pass around joints. They can also undergo high axial or orthogonal (perpendicular) tensile stress during high-energy,

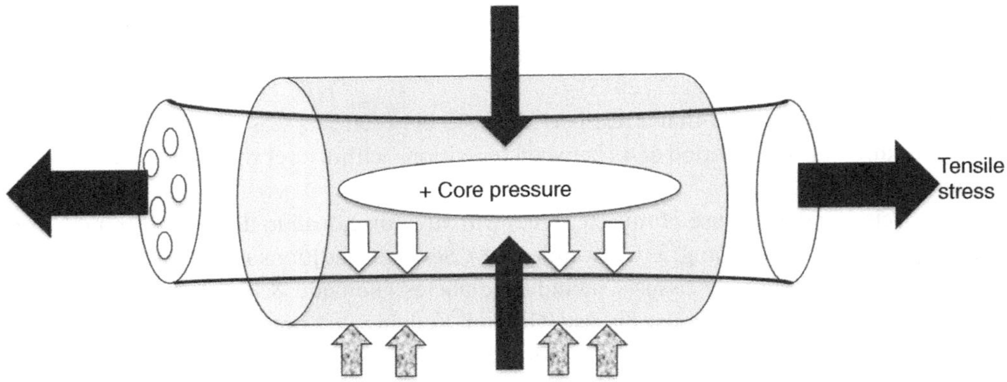

Figure 6.12 Physical stresses placed on peripheral nerves. Tensile stress applied longitudinally elongates the nerve (and increases the strain). The transverse contraction that occurs during this elongation is greatest in the middle of the section undergoing tensile stress. Positive core pressure is constrained by the outer denser fascial sheaths of the nerve. Modified from Topp, K. S., & Boyd, B. S. (2006). Structure and biomechanics of peripheral nerves: Nerve responses to physical stresses and implications for physical therapist practice. *Physical Therapy*, 86(1), 92–109. https://doi.org/10.1093/ptj/86.1.92 and Walbeehm, E. T., Afoke, A., Wit, T., Holman, F., Hovius, S. E., & Brown, R. A. (2004). Mechanical functioning of peripheral nerves: Linkage with the "mushrooming" effect. *Cell Tissue Research*, 316(1), 115–121. https://doi.org/10.1007/s00441-004-0867-9.

rapid-stretch injuries. Under tensile loading, whole nerves elongate axially and compress across the circumference nonlinearly (Wilcox, Gregory, Powell, Quick, & Phillips, 2020). This results in transverse contraction of the middle regions of nerves (Figure 6.11) (Beel et al., 1984). Nerves have also been described as pressured garden hoses (Walbeehm et al., 2004) because their central core of endoneurium and axons has a positive fluid pressure that resists compression, while the surrounding meshwork of collagen in the epi- and perineurial sheaths provides core constraint, with all layers working together to maintain nerve integrity (Figure 6.12) (Georgeu et al., 2005).

Strength

Whole nerves

Understanding the upper limit to which a nerve can be stretched before anatomical damage occurs is often examined *ex vivo* by removing a nerve segment from a cadaveric human or animal, and measuring the cross-sectional area before placing it into the clamps of a tensile testing instrument (Luttges, Stodieck, & Beel, 1986). The nerve segment is then elongated while recording the forces on the nerve until it ruptures. As shown in Table 6.6, with short-term static or gradual stretching, the ultimate tensile strength of nerves, clamped *ex vivo* at 1–12 hr post-mortem, ranges between 2.7 and 30.40 MPa and occurs at strain rates of 7–32% (Table 6.6) (Borschel, Kia, Kuzon Jr., & Dennis, 2003; Rydevik et al., 1990; Sunderland & Bradley, 1961; Walbeehm et al., 2004). Differences in strength between the various nerves include variations in their cross-sectional area. As a nerve diameter increases, the number of fascicles increase, which leads to an increase in tensile strength (Sunderland, 1990). In contrast to *ex vivo* clamping, when nerve segments are clamped *in situ* before excision, so that the internal organization, length, and diameter of the nerve segment is preserved before removal, an 18% increase in ultimate strength is observed, compared to nerves

Table 6.6 Ultimate Tensile Strength and Other Characteristics After Tensile Testing

Species and structure tested	Type of stretch and rate	Maximum loads, N (burst strength)	Ultimate strength, (Mpa)	% elongation to rupture	Histology after reaching ultimate strength (US) and post rupture (post R)
Human, whole median, ulnar or popliteal nerves	Short-term (0.05 ips) static loading	2.06–33.6	9.80–30.40	7–32%	US: Partial axon failure (~20%). Post R: Failure of all elements (~32%).
Rabbit, whole tibial nerves	0.16 mm/s 0.5%/s strain rate	6.28	11.7 ± 0.7	27%	Post R: Multiple ruptures in perineurial sheaths, axons herniated through defects. Epineurium seemed intact although occasionally coiled.
Rat, whole sciatic nerves, untreated or after acellularization	0.11 mm/s; 1%/s strain rate	Untreated: 2.14 ± 0.76 After acellularization: 1.10 ± 0.23	Untreated: 2.72 ± 0.97 After acellularization: 1.40 ± 0.29	Not provided	Acellularization using detergents resulted in a loss of axons, Schwann cell bodies, and myelin.
Rat, whole sciatic nerves clamped *in situ* versus *ex vivo*	0.03 mm/s	Not examined	*In situ*: 7.2 ± 0.5 *ex vivo*: 6.15 ± 0.6	Not examined	Not examined

Based on Borschel, G. H., Kia, K. F., Kuzon, W. M., Jr., & Dennis, R. G. (2003). Mechanical properties of acellular peripheral nerve. Journal of Surgical Research, 114(2), 133–139. 10.1016/s0022-4804(03)00255-5; Rydevik, B. L., Kwan, M. K., Myers, R. R., Brown, R. A., Triggs, K. J., Woo, S. L., & Garfin, S. R. (1990). An in vitro mechanical and histological study of acute stretching on rabbit tibial nerve. Journal of Orthopaedic Research, 8(5), 694–701. 10.1002/jor.1100080511; Sunderland, S., & Bradley, K. C. (1961). Stress–strain phenomena in human peripheral nerve trunks. Brain, 84(1), 102–119. 10.1093/brain/84.1.102; Walbeehm, E. T., Afoke, A., Wit, T., Holman, F., Hovius, S. E., & Brown, R. A. (2004). Mechanical functioning of peripheral nerves: Linkage with the "mushrooming" effect. Cell Tissue Research, 316(1), 115–121. 10.1007/s00441-004-0867-9.

allowed to relax at room temperature for an hour before testing (Table 6.6) (Walbeehm et al., 2004). Histologically, just before the point of rupture, there is the partial failure of axonal elements and endoneurial narrowing, then perineurial sheath ruptures, followed by the failure of nearly all nerve elements (Table 6.6).

Nerve components

It is important to note that nerves are heterogeneous structures, and each structure contributes differently to the material properties. The primary load-bearing portion of the nerve that provides mechanical strength is the perineurium due to its layers of collagen and perineurial cells (Topp & Boyd, 2006). The perineurium is formed by up to 15 layers of flat perineurial cells interspersed with layers of type I and II collagen fibrils and elastic fibers that are organized in circumferential, oblique, and longitudinal orientations. Each perineurial cell layer has a nearly complete basal lamina, with the innermost layer containing laminin, heparin sulfate proteoglycan, and fibronectin. Adjacent perineurial cells are held together by tight junctions so that a perineurial diffusion barrier is formed that controls the endoneurial environment. There is also abundant epineurial connective tissue surrounding the entire nerve and interfascicular epineurium separating nerve fascicles. These epineurial fascial tissues facilitate the dispersion of compressive forces (Sunderland, 1965; Topp & Boyd, 2006).

Nerve mechanical strength via the fascial layers is further supported by experiments in which whole nerves underwent acellularization using detergents in order to examine the strength properties of the fascicular tissues versus neuronal elements (Borschel et al., 2003). The acellularization process removed axons, Schwann cell bodies and myelin, and perhaps some extracellular components, which reduced the amount of energy that could be absorbed before tensile failure. As shown in Table 6.6, the acellularization significantly decreased ultimate tensile strength and load at failure (burst strength) as compared to whole untreated rat sciatic nerves.

Additionally, the morphological organization of axons and fascicles also contributes to mechanical strength. Individual axon fibers and fascicles do not run parallel courses within nerves. Instead, they fuse repeatedly and engage in plexus formations in intimately knit bundles that add tensile strength in a variable manner along the length of a nerve (Topp & Boyd, 2006). While this interchange of axons between fascicles may help to minimize functional deficits following partial injury to nerves, this organization leads to the development of multiple ruptures along a nerve as it reaches the point of ultimate tensile strength.

Strain

Whole nerves

Similar to tendons, nerves show toe, linear, and nonlinear regions during *ex vivo* strain testing. The toe region is typically observed at the initial portion of the force-elongation curve during which the nerve lengthens with no increase in load. Although this toe region is not always observed during *in situ* testing (Walbeehm et al., 2004), the toe region is generally thought to be present because axons have a greater length than the nerve itself as a result of an undulating path (a zig-zag wavy path within nerves; Figure 4.5c). This extra length of axons provides the nerve with a lengthening reserve before the nerve begins to be loaded. The average load carriage point begins between 6 and 8% after the initial nerve elongation (Grewal, Xu, Sotereanos, & Woo, 1996; Walbeehm et al., 2004). Thereafter, during short-term static loading, if the loading is gradual, the materials remain in equilibrium and nerves can sustain nearly linear increments in loading until the proportional limit is reached. At the proportional limit, the ultimate strain ranges from 29.8 to 38% with elongations of

27–40% (Beel et al., 1984; Luttges et al., 1986; Rydevik et al., 1990). Different strain rates are detected when testing *in situ* clamped nerves versus *ex vivo* relaxed nerves (29.8 versus 41.4%) (Walbeehm et al., 2004), and when tested *in vivo* when nerves still have attached branches and perineural tissue connections (both heavily increasing nerve strain) versus excised nerves (Ma et al., 2013). Loading of normal nerves beyond their proportional limit results in rapid alterations of mechanical characteristics. Large reductions in diameter first occur at one or more points along the nerve segment, occasional immediate large elongations, and occasional tearing (typically as a result of epineural failure). Continued loading ends in rupture (Beel et al., 1984).

Histologically, when nerves begin to take on load, undulations in the axons first straighten and then start to stretch (as does the perineurium). As loading increases, some axons rupture while others continue to elongate. With further loading, more axons and fascicles rupture until most fail. Intraneural blood vessels tear prior to rupture of all axonal elements. After this, the nerve elongates as a plastic structure until the perineurium ruptures (elastic properties are retained as long as the perineurium remains intact) (Sunderland & Bradley, 1961).

Clinically, severe nerve trauma occurs more often with a rapid-stretch trauma during a fall or a high-speed injury than with the slow stretching discussed earlier. Biomechanical responses of nerves to rapid stretch have been performed using variable weights and excursions (Mahan, Yeoh, Monson, & Light, 2019; Warner, Yeoh, Light, Zhang, & Mahan, 2020; Yeoh, Warner, Eli, & Mahan, 2020). Nerve rupture after rapid stretch occurs at threshold conditions. Heavier weights at longer excursions result in higher rupture odds (Table 6.7), as do more severe strains at faster stretches, compared to slow stretches. Three biomechanical-derived patterns have been identified: (a) injury within the elastic limit (<0.50 strain, <15% length change), (b) inelastic injury (0.50–1.00 strain, >15% length change), and (c) rupture (mechanical failure) (Warner et al., 2020). Loading direction is also key. A high-speed pull occurring in parallel with a nerve's axis results in ruptures at lower strains than with orthogonal loading. This is likely because orthogonal loading is performed *in situ* when there are still intact nerve branch points (which show higher strain and rupture risk than nerve without branches). In contrast, parallel loading results in ruptures in more distal regions, or proximally with avulsion of the spinal root that are mechanically frail due to their lack of epineurium and reduce perineurium (spinal roots are 10-fold lower stress tolerance than peripheral nerves, although they each exhibit similar elongation limits) (Luttges et al., 1986).

Histologically, the first change in nerves after these rapid-stretch injuries is the straightening of axons and then graded microruptures of the endoneurium that correlate strongly and positively with the severity of the strain (Figure 6.13) (Warner et al., 2020). Microruptures of the endoneurium

Table 6.7 Rupture Probability for Weights and Excursions Tested

	Rupture incidence			
Weight (g)	**5 mm**	**10 mm**	**20 mm**	**30 mm**
50	0	0	0	0
100	0	0	0	0
220	0.2	0.67	0.71	1.00
550	0.17	1.00	1.00	1.00

Mahan, M. A., Yeoh, S., Monson, K., & Light, A. (2019). Rapid stretch injury to peripheral nerves: biomechanical results. *Neurosurgery*, 85(1), 137–144. https://doi.org/10.1093/neuros/nyy423.

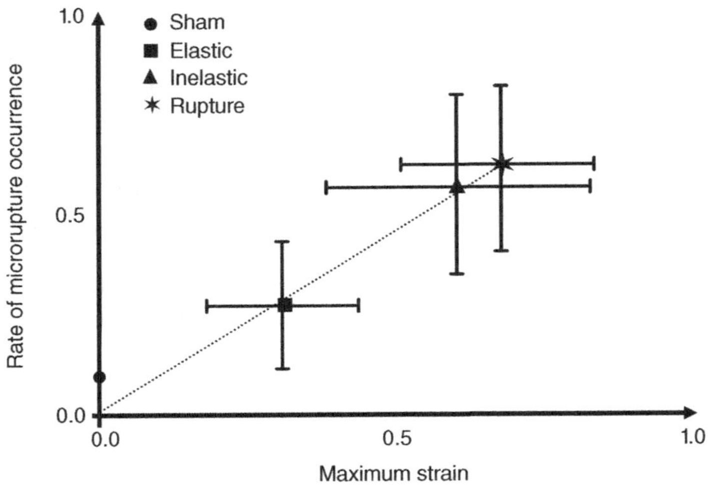

Figure 6.13 Correlation between biomechanical strain and incidence of endoneurial microrupture (Pearson's $r = 0.98$) across the four biomechanical levels of rapid-stretch injury severity (error bars indicate standard deviation). The inelastic condition is essentially only a thin transition state toward complete rupture. Modified from Warner, W. S., Yeoh, S., Light, A., Zhang, J., & Mahan, M. A. (2020). Rapid-stretch injury to peripheral nerves: Histologic results. *Neurosurgery*, 86(3), 437–445. https://doi.org/10.1093/neuros/nyz194.

were distributed along the length of the nerve and were more severe and involved greater nerve volume at higher biomechanical severity. Disruption of the epineurium and perineurium increased in frequency with progressive injury severity but were not a prediction of the grade of injury.

Nerve strain also varies with differences in the amount of extracellular matrix per unit volume, with smaller nerves typically having less extracellular matrix which results in a more pliable composite material over the test strain) (Borschel et al., 2003). Strain increases with increased collagenous connectivity to the surrounding perineural and myofascial structures when tested *in situ* (Ma et al., 2013; Stecco et al., 2020) and the presence of nerve branches (Mahan et al., 2019; Sunderland & Bradley, 1961). Nerves also show local strain differences, albeit opposite differences, in periarticular regions, with twofold reduction (more compliance) within the median nerve and three- to fivefold reduction within the sciatic nerve at joint versus non-joint regions (Phillips, Smit, De Zoysa, Afoke, & Brown, 2004). This difference in nerve compliance is partially influenced by internal neural structure and the amount of connective tissues around nerves at joint regions, although more research is needed on this topic. There are also differences in paraneural and myofascial connections, with areas with more collagenous connections heavily influencing elongation loads.

Nerve components

Although the microanatomy and collagenous composition of peripheral nerve structures are well known (Section "Peripheral Nerve Histology"), even after over 100 years of research, uncertainty persists regarding the contributions of each individual structure to the mechanical resilience of nerves (Rosso & Guck, 2019; Umansky and Midha, 2020). Chemical acellularization that removes all but connective tissues reduces the ultimate strain in rat sciatic nerves by almost half (Borschel et al., 2003). Further clarification has come from studies in which the core is separated from the sheath using methods shown in Figure 6.14 during mechanical testing. These experiments have shown that an intact nerve acts as a pressurized system, with a continuous dense connective tissue surrounding and constraining a pressurized core that is analogous to a reinforced water hose (Figure 6.11). Several findings support this idea. After nerve transection, fascial sheaths retract

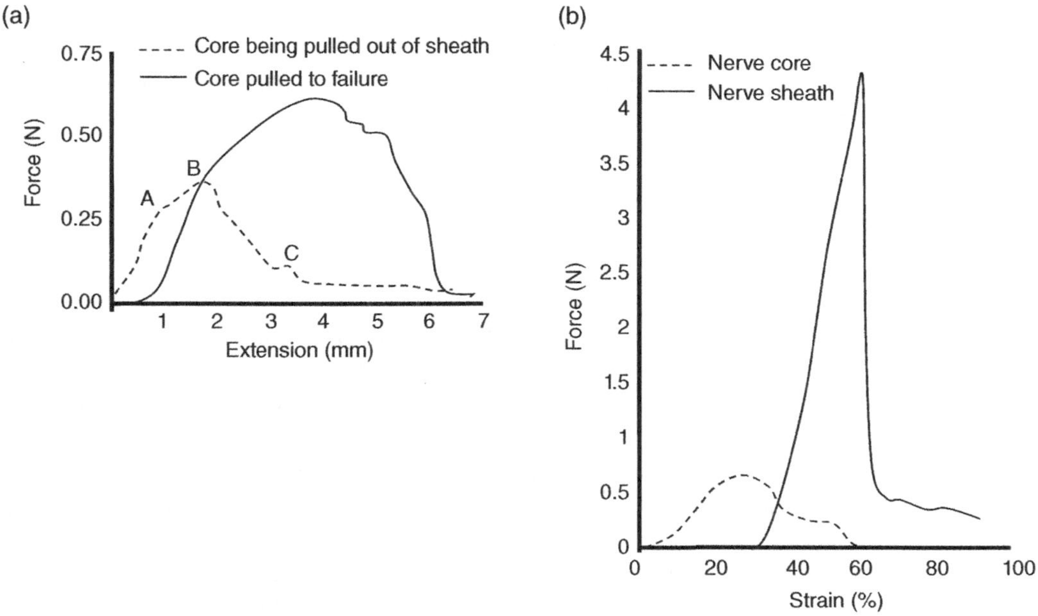

Figure 6.14 Core pullout and force-strain profiles of core versus sheath. (a) Typical curves of force against the extension of the core being pulled out of its sheath and the core being pulled to failure. The three phases of the pullout profile are shown (*A = elastic extension, B = yield or break of the core-sheath interface, C = free gliding of the core*). (b) Force–strain curves for nerve core and outer sheath. Modified from Tillett, R. L., Afoke, A., Hall, S. M., Brown, R. A., & Phillips, J. B. (2004). Investigating mechanical behaviour at a core-sheath interface in peripheral nerve. *Journal of the Peripheral Nervous System*, 9(4), 255–262. https://doi.org/10.1111/j.1085-9489.2004.09411.x.

quickly, and the endoneurial core swells slowly (mushrooms). When nerves are clamped *in situ* before testing (Table 6.6), the strain to maximum strength is 30% reduced and the stiffness modulus increases by 21%, compared to nerve segments allowed to relax (i.e., retract) before testing (Walbeehm et al., 2004). The retraction rate is slow (11%), making elastic recoil an unlikely mechanism. When the core is extracted (pulled out) from sheaths, and placed into water, there is a slow 5.7-fold increase in weight over time, compared to a 2.4-fold increase in the core-intact sheath composite. Electron microscopy reveals that the extracted core is composed of axons, myelin sheaths, endoneurium, and the innermost perineurial cell layer, while the separated sheath is composed of epineurium and most of the perineurium (Tillett, Afoke, Hall, Brown, & Phillips, 2004).

In another experiment in which retraction responses were examined, nerves were clamped at their *in situ* tension (Georgeu et al., 2005) before undergoing: (a) transection of the whole nerve and measurement of retraction, (b) transection of the outer sheath, and (c) measurement of retraction of the outer sheath or the inner core (Figure 6.14c). Retraction was measured within 5 min of transection and then again after 45 min (to allow full retraction), while postmortem loss of retraction was tested at 0 or 60 min after *in situ* clamping (fresh versus stored nerves). As shown in Table 6.8, there was an immediate retraction of each element in the fresh nerves tested at 5 min (the whole nerve showed an immediate retraction of 12.68%, representing 84% of the total retraction of the nerve of 15.13% by 45 min). In stored nerves, there was only a small amount of whole nerve retraction and the core extended rather than retracting after excision. The disappearance of tension in the stored nerves is consistent with its maintenance by an energy-dependent process (perhaps an ion-pumping mechanism) that quickly winds down postmortem.

Nerves were tested fresh or after being stored for 60 min before transection and testing.

Table 6.8 Percent Retraction of Whole Nerve, Sheath, and Core

Time after transection	Whole nerve retraction	Sheath retraction	Core retraction	Core extension
Fresh nerve – 5 min	12.68%	5.35%	4%	—
Fresh – 45 min	15%	7.21%	5.26%	—
Stored – 5 min	5.33%	5.87%	—	0.78%
Stored – 45 min	6.71%	7.87%	—	1.74%

Further core-sheath separation experiments revealed that the core-sheath interaction is a physical connection rather than a viscous fluid interface (Tillett et al., 2004). Force-elongation assays during the core-sheath pullout showed that the interface break strength is considerably less than the break strength of the core itself (Figure 6.14a) and that the core breaks at a much lower force than the sheath (Figure 6.14b). These findings support a hierarchy of mechanical break strengths that would, under increasing tensile loading, result in first interface breaking, next core rupture, and then sheath rupture.

Thus, nerves can be considered as a two-component system, biomechanically, with the stronger outer sheaths serving to protect the weaker core material from stretch injury, and that the interface between these layers is actively maintained. As the elastic limit of the nerve is exceeded, the weaker nerve fibers within the endoneurium usually fail before the elastic limit of the nerve trunk is reached, and rupture of the perineurium or epineurium occurs.

Elastic Modulus

Whole nerves

Peripheral nerve trunks elongate proportionally to a certain point under increasing load; until this point, the nerve trunk behaves like an elastic structure and after this loading, the original shape resumes. The elastic modulus for whole nerves has been calculated as approximately 0.58 MPa (Borschel et al., 2003). Beyond this elastic limit, the nerve behaves like a semi-plastic material and stress is no longer proportional to strain, until mechanical failure occurs. Beyond the elastic limit, a nerve elongates quickly without further increase in load until complete separation occurs (Figure 6.12b, c). Human cadaveric nerves show mean elastic limits of 15% (ulnar nerve) or 14% (median nerve) after elongations of 8–21% or 6–22%, respectively. Rabbit nerves stretched to 6% fully recover to normal length, whereas a 12% stretch shows an incomplete recovery (Kwan, Wall, Massie, & Garfin, 1992). It has been concluded that nerves have at least a 6% ability to elongate before damage (Fazekas, Kosa, Jobba, Szendrenyi, & Bajnoczky, 1972; Kwan et al., 1992; Sunderland & Bradley, 1961), with variations between nerves based on their axon wave size, shape, alignment, and packing density (Alvey, Jones, Tobin-O'Brien, & Pickering, 2019).

Nerve components

Atomic force microscopy has been used to study the elastic modules of peripheral nerves *ex vivo* in juvenile, young adult, and mature adult mice (Rosso & Guck, 2019). The apparent elastic modulus evolves biphasically during maturation, with the higher apparent Young's modulus in young mice, compared to juvenile and adult mice, and the lowest in juvenile mice. Collagen type IV levels in the endoneurium decrease significantly with nerve maturation. Collagen type IV is one of the most abundant types of collagen in the Schwann cell's basal lamina, where it forms an interlaced network (Chernousov & Carey, 2000). It is known to form covalent bonds with other components of the extracellular matrix to help stabilize the polymer network of the basal lamina (Yurchenco & Schittny, 1990). Since single nerve fibers are vulnerable to compression, this increased secretion of collagen type IV by Schwann cells may provide an "inside-out" protection during early nerve development. Collagen type I levels show biphasic levels, with increased levels in the endoneurium of young nerves, and then again increased levels in the perineurium and epineurium of adults and low levels in all sheath levels in juveniles. The high levels of collagen I in the fascial sheaths may provide an "outside-in" type mechanical protection in adult nerves. Collagen digestion experiments have substantiated these results and shown significant reductions in the apparent elastic modulus post-digestion, highlighting the importance of collagen to nerve elasticity. Nocodazole treatment has been used to disrupt microtubules and revealed that the microtubule cytoskeleton within axons also contributes to local nerve tissue stiffness, as do axonal membranes (which includes the Schwann cell basal lamina) (Montanino, Deryckere, Famaey, Seuntjens, & Kleiven, 2019). Only nerve cell density and myelin content have been ruled out as contributors to nerve stiffness (Rosso & Guck, 2019).

Anisotropy in peripheral nerves

Anisotropy in nerves does not refer to their biomechanical strength, but instead to their characteristics during optical imaging, such as sonography (Soong, Schafhalter-Zoppoth, & Gray, 2005). Specifically, anisotropy in nerves refers to the backscatter echoes from a specimen that depends on the directional orientation of the ultrasound field (i.e., the angle of insonation). Tendons and ligaments also have a fibrillar echotexture that is highly sensitive to ultrasound transducer manipulation (Gray, 2019).

Age

As described in Section "Nerve components," there are significant maturation changes (juveniles into mature adulthood) in collagen types I and IV that contribute to age-related differences in the elastic modulus of nerves (Rosso & Guck, 2019). The mean ultimate tensile strength of nerves is only slightly less (90%) before 20–29 years of age than the mean adult nerve strength (Yamada, 1970), and there are no age-related changes in nerve strength and ultimate percent elongation from the first decade of life up to 60–69 years of age (Yamada, 1970). However, in the older people, there are age-related changes in the mean cross-sectional area of nerves that could reduce their strength. In a study in which ultrasound was used to assess nerve area, the median nerves of aged men had larger mean cross-sectional areas and diameters during wrist deviation from neutral positions, compared to young adult men (Loh, Yeoh, & Muraki, 2019). In another study in which sciatic nerves from 27- to 93-year-old human cadavers were examined microscopically, progressive age-related increases in whole nerve cross-sectional areas were seen simultaneously with increasing intraneural connective tissue sheath areas (epineurial, perineurial, and endoneurial) and intraneural adipose tissue (Sladjana, Ivan, & Bratislav, 2008). As this was occurring, the number of myelinated nerve fibers decreased (Sladjana et al., 2008). The intraneural connective tissue increases may be the result of chronic trauma to which nerves are exposed during the course of aging (Tohgi, Tsukagoshi, & Toyokura, 1977). Alternatively, these increases may be a nonspecific compensatory phenomenon elicited by the loss of myelinated nerve fibers (as would be the increased intraneural adipose tissue) that could affect nerve elasticity (Sladjana et al., 2008).

Effects of Exercise

Exercise has also been shown to enhance axonal regeneration after nerve injury, as evaluated by recovery of compound motor action potentials and larger myofiber size in the nerve's target muscles, and to increase axon numbers and Schwann cell proliferation within nerves (Cooper, Kluding, & Wright, 2016; Park & Hoke, 2014; Sabatier, Redmon, Schwartz, & English, 2008; Wood et al., 2012). Whether these particular changes improve the nerves' biomechanical properties has not been examined. However, it has been shown that a 12-week nerve-directed stretching intervention, performed by 20-year-old human subjects, increased the range of motion of lower limbs and decreased sciatic nerve shear wave velocity (used as an *in vivo* estimate of stiffness) (Andrade et al., 2020). The latter indicates that the stiffness of peripheral nerves can adapt to the long-term loading stimuli elicited by nerve-directed stretching.

Effects of Injury and Repair

Complete stretch rupture injuries leave a large critical gap in nerves that substantially reduce strength due to the loss of continuity of all axonal and fascial elements. With time, prominent fibrotic changes take place in the peri- and epineurium that increase strain and stiffness (Yeoh et al., 2020). Even lesser mechanical insults lead to morphological changes at the cellular and subcellular changes in the nerve fibers, Schwann cell basal lamina, and fascial sheaths, which alter a nerve's tensile strength and ability to withstand stress. When peripheral nerves are tested biomechanically following experimentally induced crush injuries, injured nerves show 17% larger cross-sectional areas and 30% greater mass per unit length (presumably due to edema, immune cell infiltration into the peri- and endoneurial layers, and fibroblast proliferation (Lam Van Ba et al., 2018; Ruggieri et al., 2006)). Although injured nerves can sustain similar loads as normal uninjured nerves, they are 7% more stiff and 19% more elastic. Beyond the proportional limit, injured nerves exhibit more complex plastic deformation at the nerve-crush site and distally (due to nerve dieback), more sites of cross-sectional area reduction, and more epineurium tearing. As a function of time, post-crush nerve strength and stiffness increase from subnormal to normal levels around 6 days post-crush, to supranormal levels at 12 days (where values remain for the rest of the 3-week experiment). In contrast, nerve elasticity increases by almost a factor of 2 within 2–4 days of injury, and then decreases to near normal levels by 24 days post-crush.

After nerve injury repair, the fascial layers are fundamentally different (Luttges et al., 1986). The endoneurium contains many more cells, such as increased numbers of Schwann cells and altered internodal myelin sheath spacing that remains altered over a year in mice (equivalent to one-half of their lifetime). There is often an increase in epi- and perineurial fibrosis that may lead to nerve compression (and therefore function) (Barbe et al., 2021; Bove et al., 2019) to the extent that surgery may be required to decompress the fibrotic nerve (the fibrotic perineurium or epineurium is sliced longitudinally for decompression) (Mazal & Millesi, 2005). Post-injury scars, even those from lesser injuries, may tether the perineural sheath to myofascial structures (Smith et al., 2020), thereby limiting nerve displacement (gliding/sliding movement through the tissues, typically in the longitudinal plane) (Stecco et al., 2020). Such fibrosis results in steeper stress–strain curves and impairment of the elastic limit (Millesi, Zoch, & Reihsner, 1995).

Summary

A summary of ultimate strength, strain, and elastic modulus for each tissue is provided in Table 6.9.

The musculoskeletal system comprises several unique biological materials, each having its own distinctive role to play in providing the body the capability to move. All these materials exhibit viscoelastic properties and the remarkable capability of self-repair. The self-repair capability is critical, as all materials demonstrate fatigue damage when they are repetitively stressed. If

Table 6.9 A Summary of the Material Properties of Musculoskeletal Tissues

	Strength (MPa)	Failure strain (%)	Elastic modulus
Tendon	100	8–10%	200–2,000 MPa, with an average of 1 GPa
Ligament	40	10–15% (most common)	200–2,000 MPa, 1 GPa
Articular cartilage			
Superior layers	21–50	25–30%	2.2–7 GPa
Deep layers	13–32	25–30%	4.91–5.64 GPa
Bone, cortical	160	1.41–1.59%	20 GPa
Skeletal muscle	0.44 MPa	60%	10 kPa
Whole nerves	2.7–30.41	29–38%	0.58 MPa

self-repair were not possible, our tissues would not last very long. However, the quality of the self-repair varies tremendously according to the specific tissue involved. Bone and muscle have the greatest ability to perform restorative or adaptive repair since these materials have an excellent blood supply. Tendons, ligaments, and cartilage are poorly perfused and the repair processes for these materials are both lengthier and have poorer repair results. Subsequent chapters will explore the upshots of the damage and repair capacities of musculoskeletal tissues and discuss the ramifications in terms of maintenance of musculoskeletal health.

Bibliography

Alvey, L. M., Jones, J. F. X., Tobin-O'Brien, C., & Pickering, M. (2019). Bands of Fontana are caused exclusively by the sinusoidal path of axons in peripheral nerves and predict axon path; evidence from rodent nerves and physical models. *Journal of Anatomy, 234*(2), 165–178. https://doi.org/10.1111/joa.12910

Amis, A. (2004). *The biomechanics of ligaments*. Springer.

Andonian, P., Viallon, M., Le Goff, C., De Bourguignon, C., Tourel, C., Morel, J., . . . Croisille, P. (2016). Shear-wave elastography assessments of quadriceps stiffness changes prior to, during and after prolonged exercise: A longitudinal study during an extreme mountain ultra-marathon. *PLoS One, 11*, 0161855.

Andrade, R. J., Freitas, S. R., Hug, F., Le Sant, G., Lacourpaille, L., Gross, R., & Nordez, A. (2020). Chronic effects of muscle and nerve-directed stretching on tissue mechanics. *Journal of Applied Physiology, 129*(5), 1011–1023. https://doi.org/10.1152/japplphysiol.00239.2019

Armstrong, R. (1984). Mechanisms of exercise-induced delayed onset muscle soreness: A brief review. *Medicine and Science in Sports and Exercise, 16*, 529–538.

Arnoczky, S., Adams, M., Dehaven, K., Eyre, D., & Mow, V. (1988). Meniscus. In S.-Y. Woo & J. A. Buckwalter (Eds.), *Injury and repair of the musculoskeletal soft tissues* (pp. 487–537). American Academy of Orthopaedic Surgeons.

Aubert, X., Roquet, M. L., & Van Der Elst, J. (1951). The tension-length diagram of the frog's sartorius muscle. *Archives internationales de physiologie, 59*, 239–241.

Barbe, M., Gallagher, S., Massicotte, V., Tytell, M., Popoff, S., & Barr-Gillespie, A. (2013). The interaction of force and repetition on musculoskeletal and neural tissue responses and sensorimotor behavior in a rat model of work-related musculoskeletal disorders. *BMC Musculoskeletal Disorders, 14*, 303.

Barbe, M. F., Harris, M. Y., Cruz, G. E., Amin, M., Billett, N. M., Dorotan, J. T., & Bove, G. M. (2021). Key indicators of repetitive overuse-induced neuromuscular inflammation and fibrosis are prevented by manual therapy in a rat model. *BMC Musculoskeletal Disorders, 22*(1), 417. https://doi.org/10.1186/s12891-021-04270-0

Bayraktar, H., Morgan, E., Niebur, G., Morris, G., Wong, E., & Keaveny, T. (2004). Comparison of the elastic and yield properties of human femoral trabecular and cortical bone tissue. *Journal of Biomechanics, 37*, 27–35.

Beel, J. A., Groswald, D. E., & Luttges, M. W. (1984). Alterations in the mechanical properties of peripheral nerve following crush injury. *Journal of Biomechanics, 17*(3), 185–193. https://doi.org/10.1016/0021-9290(84)90009-5

Benjamin, M., & Evans, E. (1990). Fibrocartilage. *Journal of Anatomy, 171*, 1–15.

Bentolila, V., Boyce, T., Fyhrie, D., Drumb, R., Skerry, T., & Schaffler, M. (1998). Intracortical remodeling in adult rat longbones after fatigue loading. *Bone, 23*, 275–281.

Best, T., Gharaibeh, B., & Huard, J. (2013). Stem cells, angiogenesis and muscle healing: A potential role in massage therapies? *British Journal of Sports Medicine, 47*, 556–560.

Black, J. (1988). *Orthopaedic biomaterials in research and practice*. Churchill-Livingstone.

Black, J., & Hastings, G. (1998). Fibrocartilage. In *Handbook of biomaterials properties* (pp. 48–52). Chapman & Hall.

Bogduk, N. (1997). *Clinical anatomy of the lumbar spine and sacrum*. Churchill Livingstone.

Bonaldo, P., & Sandri, M. (2013). Cellular and molecular mechanisms of muscle atrophy. *Disease Models and Mechanisms, 6*, 25–39.

Borde, R., Hortobágyi, T., & Granacher, U. (2015). Dose–response relationships of resistance training in healthy old adults. A systematic review and meta-analysis. *Sports Medicine, 45*, 1693–1720.

Borschel, G. H., Kia, K. F., Kuzon, W. M., Jr., & Dennis, R. G. (2003). Mechanical properties of acellular peripheral nerve. *Journal of Surgical Research, 114*(2), 133–139. https://doi.org/10.1016/s0022-4804(03)00255-5

Bourrin, S., Genty, C., Palle, S., Gharib, C., & Alexandre, C. (1994). Adverse effects of strenuous exercise: A densitometric and histomorphometric study in the rat. *Journal of Applied Physiology, 76*(5), 1999–2005. https://doi.org/10.1152/jappl.1994.76.5.1999

Bove, G. M., Delany, S. P., Hobson, L., Cruz, G. E., Harris, M. Y., Amin, M., & Barbe, M. F. (2019). Manual therapy prevents onset of nociceptor activity, sensorimotor dysfunction, and neural fibrosis induced by a volitional repetitive task. *Pain, 160*(3), 632–644. https://doi.org/10.1097/j.pain.0000000000001443

Brinckmann, P., Biggemann, M., & Hilweg, D. (1988). Fatigue fracture of human lumbar vertebrae. *Clinical Biomechanics, 3*(Suppl. 1), 1–23.

Brown, S. (2020). How to speed fracture healing. https://www.betterbones.com/fractures-and-healing/speed-up-fracture-healing/

Brumitt, J., & Cuddeford, T. (2015). Current concepts of muscle and tendon adaptation to strength and conditioning. *The International Journal of Sports Physical Therapy, 10*, 748–759.

Buchanan, C., & Marsh, R. (2001). Effects of long-term exercise on the biomechanical properties of the Achilles tendon of guinea fowl. *Journal of Applied Physiology, 90*, 164–171.

Buckwalter, J. (1995). Aging and degeneration of the human intervertebral disc. *Spine, 20*, 1307–1314.

Bullough, P., Munuera, L., Murphy, J., & Weinstein, A. (1970). The strength of menisci of the knee as it relates to their fine structure. *Journal of Bone and Joint Surgery (British), 52*, 564–567.

Butler, D., Grood, E., Noyes, F., & Zernicke, R. (1978). Biomechanics of ligaments and tendons. *Exercise and Sport Sciences Reviews, 6*, 125–181.

Carroll, C., Dickinson, J., Haus, J., Lee, G., Hollon, C., Aagaard, P., & Trappe, T. (2008). Influence of aging on the in vivo properties of human patellar tendon. *Journal of Applied Physiology, 105*, 1907–1915.

Carter, D., Beaupré, G., Giori, N., & Helms, J. (1998). Mechanobiology of skeletal regeneration. *Clinical Orthopaedics and Related Research, 355*, 41–55.

Carter, D., Wong, M., & Orr, T. (1991). Musculoskeletal ontogeny, phylogeny, and functional adaptation. *Journal of Biomechanics, 24*(Suppl. 1), 3–16.

Chalchat, E., Gennisson, J.-L., Peñailillo, L. O., Malgoyre, A., Charlot, K., Bourrilhon, C., & Garcia-Vicencio, S. (2020). Changes in the Viscoelastic Properties of the Vastus Lateralis Muscle With Fatigue. *Frontiers in Physiology, 11*, 307.

Chanda, A., & Callaway, C. (2018). Computational modeling of blast induced whole-body injury: a review. *Journal of Medical Engineering Technology, 42*(2), 88–104.

Chernousov, M. A., & Carey, D. J. (2000). Schwann cell extracellular matrix molecules and their receptors. *Histology and Histopathology, 15*(2), 593–601. https://doi.org/10.14670/HH-15.593

Choi, K., Fyhrie, D., & Schaffler, M. (1994). Failure mechanisms of compact bone in bending: A microstructural analysis. *Transactions of the 40th Orthopaedic Research Society, 425*.

Claes, L., & Heigele, C. (1999). Magnitudes of local stress and strain along bony surfaces predict the course and type of fracture healing. *Journal of Biomechanics, 32*, 255–266.

Clarkson, P., & Hubal, M. (2002). Exercise-induced muscle damage in humans. *American Journal of Physical Medicine and Rehabilitation, 81*, 52–69.

Clarkson, P., & Tremblay, I. (1988). Exercise induced muscle damage, repair and adaptation in humans. *Journal of Applied Physiology, 65*, 1–6.

Cleak, M., & Eston, R. (1992). Muscle soreness, swelling, stiffness and strength loss after intense eccentric exercise. *British Journal of Sports Medicine, 26*, 267–272.

Cole, B., & Malek, M. (2004). *Articular cartilage lesions: A practical guide to assessment and treatment*. Springer.

Collins, C. (2006). Satellite cell self-renewal. *Current Opinion of Pharmacology, 6*, 301–306.

Convery, F., Akeson, W., & Keown, G. (1972). The repair of large osteochondral defects. *Clinical Orthopaedics, 86*, 193–205.

Cooper, M. A., Kluding, P. M., & Wright, D. E. (2016). Emerging relationships between exercise, sensory nerves, and neuropathic pain. *Frontiers in Neuroscience, 10*, 372. https://doi.org/10.3389/fnins.2016.00372

Couppe, C., Kongsgaard, M., Aagaard, P., Hansen, P., Bojsen-Moller, J., Kjaer, M., & Magnusson, S. (2008). Habitual loading results in tendon hypertrophy and increased stiffness of the human patellar tendon. *Journal of Applied Physiology, 105*, 805–810.

Crameri, R., Aagaard, P., Qvortrup, K., Langberg, H., Olesen, J., & Kjaer, M. (2007). Myofibre damage in human skeletal muscle: Effects of electrical stimulation versus voluntary contraction. *Journal of Physiology, 583*, 365–380.

Davy, D., & Jepsen, K. (2001). Bone damage mechanics. In Stephen C. Cowin Bone mechanics handbook (2nd ed., p. 181–18125). CRC Press.

Ding, M., Day, J. S., Burr, D. B., Mashiba, T., Hirano, T., Weinans, H., & Hvid, I. (2003). Canine cancellous bone microarchitecture after one year of high-dose bisphosphonates. *Calcified Tissue International, 72*(6), 737–744. https://doi.org/10.1007/s00223-002-2066-6

Ding, M., Odgaard, A., & Hvid, I. (2003). Changes in the three-dimensional microstructure of human tibial cancellous bone in early osteoarthritis. *The Journal of Bone and Joint Surgery British Volume, 85*(6), 906–912.

Doblaré, M., García, J., & Gómez, M. (2004). Modelling bone tissue fracture and healing: A review. *Engineering Fracture Mechanics*, *71*, 1809–1840.

Doschak, M., & Zernicke, R. (2005). Structure, function and adaptation of bone-tendon and bone-ligament complexes. *Journal of Musculoskeletal and Neuronal Interaction*, *5*, 35–40.

Ebbeling, C., & Clarkson, P. (1989). Exercise-induced muscle damage and adaptation. *Sports Medicine*, *7*, 207–234.

Eckstein, F., Hudelmaier, M., & Putz, R. (2006). The effects of exercise on human articular cartilage. *Journal of Anatomy*, *208*, 491–512.

Einhorn, T., & Gerstenfeld, L. (2015). Fracture healing: Mechanisms and interventions. *Nature Reviews Rheumatology*, *11*, 45–54.

Elliott, D. (1965). Structure and function of mammalian tendon. *Biological Reviews of the Cambridge Philosophical Society*, *40*, 392–421.

Encyclopedia, N. W. (2017). Cartilage. http://www.newworldencyclopedia.org/entry/Cartilage

Epari, D., Duda, G., & M.S., T. (2010). Mechanobiology of bone healing and regeneration: in vivo models. Proc. *Institution of Mechical Engineering, Part H: Journal of Engineering in Medicine*, *224*, 1543–1553.

Fazekas, I. G., Kosa, F., Jobba, G., Szendrenyi, J., & Bajnoczky, I. (1972). Tensile strength of nerve trunks of the upper extremities. *Zeitschrift fur Rechtsmedizin*, *70*(4), 229–234. https://doi.org/10.1007/BF02079687

Frankel, V. H., & Nordin, M. (2012). *Basic biomechanics of the skeletal system* (4th ed.). Wolters Kluwer/Lippincott Williams & Wilkins Health.

Friden, J., Sjostrom, M., & Ekblom, B. (1981). A morphological study of delayed muscle soreness. *Experimentia*, *37*, 506–507.

Friden, J., Sjostrom, M., & Ekblom, B. (1983). Myofibrillar damage following intense exercise in man. *International Journal of Sports Medicine*, *4*, 170–176.

Fung, D., Wang, W., Laudier, D., Shine, J., Basta-Pljakic, J., Jepsen, K. S., & Flatow, E. (2009). Subrupture tendon fatigue damage. *Journal of Orthopaedic Research*, *27*, 264–273.

Gallagher, S., Marras, W., Litsky, A., & Burr, D. (2006). An exploratory study of loading and morphometric factors associated with specific failure modes in fatigue testing of lumbar motion segments. *Clinical Biomechanics*, *21*, 228–234.

Gallagher, S., Marras, W., Litsky, A., Burr, D., Landoll, J., & Matkovic, V. (2007). A comparison of fatigue failure responses of old versus middle-aged lumbar motion segments in simulated flexed lifting. *Spine*, *32*, 1832–1839.

Gallo, L., Nickel, J., Iwasaki, L., & Palla, S. (2000). Stress-field translation in the healthy human temporomandibular joint. *Journal of Dental Research*, *79*, 1740–1746.

Gao, Y., Arfat, Y., Wang, H., & Goswami, N. (2018). Muscle atrophy induced by mechanical unloading: Mechanisms and potential countermeasures. *Frontiers in Physiology*, *9*, 235.

Gelberman, R., Goldberg, V., An, K.-N., & Banes, A. (1987). Tendon. In S.-Y. Woo & J. Buckwalter (Eds.), *Injury and repair of the musculoskeletal soft tissues* (pp. 1–40). American Academy of Orthopaedic Surgeons.

Gennisson, J. L., Deffieux, T., Mace, E., Montaldo, G., Fink, M., & Tanter, M. (2010). Viscoelastic and anisotropic mechanical properties of in vivo muscle tissue assessed by supersonic shear imaging. *Ultrasound in Medicine and Biology*, *36*, 789–801.

Georgeu, G. A., Walbeehm, E. T., Tillett, R., Afoke, A., Brown, R. A., & Phillips, J. B. (2005). Investigating the mechanical shear-plane between core and sheath elements of peripheral nerves. *Cell and Tissue Research*, *320*(2), 229–234. https://doi.org/10.1007/s00441-004-1031-2

Gharpuray, V. (1998). Fibrocartilage. In J. B. G. Hastings (Ed.), *Handbook of biomaterial properties* (pp. 48–58). Chapman & Hall.

Ghiasi, M., Chen, J., Vaziri, A., Rodriguez, E., & Nazarian, A. (2017). Bone fracture healing in mechanobiological modeling: A review of principles and methods. *Bone Reports, 6*, 87–100.

Ghosh, P., & Taylor, T. (1987). The knee joint meniscus: A fibrocartilage of some distinction. *Clinical Orthopaedics and Related Research, 224*, 52–63.

Ginebra, M., Planell, J., Ontañón, M., & Aparicio, C. (2000). Structure and mechanical properties of cortical bone. In M. Elices (Ed.), *Structural biological materials* (pp. 33–71). Pergamon Press.

Goodship, A., Cunningham, J., & Kenwright, J. (1998). Strain rate and timing of stimulation in mechanical modulation of fracture healing. *Clinical Orthopaedics and Related Research, 355*, 105–115.

Gordon, B., Kelleher, A., & Kimball, S. (2013). Regulation of muscle protein synthesis and the effects of catabolic states. *International Journal of Biochemistry and Cell Biology, 45*, 2147–2157.

Gray, A. T. (2019). Chapter 6—Anisotropy. In Atlas of ultrasound-guided regional anesthesia (3rd ed., pp. 13–16). Elsevier.

Grewal, R., Xu, J., Sotereanos, D. G., & Woo, S. L. (1996). Biomechanical properties of peripheral nerves. *Hand Clinics, 12*(2), 195–204.

Hall, J. (2011). *Textbook of medical physiology* (12th ed.). Elsevier.

Hauser, R., & Dolan, E. (2011). Ligament injury and healing: An overview of current clinical concepts. *Journal of Prolotherapy, 3*, 836–846.

Haut, R., Lancaster, R., & DeCamp, C. (1992). Mechanical properties of the canine patellar tendon: Some correlations with age and the content of collagen. *Journal of Biomechanics, 25*, 163–173.

Havaldar, R., Pilli, S., & Putti, B. (2014). Insights into the effects of tensile and compressive loadings on human femur bone. *Advanced Biomedical Research, 3*, 101.

Hayes, D. J., Brower, R., & John, K. (2001). Articular cartilage. Anatomy, injury, and repair. *Clinics in Podiatric Medicine and Surgery, 18*, 35–53.

Hayes, W., & Bodine, A. (1978). Flow independent viscoelastic properties of articular cartilage matrix. *Journal of biomechanics, 11*, 407–419.

Hazelwood, S., Martin, R., Rashid, M., & Rodrigo, J. (2001). A mechanistic model for internal bone remodeling exhibits different dynamic responses in disuse and overload? *Journal of Biomechanics, 34*, 299–308.

Helgason, B., Perilli, E., Schileo, E., Taddei, F., Brynjolsson, S., & Viceconti, M. (2008). Mathematical relationships between bone density and mechanical properties: A literature review. *Clinical Biomechanics, 23*, 135–146.

Hente, R., Füchtmeier, B., Schlegel, U., Ernstberger, A., & Perren, S. (2004). The influence of cyclic compression and distraction on the healing of experimental tibial fractures. *Journal of Orthopaedic Research, 22*, 709–715.

Heroux, M., & Gandevia, S. (2013). Human muscle fatigue, eccentric damage and coherence in the EMG. *Acta Physiology (Oxford), 208*, 294–295.

Hildebrand, T., & Ruegsegger, P. (1997). Quantification of bone microarchitecture with the structure model index. *Computer Methods in Biomechanics and Biomedical Engineering, 1*(1), 15–23. https://doi.org/10.1080/01495739708936692

Hollister, S.J. (2021). BME 332: Introduction to biosolid mechanics, section 9: ligament/tendon structure-function. http://websites.umich.edu/~bme332/ch10ligten/bme332ligamenttendon.htm

Holmes, A., & Hukins, D. (1994). Fatigue failure at the disc-vertebra interface during cyclic axial compression of cadaveric specimens. *Clinical Biomechanics, 9*, 133–134.

Huber, G., Nagel, K., Skrzypiec, D., Klein, A., Püschel, K., & Morlock, M. (2016). A description of spinal fatigue strength. *Journal of Biomechanics, 49*, 875–880.

Huber, G., Skrzypiec, D., Klein, A., Puschel, K., & Morlock, M. (2010). High cycle fatigue failure behavior of functional spinal units. *Industrial Health, 48*, 550–556.

Hudelmaier, M., Glaser, C., Hohe, J., Englmeier, K. -H., Reiser, M., Putz, R., & Eckstein, F. (2001). Age-related changes in the morphology and deformational behavior of knee joint cartilage. *Arthritis and Rheumatology, 44*, 2556–2561.

Isaksson, H. (2012). Recent advances in mechanobiological modeling of bone regeneration. *Mechanics Research Communications, 42*, 22–31.

James, R., Kesturu, G., Balian, G., & Chhabra, A. (2008). Tendon: Biology biomechanics, repair, growth factors and evolving treatment options. *Journal of Hand Surgery, 33*, 102–112.

Jamurtas, A., Theocharis, V., Tofas, T., Tsiokanos, A., Yfanti, C., Paschalis, V., & Nosaka, K. (2005). Comparison between leg and arm eccentric exercises of the same relative intensity on indices of muscle damage. *European Journal of Applied Physiology, 95*, 179–185.

Johnson, G., Dowson, D., & Wright, V. (1976). The fracture of articular cartilage under impact loading. *Proceedings of the 3rd Leeds—Lyons Symposium on Tribology*.

Johnson, G., Tramaglini, D., Levine, R., Ohno, K., Choi, N., & Woo, S. (1994). Tensile and viscoelastic properties of human patellar tendon. *Journal of Orthopaedic Research, 12*, 796–803.

Jozsa, L., & Kannus, P. (1997). Human tendons: Anatomy, physiology, and pathology. *Human Kinetics, 164*, 185–186.

Kamalanathan, S., & Broom, N. (1993). The biomechanical ambiguity of the articular surface. *Journal of Anatomy, 183*, 567–577.

Kardon, G. (2011). Development of the musculoskeletal system: Meeting the neighbors. *Development, 138*, 2855–2859.

Kaya, M., Karahan, N., & Yilmer, B. (2019). *Tendon structure and classification, tendons, Hasan Sözen*. IntechOpen. https://www.intechopen.com/books/tendons/tendon-structure-and-classification

Keaveny, A., Morgan, E., & Yeh, O. (2003). *Bone Mechanics*. McGraw-Hill.

Kempson, G. (1979). Mechanical properties of articular cartilage. In M. Freeman (Ed.), *Adult articular cartilage* (pp. 333–414). Pitman Medical.

Kempson, G. (1982). Relationship between the tensile properties of articular cartilage from the human knee and age. *Annals of the Rheumatic Diseases, 41*, 508–511.

Kempson, G. E., Muir, H., Pollard, C., & Tuke, M. (1973). The tensile properties of the cartilage of human femoral condyles related to the content of collagen and glycosaminoglycans. *Biochimica et Biophysica Acta, 297*, 456–472.

Ker, R. (2002). The implications of the adaptable fatigure quality of tendons for their construction, repair, and function. *Comparative Biochemistry and Physiology (Part A), 133*, 987–1000.

Kirkendall, D., & Garrett, W. (1997). Function and biomechanics of tendons. *Scandivian Journal of Medical Science and Sports, 7*, 62–66.

Komi, P., Fukashiro, S., & Jarvinen, M. (1992). Biomechanical loading of Achilles tendon during normal locomotion. *Clinics in Sports Medicine, 11*, 521–531.

Kubo, K., Kanehisa, H., Kawakami, Y., & Fukunaga, T. (2000). Elastic properties of muscle–tendon complex in long-distance runners. *European Journal of Applied Physiology, 81*, 181–187.

Kubo, K., Kanehisa, H., Miyatani, M., Tachi, M., & Fukunaga, T. (2003). Effect of low-load resistance training on the tendon properties in middle-aged and elderly women. *Acta Physiologica Scandinavica, 178*, 25–32.

Kuthe, C., Uddanwadiker, R., & Ramteke, A. (2014). Experimental evaluation of fiber orientation based material properties of skeletal muscle in tension. *Molecular and Cellular Biomechanics, 11*, 113–128.

Kwan, M. K., Wall, E. J., Massie, J., & Garfin, S. R. (1992). Strain, stress and stretch of peripheral nerve. Rabbit experiments in vitro and in vivo. *Acta Orthopaedica Scandinavica*, *63*(3), 267–272. https://doi.org/10.3109/17453679209154780

Lacourpaille, L., Nordez, A., Hug, F., Couturier, A., Dibie, C., & Guilhem, G. (2014). Time-course effect of exercise-induced muscle damage on localized muscle mechanical properties assessed using elastography. *Acta Physiology*, *211*, 135–146.

Lakes, R., & Saha, S. (1979). Cement line motion in bone. *Science*, *204*, 501–503.

Lam Van Ba, O., Barbe, M. F., Caremel, R., Aharony, S., Loutochin, O., Jacques, L., & Ruggieri, M. R., Sr. (2018). Lumbar to sacral root rerouting to restore bladder function in a feline spinal cord injury model: Urodynamic and retrograde nerve tracing results from a pilot study. *Neurourology Urodynamics*, *37*(1), 153–162. https://doi.org/10.1002/nau.23394

Laumonier, T., & Menetrey, J. (2016). Muscle injuries and strategies for improving their repair. *Journal of Experimental Orthopaedic*, *3*, 15.

Legerlotz, K., Schjerling, P., Langberg, H., Bruggemann, G., & Niehoff, A. (2007). The effect of running, strength, and vibration strength training on the mechanical, morphological, and biochemical properties of the Achilles tendon in rats. *Journal of Applied Physiology*, *102*, 564–572.

Levangie, P., & Norkin, C. (2005). *Joint structure and function: A comprehensive analysis* (4th ed.). F.A Davis Co.

Li, X. J.-Y. (1990). Adaptation of cancellous bone to aging and immobilization in the rat: A single photon absorptiometry and histomorphometry study. *The Anatomical Record*, *227*, 12–24.

Liberman, K., Fortia, L., Beyer, I., & Bautmans, I. (2017). The effects of exercise on muscle strength, body composition, physical functioning and the inflammatory profile of older adults: A systematic review. *Current Opinion in Clinical Nutrition & Metabolic Care*, *20*, 30–53.

Lieber, R. (2002). *Skeletal muscle structure, function, and plasticity*. Lippincott Williams & Wilkins.

Lipps, D. (2012). *Effect of gender-related differences in knee morphology on peak ACL strain during repeated simulated pivot landings: An in vitro investigation*. The University of Michigan.

Lipps, D., Wojtys, E., & Ashton-Miller, J. (2013). Anterior cruciate ligament fatigue failures in knees subjected to repeated simulated pivot landings. *The American Journal of Sports Medicine*, *41*, 1058–1066.

Litsky, A., & Spector, M. (1994). Biomaterials. In S. Simon (Ed.), *Orthopaedic basic science* (pp. 447–486). American Orthopaedic Society for Sports Medicine.

Liu, X. S., Cohen, A., Shane, E., Stein, E., Rogers, H., Kokolus, S. L., & Guo, X. E. (2010). Individual trabeculae segmentation (ITS)-based morphological analysis of high-resolution peripheral quantitative computed tomography images detects abnormal trabecular plate and rod microarchitecture in premenopausal women with idiopathic osteoporosis. *Journal of Bone Mineral Research*, *25*(7), 1496–1505. https://doi.org/10.1002/jbmr.50

Loh, P. Y., Yeoh, W. L., & Muraki, S. (2019). An overview of hand postures and aging on morphological changes of the median nerve. *Journal of Physiological Anthropology*, *38*(1), 9. https://doi.org/10.1186/s40101-019-0201-6

Lu, X., & Mow, V. (2008). Biomechanics of articular cartilage and determination of material properties. *Medicine and Science in Sports and Exercise*, *40*, 193–199.

Luttges, M. W., Stodieck, L. S., & Beel, J. A. (1986). Postinjury changes in the biomechanics of nerves and roots in mice. *Journal of Manipulative and Physiological Therapeutics*, *9*(2), 89–98.

Lynch, H., Johannessen, W., Wu, J., Jawa, A., & Elliott, D. (2003). Effect of fiber orientation and strain rate on the nonlinear uniaxial tensile material properties of tendon. *Journal of Biomechical Engineering*, *125*, 726–773.

Ma, Z., Hu, S., Tan, J. S., Myer, C., Njus, N. M., & Xia, Z. (2013). In vitro and in vivo mechanical properties of human ulnar and median nerves. *Journal of Biomedical Materials Research Part A, 101*(9), 2718–2725. https://doi.org/10.1002/jbm.a.34573

Maganaris, C., & Paul, J. (1999). In vivo human tendon mechanical properties. *Journal of Physiology, 521*(Part 1), 307–313.

Mahan, M. A., Yeoh, S., Monson, K., & Light, A. (2019). Rapid stretch injury to peripheral nerves: Biomechanical results. *Neurosurgery, 85*(1), 137–144. https://doi.org/10.1093/neuros/nyy423

Malm, C., Sjödin, T., Sjöberg, B., Lenkei, R., Renström, P., Lundberg, I., & Ekblom, B. (2004). Leukocytes, cytokines, growth factors and hormones in human skeletal muscle and blood after uphill or downhill running. *Journal of Physiology, 556*, 983–1000.

Mammone, J., & Hudson, S. (1993). Micromechanics of bone strength and fracture. *Journal of Biomechanics, 26*, 439–446.

Mansour, J. (2004). *Biomechanics of cartilage* (C. Oatis ed., Vol. 2). Lippincott, Williams & Wilkins.

Martin, B. (1993). Aging and strength of bone as a structural material. *Calcified Tissue Research, 53*, 34–40.

Martin, R., Burr, D., Sharkey, N., & Fyhrie, D. (2015). *Mechanical properties of ligament and tendon.* Springer-Verlag.

Massicotte, V. S., Frara, N., Harris, M. Y., Amin, M., Wade, C. K., Popoff, S. N., & Barbe, M. F. (2015). Prolonged performance of a high repetition low force task induces bone adaptation in young adult rats, but loss in mature rats. *Experimental Gerontology, 72*, 204–217. https://doi.org/10.1016/j.exger.2015.10.014

Matson, A., Konow, N., Miller, S., Konow, P., & Roberts, T. (2012). Tendon material properties vary and are interdependent among turkey hindlimb muscles. *Journal of Experimental Biology, 215*, 3552–3558.

Mazal, P. R., & Millesi, H. (2005). Neurolysis: Is it beneficial or harmful? *Acta Neurochirurgica Supplement, 92*, 3–6. https://doi.org/10.1007/3-211-27458-8_1

McCormack, T., & Mansour, J. (1997). Reduction in tensile strength of cartilage precedes surface damage under repeated compressive loading in vitro. *Journal of Biomechanics, 31*, 55–61.

McNulty, A., & Guilak, F. (2015). Mechanobiology of the meniscus. *Journal of Biomechanics, 48*, 1469–1478.

Melton, L., Lane, A., Cooper, C., Eastell, R., O'Fallon, W., & Riggs, B. (1993). Prevalence and incidence of vertebral deformities. *Osteoporosis International, 3*, 113–119.

Meyers, M., Chen, P.-Y., Lin, A. Y.-M., & Seki, Y. (2008). Biological materials: Structure and mechanical properties. *Progress in Materials Science, 53*, 1–206.

Mikic, Z. (1978). Age changes in the triangular fibrocartilage of the wrist joint. *Journal of Anatomy, 126*, 367–384.

Millesi, H., Zoch, G., & Reihsner, R. (1995). Mechanical properties of peripheral nerves. *Clinical Orthopaedics and Related Research, 314*, 76–83.

Mirhadi, S., Ashwood, N., & Karagkevrekis, B. (2013). Factors influencing fracture healing. *Journal of Trauma, 15*, 1–16.

Mitchell, H., Hamilton, T. S., Steggerda, F., & Bean, H. (1945). The chemical composition of the adult human body and its bearing on the biochemistry of growth. *Journal of Biological Chemistry, 158*, 625–637.

Montanino, A., Deryckere, A., Famaey, N., Seuntjens, E., & Kleiven, S. (2019). Mechanical characterization of squid giant axon membrane sheath and influence of the collagenous endoneurium on its properties. *Scientific Reports, 9*(1), 8969. https://doi.org/10.1038/s41598-019-45446-y

Moon, M.-S., Kim, J.-M., & Ok, I.-Y. (1984). The normal and regenerated meniscus in rabbits. Morphologic and histologic studies. *Clinical Orthopaedics and Related Research, 182*, 264–269.

Morrow, J. D. (1964). *ASTM STP 378* (pp. 45). Philadelphia: ASTM.

Mow, V., & Huiskes, R. (2005). *Basic orthopaedic biomechanics and mechanobiology*. Lippincott Williams & Wilkins.

Mukund, K., & Subramaniam, S. (2020). Skeletal muscle: A review of molecular structure and function, in health and disease. *Wiley Interdisciplinary Reviews: Systems Biology and Medicine, 12*, e1462.

Nagel, T., & Kelly, D. (2010). Mechano-regulation of mesenchymal stem cell differentiation and collagen organisation during skeletal tissue repair. *Biomechanics and Modeling in Mechanobiology, 9*, 359–372.

Neviaser, A., Andarawis-Puri, N., & Flatow, E. (2012). Basic mechanisms of tendon fatigue damage. *Journal of Shoulder and Elbow Surgery, 21*, 158–163.

Nordin, M., & Frankel, V. (2012). *Basic biomechanics of the musculoskeletal system*. Lippincott, Williams & Wilkins.

O'Brien, M. (1997). Structure and metabolism of tendons. *Scandinavian Journal of Medicine & Science in Sports, 7*, 55–61.

O'Brien, T., Reeves, N., Baltzopoulos, V., Jones, D., & Maganaris, C. (2010). Mechanical properties of the patellar tendon in adults and children. *Journal of Biomechanics, 43*, 1190–1195.

Oda, J., Tanaka, H., & Tsuzuki, N. (1988). Intervertebral disc changes with aging of human cervical vertebra. From the neonate to the eighties. *Spine, 13*, 1205–1211.

Ozkaya, N., Leger, D., Goldsheyder, D., & Nordin, M. (2017). *Fundamentals of biomechanics*. Springer.

Park, J. S., & Hoke, A. (2014). Treadmill exercise induced functional recovery after peripheral nerve repair is associated with increased levels of neurotrophic factors. *PLoS One, 9*(3), 90245. https://doi.org/10.1371/journal.pone.0090245

Parkkinen, J., Lammi, M., Helminen, H., & Tammi, M. (1992). Local stimulation of proteoglycan synthesis in articular cartilage explants by dynamic compression in vitro. *Journal of Orthopaedics Research, 10*, 610–620.

Parry, D. B., & Craig, A. (1978). A comparison of the size distribution of collagen fibers in connective tissue as a function of age and a possible relation between fibril size and mechanical properties. *Proceedings of the Royal Society of London. Series B, 203*, 305–321.

Paulsen, G., Crameri, R., Benestad, H., Fjeld, J., Mørkrid, L., Hallén, J., & Raastad, T. (2010). Time course of leukocyte accumulation in human muscle after eccentric exercise. *Medicine & Science in Sports and Exercise, 42*, 75–85.

Paulsen, G., Egner, I., Drange, M., Langberg, H., Benestad, H., Fjeld, J., & Raastad, T. (2010). A COX-2 inhibitor reduces muscle soreness, but does not influence recovery and adaptation after eccentric exercise. *Scandinavian Journal of Medicine & Science in Sports, 20*, 195–207.

Peake, J., Neubauer, O., Della Gatta, P., & Nosaka, K. (2017). Muscle damage and inflammation during recovery from exercise. *Journal of Applied Physiology, 122*, 559–570.

Phillips, J. B., Smit, X., De Zoysa, N., Afoke, A., & Brown, R. A. (2004). Peripheral nerves in the rat exhibit localized heterogeneity of tensile properties during limb movement. *Journal of Physiology, 557*(Pt 3), 879–887. https://doi.org/10.1113/jphysiol.2004.061804

Pike, A., Ker, R., & Alexander, R. (2000). The development of fatigue quality in high- and low-stressed tendons in sheep. *Journal of Experimental Biology, 39*, 2187–2193.

Prendergast, P., Huiskes, R., & Søballe, K. (1997). Biophysical stimuli on cells during tissue differentiation at implant interfaces. *Journal of Biomechanics, 30*, 539–548.

Procter, C., Schmidt, M., Whipple, R., Kelly, M., & Mow, V. (1989). Material properties of the normal medial bovine meniscus. *Journal of Orthopaedic Research*, *7*, 771–782.

Proske, U., & Morgan, D. (2001). Muscle damage from eccentric exercise: Mechanism, mechanical signs, adaptation and clinical applications. *The Journal of Physiology*, *537*, 333–345.

Provenzano, P., Lakes, R., Keenan, T., & Vanderby, R. (2001). Nonlinear ligament viscoelasticity. *Annals of Biomedical Engineering*, *29*, 908–914.

Quapp, K., & Weiss, J. (1998). Material characterization of human medial collateral ligament. *Journal of Biomechanical Engineering*, *1*, 757–763.

Rasool, G., Wang, A., Rymer, W., & Lee, S. (2018). Shear waves reveal viscoelastic changes in skeletal muscles after hemispheric stroke. *IEEE Transactions on Neural Systems and Rehabilitation Engineering*, *26*, 2006–2014.

Reeves, N., Magnaris, C., & Narici, M. (2003). Effect of strength training on human patellar tendon mechanical properties of older individuals. *Journal of Physiology*, *548*, 971–981.

Reilly, D., & Burstein, A. (1975). The elastic and ultimate properties of compact bone tissue. *Journal of Biomechanics*, *8*, 393–405.

Reilly, G. (2000). Observations of microdamage around osteocyte lacunae in bone. *Journal of Biomechanics*, *33*, 1131–1134.

Robi, K., Jakob, N., Matevz, K., & Matjaz, V. (2013). The physiology of sports injuries and repair processes. In M. Hamlin (Ed.), *Current issues in sports and exercise medicine* (pp. 43–86). Intech Open Science.

Rogers, M., & Evans, W. (1993). Changes in skeletal muscle with aging: Effects of exercise training. *Exercise and Sport Sciences Reviews*, *21*, 65–102.

Rosso, G., & Guck, J. (2019). Mechanical changes of peripheral nerve tissue microenvironment and their structural basis during development. *APL Bioengineering*, *3*(3), 036107. https://doi.org/10.1063/1.5108867

Rubin, C., & Lanyon, L. (1985). Regulation of bone mass by mechanical strain magnitude. *Calcified Tissue International*, *37*, 411–417.

Rubin, C., Recker, R., Cullen, D., Ryaby, J., McCabe, J., & McLeod, K. (2004). Prevention of postmenopausal bone loss by a low-magnitude, high-frequency mechanical stimuli: A clinical trial assessing compliance, efficacy, and safety. *Journal of Bone and Mineral Research*, *19*, 343–351.

Ruggieri, M. R., Braverman, A. S., D'Andrea, L., Simpkiss, B., Kozin, S. H., Pontari, M. A., & Barbe, M. F. (2006). Functional reinnervation of the canine bladder after spinal root transection and immediate end-on-end repair. *Journal of Neurotrauma*, *23*(7), 1125–1136. https://doi.org/10.1089/neu.2006.23.1125

Russo, C. (2009). The effects of exercise on bone. Basic concepts and implications for the prevention of fractures. *Clinical Cases in Mineral and Bone Metabolism*, *6*, 223–228.

Rydevik, B. L., Kwan, M. K., Myers, R. R., Brown, R. A., Triggs, K. J., Woo, S. L., & Garfin, S. R. (1990). An in vitro mechanical and histological study of acute stretching on rabbit tibial nerve. *Journal of Orthopaedic Research*, *8*(5), 694–701. https://doi.org/10.1002/jor.1100080511

Sabatier, M. J., Redmon, N., Schwartz, G., & English, A. W. (2008). Treadmill training promotes axon regeneration in injured peripheral nerves. *Experimental Neurology*, *211*(2), 489–493. https://doi.org/10.1016/j.expneurol.2008.02.013

Salmon, P. L., Ohlsson, C., Shefelbine, S. J., & Doube, M. (2015). Structure model index does not measure rods and plates in trabecular bone. *Frontiers of Endocrinology (Lausanne)*, *6*, 162. https://doi.org/10.3389/fendo.2015.00162

Sandri, M. (2010). Autophagy in skeletal muscle. *FEBS Letters*, *584*, 1411–1416.

Sanyal, A. G., Bayraktar, H. H., Kwon, R. Y., & Keaveny, T. M. (2012). Shear strength behavior of human trabecular bone. *Journal of Biomechanics, 45*, 2513–2519.

Sasazaki, Y., Shore, R., & Seedhom, B. (2006). Deformation and failure of cartilage in the tensile mode. *Journal of Anatomy, 208*, 681–694.

Saunier, J., & Chapurlat, R. (2018). Stress fracture in athletes. *Joint Bone Spine, 85*(3), 307–310. https://doi.org/10.1016/j.jbspin.2017.04.013

Schaffler, M., Radin, E., & Burr, D. (1989). Mechanical and morphological effects of strain rate on fatigue of compact bone. *Bone, 10*, 207–214.

Schapery, R. (1975). Theory of crack initiation and growth in viscoelastic media. 2. Approximate methods of analysis. *International Journal of Fracture, 11*, 369–388.

Schechtman, H., & Bader, D. (1997). In vitro fatigue of human tendons. *Journal of Biomechanics*, 829–835.

Schleifenbaum, S., Schmidt, M., Möbius, R., Wolfskämpf, T., Schröder, C., Grunert, R., & Prietzel, T. (2016). Load and failure behavior of human muscle samples in the context of proximal femur replacement. *BMC Musculoskeletal Disorders, 17*, 149.

Schmidt-Nielsen, K. (1984). *Scaling: Why is animal size so important?* Cambridge University Press.

Schneider, H. (1956). Zie struktur der sehnenansatzzonen. *Zeitschrift der anatomie und entwicklungsgeschichte, 119*, 431–456.

Sela, J., & Bab, I. (2012). *Principles of bone regeneration*. Springer.

Shadwick, R. (1990). Elastic energy storage in tendons: Mechanical differences related to function and age. *Journal of Applied Physiology, 68*, 1033–1040.

Sharir, A., Barak, M., & Shahar, R. (2008). Whole bone mechanics and mechanical testing. *The Veterinary Journal, 177*, 8–17.

Sharma, P., & Maffulli, N. (2005). Tendon injury and tendinopathy: Healing and repair. *Journal of Bone and Joint Surgery (American), 87*, 187–202.

Shepherd, J., & Screen, H. (2013). Fatigue loading of tendon. *International Journal of Experimental Pathology, 94*, 260–270.

Shepherd, J. H., & Legerlotz, K. (2012). The fatigue behaviour of functionally distinct bovine tendons. BSMB special meeting – tendinopathy – from basic science to treatment.

Silver, F., Bradica, G., & Tria, A. (2001). Viscoelastic behavior of osteoarthritic cartilage. *Connective Tissue Research, 42*, 223–233.

Silver, F., Bradica, G., & Tria, A. (2002). Elastic energy storage in human articular cartilage: Estimation of the elastic modulus for type II collagen and changes associated with osteoarthritis. *Matrix Biology, 21*, 129–137.

Simon, W., Mak, A., & Spirt, A. (1989). The effect of shear fatigue on bovine articular cartilage. *Journal of Orthopaedics Research, 8*, 86–93.

Siracusa, J., Charlot, K., Malgoyre, A., Conort, S., Tardo-Dino, P., Bourrilhon, C., & Garcia-Vicencio, S. (2019). Resting muscle shear modulus measured with ultrasound shear-wave elastography as an alternative tool to assess muscle fatigue in humans. *Frontiers in Physiology, 10*, 626.

Sladjana, U. Z., Ivan, J. D., & Bratislav, S. D. (2008). Microanatomical structure of the human sciatic nerve. *Surgical and Radiologic Anatomy, 30*(8), 619–626. https://doi.org/10.1007/s00276-008-0386-6

Smith, N. (2019). *In vitro tensile fatigue of human flexor digitorum profundus and superficialis tendons* (Doctoral Dissertation). Auburn University.

Smith, T. T. G., Barr-Gillespie, A. E., Klyne, D. M., Harris, M. Y., Amin, M., Paul, R. W., & Barbe, M. F. (2020). Forced treadmill running reduces systemic inflammation yet worsens upper limb discomfort in a rat model of work-related musculoskeletal disorders. *BMC Musculoskeletal Disorders, 21*(1), 57. https://doi.org/10.1186/s12891-020-3085-z

Soong, J., Schafhalter-Zoppoth, I., & Gray, A. T. (2005). The importance of transducer angle to ultrasound visibility of the femoral nerve. *Regional Anesthesia & Pain Medicine*, *30*(5), 505. https://doi.org/10.1016/j.rapm.2005.05.012

Sophia Fox, A., Bedi, A., & Rodeo, S. (2009). The basic science of articular cartilage: Structure, composition, and function. *Sports Health*, *1*, 461–468.

Stauber, W., Clarkson, P., Fritz, V. K., & Evans, W. J. (1990). Extracellular matrix disruption and pain after eccentric muscle action. *Journal of Applied Physiology*, *69*, 868–874.

Stecco, C., Giordani, F., Fan, C., Biz, C., Pirri, C., Frigo, A. C., & De Caro, R. (2020). Role of fasciae around the median nerve in pathogenesis of carpal tunnel syndrome: Microscopic and ultrasound study. *Journal of Anatomy*, *236*(4), 660–667. https://doi.org/10.1111/joa.13124

Stenroth, L., Peltonen, J., Cronin, N., Sipila, S., & Finni, T. (2012). Age-related differences in Achilles tendon properties and triceps surae muscle architecture in vivo. *Journal of Applied Physiology*, *113*, 1537–1544.

Stephens, N., Gallagher, I., Rooyackers, O., Skipworth, R., Tan, B., Marstrand, T., et al. (2010). Using transcriptomics to identify and validate novel biomarkers of human skeletal muscle cancer cachexia. *Genome Med*, *2*(1), 1.

Sun, H., Andarawis-Puri, N., Li, Y., Fung, D., Lee, J., Wang, V., & Flatow, E. L. (2010). Cycle-dependent matric remodeling gene expression response in fatigue-loaded rat patellar tendons. *Journal of Orthopaedic Research*, *28*, 1380–1386.

Sunderland, S. (1965). The connective tissues of peripheral nerves. *Brain*, *88*(4), 841–854. https://doi.org/10.1093/brain/88.4.841

Sunderland, S. (1990). The anatomy and physiology of nerve injury. *Muscle Nerve*, *13*(9), 771–784. https://doi.org/10.1002/mus.880130903

Sunderland, S., & Bradley, K. C. (1961). Stress–strain phenomena in human peripheral nerve trunks. *Brain*, *84*(1), 102–119. https://doi.org/10.1093/brain/84.1.102

Svensson, R., Heinemeier, K., Couppé, C., Kjaer, M., & Magnusson, S. (2016). Effect of aging and exercise on the tendon. *Journal of Applied Physiology*, *121*, 1353–1362.

Takaza, M., Moerman, K., Gindre, J., Lyons, G., & Simms, C. (2013). The anisotropic mechanical behavior of passive skeletal muscle tissue subjected to large tensile strain. *Journal of the Mechanical Behavior of Biomedical Materials*, *17*, 209–220.

Thornton, G., Oliynyk, A., & Frank, C., & Shrive, N. (1997). Ligament creep cannot be predicted from stress relaxation at low stress: A biomechanical study of the rabbit medial collateral ligament. *Journal of Orthopaedic Research*, *5*, 652–656.

Thornton, G. M., Schwab, T., & Oxland, T. (2007). Cyclic loading causes faster rupture and strain rate than static loading in medial collateral ligament at high stress. *Clinical Biomechanics*, *22*, 932–940.

Tidball, J. (2011). Mechanisms of muscle injury, repair, and regeneration. *Comprehensive Physiology*, *1*, 2029–2062.

Tillett, R. L., Afoke, A., Hall, S. M., Brown, R. A., & Phillips, J. B. (2004). Investigating mechanical behaviour at a core-sheath interface in peripheral nerve. *Journal of the Peripheral Nervous System*, *9*(4), 255–262. https://doi.org/10.1111/j.1085-9489.2004.09411.x

Tillman, B., & Tondury, G. (1987). Bewegungsapparat. In *Rauber/Kopsch, Anatomie des Menschen* (Vol. 1, pp. 152–155). Georg Thieme.

Tohgi, H., Tsukagoshi, H., & Toyokura, Y. (1977). Quantitative changes with age in normal sural nerves. *Acta Neuropathology*, *38*(3), 213–220. https://doi.org/10.1007/BF00688067

Topp, K. S., & Boyd, B. S. (2006). Structure and biomechanics of peripheral nerves: Nerve responses to physical stresses and implications for physical therapist practice. *Physical Therapy*, *86*(1), 92–109. https://doi.org/10.1093/ptj/86.1.92

Toumi, H., & Best, T. (2003). The inflammatory response: Friend or enemy for muscle injury? *British Journal of Sports Medicine*, *37*, 284–286.

Turner, C. (2006). Bone strength: Current concepts. *Annals of the New York Academy of Sciences*, *1068*, 429–446.

Turner, C., Rho, J., Takano, Y., Tsui, T., & Pharr, G. (1999). The elastic properties of trabecular bone and cortical bone tissues are similar: Results from two microscopic measurement techniques. *Journal of Biomechanics*, *32*, 437–441.

Turner, C. H. (2007). Aging and fragility of bone. *Journal of Musculoskeletal Neuronal Interactions*, *7*(4), 342–343.

Umansky, D., & Midha, R. (2020). Commentary: The presence and persistence of unrealistic expectations in patients undergoing nerve surgery. *Neurosurgery*, *86*(6), E522+.

Umemura, Y., Ishiko, T., Yamauchi, T., Kurono, M., & Mashiko, S. (1997). Five jumps per day increase bone mass and breaking force in rats. *Journal of Bone Mineral and Research*, *12*(9), 1480–1485. https://doi.org/10.1359/jbmr.1997.12.9.1480

Verdijk, L., Dirks, M., Snijders, T., Prompers, J., Beelen, M., Jonkers, R., . . . Van Loon, L. J. C. (2012). Reduced satellite cell numbers with spinal cord injury and aging in humans. *Medicine & Science in Sports and Exercise*, *44*, 2322–2330.

Viidik, A. (1969). Tensile strength properties of Achilles tendon systems in trained and untrained rabbits. *Acta Orthopaedica Scandinavica*, *40*, 261–272.

Walbeehm, E. T., Afoke, A., Wit, T., Holman, F., Hovius, S. E., & Brown, R. A. (2004). Mechanical functioning of peripheral nerves: Linkage with the "mushrooming" effect. *Cell Tissue Research*, *316*(1), 115–121. https://doi.org/10.1007/s00441-004-0867-9

Wang, J. (2006). Mechanobiology of tendon. *Journal of Biomechanics*, *39*, 1563–1582.

Wang, X., Ker, R., & Alexander, R. (1995). Fatigue rupture of wallaby tail tendons. *Journal of Experimental Biology*, *198*, 847–852.

Warner, W. S., Yeoh, S., Light, A., Zhang, J., & Mahan, M. A. (2020). Rapid-stretch injury to peripheral nerves: Histologic results. *Neurosurgery*, *86*(3), 437–445. https://doi.org/10.1093/neuros/nyz194

Warren, G., Lowe, D., & Armstrong, R. (1999). Measurement tools used in the study of eccentric contraction-induced injury. *Sports Medicine*, *27*, 43–59.

Weightman, B. (1976). Tensile fatigue of human articular cartilage. *Journal of Biomechanics*, *9*, 193–200.

Weightman, B., Chappell, D., & Jenkins, E. (1978). A second study of tensile fatigue properties of human articular cartilage. *Annals of the Rheumatic Diseases*, *37*, 58–63.

Weisman, G., Pope, M., & Johnson, R. (1980). Cyclic loading in knee ligament injuries. *American Journal of Sports Medicine*, *8*, 24–30.

West, R., & Fu, F. (2005). *Soft tissue physiology and repair*. American Academy of Orthopaedic Surgeons.

Wilcox, M., Gregory, H., Powell, R., Quick, T. J., & Phillips, J. B. (2020). Strategies for peripheral nerve repair. *Current Tissue Microenvironment Reports*, *1*(2), 49–59. https://doi.org/10.1007/s43152-020-00002-z

Wojtys, E., Beaulieu, M., & Ashton-Miller, J. (2016). New perspectives on ACL injury: On the role of repetitive sub-maximal knee loading in causing acl fatigue failure. *Journal of Orthopaedic Research*, *34*, 2059–2068.

Wolfe, R. (2006). The underappreciated role of muscle in health and disease. *American Journal of Clinical Nutrition*, *84*, 475–482.

Woo, S., Gomez, M., Woo, Y. K., & Akeson, W. (1982). Mechanical properties of tendons and ligaments. II. The relationships of immobilization and exercise on tissue remodeling. *Biorheology*, *19*, 397–408.

Woo, S., Hildebrand, K., Watanabe, N., Fenwick, J., Papageorgiou, C., & Wang, J. (1999). Tissue engineering of ligament and tendon healing. *Clinical Orthopaedics*, 312–323.

Woo, S., Ritter, M., Amiel, D., Sanders, T., Gomez, M., Kuei, S., & W.H., A. (1980). The biomechanical and biochemical properties of swine tendons—Long-term effects of exercise on the digital extensors. *Connective Tissue Research*, *7*, 177–183.

Woo, S.-Y., & Buckwalter, J. (Eds.) (1988). Skeletal muscle. In *Injury and repair of the musculoskeletal soft tissues* (pp. 213–291). American Academy of Orthopaedic Surgeons.

Woo, S.-Y., Orlando, C., Camp, J., & Akeson, W. (1986). The effect of postmortem storage by freezing on ligament tensile behavior. *Journal of Biomechanics*, *19*, 399–404.

Wood, K., Wilhelm, J. C., Sabatier, M. J., Liu, K., Gu, J., & English, A. W. (2012). Sex differences in the effectiveness of treadmill training in enhancing axon regeneration in injured peripheral nerves. *Developmental Neurobiology*, *72*(5), 688–698. https://doi.org/10.1002/dneu.20960

Wren, T., Lindsay, D., Beaupre, G., & Carter, D. (2003). Effects of creep and cyclic loading on the mechanical properties and failure of human Achilles tendons. *Journal of Biomedical Engineering*, *31*, 710–717.

Wu, Z., Ovaert, T., & Niebur, G. (2012). Viscoelastic properties of human cortical bone tissue depend on gender and elastic modulus. *Journal of Orthopaedic Research*, *30*, 693–699.

Yamada, H. (1970). *Strength of biological materials*. Williams & Wilkins.

Yang, L., Werf, K., Dijkstra, P., Feijen, J., & Bennink, M. (2012). Micromechanical analysis of native and cross-linked collagen type I fibrils supports the existence of microfibrils. *Journal of the Mechanical Behavior of Biomedical Materials*, *6*, 148–158.

Yeoh, S., Warner, W. S., Eli, I., & Mahan, M. A. (2020). Rapid-stretch injury to peripheral nerves: Comparison of injury models. *Journal of Neurosurgery*, 1–11. https://doi.org/10.3171/2020.5.JNS193448

Yingling, V., Callaghan, J., & McGill, S. (1997). Dynamic loading affects the mechanical properties and failure sites of lumbar spines. *Clinical Biomechanics*, *12*, 301–305.

Yurchenco, P. D., & Schittny, J. C. (1990). Molecular architecture of basement membranes. *FASEB Journal*, *4*(6), 1577–1590. https://doi.org/10.1096/fasebj.4.6.2180767

Zioupos, P. (2001). Ageing human bone: Factors affecting its biomechanical properties and the role of collagen. *Journal of Biomaterials Applications*, *15*, 187–229.

Zioupos, P., & Currey, J. (1998). Changes in the stiffness, strength, and toughness of human cortical bone with age. *Bone*, *22*, 57–66.

Zitnay, J., & Weiss, J. (2018). Load transfer, damage and failure in ligaments and tendons. *Journal of Orthopaedic Research*, *36*, 2093–3104.

7

Fatigue Failure of Musculoskeletal Tissues

Introduction

At the microscopic level, even seemingly pristine materials contain ubiquitous flaws of various shapes and sizes (Hamed, 1994). For this reason, even if a global stress imposed on the material is evenly applied, the internal stress field will not be uniformly distributed within the material. Instead, stress will become concentrated at areas of material imperfection to the point where the localized stress may be many times higher than the average applied stress. It is at points where stress is so concentrated that the material is vulnerable to the nucleation of microscopic damage (microdamage). When such damage occurs, it weakens the strength of the material in this region and may lead to additional stress concentrations. Irrespective of the material involved, atomic bonds in the material will be broken in this process given sufficient strain (Bitzek, Kermode, & Gumbsch, 2015). Since all materials (including musculoskeletal tissues) are made up of atoms, fatigue failure can be thought of as a fundamental characteristic of the specific atomic makeup of a material interacting with repetitive stress and strain. Variations in the atomic makeup of materials will lead to different failure responses in the face of loading, but all materials will eventually fail in the presence of sufficient repeated stress.

The previous chapter detailed the material properties of the specialized materials that comprise the musculoskeletal system. These materials are remarkable for their strength and resilience, some capable of millions of loading cycles throughout a lifetime of use. However, unlike most engineering materials, the inner workings of the musculoskeletal system are largely hidden from view, making it difficult to obtain direct tissue measurements that would be useful in demonstrating the presence of a fatigue failure process *in vivo*. As a result, we must rely upon evidence that though useful and informative, has attendant limitations. Thus, it is helpful to examine various lines of evidence that need to be examined to evaluate the likelihood that fatigue failure is a mechanism important in the development of MSDs. This chapter will review some of these lines of evidence.

One important source of information is studies that have examined the fatigue failure response of musculoskeletal tissues when tested *ex vivo*. Such fatigue failure studies are available for many musculoskeletal system components, including tendons, ligaments, cartilage, bone, as well as more complex structures such as spinal motion segments. While these studies provide useful information on material responses to repeated loading, they do so outside of the living physiological environment. However, several authors have examined the responses of musculoskeletal tissues to repeated loading in animal models, which are useful in understanding both tissue and

Musculoskeletal Disorders: The Fatigue Failure Mechanism, First Edition. Sean Gallagher and Mary F. Barbe.

physiological responses to loading. Since these animal models are not human, it would be useful to have data to show evidence of a fatigue failure process in living humans. Examination of epidemiologic evidence can provide some useful (though indirect) information in this regard. Finally, three recent fatigue-failure-based risk assessment tools have been developed to assess the risk associated with various occupational exposures. These include a tool to assess the risk of low back disorders from lifting and lowering tasks (Gallagher, Sesek, Schall Jr, & Huangfu, 2017), a tool to assess MSD risk to the distal upper extremity due to hand intensive tasks (Gallagher, Schall Jr, Sesek, & Huangfu, 2018), and a tool to assess shoulder MSD risk from shoulder intensive tasks (Bani Hani et al., 2021). If these tools demonstrate strong associations with MSD outcomes, they will provide further evidence that MSDs are the result of a fatigue failure process.

The number of studies examining fatigue failure of musculoskeletal tissue is not as extensive as one might imagine, with most studies performed within the last 25 years. In some cases, our knowledge of material characteristics is predicated on the responses of musculoskeletal tissues from other mammalian or even marsupial species (e.g., rats, rabbits, sheep, cows, and wallabies). However, it appears that evolution has largely settled on the materials that make up the musculoskeletal systems for a broad range of species, and it appears generally that muscle is muscle, tendon is tendon, etc. across different species. There are some differences such as the rat tendon does not possess an analog to the human matrix metalloproteinase-1 (MMP-1) gene (Shepherd & Screen, 2013). In general, however, materials making up the musculoskeletal system are quite similar. We will begin our evaluation of the evidence with the response of musculoskeletal tissues to repeated stress in the *ex vivo* state.

Ex Vivo Studies of Fatigue Failure in Musculoskeletal Tissues

Tendon

Studies examining the fatigue loading responses of tendons remain a relatively recent phenomenon, with the earliest studies being reported in the mid-1990s (Shepherd & Screen, 2013). One study was performed by Wang and colleagues on wallaby tail tendons under sinusoidal loading (Wang, Ker, & Alexander, 1995). A variety of loading frequencies were used, ranging from 1.1 to 50 Hz. The minimum stress applied in these tests was 11.5 MPa, with maximum levels of stress ranging from 20 to 80 MPa. Results demonstrated relationships between the logarithm of fatigue life and the level of stress imposed. The following relationship was demonstrated between stress and median cycles to failure:

$$S = 96.5 - 15.8\log(N)$$

in which S is the normalized stress relative to the estimated Ultimate Tensile Strength (UTS, reported as 144 MPa), and N is the number of cycles to failure.

Schechtman and Bader provided an excellent model as to how an S–N curve could be derived for musculoskeletal tissue (Schechtman & Bader, 1997). This study examined the fatigue life response of 90 human extensor digitorum longus (EDL) tendons under stress levels ranging from 10 to 90% UTS. Ten tendons were tested at each of the nine stress deciles. Twelve specimens were tested to determine the average UTS for the EDL, which averaged 99.9 (~ 100) MPa. The minimum stress range was 1 MPa and cycled to the appropriate stress level (e.g., 40 MPa for the 40% UTS condition) using a square cyclic loading waveform to represent a typical *in vivo* loading pattern (Komi, Fukashiro, & Jarvinen, 1992). Results of this study demonstrated a log-normal relationship between normalized stress level and the number of cycles to failure. The relationship observed is described by the following equation:

$$S = 101.3 - 14.8 * \log(N)$$

where S represents the normalized stress and N is the number of cycles to failure. Data obtained in this study suggested that tendon failure may have been dictated by the amount of strain experienced by the tendon. In general, tendons tended to fail at approximately 15% strain, irrespective of the level of stress. However, lower levels of stress took many more repetitions to get to this point than higher levels of stress. Data from the Schechtman & Bader (1997) study are shown in Figure 7.1.

In another study examining biopsied human tendons *ex vivo*, Wren and colleagues used 25 Achilles tendons to examine fatigue responses to a loading regimen having minimum stress of 10 MPa and maximum stresses ranging from 35–80 MPa (Wren, Lindsay, Beaupre, & Carter, 2003). In line with the previously mentioned studies, higher peak stresses were associated with decreased fatigue life and vice versa. The initial strain exhibited by the tendons was strongly associated with fatigue life, a finding they also found true for separate tests of creep loading (prolonged static loading) (Wren et al., 2003). These results point to strain as a mechanical factor that may help dictate damage development and tendon failure (Shepherd & Screen, 2013).

Pike and colleagues examined fatigue loading of the extensor digitorum lateralis and plantaris tendons in sheep (Pike, Ker, & Alexander, 2000). The former tendon is believed to experience less stress, while the latter experiences more stress. Both demonstrate an exponential decrease in cycles to failure with increasing stress; however, the authors noted that the more highly stressed tendons demonstrated a somewhat enhanced resistance to fatigue damage, compared to those that

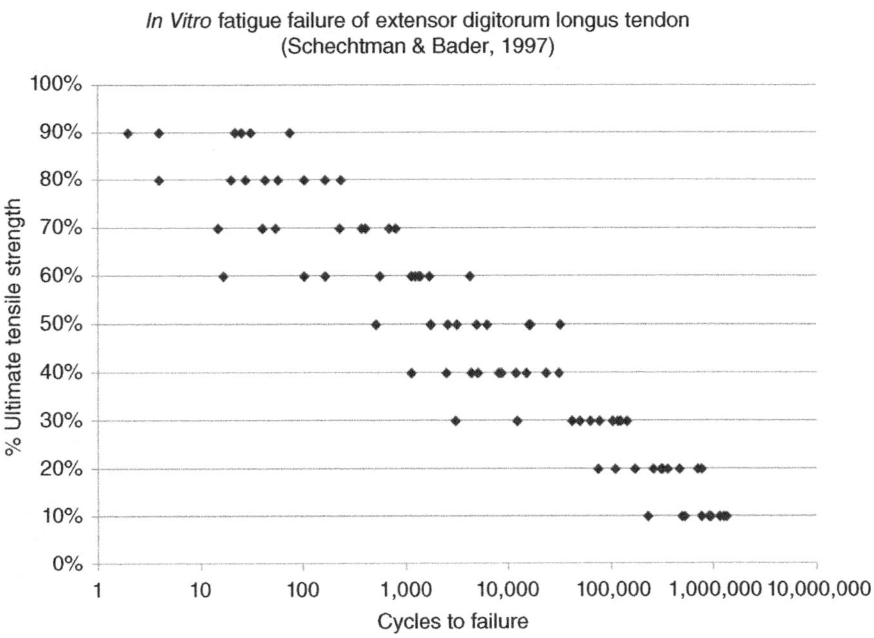

Figure 7.1 Fatigue failure data from *ex vivo* testing of human extensor digitorum longus tendons (Schechtman & Bader, 1997). Data courtesy of Dr. Helio Schechtman.

Table 7.1 Cumulative Damage Observed in *Ex Vivo* Tested Tendons at Different Levels of Fatigue.

Level of fatigue	Collagen fiber architecture	Mechanics
No fatigue	Organized alignment of collagen fibrils	
Low-level fatigue	Kinks appear in the fibers	Increased stiffness, decreased hysteresis
Moderate fatigue	Kinked fibers plus the appearance of gaps between fibers	Same as low-level fatigue
High-level fatigue	Severe matrix degeneration, fiber thinning, angulations, fiber discontinuities	Decreased stiffness, increased strain, increased energy dissipation

Modified from Shepherd, J., & Screen, H. (2013). Fatigue loading of tendon. *International Journal of Experimental Pathology, 94*, 260–270.

experienced lower stresses in life (Pike et al., 2000). Ker and colleagues demonstrated that if one normalized the data according to the expected mechanical stress of life, similar fatigue failure patterns were observed across the tendons (Ker, Wang, & Pike, 2000).

In a later study, fatigue responses of human semitendinosus versus two bovine tendons (deep digital flexor tendon and extensor tendon) were measured (Shepherd et al., 2014). Cyclic loading was performed at 60% of the UTS of these tendons for 300, 900, or 1800 cycles, and the samples were examined for collagen fascicle organization at each level of the loading cycle. At this level of loading, little damage was observed in any of the three tendon varieties after 300 cycles; however, significant damage was observed in all tendons at 900 and 1200 cycles. Fibril kinking and a loss of collagen alignment were observed in all samples at all levels, and findings of fibril disruption and increased inter-fiber space were particularly evident in samples loaded to 1200 cycles.

This pattern of progressive damage development indicative of fatigue failure processes has been observed by multiple authors and the progression of damage typically seen in tendons at different levels of fatigue is shown in Table 7.1 (Shepherd et al., 2014). Also of interest in these studies is that early stages of damage (e.g., low-level fatigue exhibiting kinked fibers) often do not display large changes in the mechanical characteristics of the tendons. However, as damage progresses, mechanical changes start to emerge.

The progression of tendon damage observed during *ex vivo* fatigue experiments has been compared with that seen in biopsied tendons (e.g., those from Achilles' tendons in patients experiencing significant tendinopathy) (Jarvinen et al., 2004; Jozsa & Kannus, 1997; Magnusson et al., 2002; Movin, Gad, Reinholt, & Rolf, 1997). Though specific changes observed varied to a degree across studies, all studies demonstrated microstructural changes consistent with the structural degradation of the tendon during *ex vivo* fatigue testing (Shepherd & Screen, 2013). Early microstructural changes observed in patellar tendons tended to show little in the way of changes in mechanical properties (Kongsgaard et al., 2010).

The structural changes observed in *ex vivo* fatigue failure testing of tendons appear to correlate well with findings of biopsies performed in late-stage tendinopathy. Shepherd & Screen (2013) reported that microstructural changes in tendon morphology similar to those observed in fatigue failure tests have been found in multiple studies examining tendinopathic tissues (Jozsa & Kannus, 1997; Kongsgaard et al., 2010; Movin et al., 1997; Tallon, Maffulli, & Ewen, 2001). These studies include findings of separated tendon fibers with increased waviness in slight and moderate achillodynia, and severe disruption of tendon fiber structure in extreme cases (Movin et al., 1997). Decreased collagen thickness and disrupted crimp continuity in tendons experiencing rupture

(Jarvinen et al., 2004), and fragmentation and fraying of collagen fibers in tendon rupture samples have also been reported (Jozsa & Kannus, 1997).

There is evidence that the morphology changes caused by fatigue loading precede certain mechanical, molecular, and cellular changes (Shepherd & Screen, 2013). Among these changes is a decrease in tenocyte numbers when damage has reached a moderate stage of tendinopathy (Tallon et al., 2001). As pathological changes progress to more extreme damage, nuclei become progressively more rounded (due to a decrease in cytoplasmic organelles and decreased metabolic activity). Late-stage tendinopathy has been associated with increased non-collagenous extracellular matrix and increased inter-fiber glycosaminoglycans (Astrom & Rausing, 1995; Jozsa & Kannus, 1997; Movin et al., 1997). However, early-stage fatigue damage may not have a noticeable impact on *in vivo* tendon mechanical properties (Kongsgaard et al., 2010).

As described further in Chapter 11, it is generally thought that inflammation plays a role in the development of tendinopathy and/or in subsequent tendon failure. One study found signs of acute inflammation in each tendon in a sampling of 60 ruptured tendons using histological staining techniques (Cetti, Junge, & Vyberg, 2003). Typically though, results from tissue biopsies of tendinopathic and ruptured tendons have generally revealed the lack of inflammatory cells at the time of surgery post rupture, reflective of late-stage tendinopathy (Jozsa, Reffy, Kannus, Demel, & Elek, 1990; Kannus & Jozsa 1991; Fredberg & Stengaard-Pedersen, 2008).

Ligaments

As discussed in Chapter 3, ligaments are structurally similar to tendons because they contain a high percentage of collagen. However, ligaments have higher levels of elastin, which provides increased flexibility allowing a greater amount of joint movement, while still maintaining important structural support for the joint. There are few studies of fatigue failure of ligaments. We will discuss two *ex vivo* studies that examined fatigue failure of knee ligaments, one in humans and one in rabbits.

In a study of low cycle fatigue failure in human cadaveric anterior cruciate ligaments (ACLs), Lipps and colleagues demonstrated that repeated loading at 3-4 times body weight (3 to 4*BW) led to relatively rapid damage of ACLs (Lipps, Wojtys, & Ashton-Miller, 2013). At 4*BW, eight of 10 knees failed (mean cycles to failure was 21 $\pm$ 18 SD), and when subjected to the 3*BW load, five of 10 knees failed (mean cycles to failure was 52 $\pm$ 10 SD). Cox regression analysis demonstrated that increased simulated landing force and decreased ACL cross-sectional area were the factors significantly related to cycles to failure; these findings are congruent with a fatigue process. Observed damage modes included complete or partial ACL tears, tibial avulsions, and increased anterior tibial translation. Increased tensile stress in ligaments was associated with more rapid damage accumulation and a reduction in the modulus of elasticity (Lipps, 2012). Figure 7.2 provides the inferred relationship with respect to fatigue failure of male versus female ACLs (Lipps, 2012).

Thornton and colleagues studied cyclic loading of rabbit medial collateral ligament (MCL) specimens, stressed to 15, 30, and 60% of their predicted ultimate tensile strength (%UTS) (Thornton, Schwab, & Oxland, 2007). Sinusoidal loading with a 1 Hz cycle ranging from 1 N to the assigned %UTS was employed, and fatigue testing was continued until ligament rupture (or stopped at a predetermined time). For comparison with the previously discussed tendon tests, data on ruptured tendons reported by Thornton et al. (2007) were analyzed by the current authors in the present study using a lognormal regression. The following equation was obtained:

$$S = 115.3 - 7.94\, log\, (N)$$

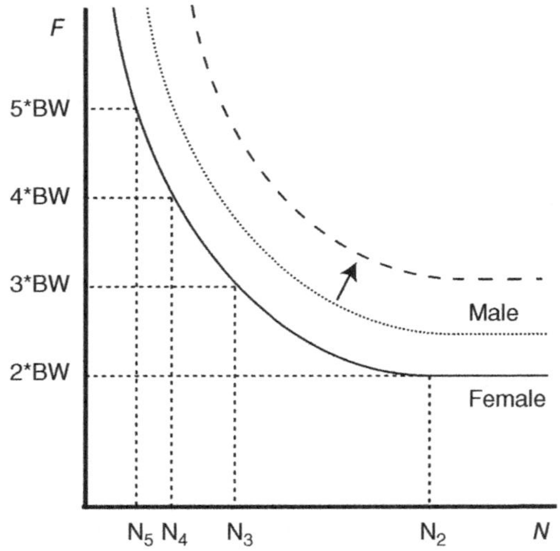

Figure 7.2 Inferred relationship between the knee pivot landing force (*F*) in multiples of body weight and the number of loading cycles to ACL failure (*N*). The number of cycles to ACL failure increases as the repetitive landing force is decreased. Authors suggested that the gender difference in this fatigue failure behavior may explain the higher ACL injury risk observed in females (Lipps, 2012). This figure is taken from a dissertation copyrighted by David Benjamin Lipps, University of Michigan, 2012.

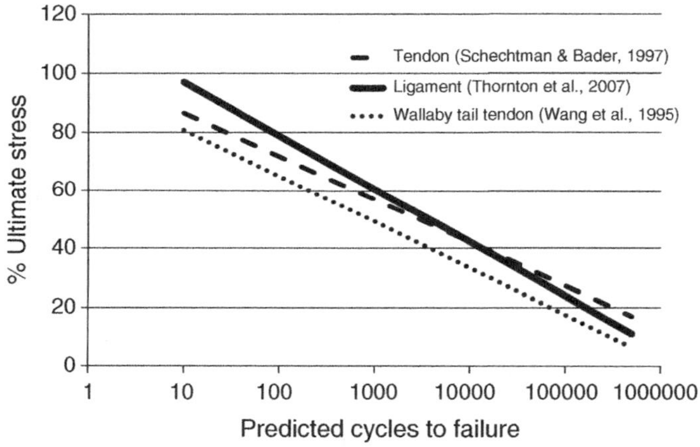

Figure 7.3 Comparison of *S–N* curves from studies assessing fatigue failure of tendons. (Schechtman, H., & Bader, D. (1997). In vitro fatigue of human tendons. *Journal of Biomechanics, 30*, 829–835; Wang, X., Ker, R., & Alexander, R. (1995). Fatigue rupture of wallaby tail tendons. *Journal of Experiemental Biology, 198*, 847–852) and ligaments (Thornton, G., Schwab, T., & Oxland, T. R. (2007). Cyclic loading causes faster rupture and strain rate than static loading in medial collateral ligament at high stress. *Clinical Biomechanics, 22*, 932–940).

where *S* is the stress normalized to a percentage of UTS (100 MPa for rabbit MCL) and *N* is the number of cycles to failure. Thornton and Bailey also examined the fatigue life of healing ligaments and demonstrated greatly reduced fatigue life and increased strain rates during healing, compared to healthy tendons (Thornton & Bailey, 2013).

The results of studies on *ex vivo* tendon and ligament fatigue failure indicate that both these collagen-based structures demonstrate fatigue failure responses when exposed to cyclic loading at different levels of stress. Figure 7.3 provides a summary of the fatigue failure responses from three studies that used a relatively wide range of repeated stress exposure (Schechtman & Bader, 1997; Thornton et al., 2007; Wang et al., 1995). These three studies demonstrate general agreement in terms of the fatigue life of these materials at different levels of the material ultimate stress.

Spinal Motion Segments

Several researchers have examined the effects of repetitive stress on damage development in spinal motion segments *ex vivo*, both in human (Adams & Hutton, 1985; Brinckmann, Biggemann, & Helweg, 1988; Gallagher et al., 2007; Hansson, Keller, & Spengler, 1987; Huber et al., 2016) and animal (Yingling, Callaghan, & McGill, 1997) models. In all cases, a strong relationship was demonstrated between the magnitude of the load imposed on the specimens and the number of cycles to failure experienced by spinal motion segments.

A classic study on fatigue failure of lumbar spine motion segments was performed by Brinckmann and colleagues (Brinckmann et al., 1988). These authors dissected out cadaveric lumbar and lower thoracic motion segments from individual spines and randomly selected one segment from each spine for an ultimate compressive strength test. The ultimate compressive strength of adjacent motion segments was estimated using previous estimates of the difference in strength between levels of the lumbar spine (Hansson et al., 1987). These motion segments were then assigned to be loaded at a percentage (20–70%) of their predicted ultimate compressive strength (UCS). The number of cycles to failure of the vertebral endplate (a structure composed of fibrocartilage) was then recorded. A maximum of 5,000 loading cycles were performed, and if specimens did not meet the failure criterion by this point, their data were censored.

Table 7.2 provides the results of the current study. The magnitude of loading is shown on the left and the number of loading cycles to failure at the various loading levels is along the bottom. The bars represent the percentage of specimens failing according to load level and the number of cycles experienced. At the end of 5,000 loading cycles, only 8% of specimens loaded at 20–30% of the UCS failed, while 100% of specimens loaded at 60–70% UCS failed. The progressive decrease in fatigue life with increasing load demonstrates that lumbar motion segments are subject to a fatigue failure process when subjected to compressive loading.

The study by Brinckmann et al. (1988) provide useful fatigue data; however, the limited number of loading cycles performed is a significant limitation with respect to understanding the responses of spinal segments at low load levels. This study would be characterized as one investigating "low cycle" fatigue responses to compression (i.e., cycles < 10,000). Additional data on high cycle (up to 300,000 cycles) fatigue of lumbar motion segments have been reported by Huber and colleagues (Huber et al., 2016; Huber, Skrzypiec, Klein, Puschel, & Morlock, 2010). Figure 7.4 provides a

Table 7.2 Percentage of Motion Segments Failing at Different Numbers of Loading Cycles for Different Percentages of Ultimate Strength

	Load Cycles				
% Ultimate Strength	**10**	**100**	**500**	**1000**	**5000**
60–70	9%	63%	91%	91%	100%
50–60	0%	39%	62%	85%	92%
40–50	0%	36%	55%	55%	68%
30–40	0%	0%	18%	18%	27%
20–30	0%	0%	0%	0%	8%

Brinckmann, P., Biggemann, M., & Helweg, D. (1988). Fatigue fracture of human vertebrae. *Clinical Biomechanics, 3* (Suppl 1), S1–S23.

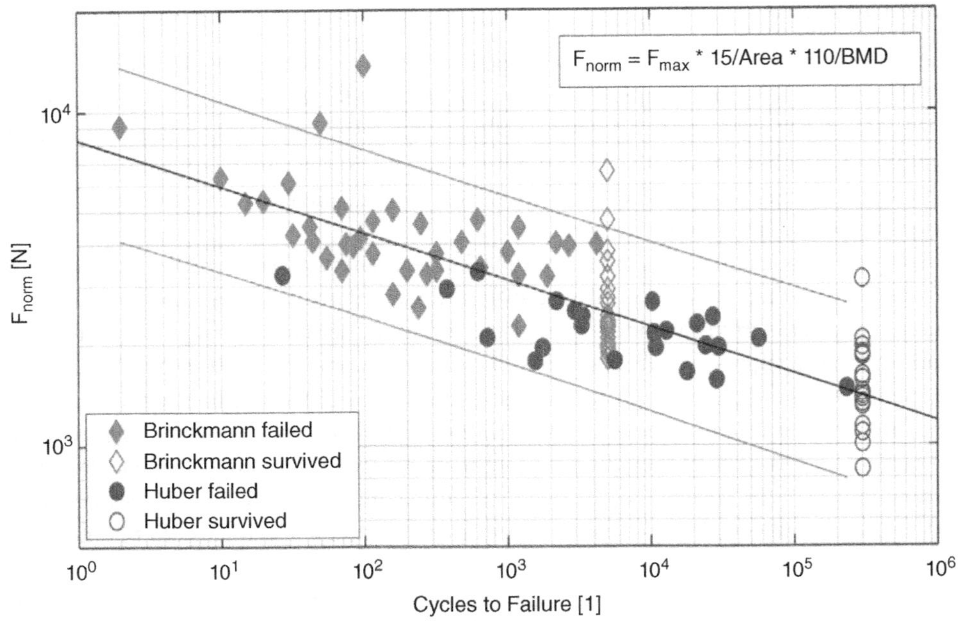

Figure 7.4 Fatigue failure responses of spinal motion segments using combined data from Huber, G., Nagel, K., Skrzypiec, D., Klein, A., Püschel, K., & Morlock, M. (2016). A description of spinal fatigue strength. *Journal of Biomechanics*, 49, 875–880/with permission of Elsevier. Filled grey diamonds represent failed specimens from Brinckmann et al.'s data, while open grey diamonds represent censored data. Black circles represent failed specimens from Huber et al.'s data and open circles represent censored observations. F = force, BMD = bone mineral density.

fatigue failure relationship developed by combining the low cycle data provided by Brinckmann et al. (1988) with the new high cycle fatigue data generated by Huber et al. (2016).

This graph provides evidence that the fatigue failure relationship for low-cycle fatigue appears to follow the same trend when one adds the high-cycle data to it. In this figure, the compressive load is normalized by both the area and the bone mineral density (BMD) of the specimen. The area of the specimen is normalized to 15 cm^2 and the BMD is normalized to 110 mg of K_2HPO_4 per milliliter. As can be seen, as the normalized force increases, fatigue life decreases, and as the normalized force decreases, fatigue life becomes increasingly extended.

As indicated in the studies above, BMD and the size of vertebrae are important factors in determining the fatigue life of lumbar motion segments. Increased BMD and vertebral volume have been associated with increased fatigue life (Gallagher et al., 2007; Huber et al., 2016). Bone mineral content combines these two factors into a single metric that is highly related to both the ultimate compressive strength of spinal motion segments (Hansson & Roos, 1981), and the fatigue life observed under repetitive stress (Gallagher et al., 2007). A loss of bone mineral with aging (especially among post-menopausal women) suggests increased susceptibility to the effects of repetitive loading among these populations.

While the earlier studies have focused primarily on the role of compressive loading and fatigue failure of the lumbar spine, a few studies have examined fatigue loading of the spine in shear (Cyron & Hutton, 1978; Cyron, Hutton, & Troup, 1976). These studies demonstrated that the application of repetitive shear loads resulted in damage similar to that seen in spondylitic fractures. The range of the shear loads applied in Cyron et al. (1976) was fairly low compared to the ultimate shear stress limits observed in previous studies, and unsurprisingly, the vertebrae were generally able to withstand tens or hundreds of thousands of cycles. Only a few working-age specimens (9 out of 50) lasted less than 10,000 cycles, and only 3 out of 50 lasted less than 1,500 cycles. However, additional data provided by Cyron & Hutton (1978) allowed for a greater range of stress levels to assess shear fatigue life (30–70% ultimate shear strength). The combination of these shear fatigue failure data sets were used to recommend occupational limits for repetitive spinal shear loading (Gallagher & Marras, 2012). These authors recommended shear loads of less than 700 N shear for tasks involving up to 1,000 daily cycles, and 1,000 N shear for tasks involving less than 100 daily cycles.

In addition, there is evidence that damage to structures associated with back pain is likely the result of a fatigue failure process. One model of etiology of chronic low back pain suggests that fractures of the vertebral endplate initiate changes in the mechanics of the intervertebral disc that lead to disc degradation (Bogduk, Aprill, & Derby, 2013). As discussed in greater detail below, there is evidence to suggest that a fatigue failure process may be responsible for damage associated with both endplates fractures and disc disruption, both of which have been associated with low back pain (Bogduk, 1997).

As mentioned above, studies have demonstrated that failure to vertebral endplates follows fatigue failure principles (Brinckmann et al., 1988; Gallagher et al., 2007; Huber et al., 2016). The combination of loading magnitude and cycles appear to be well within the loads that can occur during the course of occupational activities or even in the course of normal daily living. Fracture of the endplates has been shown to lead to so-called Modic changes. Modic changes are observed on magnetic resonance images (MRI) and occur in three types (Rhame & Mouss, 2008). Type 1 changes are associated with endplate damage and represent the presence of inflammatory edema and are associated with the presence of inflammatory cytokines, including interleukin (IL) 6, IL 8, and prostaglandin E2. Type 2 Modic changes occur after Type 1 and indicate the deposition of fatty tissue subsequent to the resolution of the inflammatory process. Type 3 Modic changes are thought to be associated with sclerotic changes in the vertebral body. Studies have shown that Type 1 and 2 Modic changes (but not Type 3) have been significantly associated with patients experiencing low back pain, compared to asymptomatic patients (Jensen, Karpinnen, Sorensen, Niinimäki, & Lebeouf-Yde, 2008; Rhame & Mouss, 2008).

Endplate fracture appears to profoundly disrupt the biomechanics of the disc, including significant alterations in the distribution of stress in different disc regions. In general, the stress in the central area of the disc is decreased, while increased stress is observed in posterior regions of the disc (Adams, McNally, Wagstaff, & Goodship, 1993). These results have been confirmed in animal studies in which degradation of the nuclear matrix has been initiated by producing fractures of the vertebral endplate (Cinotti et al., 2005; Holm, Kaigle-Holm, Ekstrom, Karladani, & Hansson, 2004). Internal disruption of the disc is associated with the development of tears in fibers located in the central region of the disc (Figure 7.5, Grade I). Failure of these initial fibers leads to increased stress concentration in this region and increased strain on adjacent fibers. As the injured region becomes exposed to further repeated stress, the fissure starts to expand. As repeated stress continues, the fissure may extend to the outer reaches of the disc where pain receptors will be encountered resulting in back pain (Bogduk et al., 2013). In patients experiencing chronic low back pain (CLBP), the occurrence of internal disc disruption is at least 39% (Schwarzer, Aprill, Derby, Bogduk, & Kine, 1995), which represents the highest association of a measure of spinal degradation with CLBP that has yet been demonstrated.

Thus, there is evidence that the process of disc degeneration may be composed of two fatigue failure processes, the first of which involves the development of a vertebral endplate fracture resulting from exposure to repeated stress. When this fracture occurs, the mechanics of the

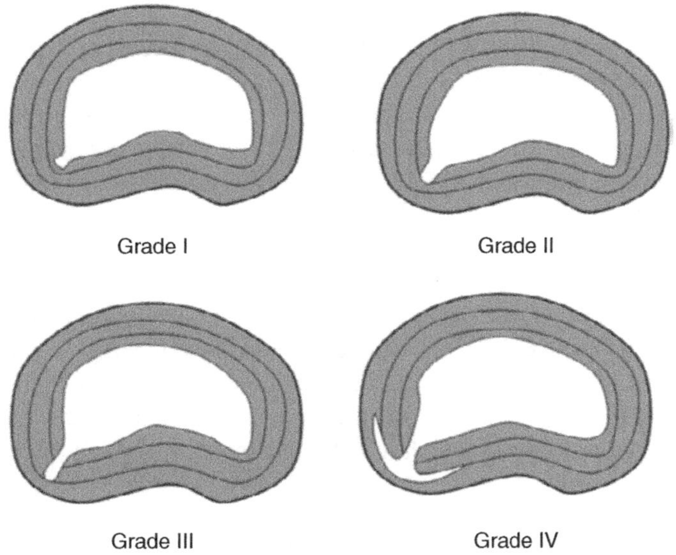

Figure 7.5 Grades of progressive internal disc disruption. Bogduk, N., Aprill, C., & Derby, R. (2013). Lumbar discogenic pain: State-of-the-art review. *Pain Medicine, 14*, 813–836.

intervertebral disc are disrupted, leading to a second fatigue failure process in which a small defect in the annular material occurs in the central portion of the disc. With continued exposure to repeated stress, the area of damage continues to expand until the damage reaches the outmost layers of the disc.

Cartilage

Cartilage is present throughout the body and is an important component in the musculoskeletal system. As detailed in Chapters 3 and 11, it has several unique aspects compared to other musculoskeletal tissues in that it is totally avascular, aneural, and alymphatic (Chang, Marston, & Martin, 2021). The primary cell type within the cartilage matrix is the chondrocyte, which produces a matrix made up of collagen, elastin, and proteoglycans. These materials make up the supporting structure of the collagen, and most of the remainder is made up of water. Since there are no blood vessels, the chondrocytes derive most of their nutrition through diffusion.

In some of the earliest *ex vivo* fatigue failure studies of musculoskeletal tissues, Weightman and colleagues performed tensile fatigue failure tests on articular cartilage specimens from the superior surface of the head of the femur (Weightman, 1976; Weightman, Chappell, & Jenkins, 1978). These authors believed repeated tensile loading of cartilage to be a cause of collagen fibrillation. In the latter (and most comprehensive) investigation, 115 articular cartilage specimens from 20 donors were tested over a wide range of stress levels. Specimens were obtained from 11 men and 9 women aged 9–82 years. Figure 7.6 provides data derived from this study demonstrating the fatigue responses of the superficial layer of articular cartilage when normalizing the results to the predicted ultimate tensile strength of each specimen. This figure exhibits an exponential increase in the fatigue life of articular cartilage with lower loads, congruent with fatigue failure theory. As expected, the fatigue strength was found to be reduced in older specimens. Older specimens tend to show the onset of osteoarthritic fibrillation, which may be associated with the decreased fatigue life observed in these specimens. Weightman and colleagues concluded that fatigue failure could occur in life, particularly in those individuals experiencing high contact

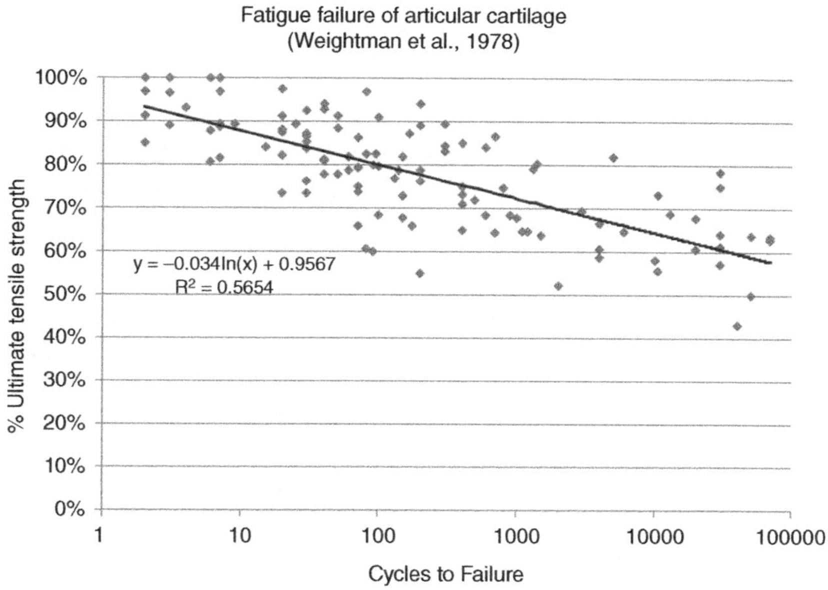

Figure 7.6 Tensile fatigue failure responses of articular cartilage samples from the femoral head. Based on Weightman, B., Chappell, D., & Jenkins, E. (1978). A second study of tensile fatigue properties of human articular cartilage. *Annals of the Rheumatic Diseases, 37*, 58–63.

pressures and those having cartilage with lower than average fatigue tolerance (Weightman et al., 1978). In hips joints, abnormally high contact pressures are most likely to occur at the zenith of the femoral head, which is typically the site that showed progressive osteoarthritic changes (Byers, Contepomi, & Farkas, 1970)

Fibrocartilage is also relevant to the current discussion. Fibrocartilage plays an important role in the provision of a stable interface between ligaments, tendons, and bones (Gharpuray, 1998). This type of cartilage has a higher dry weight of collagen and less water content, making it tougher but less resilient than hyaline cartilage. Vertebral endplates are made of fibrocartilage. As discussed, multiple studies have shown fatigue damage of vertebral endplates as a result of repetitive loading of lumbar motion segments (Brinckmann et al., 1988; Gallagher et al., 2007; Hansson et al., 1987). Other fibrocartilage structures also demonstrate classic fatigue failure responses to repeated stress, e.g., the temporomandibular joint (Gallo, Nickel, Iwasaki, & Palla, 2000). Repetitive loading of this joint results in microscopic crack development, consistent with fatigue failure principles.

Bone

The literature on fatigue failure in bone is more extensive than for any other musculoskeletal tissue, likely because of the relative ease of testing of this material, and perhaps because of its greater similarity to traditional engineering materials (compared to other musculoskeletal tissues). The development of fatigue failure in bone has been observed clinically in overuse stress fractures in young adults exposed to repetitive loading (Bargren & Tilson, 1971; Devas, 1958; Matheson et al., 1987; McBryde, 1976; Milgrom et al., 1985) as well as to bone fractures (e.g., femoral neck fractures) in the elderly (Freeman, Todd, & Pirie, 1974; Griffiths, Swanson, & Freeman, 1971; Martin, 1993).

Several studies have shown that bone behaves as a typical composite material, demonstrating a gradual loss of stiffness and strength with repetitive loading (Carter & Hayes, 1976; Pattin,

Carter, & Caler, 1990; Schaffler, Radin, & Burr, 1989). Damage development has been observed in commonly experienced physiological stress ranges (Freeman et al., 1974; Frost, 1960; Schaffler et al., 1989), and it is believed by some that fatigue damage development may play an important role in regulating the bone remodeling mechanism (Burr, Martin, Schaffler, & Radin, 1985). Several studies have been performed to understand the fatigue life of both compact and trabecular bone exposed to fatigue loading, and several authors have examined the process of microdamage accumulation in bone subjected to fatigue loading (Boyce, Fyhrie, Radin, & Schaffler, 1998; Martin & Burr, 1982). We will briefly review the relationship of repeated stress in relation to fatigue life and examine research that has evaluated the nature of damage accumulation in bone.

Carter and Hayes tested bovine compact bone specimens at five separate stress amplitudes, ranging from 65–108 MPa, and at four temperature levels (21–45°C) (Carter & Hayes, 1976). Results demonstrated a significant negative correlation between the magnitude of stress and the number of cycles to material failure. Increased bone mineral content was found to significantly increase fatigue life, a finding echoed in studies of spinal motion segment tests (Gallagher et al., 2007; Hansson & Roos, 1981). Increased ambient temperature led to decreased cycles to failure, a finding common to fatigue failure in other materials (Stephens, Fatemi, Stephens, & Fuchs, 2001). Post-test microstructural analysis of the specimens indicated that the outer cortical bone regions containing Haversian canals failed more quickly than cortical bone with few (or a total lack of) Haversian canals. This research also determined that cortical bone was susceptible to microdamage and fatigue failure at relatively low-stress levels, indicating the absence of an endurance limit for this material (Carter & Hayes, 1976). These authors compared the regression equation derived from their own data to data obtained in two previous studies (King & Evans, 1967; Swanson, Freeman, & Day, 1971), as shown in Figure 7.7.

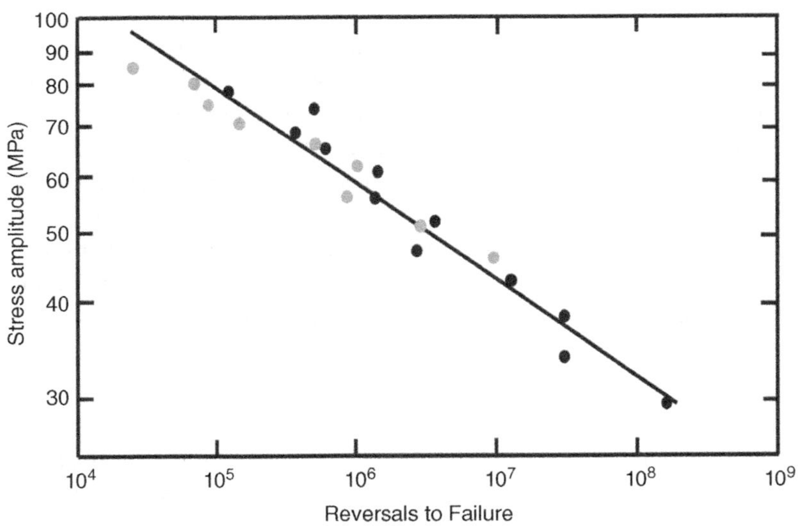

Figure 7.7 Multiple regression lines obtained by Carter, D., & Hayes, W. (1976). Fatigue life of compact bone--I. Effects of stress amplitude, temperature and density. *Journal of Biomechanics, 9*, 27–34. compared against previous data of fatigue of human cortical bone from King, A., & Evans, F. (1967). Analysis of fatigue strength of human compact bone by the Weibull method. In: Bertil Jacobson *Digest of the Seventh International Conference on Medical and Biological Engineering* (p. 514). Stockholm: The Organizing Committee of the Conference (black dots) and Swanson, S., Freeman, M., & Day, W. (1971). The fatigue properties of human cortical bone. *Medical and Biological Engineering, 9*, 23–32 (gray dots).

Carter and colleagues also evaluated the fatigue life of adult cortical bone as a function of the strain range and the mean strain experienced in repeated stress (Carter, Caler, Spengler, & Frankel, 1981). Tests were performed in a humidified environmental chamber at 37 °C. Failure was defined as the point when the total stress range was diminished to 70% of that observed on the first cycle. The magnitude of the strain range experienced was most predictive of the fatigue life of compact bone. Figure 7.8 provides the fatigue life data as a function of the strain range of the loading and relates the findings to predicted strain ranges associated with different levels of physical activity.

The response of bone to fatigue damage is dependent on the specifics of the loading experienced. Carter and Hayes reported that microdamage development in compact bone varies significantly based on whether the repeated load is compressive or tensile (Carter & Hayes, 1976). Compressive fatigue leads to the nucleation and growth of microscopic cracks on planes of maximum shear (Carter & Hayes, 1976; Chamay & Tschantz, 1972), a phenomenon also observed in metals (Stephens et al., 2001). Of course, bone is weaker in shear compared to other loading modalities, which may further promote crack growth in this loading plane. Tensile fatigue loading results in osteon cement lines and results in the debonding of osteons from interstitial bone (Carter & Hayes, 1976).

The development of fatigue in compact bone results in significant material changes, which include a decrease in material properties such as elastic modulus, fracture toughness, and strength, thereby leading to increased deformation of the bone (Boyce et al., 1998). Depending on the specific type of loads experienced locally, a variety of damage morphologies may be observed. This suggests that compact bone has an array of fatigue damage mechanisms that help to dissipate the mechanical energy of the repetitive load, some of which may help reduce the rate of crack propagation (Morgan, Unnikrisnan, & Hussein, 2018). Due to the anisotropic nature of bone, tensile loading and compressive loading are initiated at different magnitudes of strain, with damage starting at the lower strain in tensile loading as compared to compressive loading (Boyce et al., 1998). Fatigue failure of bone subjected to repetitive shear occurs at much lower stress levels than in tensile or compressive loading. The *S-N* curve for cortical bone in shear is provided in Figure 7.9 (Turner et al., 2001).

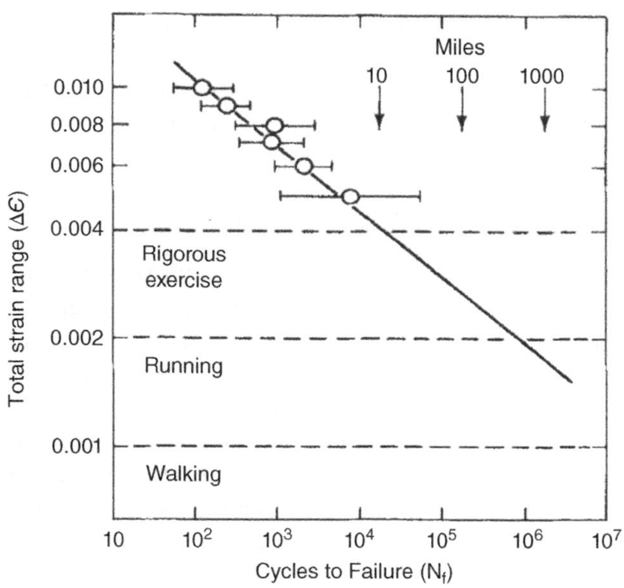

Figure 7.8 The relationship between strain range and cycles to failure for bone in relation to estimated strain associated with different levels of exercise. Carter, D., Caler, W., Spengler, D., & Frankel, V. (1981). Fatigue behavior of adult cortical bone: The influence of mean strain and strain range. *Acta Orthopaedica Scandinavica, 52*, 481–490.

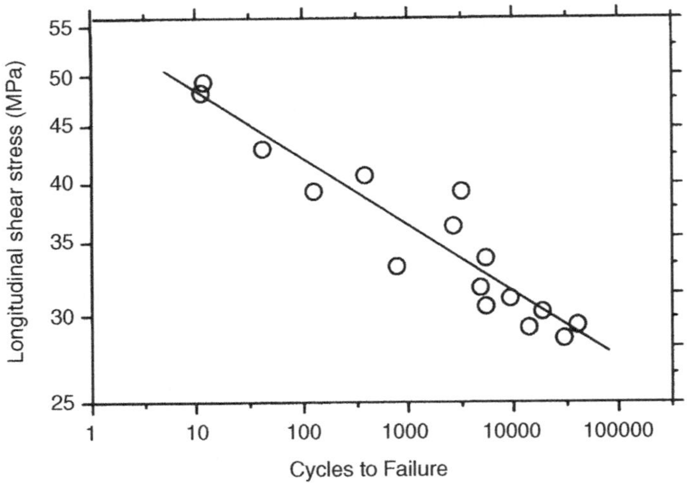

Figure 7.9 Fatigue life of cortical bone in shear ($R^2 = 0.89, p < 0.00001$). Turner, C., Wang, T., & Burr, D. (2001). Shear strength and fatigue properties of human cortical bone determined from pure shear tests. *Calcified Tissue International, 69*, 373–378.

Trabecular bone has a similar material makeup as cortical bone; however, trabecular bone is considerably more porous (40–90% porosity versus 5–15% for cortical bone), yet has a slightly higher density. The elastic modulus of trabecular bone is 10% lower, tensile yield strain is 15% lower, and tensile/compressive strength is 25% less than cortical bone. A comparison of the fatigue failure response of cortical versus trabecular bone in a four-point bending protocol was performed by Choi and Goldstein (Choi & Goldstein, 1992). In this study, similar-sized rectangular beam specimens of cortical and trabecular bone from the tibia were tested to fatigue. The rectangular beams for trabecular bone were created by sectioning and milling samples of trabecular bone (group 1). Cortical bone beams were created using two methods: sectioning and milling (group 2) or a two-phase sectioning approach (group 3). Trabecular bone was tested at five different stress levels (100–140 MPa), while cortical bone was tested at four stress levels (150–180 MPa). Tests were discontinued after 200,000 cycles if no failure occurred. Results can be seen in Figure 7.10. As illustrated in this figure, both materials demonstrated typical fatigue failure S-N curves; however, the curve for trabecular bone is approximately 30–50 MPa below that of cortical bone for an equivalent number of cycles to failure (Choi & Goldstein, 1992).

Summary of *Ex Vivo* Fatigue Testing

Studies of *ex vivo* fatigue testing of musculoskeletal tissues demonstrate that all exhibit a characteristic fatigue failure response when exposed to repeated stress. Moreover, the tissue damage patterns exhibited in laboratory tests often match the pattern of damage seen in various musculoskeletal outcomes. The evidence described in this section is clearly supportive of the notion that musculoskeletal tissues experience fatigue failure damage when exposed to repeated stress. Of course, there are limitations associated with *ex vivo* testing. Notably, there are many complex systems in the biological environment that may modify the response of these tissues to repeated stress, compared to the laboratory setting where more controlled experimentation can take place. Among these aspects, one might include the healing and remodeling processes, possible changes in certain material properties in the *in vivo* state, different stress distributions experienced by

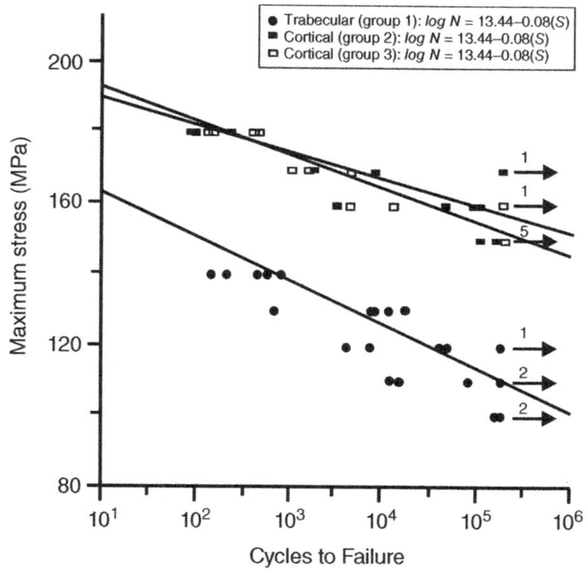

Figure 7.10 Comparison of the fatigue characteristics of trabecular (group 1) and cortical (groups 2 and 3) bone. Arrows represent the number of censored observations (no failure observed as of 200,000 cycles) at given stress levels. Choi, K., & Goldstein, S. (1992). A comparison of the fatigue behavior of human trabecular and cortical bone tissue. *Journal of Biomechanics, 25*, 1371–1381/with permission of Elsevier.

tissues, etc. However, while these and other differences may clearly modify some responses to tissue loading, it is difficult to imagine that anything in the *in vivo* state would somehow nullify the fundamental relationship between exposure to repeated stress and the development of damage in materials.

There are, however, methods to examine whether fatigue failure occurs in the physiological state (*in vivo*). For example, several animal studies have been performed repetitive stress in tendons and other structures *in vivo* to understand both the resulting physical damage and cellular biological responses. The following section reviews some animal models and human subject studies that have examined the effects of loading on musculoskeletal tissues *in vivo* along with related physiological responses.

In Vivo Studies of Fatigue Failure

Tendons

A comprehensive analysis of the responses of Sprague-Dawley rats exposed to various levels of force and repetition has been provided by Barbe and colleagues (Barbe et al., 2013). Rats were exposed to either low force, low repetition (LFLR), low-force, high-repetition (LFHR), high-force, low-repetition (HFLR), or high-force, high-repetition (HFHR) exertions (Figure 7.11d). Rats were randomly assigned to one of these treatment conditions and exposed to a repetitive reaching and grasping task for a 12-week period before evaluation of tissue pathology in all involved musculoskeletal tissues of the upper extremity (tendon, cartilage, bone, and muscle) as well as certain physiological responses (e.g., cytokine responses in these tissues and in serum). As shown in Figure 7.11a, the observed tendon pathology demonstrated a significant force-repetition interaction in terms of the degree of tendon damage determined using a Bonar scoring system. Interaction between force and repetition showed a pattern indicative of an underlying fatigue failure process

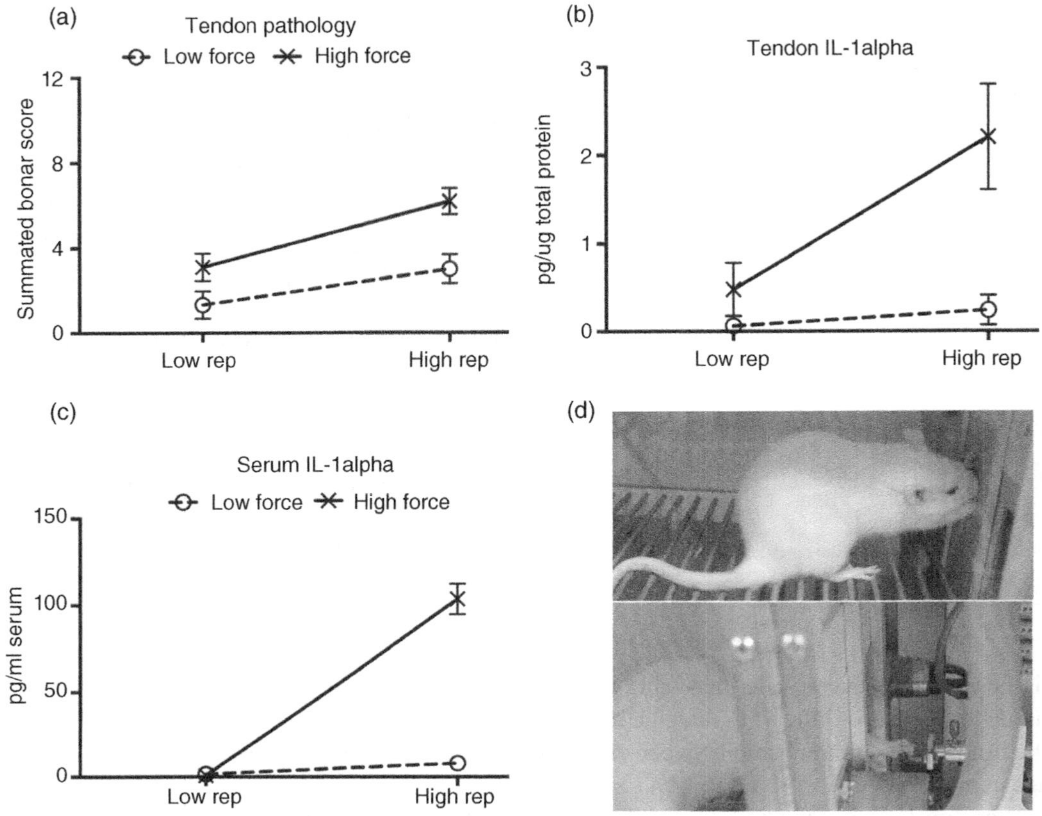

Figure 7.11 Tendon and serum responses to performance of reaching and grasping task at low or high repetition (Rep), or low or high force requirements. (a) Tendon Bonar scores demonstrate a significant ($p = 0.0005$) force-repetition interaction pattern that is indicative of a fatigue failure process. (b) Tendon levels of IL-1alpha (Force $p = 0.01$, Repetition $p = 0.03$). (c) Serum levels of IL-1alpha ($p < 0.0001$ interaction). (d) Experimental setup of a rat pulling on a lever bar. Modified from Barbe, M., Gallagher, S., Massicotte, V., Tytell, M., Popoff, S., & Barr-Gillespie, A. (2013). The interaction of force and repetition on musculoskeletal and neural tissue responses and sensorimotor behavior in a rat model of work-related musculoskeletal disorders. *BMC Musculoskskeletal Disorders,* 14/CC BY 2.0.

(Gallagher & Heberger, 2013). Several cytokines in the tissues also demonstrated significant force-repetition interactions, including interleukin 1-alpha (IL-1alpha) in tendons and serum (Barbe et al., 2013). Muscle showed similar significant force-repetition interactions (Barbe et al., 2013). The magnitude of the inflammatory response appears to be consistent with the magnitude of damage in tissues subjected to repeated stress, and the serum cytokine responses resembled those seen in human subjects with upper extremity repetition motion injuries (Carp, Barbe, Winter, Amin, & Barr, 2007), each supporting the presence of a fatigue failure process.

Nakama and colleagues performed an *in vivo* study to evaluate the development of microtears in tendons of New Zealand white rabbits due to cyclic loading (Nakama, King, Abrahamsson, & Rempel, 2005). The flexor digitorum profundus (FDP) muscles of nine rabbits were stimulated to contract repetitively for 80 hours over a 14-week-period, with the contralateral limb serving as a control. Microtears were quantified using image analysis techniques in four regions of the tendon at the medial epicondyle insertion site. The tear density and mean tear size were compared in the four regions of the tendons in both loaded and unloaded limbs. Results showed that both the mean tear sizes and tear densities in the tendons were significantly greater in the limbs experiencing repetitive stress loading, compared to the unloaded limbs. The authors concluded that the finding of increased size and density of microtears in tendons experienced with repeated loading might be focal points for the development of further tissue degeneration that lead to tendinosis, a result that implicates a fatigue failure process.

An interesting series of *in vivo* fatigue studies on rat patellar tendons have been performed (Andarawis-Puri & Flatow, 2011; Fung et al., 2009; Fung et al., 2010; Sun et al., 2010). These studies allowed the controlled assessment of the physical and biological responses of tendons at various stages of the fatigue failure process. Figure 7.12 illustrates the experimental setup for the study performed by Fung and colleagues (Fung et al., 2010). Tendon structural responses to fatigue loading demonstrated a pattern of degradation that could be divided into phases, as seen in Figure 7.13. In controls, the tendon exhibited an organized structure in which collagen fibers were tightly aligned linearly without any noticeable deformations (Figure 7.13a). Tendons exposed to low-level fatigue developed kinked fibers in some tendon areas that were the first notable deformation observed in the tendon fiber structure (Figure 7.13b). When fatigue loading continued to a moderate level, a greater number of fibers demonstrated the kinked deformations,

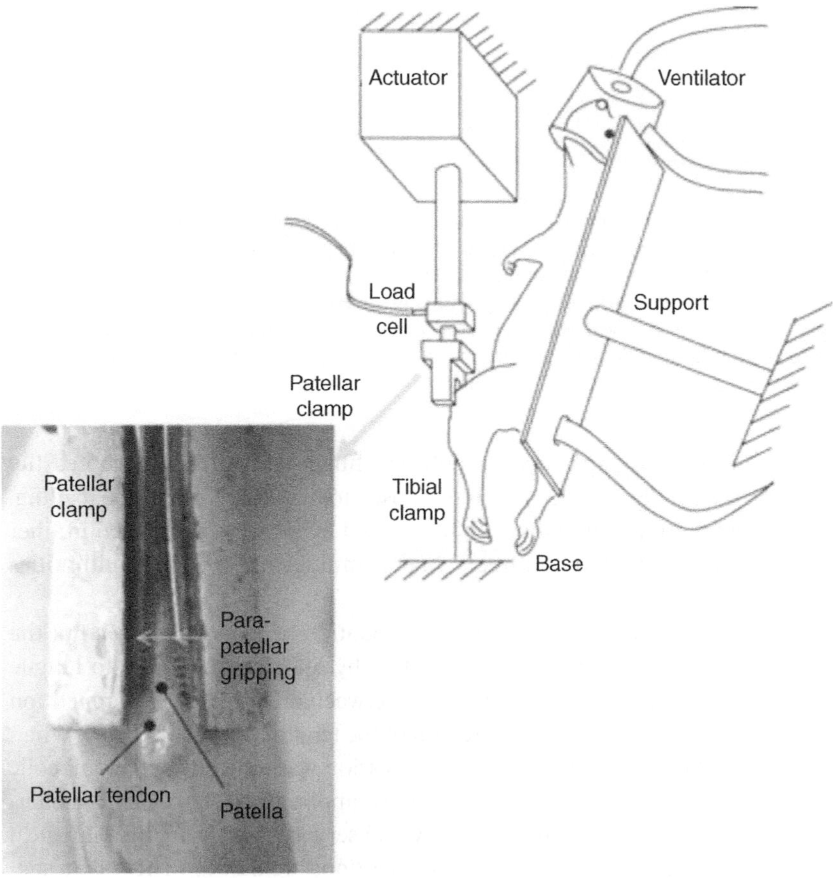

Figure 7.12 Experimental setup used by Fung et al. (2009) in their study of controlled *in vivo* fatigue loading. Based on Fung, D., Wang, W., Laudier, D., Shine, J., Basta-Pljakic, J., Jepsen, K. S., & Flatow, E. (2009). Subrupture tendon fatigue damage. *Journal of Orthopaedic Research, 27*, 264–273.

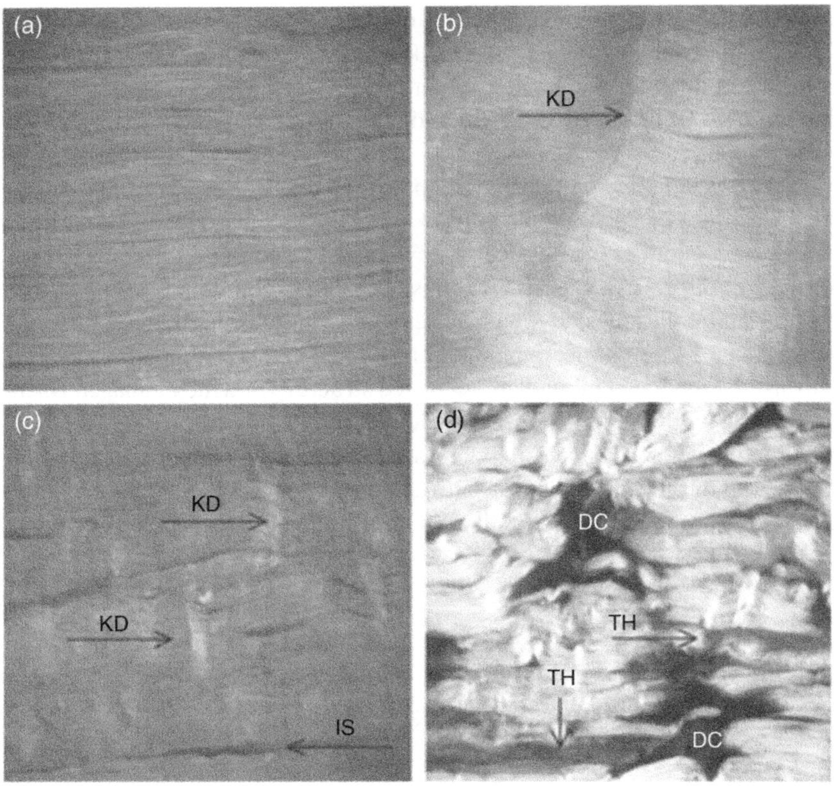

Figure 7.13 Imaging of the progressive tendon damage resulting from exposure to repeated stress *in vivo*: (a) Control tendons showing aligned fibers, (b) low fatigue loading results in appearance of kinked fiber deformation, (c) moderate fatigue loading results in additional kinked fiber deformations and the development of inter-fiber spaces, (d) high fatigue loading results in severe matrix discontinuities (DC) and fiber thinning (TH). Fung, D., Wang, V., Andarawis-Puri, N., Basta-Pljakic, J., Li, Y., Laudier, D., . . . Flatow, E. (2010). Early response to tendon fatigue damage accumulation in a novel in vivo model. *Journal of Biomechanics, 43*, 274–279.

as well as the onset of separations or gaps between collagen fibers that further disrupted the organization of the collagen fibers (Figure 7.13c). When exposed to high levels of fatigue loading, the tendons exhibited extreme matrix degradation, characterized by a severe disruption in fiber alignment, more numerous separations between fibers, fiber thinning, and frank discontinuities in the matrix (Figure 7.13d).

Not only did these studies demonstrate fatigue failure degradation of tendons *in vivo*, but the experimental model also allowed assessment of some of the physiological responses to fatigue loading. The present study sought to quantify the differences between different levels of repetition using a constant load of 40% of the predicted failure strength of the tendon (Sun et al., 2010). When this load was repetitively applied for 100 cycles, the gene expression was indicative of an anabolic response (a building up of tissues). However, when this load was applied for 7200 cycles (a moderate fatigue level), a catabolic response (tissue breakdown) was observed. This shows the biological system can develop a beneficial response to loading when repetitions are modest. These data suggest that the presence of a damage threshold, once overcome, changes the system response to stress from one that is beneficial to one that is degenerative (Andarawis-Puri & Flatow, 2011).

The early stages of the fatigue failure processes are difficult to observe in most materials, and tendons (and other musculoskeletal tissues) are no exception. However, as illustrated in Figures 7.11a and 7.13, distinct macroscopic changes become evident when tendons are repeatedly stressed. Schechtman & Bader (2002) suggested that this process may result from frictional stresses experienced among the collagenous fibers due to repeated stress. A similar process is observed in wire cables and ropes that experience friction and rubbing together of strands of these structures, leading to the development of fatigue damage in a process known as *fretting fatigue* (Suresh, 1998).

A potential mechanism has been suggested for the development of molecular-level damage to collagenous tissues. Research has demonstrated that triple-helical collagen denaturation accumulates in response to fatigue loading and that this collagen molecular "unfolding" increases in proportion to the amount of cyclic loading experienced (Zitnay et al., 2020). This process is thought to be a potential explanation for the fibril kinking that is observed in fatigue-loaded tendons (Andarawis-Puri & Flatow, 2011).

Cartilage

The 2013 study by Barbe and colleagues also examined the effects of exposure to varying levels of force and repetition on the distal articular cartilage of the radius (i.e., the wrist) in a rat model (Barbe et al., 2013). Morphological changes in the cartilage were assessed using a modified Mankin scoring system, which evaluates the structure of the cartilage, cellular abnormalities, and changes in staining (using Safranin orange and fast green). The structure subscore evaluated structural disorganization (chaotic structure, osteoclast activity, and presence of cysts), cellular abnormalities included hypo- or hyper-cellularity or abnormal cellular clusters, and staining was graded from 0 (normal) to 4 (absence of staining). Increased pathology was observed in histological scoring (Figure 7.14a), and multiple structural and cellular changes were observed in the rats exposed to high force and repetition that were not observed in control animals (Figure 7.14b). Both the force-repetition interaction observed in histopathology findings and the degenerative changes observed in the cartilage structure are consistent with a fatigue failure process.

In vivo studies of repetitive impulse loading of articular cartilage have been performed by several authors (Anderson, Brown, & Radin, 1993; Radin et al., 1972; Radin & Paul, 1971). The conclusion of these studies was that cartilage wear was associated with repetitive impulse loading. In these studies, the hind limb of New Zealand white rabbits was subjected to a repetitive impulsive load for 1 hour per day at a rate of 1 Hz. After six days of loading (a total of 21,600 cycles), a stiffening response was observed in the bone. However, after 28 days of loading (100,800 cycles), significant wear was observed in the cartilage, and the underlying bone exhibited numerous trabecular microfractures. Overall, these studies indicate that repeated compressive impact loading may lead to disruption of the interfibrillar connections between collagen fibers in the matrix leading to a weaker, less resistant structure.

Several authors have examined the hypothesis that mechanical fatigue may be a mechanism in the development of osteoarthritis (Johnson, Dowson, & Wright, 1976; Weightman, 1976; Weightman et al., 1978; Simon, Mak, & Spirt, 1989). These studies examined the effects of cyclic loading with respect to the damage caused in the articular cartilage surface using different types of loading. Fibrillation of the articular joint surface was observed. The tensile strength of the articular cartilage matrix (beneath the surface layer) is also negatively impacted by the application of repeated stress during *in vitro* testing, even in the absence of damage to the surface layer (McCormack & Mansour, 1997).

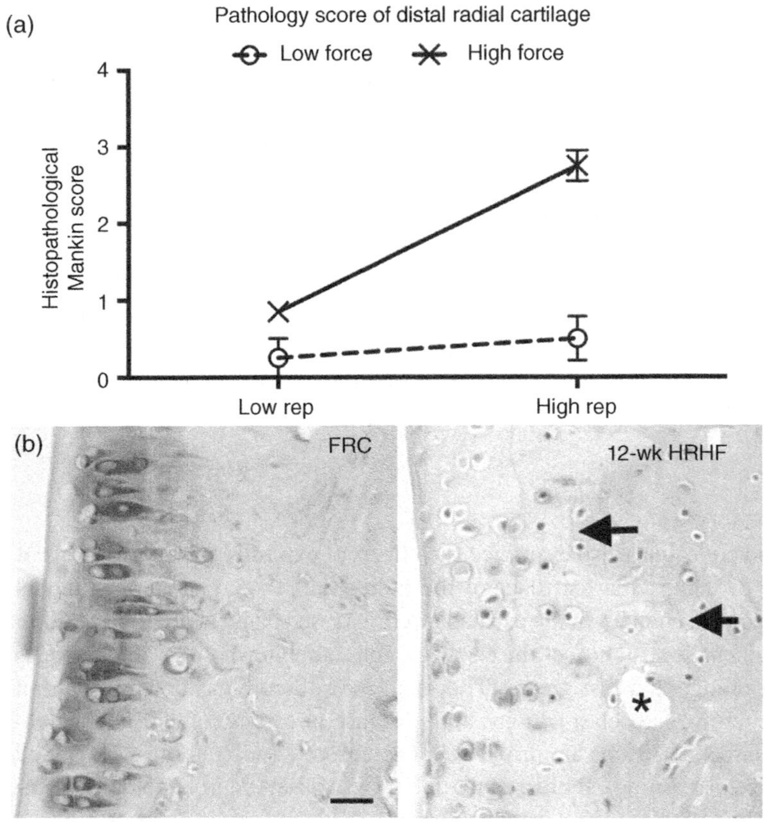

Figure 7.14 Cartilage responses in the distal radius (wrist) to the performance of reaching and grasping tasks. (a) Modified Mankin scoring demonstrated a significant (p=0.002) force-repetition interaction. (b) Comparison of food-restricted controls versus high repetition, high force (HRHF) exposed rats. The latter demonstrated loss of proteoglycan content (reduced staining), an altered tidemark region (arrows), and the presence of subchondral cysts (asterisk). Modified from Barbe, M., Gallagher, S., Massicotte, V., Tytell, M., Popoff, S., & Barr-Gillespie, A. (2013). The interaction of force and repetition on musculoskeletal and neural tissue responses and sensorimotor behavior in a rat model of work-related musculoskeletal disorders. *BMC Musculoskskeletal Disorders,* 14/CC BY 2.0.

Bone

Using their unique rat model, Barbe and colleagues examined the effects of force and repetition on the bone (Barbe et al., 2013). Forelimb bone degradation was seen particularly apparent for rats exposed to 12 weeks of HRHF loading, while forelimb bones of rats exposed to LRHF and HRLF loading responded anabolically. The HRHF rats demonstrated decreases in bone volume in the radius (Figure 7.15a) and an increase in numbers of activated osteoclasts (Figure 7.15b), suggesting that bone was being resorbed and undergoing catabolism (breakdown). In contrast, forelimb bones of the LRHF rats showed more osteoblasts than in the other groups (Figure 7.15c), a finding supportive of anabolism. Serum levels of CTX-1, a biomarker of collagen type I breakdown by osteoclasts, further supporting the prevalence of bone catabolism in the HRHF rats (Figure 7.15d). These results agree with the fatigue failure theory that predict that the combination of high force and high repetition would lead to greater material damage. These results also show the inability of the body to replace damaged bone under the HRHF loading conditions in which osteoclast activity (and numbers) outweigh those of osteoblasts.

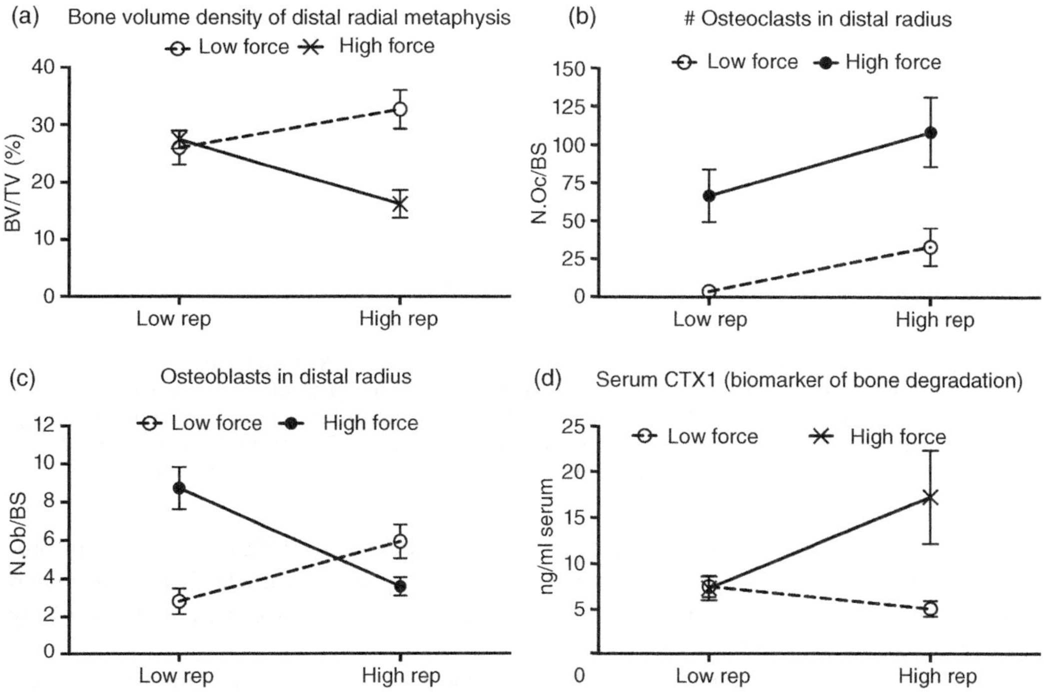

Figure 7.15 Bone responses in the distal metaphysis of the radius to performance of reaching and grasping task. (a) Bone volume density (% bone volume normalized to tissue volume, %BV/TV) demonstrated a significant (p=0.006) force-repetition interaction. (b and c) Numbers of osteoclasts and osteoblasts, each showed a significant interaction (p<0.0001). (d) Serum levels of CTX-1, a biomarker of collagen type I degradation in bone showed a significant interaction (p=0.04). Barbe, M., Gallagher, S., Massicotte, V., Tytell, M., Popoff, S., & Barr-Gillespie, A. (2013). The interaction of force and repetition on musculoskeletal and neural tissue responses and sensorimotor behavior in a rat model of work-related musculoskeletal disorders. *BMC Musculoskskeletal Disorders,* 14. Open Access/Springer Nature/CC BY 2.0.

In a study using anesthetized female New Zealand white rabbits, fatigue loading was applied to the right forelimb *in vivo* using a cyclic load ranging from 10–170 N. Left forearms were used as controls (Buettmann & Silva, 2016). This loading was continued until the apparent stiffness of the forearm increased 10% from the stiffness at the tenth cycle, indicative of the development of a stress fracture in the ulna. Two-to-five weeks after the stress fracture creation, a robust repair was observed with abundant woven bone in the region of the fatigue fracture. At five weeks, the intracortical repair was also observed, indicating that cortical bone damage provokes an intracortical repair response (Buettmann & Silva, 2016).

Skeletal Muscle

The development of damage in muscle fibers is almost always associated with repeated eccentric (rather than isometric or concentric) muscle contraction. This should not be surprising, as eccentric contractions are associated with higher muscle force generation than other contraction modes. Thus, it can be assumed that muscle tissue is closer to its ultimate strength and would be experiencing close to its highest level of strain during the performance of eccentric contractions. Such a high level of strain would likely only be able to be withstood for a limited number of cycles if fatigue failure is indeed the mechanism of muscle as well. While single eccentric exertions appear

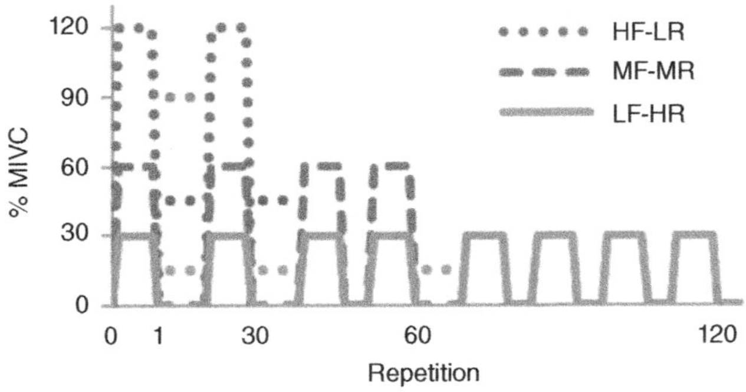

Figure 7.16 Three levels of eccentric exercise used in Huangfu et al. (2018): high force- low repetition (HF-LR), medium force-medium repetition (MF-MR), and low force-high repetition (LF-HR). Huangfu, R., Gallagher, S., Sesek, R., Schall, M., & Davis, G. (2018). Evaluating the linear integration method of estimating cumulative loading using an eccentric exercise. *Proceedings of the Human Factors and Ergonomics Society Annual Meeting*. *62*(1), pp. 882–885. Los Angeles, CA: Sage/with permission of SAGE publications.

not to lead to the development of muscle damage (Teague & Schwane, 1995), damage can be produced after a dozen or more repetitions. Thus, damage development in muscle fibers is most often associated with eccentric contractions, and these contractions need to be experienced repetitively in order for damage to manifest in the sarcomeres.

A couple of studies using human subjects provide evidence in support of a fatigue failure process underlying the development of eccentric exercise muscle damage. One study examined exposure to three separate eccentric loading conditions, all having the same "area under the curve" (Huangfu, Gallagher, Sesek, Schall, & Davis, 2018). These included eccentric loads at 30% of the subjects Maximum Isometric Voluntary Contraction (MIVC) for 120 repetitions (low force, high repetition: LF-HR), another at 60% MIVC for 60 repetitions (medium force, medium repetition: MF-MR), and the third at 120% MIVC for 30 repetitions (high force, low repetition: HF-LR). Figure 7.16 provides a graphic depicts the three loading conditions. Ten healthy male subjects were randomly assigned to these three loading conditions and the eccentric exertions were performed using an isokinetic dynamometer dynamometer.

Though the sum of the area under the curve for the eccentric loading (the work, or "volume") is equivalent, due to the exponential relationship between stress level and cycles to failure, fatigue failure theory would predict that the HF-LR condition would be expected to lead to greatest muscle damage, followed by the MF-MR group, and then the LF-HR group. Results of this study demonstrated significant differences between the HF-LR and the other groups on measures indicative of muscle damage due to eccentric exercise (Figure 7.17). A significant interaction was observed between group and day regarding the decrease in strength observed by the different groups. The HF-LR group was found to exhibit significantly decreased MIVC strength compared to the other groups through day 4 of recovery (Figure 7.17a). Prolonged strength loss is considered to be one of the most valid and reliable indirect measures of muscle damage in humans (Clarkson & Hubal, 2002; Warren, Lowe, & Armstrong, 1999); thus, this finding is indicative of significantly greater transient muscle damage in the HF-LR groups compared to the others. Figure 7.17b demonstrates that the HF-LR had a significantly decreased resting elbow angle compared to the LF-HR condition. Decreases in elbow resting angle are believed to be due to damage to the sarcoplasmic reticulum resulting from eccentric exercise, causing calcium to flood the muscle cells leading to a sustained contracture of the muscles until the healing process repairs the damage (Cleak & Eston, 1992).

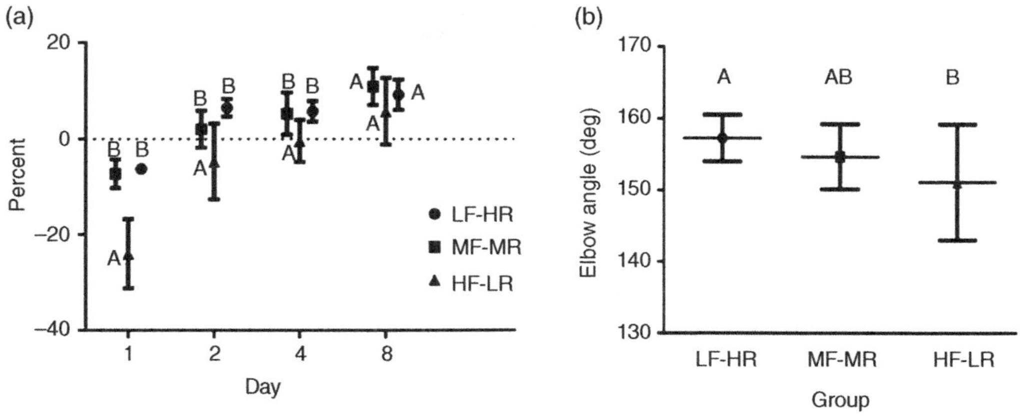

Figure 7.17 (a) The HF-LR group demonstrated significant reductions in MIVC compared to other groups from Day 1 through Day 4 of recovery. (b) The HF-LR group demonstrated a significantly lower average resting elbow angle during recovery compared to the LF-HR group. Letters next to graph conditions represent the results of Tukey HSD tests. Conditions with the same letters are not significantly different. Huangfu, R., Gallagher, S., Sesek, R., Schall, M., & Davis, G. (2018). Evaluating the linear integration method of estimating cumulative loading using an eccentric exercise. *Proceedings of the Human Factors and Ergonomics Society Annual Meeting*. 62(1), pp. 882–885. Los Angeles, CA: Sage/with permission of SAGE publications.

The results above suggest that a limited number of eccentric repetitions at high levels of stress are associated with increased damage in muscle tissues, much more so than higher levels of repetition at lower force levels. These findings are congruent with expectations of fatigue failure. Another finding that supports the assumption that muscle damage results from fatigue failure is that mechanical strain of muscle is a primary causal factor of exercise-induced muscle damage (Falkner, Brooks, & Opiteck, 1993). Damage is more prevalent when eccentric exercise is performed with the muscle at a longer length, especially when the muscle is beyond 140% of its optimal length. This appears true in both human and animal studies (Clarkson & Hubal, 2002).

Summary of *In Vivo* Studies

The studies discussed above demonstrate that animals and even human subjects experiencing repetitive loading display significant tissue damage that conforms with a fatigue failure process of material damage. Tissues that sustain this damage include tendons, cartilages, bones, and nerves. Additional studies applying controlled loading *in vivo* animal models have demonstrated that fatigue failure can occur in living biological tissues (Andarawis-Puri & Flatow, 2011; Buettmann & Silva, 2016; Nakama et al., 2005). However, the question remains as to whether fatigue failure might be implicated in the development of specific types of MSDs. For this, we can evaluate epidemiological evidence examining whether a particular pattern of interaction between force and repetition is observed in relation to the development of various MSD outcomes.

Epidemiological Data

Figure 7.18 provides an example of the pattern of the anticipated force-repetition interaction based on a standard fatigue failure *S-N* curve. In this example, we used the *S-N* curve equation for tendon fatigue shown in Figure 7.1 (Schechtman & Bader, 1997). For the low force condition, expected

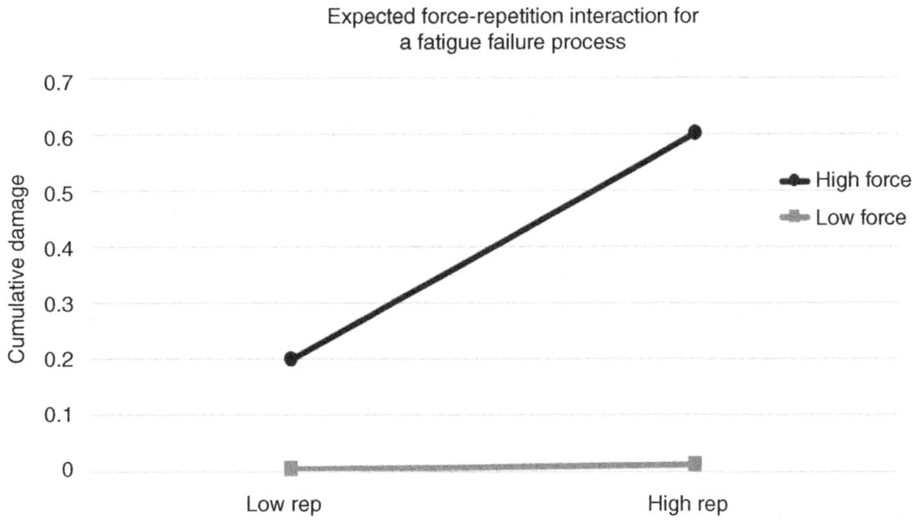

Figure 7.18 Expected force-repetition interaction pattern for cumulative damage development based on fatigue failure *S-N* curve. Modified from Schechtman, H., & Bader, D. (1997). In vitro fatigue of human tendons. *Journal of Biomechanics, 30*, 829–835.

cycles to failure were set as the predicted life of a tendon at 25% of the UTS, and the cumulative damage per cycle equaled 0.0000067. The high force cycles to failure represent the predicted tendon life at 50% UTS, giving a damage per cycle of 0.00033. A low repetition task was considered as 600 cycles per work shift, and high repetition was considered 1,800 cycles per shift, and these were multiplied by the appropriate damage per cycle for each condition. Based on these assumptions, the expected cumulative damage development for the four combinations of force and repetition is shown.

Thus, if a fatigue failure process occurs in musculoskeletal tissues, we would expect to observe a similar pattern for MSD outcomes in studies that have divided force and repetition into quadrants (combinations of high and low for each). It should be noted here that the same basic interaction pattern would be observed for any other percentages of UTS, as long as one is higher than the other.

Force-Repetition Interaction in Epidemiological Studies

A systematic review of epidemiology studies evaluating the possible presence of a force-repetition interaction with respect to MSD outcomes revealed a significant interaction in 10 of 12 studies that tested for one (Gallagher & Heberger, 2013). Seven of these studies provided sufficient data to evaluate the form of this interaction and are shown in Figure 7.19. The pattern of interaction observed in these studies is very like the pattern expected if a fatigue failure process was an underlying mechanism. In general, these graphs demonstrate a relatively low slope when examining the effects of repetition with low force. In contrast, the effect of repetition for high force cases is usually quite dramatic, resulting in a much higher slope. There is some variability in the response, but it is noteworthy that many of the studies (examining a variety of MSD outcomes) exhibit a pattern that closely mirrors the response anticipated if a fatigue failure response was present.

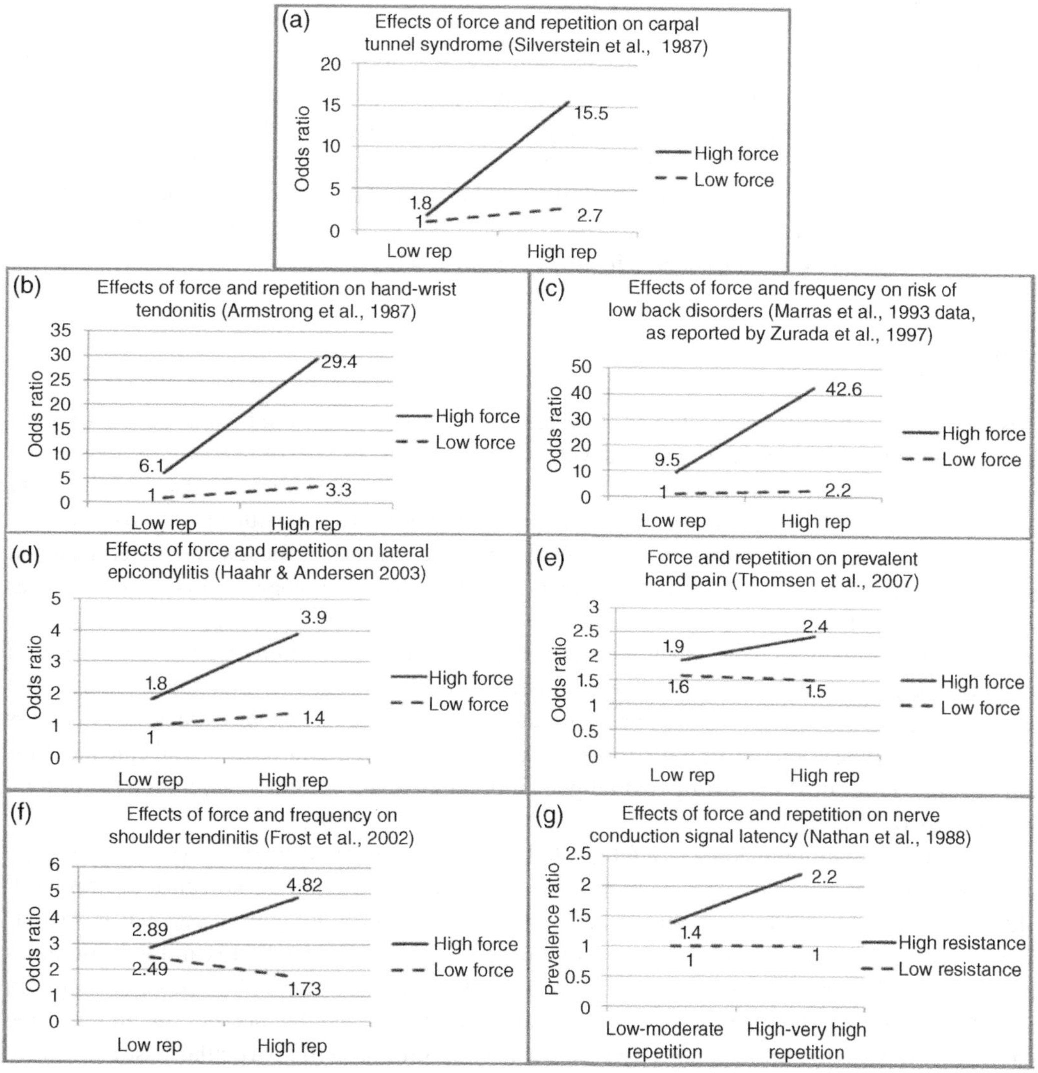

Figure 7.19 Results of seven cross-sectional epidemiological studies allowing 2 × 2 analysis of force and repetition and that exhibit a Force × Repetition interaction: (a) Based on Silverstein, B., Fine, L., & Armstrong, T. (1987). Occupational factors and carpal tunnel syndrome. *American Journal of Industrial Medicine, 11*, 343–358; (b) Based on Armstrong, T., Fine, L., Goldstein, S., Lifshitz, Y., & Silverstein, B. (1987). Ergonomic considerations in hand-wrist tendinitis. *Journal of Hand Surgery, 12A*, 830–837.; (c) Marras, W., Lavender, S., Leurgans, S., Rajulu, S., Allread, W. G., Fathallah, F., & Ferguson, S. (1993). The role of dynamic three-dimensional motion in occupationally-related low back disorders: The effects of workplace factors, and trunk motion characteristics on risk of injury. *Spine, 18*, 617–628.; data reported in Zurada, J., Karwowski, W., & Marras, W. (1997). A neural network-based system for classification of industrial jobs with respect to risk of low back disorders due to workplace design. *Applied Ergonomics, 28*, 49–58; (d) Based on Haahr, J., & Andersen, J. (2003). Physical and psychosocial risk factors for lateral epicondylitis: A population based case- referent study. *Occupational and Environmental Medicine, 60*, 322–329.; (e) Based on Thomsen, J., Mikkelsen, S., Andersen, J., Fallentin, N., Loft, I., Frost, P., ... Overgaard, E. (2007). Risk factors for hand-wrist disorders in repetitive work. *Occupational and Environmental Medicine, 64*, 527–533.; (f) Based on Frost, P., Bonde, J., Mikkelsen, S., Andersen, J., Fallentin, N., Kaergaard, A., & Thomsen, J. (2002). Risk of shoulder tendinitis in relation to shoulder loads in monotonous repetitive work. *American Journal of Industrial Medicine, 41*, 1118.; (g) Based on Nathan, P., Meadows, K., & Doyle, L. (1988). Occupation as a risk factor for impaired sensory nerve conduction of the median nerve at the carpal tunnel. *Journal of Hand Surgery, 13B*, 167–170.

Fatigue Failure-Based Risk Assessment Tools

Another source of epidemiological data that supports the notion that a fatigue failure process underlies MSD development is that three newly developed risk assessment tools based on fatigue failure principles have demonstrated dose-response relationships with multiple MSD outcomes. This is true for a tool examining lifting/lowering tasks and the prevalence of low-back disorders (Gallagher, Sesek, et al., 2017), a tool examining hand intensive tasks and (Gallagher et al., 2018), and a tool evaluating shoulder intensive tasks (Hani et al., 2019). These tools, and the results of their validation studies, will be covered in greater detail in Chapter 13.

Summary

This chapter has presented several lines of evidence supporting the notion that fatigue failure may be an important etiological factor in the development of MSDs. *Ex vivo* testing of musculoskeletal tissues indicates that a classic fatigue failure in response to repeated stress is observed for every system component tested. Comparisons of the damage patterns observed during *ex vivo* studies are also found to correlate well with damage observed in tissue biopsies of these same materials when MSDs are experienced. Animal studies have demonstrated tissue pathology and cytokine responses congruent with a fatigue failure process, including as a result of controlled fatigue loading during *in vivo* studies. Finally, epidemiological studies examining the interaction of force and repetition demonstrate an interaction between force and repetition mirroring the interaction pattern that would be expected if a fatigue failure process were present. These responses were observed across a wide range of MSDs, including low back disorders, carpal tunnel syndrome, lateral epicondylitis, and shoulder tendinitis, suggesting that fatigue failure may be a common precipitating factor for a wide variety of MSDs.

Of course, the traditional domain of fatigue failure has been in the realm of inert (non-biological) materials. The fact that musculoskeletal tissues are immersed in a dynamic biological environment adds considerable complexity to an already complicated material fatigue process. Of particular significance is the unique capacity of musculoskeletal tissues to self-heal. This ability is undoubtedly a critical factor in the longevity of musculoskeletal tissues. The body's effort to maintain homeostasis in these tissues must attempt to heal any daily damage that accrues due to repetitive loading. However, this healing capacity varies widely according to the particular tissue involved. Materials that are well vascularized tend to heal more quickly and effectively than those with inferior blood flow. Some of the unique aspects of repeated stress in biological materials will be discussed in Chapter 10.

It is important to acknowledge that while fatigue failure of musculoskeletal tissues appears to be an important etiological factor for MSDs, that damage may also result from other mechanisms. Notably, numerous physiological systems provide important roles in supporting the musculoskeletal system. A case could be made that the primary purpose of most, if not all, of these physiological (e.g., cardiovascular, respiratory, gastrointestinal) systems is to provide the support necessary to promote the body's ability to move. Any perturbation of these systems may impact the health of musculoskeletal tissues, such as issues associated with a lack of (or substantial reduction in) blood flow and/or delivery of required nutrients. Physiological factors such as these may lead to damage in and of themselves or may result in an exacerbation of damage due to repetitive loading. Thus, any issues that cause a decrease in the function of one or more of these physiological systems have the potential to lead to negative musculoskeletal consequences. Nevertheless, data presented in this chapter strongly implicate fatigue failure as a process heavily involved in the development of MSDs.

Bibliography

Adams, M., & Hutton, W. (1985). Gradual disc prolapse. *Spine, 10*, 524–531.

Adams, M., McNally, D., Wagstaff, J., & Goodship, A. (1993). Abnormal stress concentrations in lumbar intervertebral discs following damage to the vertebral bodies: A cause of disc failure? *European Spine Journal, 1*, 214–221.

Andarawis-Puri, N., & Flatow, E. (2011). Tendon fatigue in response to mechanical loading. *Journal of Musculoskeletal and Neuronal Interactions, 11*, 106–114.

Anderson, D., Brown, T., & Radin, E. (1993). The influence of basal cartilage calcification on dynamic juxtaarticular stress transmission. *Clinical Orthopaedics, 286*, 298–307.

Armstrong, T., Fine, L., Goldstein, S., Lifshitz, Y., & Silverstein, B. (1987). Ergonomic considerations in hand-wrist tendinitis. *Journal of Hand Surgery, 12A*, 830–837.

Astrom, M., & Rausing, A. (1995). Chronic Achilles tendinopathy. A survey of surgical and histopathologic findings. *Clinical Orthopaedics, 316*, 151–164.

Baker, J., Frankel, V., & Burstein, A. (1972). Fatigue fractures: Biomechanical considerations. *Journal of Bone and Joint Surgery, 54A*, 1345–1346.

Bani Hani, D., Huangfu, R., Sesek, R., Schall, M., Davis, G., & Gallagher, S. (2021). Development and validation of a cumulative exposure shoulder risk assessment tool based on fatigue failure theory. *Ergonomics, 64*(1), 39–64.

Barbe, M., Gallagher, S., Massicotte, V., Tytell, M., Popoff, S., & Barr-Gillespie, A. (2013). The interaction of force and repetition on musculoskeletal and neural tissue responses and sensorimotor behavior in a rat model of work-related musculoskeletal disorders. *BMC Musculoskskeletal Disorders, 14*, 303. https://doi.org/10.1186/1471-2474-14-303

Bargren, J., & Tilson, D. (1971). Prevention of displaced fatigue fractures of the femur. *Journal of Bone and Joint Surgery, 54A*, 1115.

Birch, H. W. (2008). Matrix metabolism rate differs in functionally distinct tendons. *Matrix Biology, 27*, 182–189.

Bitzek, E., Kermode, J., & Gumbsch, P. (2015). Atomistic aspects of fracture. *International Journal of Fracture, 191*, 13–30.

Bogduk, N. (1997). *Clinical anatomy of the lumbar spine and sacrum*. New York: Churchill Livingstone.

Bogduk, N., Aprill, C., & Derby, R. (2013). Lumbar discogenic pain: State-of-the-art review. *Pain Medicine, 14*, 813–836.

Boyce, T., Fyhrie, D. G., Radin, E., & Schaffler, M. (1998). Damage type and strain mode associations in human compact bone bending fatigue. *Journal of Orthopaedic Research, 16*, 322–329.

Brinckmann, P., Biggemann, M., & Helweg, D. (1988). Fatigue fracture of human vertebrae. *Clinical Biomechanics, 3*(Suppl 1), S1–S23.

Buettmann, E., & Silva, M. (2016). Development of an in vivo bone fatigue damage model using axial compression of the rabbit forelimb. *Journal of Biomechanics, 49*, 3564–3569.

Burr, D., Martin, R., Schaffler, M., & Radin, E. (1985). Bone remodeling in response to in vivo fatigue. *Journal of Biomechanics, 18*, 189–197.

Byers, P., Contepomi, C., & Farkas, T. (1970). A post-mortem study of the hip joint. *Annals of the Rheumatic Diseases, 29*, 15–31.

Carp, S., Barbe, M., Winter, K., Amin, M., & Barr, A. (2007). Inflammatory biomarkers increase with severity of upper-extremity overuse disorders. *Clinical Science (London), 112*, 305–314.

Carter, D., Caler, W., Spengler, D., & Frankel, V. (1981). Fatigue behavior of adult cortical bone: The influence of mean strain and strain range. *Acta Orthopaedica Scandinavica, 52*, 481–490.

Carter, D., & Hayes, W. (1976). Fatigue life of compact bone--I. Effects of stress amplitude, temperature and density. *Journal of Biomechanics, 9*, 27–34.

Cetti, R., Junge, J., & Vyberg, M. (2003). Spontaneous rupture of the Achilles tendon is preceded by widespread and bilateral tendon damage and ipsilateral inflammation: a clinical and histopathologic study of 60 patients. *Acta Orthopaedica Scandinavica, 74*(1), 78–84.

Chamay, A., & Tschantz, P. (1972). Mechanical influences in bone remodeling. *Journal of Biomechanics, 5*, 173–180.

Chang, L., Marston, G., & Martin, A. (2021, July 17). Anatomy, Cartilage. In *StatPearls [Internet]*. Treasure Island (FL): StatPearls Publishing. https://www.ncbi.nlm.nih.gov/books/NBK532964/

Choi, K., & Goldstein, S. (1992). A comparison of the fatigue behavior of human trabecular and cortical bone tissue. *Journal of Biomechanics, 25*, 1371–1381.

Cinotti, G., Della Rocca, C., Romeo, S., Vittur, F., Toffanin, R., & Trasimeni, G. (2005). Degenerative changes of porcine intervertebral disc induced by vertebral endplate injury. *Spine, 30*, 174–180.

Clarkson, P., & Hubal, M. (2002). Exercise-induced muscle damage in humans. *American Journal of Physical Medicine and Rehabilitation, 81*(Suppl), S52–S69.

Cleak, M., & Eston, R. (1992). Muscle soreness, stiffness, and strength loss after intense eccentric exercise. *British Journal of Sports Medicine, 26*, 267–272.

Cyron, B., & Hutton, W. (1978). The fatigue strength of the lumbar neural arch in spondylolysis. *Journal of Bone and Joint Surgery, 60B*, 234–238.

Cyron, B., Hutton, W., & Troup, J. (1976). Spondylitic fractures. *Journal of Bone and Joint Surgery, 58B*, 462–466.

Devas, M. (1958). Stress fracture of the tibia in athletes or "shin soreness". *Journal of Bone and Joint Surgery, 40B*, 227.

Falkner, J., Brooks, S., & Opiteck, J. (1993). Injury to skeletal muscle fibers during contractions: Conditions of occurrence and prevention. *Physical Therapy, 73*, 911–921.

Fredberg, U., & Stengaard-Pedersen, K. (2008). Chronic tendinopathy tissue pathology, pain mechanisms, and etiology with a special focus on inflammation. *Scandinavian Journal of Medicine and Science in Sports, 18*, 3–15.

Freeman, M., Todd, R., & Pirie, C. (1974). The role of fatigue in the pathogenesis of senile femoral nec fractures. *Journal of Bone and Joint Surgery, 56B*, 698–702.

Frost, H. (1960). Presence of microscopic cracks in in vivo bone. *Henry Ford Hospital Bulletin, 3*, 25–35.

Frost, P., Bonde, J., Mikkelsen, S., Andersen, J., Fallentin, N., Kaergaard, A., & Thomsen, J. (2002). Risk of shoulder tendinitis in relation to shoulder loads in monotonous repetitive work. *American Journal of Industrial Medicine, 41*, 11–18.

Fung, D., Wang, V., Andarawis-Puri, N., Basta-Pljakic, J., Li, Y., Laudier, D., . . . Flatow, E. (2010). Early response to tendon fatigue damage accumulation in a novel in vivo model. *Journal of Biomechanics, 43*, 274–279.

Fung, D., Wang, W., Laudier, D., Shine, J., Basta-Pljakic, J., Jepsen, K. S., & Flatow, E. (2009). Subrupture tendon fatigue damage. *Journal of Orthopaedic Research, 27*, 264–273.

Gallagher, S., & Heberger, J. (2013). Examining the interaction of force and repetition on musculoskeletal disorder risk: A systematic literature review. *Human Factors, 14*, 108–124.

Gallagher, S., & Marras, W. (2012). Tolerance of the lumbar spine to shear: A review and recommended exposure limits. *Clinical Biomechanics, 27*, 973–978.

Gallagher, S., Marras, W., Litsky, A., Burr, D., Landoll, J., & Matkovic, V. (2007). A comparison of fatigue failure responses of old versus middle-aged lumbar motion segments in simulated flexed lifting. *Spine, 32*, 1832–1839.

Gallagher, S., Schall Jr, M., Sesek, R., & Huangfu, R. (2017). Job rotation as a technique for the control of MSDs: A fatigue failure perspective. *Proceedings of the Human Factors and Ergonomics Society Annual Meeting* (pp. 993–994). Santa Monica, CA: Human Factors and Ergonomics Society.

Gallagher, S., Schall, M., Jr., Sesek, R., & Huangfu, R. (2018). An upper extremity risk assessment tool based on material fatigue failure theory: The Distal Upper Extremity Tool (DUET). *Human factors, 60*, 1146–1162.

Gallagher, S., Sesek, R., Schall, M., Jr., & Huangfu, R. (2017). Development and validation of an easy-to-use risk assessment tool for cumulative low back loading: The Lifting Fatigue Failure Tool (LiFFT). *Applied Ergonomics, 63*, 142–150.

Gallo, L., Nickel, J., Iwasaki, L., & Palla, S. (2000). Stress-field translation in the healthy human temporomandibular joint. *Journal of Dental Research, 79*, 1740–1746.

Gharpuray, V. (1998). Fibrocartilage. In J. Black & G. Hastings (Eds.), *Handbook of biomaterial properties* (pp. 48–52). London: Chapman and Hall.

Griffiths, W., Swanson, S., & Freeman, M. (1971). Experiemental fatigue fracture if the human cadaveric femoral neck. *Journal of Bone and Joint Surgery, 53B*, 136.

Haahr, J., & Andersen, J. (2003). Physical and psychosocial risk factors for lateral epicondylitis: A population based case-referent study. *Occupational and Environmental Medicine, 60*, 322–329.

Hamed, G. (1994). Molecular aspects of the fatigue and fracture of rubber. *Rubber Chemistry and Technology, 67*, 529–536.

Hani, D., Gallagher, S., Sesek, R., Huangfu, R., Schall, M., Jr., & Davis, J. N. (2019). Shoulder risk assessment based on fatigue failure theory. *Proceedings of the Human Factors and Ergonomics Society Annual Meeting, 63*, 1117–1121. Los Angeles, CA: SAGE Publications

Hansson, T., Keller, T., & Spengler, D. (1987). Mechanical behavior of the human lumbar spine. II. Fatigue failure under dynamic compressive loading. *Journal of Orthopaedic Research, 5*, 479–508.

Hansson, T., & Roos, B. (1981). The relationship between bone mineral content, experimental compression fractures and disc degeneration in lumbar vertebrae. *Spine, 6*, 147–153.

Holm, S., Kaigle-Holm, A., Ekstrom, L., Karladani, A., & Hansson, T. (2004). Experimental disc degeneration due to endplate injury. *Journal of Spinal Disorders Tech, 17*, 64–71.

Huangfu, R., Gallagher, S., Sesek, R., Schall, M., & Davis, G. (2018). Evaluating the linear integration method of estimating cumulative loading using an eccentric exercise. *Proceedings of the Human Factors and Ergonomics Society Annual Meeting, 62*(1), 882–885. Los Angeles, CA: Sage

Huber, G., Nagel, K., Skrzypiec, D., Klein, A., Püschel, K., & Morlock, M. (2016). A description of spinal fatigue strength. *Journal of Biomechanics, 49*, 875–880.

Huber, G., Skrzypiec, D., Klein, A., Puschel, K., & Morlock, M. (2010). High cycle fatigue failure behavior of functional spinal units. *Industrial Health, 48*, 550–556.

Jarvinen, T., Teppo, L., Jarvinen, T., Kannus, K., Jozsa, L., & Jarvinen, M. (2004). Collagen fibers of the spontaneously ruptured human tendons display decreased thickness and crimp angle. *Journal of Orthopaedic Research, 22*, 1303–1309.

Jensen, T., Karpinnen, J., Sorensen, J., Niinimäki, J., & Lebeouf-Yde, C. (2008). Vertebral endplate signal changes (Modic change): A systematic literature review of prevalence and association with non-specific low back pain. *European Spine Journal, 17*, 1407–1422.

Johnson, G., Dowson, D., & Wright, V. (1976). The fracture of articular cartilage under impact loading. In *Proceedings of the 3rd Leeds—Lyons Symposium on Tribology*. Leeds, U.K: University of Leeds.

Jozsa, L., & Kannus, P. (1997). Histopathological findings in spontaneous tendon ruptures. *Scandinavian Journal of Medicine and Science in Sports, 7*, 113–118.

Jozsa, L., Reffy, A., Kannus, P., Demel, S., & Elek, E. (1990). Pathological alterations in human tendons. *Archives of Orthopaedic and Trauma Surgery, 110*(1), 15–21.

Kannus, P., & Jozsa, L. (1991). Histopathological changes preceding spontaneous rupture of a tendon. A controlled study of 891 patients. *The Journal of Bone and Joint Surgery. American, 73*(10), 1507–1525.

Keaveny, A., Morgan, E., & Yeh, O. (2003). Bone Mechanics. In M. Kutz (Ed.), *Standard handbook of biomedical engineering and design*. New York: McGraw-Hill.

Ker, R., Wang, X., & Pike, A. (2000). Fatigue quality of mammalian tendons. *Journal of Experimental Biology, 203*, 1317–1327.

King, A., & Evans, F. (1967). Analysis of fatigue strength of human compact bone by the Weibull method. In B. Jacobson (Ed.), *Digest of the Seventh International Conference on Medical and Biological Engineering* (pp. 514). Stockholm: The Organizing Committee of the Conference.

Kjaer, M., Langberg, M., Miller, B., Boushel, R., Crameri, R., Koskinen, S., . . . Magnusson, P. (2005). Metabolic activity and collagen turnover in human tendon in response to physical activity. *Journal of Musculoskeletal and Neuronal Interaction, 5*, 41–52.

Komi, P., Fukashiro, S., & Jarvinen, M. (1992). Biomechanical loading of the Achilles tendon during normal locomotion. *Clinical Sports Medicine, 11*, 521–531.

Kongsgaard, M., Qvortrup, K., Larsen, J., Aagaard, P., Doessing, S., Hansen, P., . . . Magnusson, S. P. (2010). Fibril morphology and tendon mechanical changes in patellar tendinopathy: Effects of heavy slow resistance training. *Amercian Journal of Sports Medicine, 38*, 749–756.

Kuslich, S., Ulstrom, C., & Michael, C. (1991). The tissue origin of low back pain and sciatica: A report of pain response to tissue stimulation during operations on the lumbar spine using local anesthesia. *Orthopaedic Clinics North America, 22*, 18.

Lipps, D. (2012). *Effect of gender-related differences in knee morphology on peak ACL strain during repeated simulated pivot landings: An in vitro investigation*. The University of Michigan.

Lipps, D., Wojtys, E., & Ashton-Miller, J. (2013). Anterior cruciate ligament fatigue failures in knees subjected to repeated simulated pivot landings. *The American Journal of Sports Medicine, 41*, 1058–1066.

Magnusson, S. P., Qvortrup, K., Larson, J. O., Rosager, S., Hanson, P., Aagaard, P., . . . Kjaer, M. (2002). Collagen fibril size and crimp morphology in ruptured and intact Achilles tendons. *Matrix Biology, 21*, 369–377.

Marras, W., Lavender, S., Leurgans, S., Rajulu, S., Allread, W. G., Fathallah, F., & Ferguson, S. (1993). The role of dynamic three-dimensional motion in occupationally-related low back disorders: The effects of workplace factors, and trunk motion characteristics on risk of injury. *Spine, 18*, 617–628.

Martin, B. (1993). Aging and strength of boneas a structural material. *Calfified Tissue International, 53*(Suppl. 1), S34–S40.

Martin, R., & Burr, D. (1982). A hypothetical mechanismfor the stimulation of osteonal bone remodeling by fatigue damage. *Journal of Biomechanics, 15*, 137–139.

Matheson, G., Clement, D., McKenzie, D., Taunton, J., Lloyd-Smith, J., & MacIntyre, J. (1987). Stress fractures in athletes: A study of 320 cases. *American Journal of Sports Medicine, 15*, 46–58.

McBryde, A. (1976). Stress fractures in athletes. *Journal of Sports Medicine, 3*, 212.

McCormack, T., & Mansour, J. (1997). Reduction in tensile strength of cartilage precedes surface damage under repeated compressive loading in vitro. *Journal of Biomechanics, 31*, 55–61.

Milgrom, C., Giladi, M., Stein, M., Kashtan, H., Margulies, J., Chisin, R., . . . Aharonsen, G. (1985). Stress fractures in military recruits: a propsective study showing an unusually high incidence. *Journal of Bone and Joint Surgery [Br], 67*, 732–735.

Miller, B., Olesen, J., Hansen, M., Døssing, S., Crameri, R., Welling, R., . . . Rennie, M. (2005). Coordinated collagen and muscle protein synthesis in human patella tendon and quadriceps muscle after exercise. *The Journal of Physiology, 567*(Pt 3), 1021–1033.

Morgan, E., Unnikrisnan, G., & Hussein, A. (2018). Bone mechanical properties in healthy and diseased states. *Annual Review of Biomedical Engineering, 20*, 119–143.

Movin, T., Gad, A., Reinholt, F., & Rolf, C. (1997). Tendon pathology in long-standing achillodynia: Biopsy findings in 40 patients. *Acta Orthopaedica, 68*, 170–175.

Nakama, L., King, K., Abrahamsson, S., & Rempel, D. (2005). Evidence of microtears due to cyclic loading in an in vivo tendinopathy model. *Journal of Orthopaedic Research, 23*, 1199–1205.

Nash, C. (1966). *Fatigue of self-healing structure: A generalized theory of fatigue failure*. New York: American Society of Mechanical Engineers.

Nathan, P., Meadows, K., & Doyle, L. (1988). Occupation as a risk factor for impaired sensory nerve conduction of the median nerve at the carpal tunnel. *Journal of Hand Surgery, 13B*, 167–170.

Parent, G., Huppe, N., & Langalier, E. (2011). Low stress tendon fatigue in relatively rapid process in the context of overuse injuries. *Annals of Biomedical Engineering, 39*, 1535–1545.

Pattin, C., Carter, D., & Caler, W. (1990). Cortical bone modulus reduction in tensile and compressive fatigue. *Transaction of the 36th Meeting of the Orthopaedic Research Society*, 50.

Pike, A., Ker, R., & Alexander, R. (2000). The development of fatigue quality in high- and low-stressed tendons in sheep. *Journal of Experimental Biology, 39*, 2187–2193.

Radin, E., Parker, H., Pugh, J., Steinberg, R., Paul, I., & Rose, R. (1972). The response of joints to impact loading. III– relationship between trabecular microfractures and cartilage degeneration. *Journal of Biomechanics, 6*, 51–57.

Radin, E., & Paul, I. (1971). The response of joints to impact loading. I – in vitro wear. *Arthritis and Rheumatism, 14*, 356.

Rhame, R., & Mouss, R. (2008). The Modic vertebral endplate and marrow changes; pathologic significance and relation to low back pain and segmental instability of the lumbar spine. *American Journal of Neuroradiology, 29*, 838–842.

Schaffler, M., Radin, E., & Burr, D. (1989). Mechanical and morphological effects of strain rate on fatigue of compact bone. *Bone, 10*, 207–214.

Schechtman, H., & Bader, D. (1997). In vitro fatigue of human tendons. *Journal of Biomechanics, 30*, 829–835.

Schechtman, H., & Bader, D. (2002). Fatigue damage of human tendons. *Journal of Biomechanics, 35*, 347–353.

Schwarzer, A., Aprill, C., Derby, R., Bogduk, N., & Kine, G. (1995). The prevalence and clinical features of internal disc disruption in patients with chronic low back pain. *Spine, 20*, 1878–1883.

Sharma, P., & Maffulli, N. (2005). Tendon injury and tendinopathy: Healing and repair. *Journal of Bone and Joint Surgery (American), 87*, 187–202.

Shepherd, J., & Screen, H. (2013). Fatigue loading of tendon. *International Journal of Experimental Pathology, 94*, 260–270.

Shepherd, J. H., Legerlotz, K., Demirci, T., Klemt, C., Riley, G., & Screen, H. (2014). Functionally distinct tendon fascicles exhibit different creep and stress relaxation behaviour. *Proceedings of the Institution of Mechanical Engineers. Part H, Journal of Engineering in Medicine, 228*, 49–59.

Silverstein, B., Fine, L., & Armstrong, T. (1987). Occupational factors and carpal tunnel syndrome. *American Journal of Industrial Medicine, 11*, 343–358.

Simon, W., Mak, A., & Spirt, A. (1989). The effect of shear fatigue on bovine articular cartilage. *Journal of Orthopaedics Research, 8*, 86–93.

Stephens, R., Fatemi, A., Stephens, R., & Fuchs, H. (2001). *Metal fatigue in engineering* ((2nd ed.). New York: John Wiley & Sons.

Sun, H., Andarawis-Puri, N., Li, Y., Fung, D., Lee, J., Wang, V., . . . Flatow, E. L. (2010). Cycle-dependent matric remodeling gene expression response in fatigue-loaded rat patellar tendons. *Journal of Orthopaedic Research, 28*, 1380–1386.

Suresh, S. (1998). *Fatigue of materials* (2nd ed.). Cambridge, UK: University Press.

Swanson, S., Freeman, M., & Day, W. (1971). The fatigue properties of human cortical bone. *Medical and Biological Engineering, 9*, 23–32.

Tallon, C., Maffulli, N., & Ewen, S. W. (2001). Ruptured Achilles tendons are significantly more degenerated than tendinopathic tendons. *Medicine and Science in Sports and Exercise, 33*(12), 1983–1990.

Teague, B., & Schwane, J. (1995). Effect of intermittent eccentric contractions on symptoms of muscle microinjury. *Medicine and Science in Sports and Exercise, 27*, 1378–1384.

Thomsen, J., Mikkelsen, S., Andersen, J., Fallentin, N., Loft, I., Frost, P., . . . Overgaard, E. (2007). Risk factors for hand-wrist disorders in repetitive work. *Occupational and Environmental Medicine, 64*, 527–533.

Thornton, G., & Bailey, S. (2013). Healing ligaments have shorter lifetime and greater strain rate during fatigue than creep at functional stresses. *Journal of Biomechanical Engineering, 135*, 1713–1721.

Thornton, G., Schwab, T., & Oxland, T. R. (2007). Cyclic loading causes faster rupture and strain rate than static loading in medial collateral ligament at high stress. *Clinical Biomechanics, 22*, 932–940.

Turner, C., Wang, T., & Burr, D. (2001). Shear strength and fatigue properties of human cortical bone determined from pure shear tests. *Calcified Tissue International, 69*, 373–378.

Wang, X., Ker, R., & Alexander, R. (1995). Fatigue rupture of wallaby tail tendons. *Journal of Experiemental Biology, 198*, 847–852.

Warren, G., Lowe, D., & Armstrong, R. (1999). Measurement tools used in the study of eccentric contraction-induced injury. *Sports Medicine, 27*, 43–59.

Weightman, B. (1976). Tensile fatigue of human articular cartilage. *Journal of Biomechanics, 9*, 193–200.

Weightman, B., Chappell, D., & Jenkins, E. (1978). A second study of tensile fatigue properties of human articular cartilage. *Annals of the Rheumatic Diseases, 37*, 58–63.

Wren, T., Lindsay, D., Beaupre, G., & Carter, D. (2003). Effects of creep and cyclic loading on the mechanical properties and failure of human Achilles tendons. *Journal of Biomedical Engineering, 31*, 710–717.

Yingling, V., Callaghan, J., & McGill, S. (1997). Dynamic loading affects the mechanical properties and failure sites of lumbar spines. *Clinical Biomechanics, 12*, 301–305.

Zitnay, J., Jung, G., Lin, A., Qin, Z., Li, Y., Yu, M., . . . Weiss, J. (2020). Accumulation of collagen molecular unfolding is the mechanism of cyclic fatigue damage and failure in coll. *Science Advances, 6*, 1–10.

Zurada, J., Karwowski, W., & Marras, W. (1997). A neural network-based system for classification of industrial jobs with respect to risk of low back disorders due to workplace design. *Applied Ergonomics, 28*, 49–58.

8

MSDs as a Fatigue Failure Process

Introduction

It is interesting to note that before the term "musculoskeletal disorders" came into broad usage, musculoskeletal disorders (MSDs) were commonly referred to as "cumulative trauma disorders," "repetitive stress injuries," or "repetitive strain injuries." The latter terms invoke the language of fatigue failure theory (stress, strain, repetition, and cumulative damage), and seem to infer the presence of a fatigue failure process in the development of these disorders. Though these names have been supplanted by the more generic term "musculoskeletal disorders," the fatigue-related appellations mentioned earlier may well be more accurate descriptors of the process through which many musculoskeletal outcomes develop.

Despite the fatigue-related labels previously used to describe these disorders mentioned earlier, fatigue failure has (until recently) rarely been discussed as a potential causal mechanism in the ergonomics or sports medicine literature, and fatigue failure principles have not previously been used in the development of many risk assessment tools. In the vast musculoskeletal literature, there have been but a few exceptions. One notable example is a publication by Nash who suggested a generalized model of fatigue failure in self-healing tissues (Nash, 1966). This model suggested that total damage to biological tissues might be the result of fatigue failure, damage due to aging, and damage due to disease, minus the damage that could be repaired by healing. Another example is a 2001 article by Kumar, who examined several possible theories of MSD causation. In this article, fatigue failure was mentioned as one of the several potential causal mechanisms (Kumar, 2001).

On the other hand, researchers who have examined the responses of musculoskeletal tissues to repeated stress in laboratory settings have understood for some time that musculoskeletal tissues exhibit textbook fatigue failure damage responses when tested *ex vivo* (e.g., Brinckmann, Biggemann, & Hilweg, 1988; Carter & Hayes, 1976; Cyron & Hutton, 1978; Cyron & Hutton, 1981; Gallagher et al., 2007; Schechtman & Bader, 1997; Shepherd & Screen, 2013; Thornton, Schwab, & Oxland, 2007; Yingling, Callaghan, & McGill, 1997), as well as *in vivo* (Barbe et al., 2013; Sun et al., 2010). While laboratory studies have demonstrated musculoskeletal tissues exhibit fatigue failure damage as early as the 1950s, the development of numerous ergonomics risk assessment tools and reviews of epidemiological literature since that time does not appear to have embraced the possibility that MSDs might be the result of cumulative damage development resulting from a fatigue failure mechanism (National Research Council—Institute of Medicine, 2001; NIOSH, 1997).

Musculoskeletal Disorders: The Fatigue Failure Mechanism, First Edition. Sean Gallagher and Mary F. Barbe.

The question is "Why?" Several possible reasons come to mind. In some cases, like the Nash (1966) article cited earlier, the literature was published for a different field (mechanical engineering) and was relatively older and may not have been read by musculoskeletal researchers. Another reason may be that although fatigue failure of musculoskeletal tissues has consistently been demonstrated during *ex vivo* studies, there was healthy skepticism that the same process would necessarily occur in living tissue. Certainly, the complex biological environment could be thought to have an influence that might alter the fatigue failure process.

However, as detailed in Chapter 7, multiple lines of evidence now suggest that fatigue failure can and does occur in musculoskeletal tissues both *ex vivo* and *in vivo*. If MSDs are indeed the result of a fatigue failure process, there are numerous implications as to how we should analyze data from epidemiological studies, assess MSD risk, and design jobs and activities to reduce the likelihood of injury. This chapter will discuss these and other implications that would follow should MSDs be the result of a fatigue failure process. To address these ramifications, it may be helpful to examine some of the differences between prior MSD risk assessment models and the fatigue failure approach.

Prior Models and Approaches

Over the past several decades, numerous methods have been developed to assess the risk of MSDs. These efforts have resulted in significant advances in our understanding of MSDs and the risk factors that influence the risk associated with low back and upper extremity pain and have improved our ability to design jobs with a lower risk of injury. The number of models developed is too numerous to address in the current discussion, but we will briefly describe a few of the more prominent and frequently employed risk assessment models. The foremost models for the control of low back outcomes include the 1981 NIOSH Work Practices Guide for Manual Lifting (National Institute for Occupational Safety and Health (NIOSH), 1981) and the revised NIOSH Lifting Equation (Waters T., Putz-Anderson, Garg, & Fine, 1993); the psychophysically based Liberty Mutual Manual Materials Handing tables (Potvin, Ciriello, Snook, Maynard, & Brogmus, 2021; Snook, 1978; Snook & Ciriello, 1991); the 3-dimensional Static Strength Prediction (3DSSPP) model (Chaffin, 1997), and the Lumbar Motion Monitor model (Marras et al., 1993; Marras, Allread, Burr, & Fathallah, 2000). Notable prior models for assessment of distal upper extremity include the Strain Index (Moore & Garg, 1995) and the (ACGIH) American Conference of Governmental Industrial Hygienists -Threshold Limit Value for Hand Activity Level (TLV for HA) (ACGIH, 2019). These and other methods have greatly added to the knowledge base of MSDs, and the risk assessment techniques mentioned earlier have helped reduce the development of MSDs in occupational settings. A summary of MSD risk assessment tools and studies evaluating the efficacy of these tools can be found at the International Ergonomics Association website (https://secureservercdn.net/50.62.89.79/m4v.211.myftpupload.com/wp-content/uploads/2020/05/Musculoskeletal-Disorder-Risk-Assessment-Tools.pdf). The following sections will briefly summarize the specified methods of risk assessment, followed by a discussion of the proposed fatigue failure mechanism.

Revised NIOSH Lifting Equation

The Revised NIOSH Lifting Equation (RNLE) is a widely used method of assessing the risk associated with manual lifting tasks (Waters T., Putz-Anderson, Garg, & Fine, 1993). This tool provides an equation with seven factors to estimate the recommended weight of lift (RWL) for a given set of conditions. An applications manual for the RNLE is available (Waters, Putz-Anderson, & Garg, 1994). The RNLE equation is as follows:

$$RWL = LC \times HM \times VM \times DM \times AM \times FM \times CM$$

where LC represents a load constant (set at 23 kg or 51 lbs.), HM is a horizontal multiplier, VM is the vertical multiplier, DM is the distance multiplier, AM is the asymmetry multiplier, FM is the frequency multiplier, and CM is the coupling multiplier. Further, the RWL denotes the object weight considered safe for nearly all healthy persons to handle for the given conditions. The Lifting Index (LI) can be calculated to assess the relative amount of risk associated with a particular task. For example, if the RWL for a task is 15 pounds and the actual weight being handled for this task is 30 pounds, the LI would equal 2.0.

The preceding equation can be used for mono-task jobs in which the same lifting task is performed by the worker for an entire shift. However, when multi-task job assessments are performed, additional procedures are required. For example, calculation of a composite lifting index (CLI) involves the calculation of Frequency-Independent Recommended Weight Limit (FIRWL), Single-Task Recommended Weight Limit (STRWL) for each additional lifting task (STRWL = FIWRL × FM), the Frequency Independent Lifting Index (FILI), and the Single Task Lifting Index (STLI). Tasks are subsequently reordered from the highest to lowest STLI value and thus CLI is calculated (Waters et al., 1994). Calculators are available online to facilitate the assessment of RNLE, including multi-task jobs. Similar procedures have been developed to analyze sequential and variable multi-task jobs (Waters, Lu, & Occhipinti, 2007; Waters, Occhipinti, Colombini, Alvarez-Casado, & Fox, 2016).

The Psychophysical Method

The psychophysical method developed by Snook and colleagues at the Liberty Mutual Insurance Company is based on the subjective judgments of study participants regarding the amount of load they can handle (or exert) under various conditions (Snook, 1978; Snook & Ciriello, 1991). Tables of acceptable loads and forces were developed for lifting, lowering, and carrying manual handling tasks, as well as initial and sustained forces for tasks involving pushing and pulling. These tasks were based on the loads that the participants estimated would be acceptable if performed over an 8-hr workday. Results of psychophysical studies of lifting tasks contributed significantly to the development of both the original and revised NIOSH lifting recommendations (National Institute for Occupational Safety and Health (NIOSH), 1981; Waters T., Putz-Anderson, Garg, & Fine, 1993).

It has been shown that if tasks are designed in accordance with psychophysically loads acceptable to 75% of females that low back incidence rates are reduced when compared to loads that exceed this criterion (Snook, Campanelli, & Hart, 1978). However, certain caveats exist with respect to the design of manual lifting jobs according to psychophysical criteria. For example, Snook and Ciriello noted that psychophysical estimates of acceptable loads at higher lifting frequencies may exceed recommended physiological energy expenditure criteria for an 8-hr workday (Snook & Ciriello, 1991). The psychophysical approach also does not allow for the assessment of situations in which a variety of different manual handling tasks are performed (Potvin et al., 2021). When the maximum acceptable loads for combined tasks (e.g., lifting, carrying, and lowering) have been examined, the loads acceptable to participants are less than the psychophysical recommendations for each individual task. Thus, while the psychophysical limits are quite useful for the analysis and design of individual manual handling tasks, the assessment of the acceptable loads for tasks involving high-frequency lifting and multi-task manual handling activities (e.g., situations commonly experienced in occupational settings) are not currently amenable to the psychophysical approach (Potvin et al., 2021).

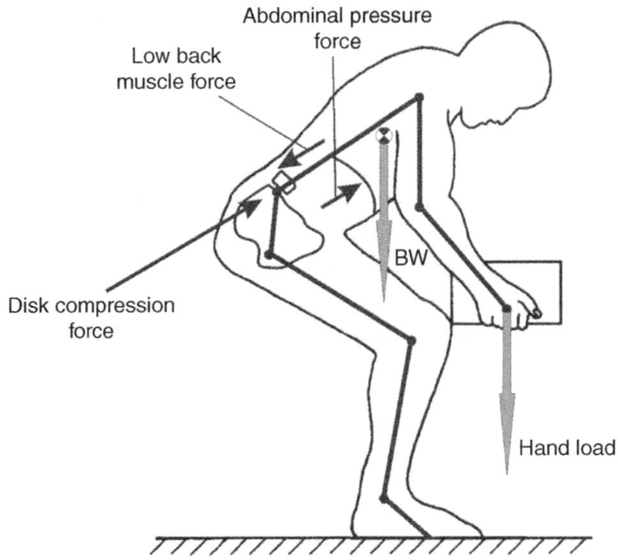

Figure 8.1 Biomechanical factors used in static biomechanical analysis models such as the 3D Static Strength Prediction Program (3DSSPP). Chaffin, D. (1997). Development of computerized human static strength simulation model for job design. *Human Factors and Ergonomics in Manufacturing*, 7, 305–322.

Static Biomechanical Modeling

Modeling the biomechanical loads experienced by an individual during lifting tasks is an important factor in assessing the risk of MSDs. Several approaches have been used to estimate spinal loads on individuals performing manual lifting tasks. One popular method of assessing the biomechanical load is the 3D Static Strength Prediction Program (3DSSPP) (Chaffin, 1997). This computer program is applicable to the analysis of materials handling tasks that do not involve significant acceleration or momentum (Figure 8.1). Such tasks can be analyzed as a sequence of postures throughout a manual handling task, and the program provides estimates of forces and moments on the low back and other joints based on static biomechanical calculations.

While an understanding of the biomechanical loads on the body is a critical factor in the understanding of the risk of MSD development, a 3DSSPP model does not provide guidance regarding the effect of repetition on injury risk. It can be readily appreciated that a lifting task resulting in a 3,000 N compression load on the L5-S1 disk will result in a greater risk of injury if it is performed 500 times a day as opposed to a one-time lift. In addition, the cumulative effect of activities resulting in variable magnitude loading (lifting items of various weights during the workday) is not addressed in this or similar models. Thus, while the biomechanical model provides useful information regarding estimated loads on body joints, neither the effects of repetition nor the impacts of variable loading from different lifting tasks are addressed.

The Lumbar Motion Monitor Model

The Lumbar Motion Monitor model uses an instrumented exoskeleton of the spine to estimate the three-dimensional position of the spine and permits calculation of three-dimensional dynamic characteristics of spinal motion, such as velocity and acceleration, during manual materials handling and related activities. This model has demonstrated both concurrent and prospective validity in epidemiology studies (Marras et al., 1993, 2000).

The five factors included in the model include the lifting frequency (per hour), the peak load moment (weight handled times the maximum distance of the load from the spine), the maximum sagittal angle of the trunk, the average trunk twisting velocity, and the maximum trunk lateral velocity. Factors were assumed not to interact, and the average of the individual probabilities for each factor were taken as the overall probability of high risk of a low back disorder group membership. High-risk jobs in these studies were defined as jobs in which 12 or more injuries were experienced per 200,000 hr of worker exposure, while low-risk jobs were defined as jobs in which no low back disorders were experienced and no turnover was observed over a 3-year period (Marras et al., 1993). Jobs analyzed in these validation studies were mono-task jobs (i.e., jobs in which the individual performed the same task for the entire workday). However, an algorithm is employed in the LMM software to evaluate the risk associated with multi-task jobs.

Upper Extremity Risk Assessment Tools

Two of the more popular upper extremity risk assessment models are the Strain Index (Moore & Garg, 1995) and the Threshold Limit Value for Hand Activity (TLV-HA) (American Conference of Governmental Industrial Hygienists, 2019; Latko et al., 1997). As discussed below, both methods have been validated against data from epidemiology studies.

The Strain Index

The Strain Index (SI) was developed to differentiate between jobs that exposed workers to an increased risk of injury to the distal upper extremities versus jobs in which workers were not exposed to substantial injury risk. The SI is based on the principles of physiology, biomechanics, and epidemiology, along with professional judgment (Moore & Garg, 1995). Factors considered include the intensity, duration, and frequency of exertion, the hand and wrist posture, the speed of work, and the duration of the task per day. Each of these six factors was judged on a 5-point scale. The original version of the SI addressed only mono-task jobs; however, more recent updates have provided procedures to assess multi-task jobs based on logic similar to the NIOSH Lifting Equation Cumulative Loading Index (Garg, Moore, & Kapellusch, 2017; Waters et al., 1994).

The SI model assumes that these six factors act in a multiplicative fashion with respect to upper extremity risk. Once all of the rating values have been obtained for these six factors, the multipliers are determined and the SI is calculated. An SI value of 5 or greater is considered a hazardous job, while values of 5 or less are considered a safe job. Several validation studies have been performed indicating that this tool demonstrates predictive validity for mono-task jobs (e.g., Knox & Moore, 2001; Moore & Garg, 1994; Rucker & Moore, 2002).

The Threshold Limit Value for Hand Activity

The Threshold Limit Value (TLV) for Hand Activity is a risk assessment tool for mono-task jobs that are performed for 4 or more hr a day (American Conference of Governmental Industrial Hygienists, 2019). This tool is partly based on prior research which developed a scale of hand activity that included information on both the rest periods and frequency and was based on a consensus of expert ergonomists (Latko et al., 1997). This original work addressed information regarding hand activity only but did not incorporate force as a variable. The American Conference of Governmental Industrial Hygienists took this scale and combined it with normalized peak force to develop proposed limits with respect to the combination of force and average hand activity based on the activity frequency (exertions per second), the length of activity (seconds/exertion), and forceful exertions. Both force and hand activity are rated on 10-point scales.

Data collection procedures include selecting a sampling period for job activities comprised of several complete work cycles. Videotaping of jobs is recommended for documentation as well as potential further evaluations. Based on the data obtained, the hand activity level is rated on the 10-point scale by the analyst (a team consensus is recommended), and the normalized peak force is assessed through the identification of forceful exertions and awkward postures. Additional factors such as exposures to sustained non-neutral postures, contact stresses, low temperatures, and vibration may be used to adjust the ratings according to professional judgment (American Conference of Governmental Industrial Hygienists, 2019). The 10-point scales for hand activity and normalized peak force are then plotted against a graph having two exposure lines. An Action Level line represents a limit above which "general controls, including surveillance" are recommended, while the TLV line represents a limit above which elevated MSD risk is anticipated and where immediate action is recommended.

Summary of Prior Models

The risk assessment models described earlier represent important advances in our ability to assess the risk of MSDs and to provide guidance in terms of jobs requiring intervention using ergonomic design principles. These models have received support from epidemiological studies indicating that these techniques are associated with the development of MSDs under specified circumstances (e.g., for mono-task jobs for the TLV for Hand Activity). As stated earlier, there can be no doubt that these risk assessment tools have been responsible for significantly decreasing the risk for countless workers. However, none have been based on fatigue failure theory. If fatigue failure is indeed a causal mechanism for MSDs (as the evidence in Chapter 7 suggests), it would make sense that fatigue failure methods be employed to assess risk. The following sections discuss the implications of fatigue failure as a causal mechanism, and the benefits that may accrue from application of this theory.

Considering MSD Risk Factors from the Fatigue Failure Perspective

The Consistent Emergence of Select Risk Factors

Over the past few decades, certain physical risk factors have consistently been associated with the prevalence and/or incidence of MSDs (NIOSH, 1997; National Research Council—Institute of Medicine, 2001). While listings of MSD physical risk factors can vary somewhat, the four risk factors most cited include (a) use of forceful exertions; (b) repetitive motions/actions; (c) adoption of non-neutral postures; and (d) exposure to vibration (whole-body or segmental) (NIOSH, 1997). In most epidemiology studies, these risk factors have typically been analyzed as main effects, and only rarely have studies examined interaction terms evaluating the combined effects of these factors (Gallagher & Heberger, 2013). However, while physical risk factors have often been treated as statistically independent in epidemiology studies, fatigue failure suggests an important interactive relationship exists between the critical risk factors of force and repetition. Specifically, the effect of repetition on material damage is highly dependent on the level of stress experienced by the tissue. At low levels of force or stress, each repetition results in a very small amount of damage. However, as stress increases the effect of repetition on cumulative damage development increases exponentially. In fact, compared to a very low force repetition, a very high force repetition can cause tens of thousands of times more damage per cycle in a material. The stress-dependent effect of repetition is critically important in assessing the risk of developing MSDs.

This potent interaction between force and repetition on cumulative damage growth and MSD risk in epidemiology studies has important statistical ramifications for how studies should treat the factors of force and repetition. Given the several lines of evidence supporting the notion that MSDs are the result of a fatigue failure process, it is advisable that research examining physical risk factors for MSDs should evaluate the interaction of force and repetition in their statistical models (Gallagher & Heberger, 2013). Examining only the main effects of force and repetition (without considering the interaction) may lead to misleading results and an incomplete understanding of the true interactive nature of force and repetition and MSD risk (Meyer, 1991). One benefit of fatigue failure theory is that the interaction of force and repetition can be combined into a single continuous measure of risk (cumulative damage) as described in the next section.

Adoption of Non-neutral Postures

The fatigue failure paradigm can provide us an appreciation for the interaction of force and repetition in the development of MSDs, but what about other common physical risk factors for MSDs? For example, how does the well-known risk factor of adopting non-neutral postures play into the fatigue failure paradigm? The answer is that non-neutral postures are usually associated with the imposition of increased force (and stress) on musculoskeletal tissues. A simple example is that of torso flexion. If an average man adopts a normal standing posture, it has been estimated that the compression experienced by the lumbar spine may be estimated to be 500 N. However, if he bends forward at the waist, the force on the spine may be 2–3 times higher than that experienced when standing upright (Wilke, Neef, Caimi, Hoogland, & Claes, 1999). Thus, the adoption of non-neutral postures can greatly increase the force (and stress) experienced by the spine. If such an action is repeated, each non-neutral posture adopted will lead to more cumulative damage per cycle due to the increased stress associated with the non-neutral (flexed) trunk posture.

Awkward postures can also increase musculoskeletal tissue stress in other ways. For example, when the wrist is deviated, it has been shown that frictional forces (and stress) as well as tensile forces will increase, thereby increasing the risk of tendon damage (Armstrong and Chaffin, 1979). It should be noted that awkward postures may have other effects on musculoskeletal tissues, such as reduced blood flow (Chaffin, 1999) or viscoelastic effects (Solomonow, Baratta, Banks, Freudenberger & Zhu 2003). However, a major reason that non-neutral postures are associated with increased risk may be because such postures result in increased mechanical stress on musculoskeletal tissues, leading to an acceleration of damage accumulation in accordance with fatigue failure principles.

Vibration Exposure

The final commonly observed physical risk factor for MSDs is the exposure of various human body structures to forced vibration (segmental or whole-body). Vibration is composed of rapidly repeated stress imposed on a material or structure, and unsurprisingly, material experiencing sufficient vibration exposure will experience fatigue damage. In fact, the so-called "vibration fatigue" represents a specific type of fatigue failure that describes damage development in materials exposed to the repeated stress of vibration (Dong, Wu, Xu, Welcome, & Krajnak, 2021; Lutes & Sarkani, 2004;

Wikipedia, 2010). The excitation of the vibrated material leads to a dynamic stress load in the material, and the fatigue response is the result of the shape of the excitation profile and the material response to this loading profile. Typically, profiles of excitation and response are assessed using the frequency domain (using techniques such as power spectral density), which then allow traditional fatigue life assessment methods like rainflow analysis (Matsuishi & Endo, 1968) and the Palmgren-Miner linear damage hypothesis (Miner, 1945; Palmgren, 1924) to be employed to estimate cumulative damage development and fatigue life (these techniques will be covered in Chapter 9). An important aspect of vibration fatigue life analysis is *modal analysis*, which identifies the natural modes and frequencies of the material structure under vibration that will allow accurate characterization of local stress responses for a given excitation profile. When these stress responses are understood, the fatigue life of the material under vibration loading can be reasonably estimated (Wikipedia, 2010).

MSD Physical Risk Factor Summary: Fatigue Failure as a Unifying Framework

The preceding sections suggest that the four common MSD physical risk factors, namely force, repetition, non-neutral postures, and vibration exposure may have an important organizing principle tying them together (Figure 8.2). Specifically, it is plausible that all of these MSD risk factors may have emerged due to their role in the development of cumulative damage of tissues through the mechanism of fatigue failure. Fatigue failure theory may thus provide a unifying framework within which each of these risk factors operates, ultimately resulting in the development of MSDs. This may open up the possibility of combining several of these risk factors into a single risk metric. For example, a delivery driver may be exposed to both whole-body vibrations while driving and lifting demands, both conditions resulting in repeated stress to his or her low back. Fatigue failure has the potential to assess the estimated cumulative damage associated with both activities and to use a single unifying measure of risk to assess the combined stresses of such a job.

This does not mean to imply that there may not other mechanisms that lead to (or affect the development of) certain MSDs. But for the large proportion of musculoskeletal injuries resulting from the repeated application of physical stress to tissues, fatigue failure would seem to be a major candidate as an underlying mechanism through which damage is initiated and propagated, ultimately leading to pain and disability (Zitnay et al., 2020). Fortunately, the process of fatigue failure has been studied for literally hundreds of years and a great deal is understood about this process. As a result, many analysis techniques are available that can help us understand and assess the fatigue failure process in musculoskeletal tissues, as described in greater detail in the next section.

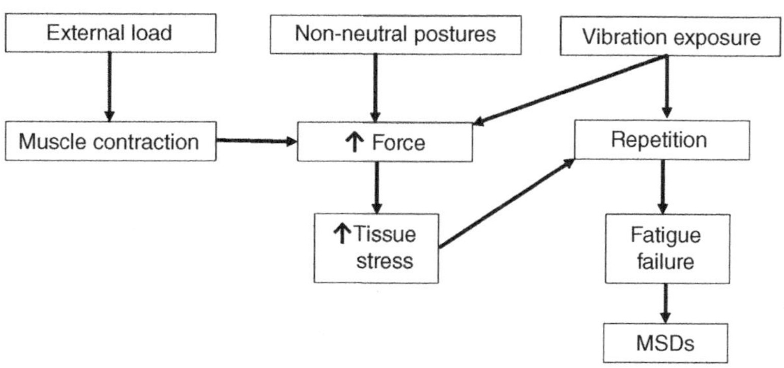

Figure 8.2 Model of physical risk factors and their role in the fatigue failure process, leading to MSDs.

Benefits of the Fatigue Failure Model

A Potential Causal Mechanism

While prior models have been shown to be useful at assessing MSD risk, none of them is based on a specific causal mechanism by which MSDs develop at the tissue level. A causal mechanism can be defined as "a process through which a certain outcome is brought into being." Identification of such mechanisms is, of course, a fundamental objective of science and helps us understand *why* things happen through an understanding of *how* they are brought about by causal mechanisms. These mechanisms can be thought to possess certain causal capacities, due to properties or powers they possess that endow them with the capacity to bring about certain events or states of being (Dupree & Cartwright, 1988). Therefore, arguments relating to causal relationships require substantive explanations regarding the causal powers or capacities that govern the responses of the entities involved (Cartwright, 1989).

The fact that inert (non-healing) materials consistently exhibit a fatigue failure process when exposed to sufficient repeated stress is beyond dispute. As a result, fatigue failure is well accepted as a causal mechanism of cumulative damage development and (ultimately) failure in these materials. As detailed in Chapter 7, all varieties of musculoskeletal tissue also demonstrate cumulative damage consistent with a fatigue failure process when repetitively stressed *ex vivo*. Are these materials immune from this process when situated in a biological setting? It would not appear so. *In vivo* evidence provided in Chapter 7 demonstrates that this mechanism is also at work in tissues in the biological setting. As we will see, there are some important differences in the response of musculoskeletal tissues to repeated mechanical stress *in vivo* (e.g., the ability of these tissues to remodel and heal). However, it is quite clear that musculoskeletal tissues experience cumulative damage development in accordance with the fatigue failure mechanism, for both *ex vivo* and *in vivo* settings. Given this evidence, it would make sense to use the long-established principles of fatigue failure as a foundation to assess the development of cumulative damage incurred in musculoskeletal tissues subjected to repeated stress.

Numerous benefits can accrue from basing risk assessment procedures on an apparent causal mechanism. In the case of the fatigue failure theory, the cumulative damage mechanism has been studied for over 175 years and a great deal is known about the process of material failure due to repeated stress (Stephens, Fatemi, Stephens, & Fuchs, 2001). As a result, a broad array of validated techniques is immediately available that can be leveraged to quantify the process of material damage in musculoskeletal tissues. As we will see, several of these techniques provide ready solutions to challenging problems that have long faced musculoskeletal researchers. As we will discuss, fatigue failure provides validated methods of summing the cumulative damage from complex loading histories (exposures commonly experienced by musculoskeletal tissues). Furthermore, a consensus method is also available that illustrates how cycles should be defined and counted when complex loading conditions are experienced. This procedure may be particularly valuable as methods of real-time or continuous exposure continue to improve. In addition to estimating the effects of cyclic loading, the effects of static (creep) loading on musculoskeletal tissues can be quantified, and there are established techniques for combining the damage development resulting from combined creep and cyclic loading. The following sections describe a few benefits that can be derived from using fatigue failure processes to assess the risk of MSDs.

If one accepts the evidence that a fatigue failure process is responsible for the development of MSDs, the efficacy of prior MSD risk assessment models would seem related to the degree to which these tools reproduce the relationships of fatigue failure theory. It is interesting to note, for example, that all of the prior models incorporate measures that estimate force (or load) and repetition in their assessment of risk. These are the fundamental factors involved in the fatigue failure process. However, the rationale for the inclusion of the frequency (repetition) factor in the NIOSH lifting equation was the physiological cost, while the fatigue failure model would suggest that the importance of repetition is that repeated stress leads to the nucleation of damage (microdamage) in musculoskeletal tissues and that continued exposure to repetitive stress causes this damage to propagate. There is little doubt that physiological demands are an important factor to consider in physically demanding jobs; however, the relationship of this factor to actual musculoskeletal tissue damage (while likely related) is not clear at this juncture.

Since prior models did not consider fatigue a mechanism of tissue injury, these models were not able to take advantage of the important benefits of fatigue failure theory. For example, it has generally been accepted that the cumulative effect of loading (often involving the performance of multiple tasks with highly variable loads) is important in the etiology of MSDs. However, some tools still have limited applicability to mono-task jobs, despite the high prevalence of multi-task jobs. Others that have developed methods for assessing the cumulative effects of multi-task jobs have developed methods that have been rather complex. However, fatigue failure theory provides a straightforward (and well-validated) method of assessing the effects of cumulative loading associated with highly variable tasks. This technique (The Palmgren-Miner Rule) also has shown the important benefit of providing the proportion of risk associated with each task, which can be useful in prioritizing tasks requiring ergonomic interventions.

Another benefit of fatigue failure assessment is its relative simplicity. To perform a basic assessment of a work task, only a measure of load or stress and a measure of repetition are needed. Some of the prior models require the assessment of six or more factors per task. If fatigue failure is (as it appears) indeed a mechanism by which MSDs develop, it is possible that certain prior risk assessment methods may overcomplicate the process of risk assessment. There are many other important implications if fatigue failure is a causal mechanism in the development of MSDs. The following sections briefly describe and discuss some of these implications.

Validated Methods of Cumulative Exposure

It has been widely recognized for some time that MSDs are the result of the cumulative exposure experienced by an individual (Coenen, Kingma, Boot, Bongers, & van Dieën, 2014; Norman, et al., 1998). However, not all current risk assessment tools permit assessment of the effects of cumulative exposure to multiple tasks, and for some of those that do, the rationale given for the method of risk accumulation is rather vague. The loading histories experienced by musculoskeletal tissues are complex and often involve highly variable stress amplitudes. For example, workers may perform multiple tasks during a workday, some of which may be high stress, some low stress, and some in between. Developing a method to estimate the *cumulative* effect of highly variable loading conditions on musculoskeletal tissues has been a challenging problem for those interested in assessing the risk of MSDs.

Methods of estimating cumulative loading for low back pain have included techniques such as taking the area under the loading curve (Norman et al., 1998), which makes intuitive sense. Such techniques, however, might suggest that high loading for a short period of time is equivalent to a low level of loading for a longer period. However, the interaction of force and repetition in fatigue failure suggests that the former may result in much more damage than the latter. Such techniques also do not address many important issues that are important in the development of a cumulative damage estimate from a fatigue failure perspective, for example, the dominant influence of the stress range in material damage development (Stephens et al., 2001).

Validated procedures derived from fatigue failure theory, on the other hand, provide a clear foundation for summing combined exposures having variable amplitude and use a risk measure that permits easy calculation (and summation) of the risk associated with multiple tasks. The most straightforward and popular method is called the Palmgren-Miner Linear Damage Rule (Miner, 1945; Palmgren, 1924; Stephens et al., 2001). Cumulative damage is typically expressed as a decimal, for example, 0.01 would represent 1% of the damage necessary to achieve some outcome of failure. A major benefit of this measure is that there are several validated techniques by which the cumulative damage for each individual task can be summed to develop total cumulative damage for the combined tasks. Another benefit of the fatigue failure approach is that the principal measure of risk is a continuous measure, specifically cumulative damage. Validated models are also available to estimate the residual strength of a material based on a variable amplitude loading history (Philippidis & Passipoularidis, 2007).

Accounting for Remodeling/Healing Impacts in Musculoskeletal Injuries

It is quite clear that musculoskeletal tissues subjected to repeated stress experience tissue damage resulting from a fatigue failure process (e.g., Barbe et al., 2013; Brinckmann et al., 1988; Carter, Caler, Spengler, & Frankel, 1981; Carter & Hayes, 1976; Fung et al., 2009; Fung et al., 2010; Gallagher et al., 2007; Schechtman & Bader, 1997; Shepherd et al., 2014; Shepherd & Screen, 2013; Sun et al., 2010; Thornton et al., 2007; Wang, 2006). Fortunately for us, musculoskeletal tissues possess the remarkable capacity to remodel and self-heal. Musculoskeletal health thus depends on a dynamic balance between the rate of damage accrual and the rate of healing that can be achieved. This balance determines whether a damaged tissue is going to heal (and maintain homeostasis), or whether damage accrual will exceed healing capacity. A benefit of the fatigue failure approach is that because the metric used is damage to the musculoskeletal tissues, the model can easily be formulated to include the effects of a healing process that accounts for the remodeling or repair of musculoskeletal tissue. Thus, the fatigue failure model is well positioned to adapt to new developments in our understanding of both damage and healing processes.

While some research has focused on both the damage accrual and healing processes, much more needs to be understood about the processes of damage accrual and healing (and their interaction) in the biological setting. However, as musculoskeletal tissues have all been shown to exhibit classic fatigue failure responses when repetitively stressed, fatigue failure techniques would be quite useful in quantifying the damage portion of the equation. The dynamics of the healing side of the equation are less well known but appear to be quite variable depending on the state of damage. As will be discussed in forthcoming chapters, there is reason to believe that conditions resulting in an impaired healing process may also increase MSD risk (Gallagher & Barbe, 2021). There are many conditions known to impair the healing process, including psychological stress, obesity, sex, and aging. Thus, the fatigue failure model may also help to explain how the presence of an impaired healing process may influence musculoskeletal health. This topic will be discussed in greater detail in Chapters 10 and 11.

Understanding the Influence of Personal Characteristics on MSD Risk

One of the essential hallmarks of the human species is its astonishing variability. This variability is partly a function of the process of Mendelian inheritance through which we obtain our own unique complement of deoxynucleic acid (DNA), and partly due to environmental factors that play an important role in shaping individual characteristics. The resulting diversity is manifest in a multitude of ways, some of which are undoubtedly important in the development of material

Table 8.1 Example of the influence of Variable Tendon Ultimate Stress on the Rate of Damage Accrual for a Task Having Constant Stress (20 MPa) and Repetition (2,000 Cycles)

Tendon ultimate stress (MPa)	Task % ultimate stress	Predicted cycles to failure	Damage accrued in 2,000 cycles
100	20%	280,000	0.007
80	25%	165,000	0.012
60	33%	70,000	0.029

damage in musculoskeletal tissues and in the healing of that damage. This variability greatly complicates the goal of controlling musculoskeletal injury risk, due to the fact that individuals will have a wide range of tissue strength and size, healing capacity, and other variables that will influence the development of tissue damage. Influential factors well known to musculoskeletal researchers include anthropometry, age, sex, and fitness. As a result of such variability, the fatigue failure theory indicates that a level of repeated stress tolerable by some individuals will unfortunately exceed the capacity of others.

A fundamental principle of fatigue failure theory is that the effect of repetitive stress on the material *is indexed to the Ultimate Strength of that material.* Unsurprisingly, the variability in material strength between individuals is enormous in humans. Thus, given the same load and rate of repetition, individuals with different tissue strengths will exhibit highly variable rates of damage development.

An example of this effect is shown in Table 8.1. One assumes a work task that results in a 20 MPa stress on a particular tendon and that the task is performed 2,000 times during a workday. The effects of this stress on three tendons with different ultimate stresses (100, 80, and 60 MPa) are evaluated. The percentage of ultimate stress for the load is 20, 25, and 33%, respectively. Based on estimated cycles to failure for the tendon (Schechtman & Bader, 1997), one can estimate the number of cycles to failure for each condition. As can be seen in Table 8.1, cycles to failure can vary quite significantly with changes in the percentage of the stress in relation to the tendon ultimate strength. We can compare the number of cycles performed (2,000) to that of cycles to failure to calculate the percentage of cycles to failure for each condition. Results of this analysis indicate that the 100 MPa tendon would experience 0.7% of its fatigue life as the result of this task, while the 80 MPa tendon experiences 1.2% of its fatigue life and the 60 MPa tendon experiences 2.9% of its fatigue life. If one compares the weakest tendon to the strongest tendon, it can be seen that the weaker tendon would accrue damage at more than four times the rate given an equivalent stress exposure.

It should be noted that the variation in tendon ultimate stress in this example might be the result of different various factors. For example, the ultimate stress variation could simply represent the tendon strength of three different workers performing the same task. The worker with the weaker tendon would be at higher risk of cumulative damage development and MSDs due to increased damage accrual rate. However, the variation in tendon strength could also be thought of as the result of tissue deterioration as a worker ages. That is, as a young worker, an individual may have a strong tendon (100 MPa) that shows a decrease in strength in middle age (80 MPa) and further declines in old age (60 MPa). Not surprisingly the degradation that occurs in the aged worker would lead to a faster accrual of damage compared to the worker's younger self. Of course, there will be a generalized decrease in the tendon's ultimate stress with age in the overall population of workers as well. The fact that older workers will exhibit a generalized decrease in tissue strength compared to younger workers (Knight, Hore, & Nigam, 2017) would suggest that stress exposures should be "stepped down" with increasing worker age.

The implications of this example should be clear. Given the highly variable nature of human beings, we must expect that workers (even of the same age) are going to exhibit enormous variability in tissue strength, which will lead to equally variable rates of damage progression, even in jobs imposing equivalent stress. Workers will inevitably present with a variety of ages, genders, anthropometry, healing capacities, and fitness levels. Thus, if 100 workers worked the same job and experienced the same tendon stress, we could easily anticipate 100 different damage accrual rates.

Obviously, we have a lot to learn regarding the influence of personal characteristics and MSD risk (a topic that will be explored further in Chapter 12). Fortunately, fatigue failure methods are well-situated with respect to the quantification of these effects and may provide essential insights into the importance of personal characteristics and the incidence of MSDs.

Combining Cumulative Damage from Dynamic and Static Loading

We have focused thus far on the effects on musculoskeletal tissues due to repeated dynamic stress exposure. However, it must be recognized that musculoskeletal tissues experience a combination of dynamic (cyclic) and static (creep) loading every day. Cyclic loading is characterized by variable stress being repeatedly imposed on material, while creep loading is caused by a constant (non-varying) stress experienced by a material. It is important to note that both methods of loading can lead to material deformation and damage (alone or in combination).

A simple example of the interaction between creep and cyclic loading experienced by humans is the following. Imagine a male worker performing a bag-palletizing task who is initially standing by a conveyor, waiting for the arrival of the bags he will soon have to lift onto the pallet. Assuming that he is an average size male, his lumbar spine will be subjected to a constant compressive force of approximately 500 N (Shirazi-Adl, El-Rich, Pop, & Parnianpour, 2005). This constant load will lead to a slow creep deformation of the materials of which the spine is made. If experienced for a sufficiently long time, such a load may lead to the development of damage in these tissues.

Imagine that the bags are now arriving on the conveyor and the worker must repeatedly lift these bags onto the pallet. The spine will now be subjected to cyclic loading in addition to the static creep load experienced by the spine. This load will lead to a substantial variation in the compressive load on the lumbar spine, perhaps cycling from 500 to 3,000 N. In general, cyclic loading will lead to damage development much more rapidly than exposure to creep loading (Thornton et al., 2007). However, it is clear that both methods of stress exposure can lead to the development of damage given sufficient repetitions or time, and the cumulative load on the spine in this example will include both creep and fatigue loading.

Fortunately, there exists a consensus method for calculating the combined effects of fatigue and creep loading, which is provided in the Code of the American Society of Mechanical Engineers (ASME). the combination of creep and fatigue should be evaluated by summing the damage fractions of both cyclic and creep loading (Wright, Carroll, Sham, Lybeck, & Wright, 2016). The following equation describes how to evaluate the interaction of creep and fatigue loading:

$$\sum_j \left(\frac{n}{N_d}\right)_j + \sum_k \left(\frac{\Delta t}{T_d}\right)_k \tag{8.1}$$

where n represents the number of cycles experienced; N_d denotes the number that will lead to failure for a particular loading condition; and Δt and T_d represent the creep loading time and the time that would lead to failure at that creep loading level, respectively. The left-hand term represents the previously mentioned Palmgren-Miner rule, used to assess cyclic damage for highly variable cyclic loading conditions (Miner, 1945; Palmgren, 1924), while the right-hand term denotes a similarly derived "time fraction" summation for creep damage. This time fraction represents the amount of creep time experienced divided by the creep time required to lead to damage initiation. As indicated by the equation, the creep component can also involve multiple levels of creep stress which would be summed to obtain the damage associated with the creep portion of loading. Prior models do not provide methods of assessing a combination of cyclic and creep loading; however, such analyses have the potential to be assessed using validated fatigue methods.

Counting Cycles in Variable Amplitude Loading

We are entering into an era in which methods of real-time exposure assessment are constantly being developed and will likely be widely available in the not-too-distant future. This is an exciting prospect, but also raises issues regarding how a highly variable loading curve should be analyzed. Questions such as "What constitutes a cycle?" in a complex loading curve require definitive answers. Fortunately, this problem was encountered long ago in the field of fatigue failure, and several validated techniques have been developed to break down highly variable amplitude loading patterns into cycles. Of these, the most commonly used technique is known as "rainflow analysis" (Matsuishi & Endo, 1968). This technique can be used to break a variable amplitude curve into cycles no matter how complicated the original loading pattern might be. The "rainflow" term refers to an analogy of rain dripping off of the roof of a pagoda. This analysis technique takes a complex set of varying stress exposures and breaks it down into a series of stress reversals. Once these stress reversals are obtained, one can apply the Goodman relationships and/or the Palmgren-Miner technique to estimate cumulative damage. Prior models do not currently have the capability to assess highly variable loading curves, but here again, fatigue failure methods are readily available to address this complex and challenging scenario. Rainflow analysis and other fatigue failure analysis techniques will be discussed in further detail in Chapter 9.

Assessment of MSD Risk Associated with Job Rotation

Fatigue failure also has the ability to evaluate the influence of job rotation strategies on MSD risk. Job rotation is an organizational strategy used by many industries that has received a great deal of attention in the ergonomics literature (Mehdizadeh et al., 2020; Padula, Comper, Sparer, & Dennerlein, 2017). Several benefits have been attributed to the use of job rotation, including the reduction of monotony and boredom for the worker, and the ability to cross-train workers. Many companies have used the technique as a method of trying to reduce MSDs by "balancing" the risk between physically demanding jobs and less demanding jobs by having workers rotate through these jobs. The implicit assumption made in this situation is that having all workers rotate through the worst job will lead to an overall decrease in risk to the entire group of workers involved in the rotation. Unfortunately, the nonlinear nature of the relationship to stress and risk suggested by fatigue failure theory indicates that the *increase* in risk to those in jobs with lighter physical demands may be greater than the *reduction* of risk for those in jobs with high physical demands (Mehdizadeh et al., 2020).

A recent study using an optimization framework to assess the effectiveness of job rotation schemes in reducing MSD risk used real injury data and employed fatigue failure-based risk assessment methods to ascertain MSD risk (Mehdizadeh et al., 2020). Results demonstrated that whenever a high-risk job was included in the job rotation pool, the overall MSD risk to the workers in the pool was increased. The concavity of the fatigue failure risk function guarantees that whenever a high-risk job is present, the increase in risk to workers in lower demand jobs will exceed the decrease in risk to the worker in the high-risk job. However, if jobs for all workers are all relatively low risk in the job rotation pool, the differences in MSD risk will be minor and the benefits of reducing monotony and increased cross-training experience would not come at the cost of increased MSD risk.

However, if high-risk jobs are present in the job rotation pool, it would be advisable to use ergonomic job redesign techniques to address the high-risk jobs rather than job rotation (Gallagher, Schall Jr, Sesek, & Huangfu, 2017).

Evaluating the Risk Reduction Due to Exoskeleton Use

Cumulative damage assessment using principles of fatigue failure does not have to measure stress directly but can use various surrogate measures including load, moment, torque, strain, and deflection (Stephens et al., 2001). The moment about a joint due to a load can be a very useful measure in the ergonomics risk assessment realm as this quantity requires only the measurement of a lever arm and the weight of the load, two things generally easy to obtain in the field. For example, The Lifting Fatigue Failure Tool (LiFFT), a fatigue failure-based risk assessment tool for low back (Gallagher, Sesek, Schall Jr, & Huangfu, 2017), for example, uses the peak load moment (weight of lifted load times the maximum horizontal distance from the load to the spine) experienced when lifting or lowering a load as a surrogate measure of stress on the spine. This measure of stress, when combined with repetition, provides an estimate of cumulative damage that exhibited a strong dose-response relationship to multiple low back outcomes in two separate studies (Marras et al., 1993; Sesek, 1999).

This relationship of cumulative damage to low back risk has spurred the development of a new tool (ExoLiFFT) that can estimate the amount of peak load moment reduction associated with back exoskeletons, as well as the estimated reduction in the risk of low back disorders associated with exoskeleton use (Zelik et al., 2021). This ability to assess the efficacy of exoskeleton use is a function of the use of a physics-based surrogate measure of stress and application of the fatigue failure cumulative damage metric and is not currently possible with other MSD risk models. The LiFFT risk assessment tool will be described in detail in Chapter 13.

Other Potential Applications of Fatigue Failure

Fatigue failure is a fundamental law describing the development of damage in all materials, and musculoskeletal tissues are not the only materials in the body to which this law would be expected to apply. Thus, fatigue failure theory may help explain phenomena (other than MSDs) in which repeated stress on bodily materials is experienced. This section provides a couple of brief examples of other health-related problems that may also result from a fatigue-failure process.

Chronic Traumatic Encephalopathy (CTE)

There has been a great deal of recent interest in the development of Chronic Traumatic Encephalopathy (CTE) in football players, boxers, military veterans, and others having a history of repetitive brain trauma. Exposure to repeated blows to the head is associated with an accumulation of phosphorylated *tau* protein in sulci and perivascular regions of the brain. Progressive debilitating neurodegeneration has been linked to such repeated trauma, which may lead to behavioral changes (aggression, depression, delusions, etc.), cognitive deficits (diminished attention, memory, and language deficits), and motor problems (poor coordination, spasticity, and Parkinson traits such as tremors) (Jordan, 2013).

It appears that CTE requires repetitive brain trauma, which may often develop over the period of many years. Evidence suggests that one injury is not sufficient to cause CTE and that subconcussive blows to the head may contribute significantly to the development of CTE (Stein, Alvarez, & McKee, 2015). In fact, 16% of those having CTE report not having a history of concussion (Stein, Alvarez, & McKee, 2015). However, it has been estimated that an offensive lineman in American football can experience over 1,000 subconcussive blows > 10 g in a single collegiate season (Crisco et al., 2010). Furthermore, it has been demonstrated that the abnormal *tau* pathology in CTE is concentrated in those regions of the brain that appear most susceptible to stress concentration associated with repeated trauma (Smith et al., 1997).

The forceful and repetitive nature of concussive and subconcussive head trauma described earlier suggests the presence of a fatigue failure damage process in brain tissue. Prevention of cumulative trauma to the brain would seem imperative in the effort to reduce the serious consequences of CTE. This is particularly true because of the poor healing capacity of brain tissue. Fatigue failure techniques may be useful in quantifying the risk of CTE due to repetitive traumatic brain injury, especially if the forces can be quantified (Guskiewicz et al., 2007).

Noise-Induced Hearing Loss

The process of hearing involves the application of a shear force on the stereocilia of the hair cells located on the lining of the cochlear basilar membrane. Sound pressure is equal to the force of sound (N) over the surface area (m^2) of a material measured perpendicular to the direction of the sound (Engineering Toolbox, 2003). Force acting over the surface area of an object is, of course known as stress and is measured in Pascals (Pa). When these pressure waves achieve moderate to high amplitude and are sufficiently repetitive, they can lead to the damage of stereocilia cells, potentially leading to their demise (Ward, Santi, Duvall, & Turner, 1981). Damage can be caused by short exposures to very high-pressure waves (known as "acoustic trauma"), or repetitive exposure to moderate or moderately high-pressure waves (i.e., repeated stress), leading to cumulative damage to auditory system components, which is known as noise-induced hearing loss (NIHL). Repeated stress leading to wear and tear (cumulative damage) of material structures are hallmarks of the fatigue failure process.

Though fatigue failure techniques do not appear to have been used to assess the risk of NIHL, there are data that suggest that such an approach might be beneficial. The extent of damage resulting from noise exposure has been shown to be associated with the total amount of noise experienced, which has typically been expressed as energy level. Energy level is defined as a function of the sound pressure level (SPL) measured in decibels (dB) and the duration of exposure over time (Konings, Van Laer, & Van Camp, 2009). Animal studies have demonstrated that similar cochlear damage appears to result in higher levels of noise for a short time or a lower level of noise experienced for a longer duration of time (Ward et al., 1981), congruent with fatigue failure principles. For example, studies on chinchillas have indicated that the hearing loss associated with a 2-hr exposure to 117 dB and a 30-min exposure to 123 dB were roughly equivalent (50–60 dB). Furthermore, a follow-up study indicated that a series of noise exposures designed to have "equal energy" from 22 min at 120 dB to 150 days at 82 dB indicated a similar average permanent hearing loss of 15–20 dB (Ward et al., 1981). This relationship indicates that lower levels of stress require exponentially greater time of exposure (thus involving an exponentially greater number of sound pressure cycles). This is the same basic relationship observed in the failure of other materials (such as musculoskeletal tissues).

The model used to assess cumulative damage resulting in NIHL is the equal energy model, which states similar damage to the cochlea will occur from loud sounds of short duration as to softer sounds of a longer duration (Konings et al., 2009). According to this model, noise is harmful to human ears when exposed to 85 dB for 8 hr, and increasing noise intensity by 3 dB doubles the energy output. Therefore, the exposure time must be reduced by half to maintain the same NIHL risk. However, the current model does not allow for the assessment of the cumulative damage using a summation of pressure wave exposure of varying amplitude and may understate the cumulative load experienced. If NIHL is indeed a result of damage to a material as the result of repetitive stress on this structure, it is possible that improved cumulative assessment of exposure may be achieved using validated fatigue failure techniques that deal with the effects of repetitive stress on damage to structures.

Summary

This chapter has discussed prior models for MSD risk assessment, and important implications regarding risk assessment should MSDs be the result of a fatigue failure process. Several prior models have demonstrated associations and predictive capability for various MSDs. However, in some cases, these relationships are limited to a specific type of job (for example, only mono-task jobs). When multi-task analyses have been developed, the methods used to assess jobs are often complicated and their basis is not always clear. As discussed, there are many potential benefits regarding the use of fatigue failure techniques in risk assessment. These include: fatigue failure is a potential causal mechanism for MSDs, fatigue failure has validated methods of easily combining the risks of a multi-task job into a cumulative measure of risk, ability to assess effects of personal characteristics and MSD risk, the capacity to assess complex loading curves using validated methods (useful as real-time exposure assessment techniques are developed), the ability to account for both damage and healing of musculoskeletal tissues, and validated techniques to combine the effects of both dynamic (cyclic) and static (creep) loading in an overall measure of cumulative risk. Many of these potential benefits are not currently available with prior models. Chapter 9 will discuss some important principles and techniques of fatigue failure analysis and their potential benefits in terms of MSD risk assessment.

Evidence suggesting that MSDs are the result of a fatigue failure process leads to a number of significant implications in terms of how we understand the risk factors for MSDs, how we should assess risk, and provides insights into work organization methods. Fatigue failure theory helps to explain why certain MSD risk factors have repeatedly emerged as significant variables in epidemiological studies and can explain why a specific pattern of interaction between force and repetition has been observed in multiple studies. If fatigue failure is truly a causal mechanism in the development of MSDs, a number of validated analysis procedures become available, many of which provide useful answers to challenging problems faced by MSD researchers. For example, fatigue failure theory has procedures to estimate the effects of cumulative loading involving variable amplitude loading conditions and methods of breaking down complex loading histories into discrete cycles to permit the use of cumulative loading models even with extremely complex load histories (or any load history). While in this circumstance, fatigue failure is occurring in a biological setting in which damage and healing may be occurring simultaneously, fatigue failure techniques provide a validated method of quantifying the damage portion of the equation, and healing rates can also be incorporated into the assessment if estimates are available. The general importance of personal characteristics (such as age, gender, and anthropometry) with respect to MSD risk has also been touched on. This chapter has served to briefly address some of the important implications associated with MSDs as a fatigue failure process. Many of these topics will be dealt with in greater detail in the coming chapters.

Bibliography

American Conference of Governmental Industrial Hygienists (2019). *Threshold limit values for chemical substances and physical agents and biological exposure indices*. Cincinnati, OH: ACGIH Worldwide.

Armstrong, T. J., & Chaffin, D. (1979). Carpal tunnel syndrome and selected personal attributes. *Journal of Occupational Medicine, 21*, 481–486.

Bani Hani, D., Huangfu, R., Sesek, R., Schall, M., Davis, G., & Gallagher, S. (2020). Development and validation of a cumulative exposure shoulder risk assessment tool based on fatigue failure theory. *Ergonomics*, 1–16.

Barbe, M., Gallagher, S., Massicotte, V., Tytell, M., Popoff, S., & Barr-Gillespie, A. (2013). The interaction of force and repetition on musculoskeletal and neural tissue responses and sensorimotor behavior in a rat model of work-related musculoskeletal disorders. *BMC Musculoskskeletal Disorders, 14*, 303.

Brinckmann, P., Biggemann, M., & Hilweg, D. (1988). Fatigue fracture of human lumbar vertebrae. *Clinical Biomechanics, 3*(Suppl. 1), S1–S23.

Carter, D., Caler, W., Spengler, D., & Frankel, V. (1981). Fatigue behavior of adult cortical bone: The influence of mean strain and strain range. *Acta Orthopaedica Scandinavica, 52*, 481–490.

Carter, D., & Hayes, W. (1976). Fatigue life of compact bone—I. Effects of stress amplitude, temperature and density. *Journal of Biomechanics, 9*, 27–34.

Cartwright, N. (1989). *Nature's capacities and their measurement*. Oxford: Oxford University Press.

Chaffin, D. (1997). Development of computerized human static strength simulation model for job design. *Human Factors and Ergonomics in Manufacturing, 7*, 305–322.

Chaffin, D. A. (1999). *Occupational Biomechanics* (3rd ed.). New York: John Wiley & Sons, Inc.

Coenen, P., Kingma, I., Boot, C., Bongers, P., & van Dieën, J. (2014). Cumulative mechanical low-back load at work is a determinant of low-back pain. *Occupational and Environmental Medicine, 71*, 332–337.

Crisco, J., Fiore, R., Beckwith, J., Chu, J., Brolinson, P., Duma, S., . . . Greenwald, R. (2010). Frequency and location of head impact exposures in individual collegiate football players. *Journal of Athletic Training, 45*, 549–559.

Cyron, B., & Hutton, W. (1978). The fatigue strength of the lumbar neural arch in spondylolysis. *Journal of Bone and Joint Surgery. British Volume (London), 60-B*, 234–238.

Cyron, B., & Hutton, W. (1981). The behavior of the lumbar intervertebral disc under repetitive forces. *International Orthopaedics, 5*, 203–207.

Dong, R., Wu, J., Xu, X., Welcome, D., & Krajnak, K. (2021). A review of hand-arm vibration studies conducted by US NIOSH since 2000. *Vibration, 4*, 482–528.

Dupree, J., & Cartwright, N. (1988). Probability and causality: Why Hume and indeterminism don't mix. *Nous, 22*, 521–536.

Engineering Toolbox. (2003). *Sound intensity, power and pressure levels.* Retrieved from https://www.engineeringtoolbox.com/sound-power-intensity-pressure-d_57.html

Fesharaki-Zadeh, A. (2019). Chronic traumatic encephalopathy: A brief overview. *Frontiers in Neurology, 10,* 713.

Fung, D., Wang, V., Andarawis-Puri, N., Basta-Pljakic, J., Li, Y., Laudier, D., . . . Flatow, E. (2010). Early response to tendon fatigue damage accumulation in a novel in vivo model. *Journal of Biomechanics, 43,* 274–279.

Fung, D., Wang, W., Laudier, D., Shine, J., Basta-Pljakic, J., Jepsen, K. S., . . . Flatow, E. (2009). Subrupture tendon fatigue damage. *Journal of Orthopaedic Research, 27,* 264–273.

Gallagher, S., & Barbe, M. (2021). The impaired healing hypothesis: A mechanism by which psychosocial stress and personal characteristics increase MSD risk? *Ergonomics.* https://doi.org/10.1080/00140139.2021.1974103

Gallagher, S., & Heberger, J. (2013). Examining the interaction of force and repetition on musculoskeletal disorder risk: A systematic literature review. *Human Factors, 14,* 108–124.

Gallagher, S., Marras, W., Litsky, A., Burr, D., Landoll, J., & Matkovic, V. (2007). A comparison of fatigue failure responses of old versus middle-aged lumbar motion segments in simulated flexed lifting. *Spine, 32,* 1832–1839.

Gallagher, S., Schall, M., Jr., Sesek, R., & Huangfu, R. (2017). Job rotation as a technique for the control of MSDs: A fatigue failure perspective. In *Proceedings of the Human Factors and Ergonomics Society Annual Meeting* (pp. 993–994). Santa Monica, CA: Human Factors and Ergonomics Society.

Gallagher, S., Schall, M., Jr., Sesek, R., & Huangfu, R. (2018). An upper extremity risk assessment tool based on material fatigue failure theory: The distal upper extremity tool (DUET). *Human Factors, 60,* 1146–1162.

Gallagher, S., Sesek, R., Schall, M., Jr., & Huangfu, R. (2017). Development and validation of an easy-to-use risk assessment tool for cumulative low back loading: The lifting fatigue failure tool (LiFFT). *Applied Ergonomics, 63,* 142–150.

Garg, A., Moore, J., & Kapellusch, J. (2017). The composite strain index (COSI) and cumulative strain index (CUSI): Methodologies for quantifying biomechanical stressors for complex tasks and job rotation using the revised strain index. *Ergonomics, 60,* 1033–1041.

Guskiewicz, K., Mihalik, J., Shankar, V., Marshall, S., Crowell, D., Oliaro, S., . . . Neurosurgery, V. (2007). Measurement of head impacts in collegiate football players: Relationship between head impact biomechanics and acute clinical outcome after concussion. *Neurosurgery, 61,* 1244–1253.

Jordan, B. (2013). The clinical spectrum of sport-related traumatic brain injury. *Nature Reviews Neurology, 9,* 222–230.

Knight, J., Hore, M., & Nigam, Y. (2017). Anatomy and physiology of ageing 10: The musculoskeletal system. *Nursing Times, 113,* 60–63.

Knox, K., & Moore, J. (2001). Predictive validity of the strain index in Turkey processing. *Journal of Occupational and Environmental Medicine, 43,* 451–462.

Konings, A., Van Laer, L., & Van Camp, G. (2009). Genetic studies on noise-induced hearing loss: A review. *Ear and Hearing, 30,* 151–159.

Kumar, S. (2001). Theories of musculoskeletal injury causation. *Ergonomics, 44,* 17–47.

Latko, W., Armstrong, T., Foulke, J., Herrin, G., Rabourn, R., & Ulin, S. (1997). Development and evaluation of an observational method for assessing repetition in hand tasks. *American Industrial Hygiene Association Journal, 58,* 278–285.

Lutes, L., & Sarkani, S. (2004). *Random vibrations: Analysis of structural and mechanical systems.* Butterworth-Heinemann, Oxford.

Marras, W., Allread, W., Burr, D., & Fathallah, F. (2000). Prospective validation of a low-back disorder risk model and assessment of ergonomic interventions associated with manual materials handling tasks. *Ergonomics, 43*, 1866–1886.

Marras, W., Lavender, S., Leurgans, S., Rajulu, S., Allread, W. G., Fathallah, F., . . . Ferguson, S. (1993). The role of dynamic three-dimensional motion in occupationally-related low back disorders: The effects of workplace factors, and trunk motion characteristics on risk of injury. *Spine, 18*, 617–628.

Mathiassen, S. (2006). Diversity and variation in biomechanical exposure: What is it, and why would we like to know? *Applied Ergonomics, 37*, 419–427.

Mathiassen, S. E., Möller, T., & Forsman, M. (2003). Variability in mechanical exposure within and between individuals performing a highly constrained industrial work task. *Ergonomics, 46*, 800–824.

Matsuishi, M., & Endo, T. (1968). *Fatigue of metals subjected to varying stress. Paper presented to the Japanese Society of Mechanical Engineers*. Fukuoka, Japan: Japanese Society of Mechanical Engineers.

Mehdizadeh, A., Vinel, A., Hu, Q., Schall, M., Jr., Gallagher, S., & Sesek, R. (2020). Job rotation and work-related musculoskeletal disorders: A fatigue-failure perspective. *Ergonomics, 63*, 461–476.

Meyer, D. L. (1991). Misinterpretation of interaction effects: A reply to Rosnow and Rosenthal. *Psychological Bulletin, 110*, 571–573.

Miner, M. A. (1945). Cumulative damage in fatigue. *Journal of Applied Mechanics, 16*, A159–A164.

Moore, J., & Garg, A. (1994). Upper extremity disorders in a pork processing plant: Relationships between job risk factors and morbidity. *American Industrial Hygiene Association Journal, 55*, 703–715.

Moore, J., & Garg, A. (1995). The strain index: A proposed method to analyze jobs for risk of distal upper extremity disorders. *American Industrial Hygiene Association Journal, 56*, 443–458.

Nash, J. C. (1966). *Fatigue of self-healing structure: A generalized theory of fatigue failure*. New York: American Society of Mechanical Engineers.

National Institute for Occupational Safety and Health (NIOSH) (1981). *Work practices guide for manual lifting*. Cincinnati: National Institute for Occupational Safety and Health.

National Research Council—Institute of Medicine (2001). *Musculoskeletal disorders and the workplace: Low back and upper extremities*. Washington, DC: National Academy Press.

NIOSH (1997). *Musculoskeletal disorders and workplace factors*. Cincinnati, OH: National Institute for Occupational Safety and Health.

Norman, R., Wells, R., Neumann, P., Frank, J., Shannon, H., Kerr, M., . . . Group, T (1998). A comparison of peak vs cumulative physical work exposure risk factors for the reporting of low back pain in the automotive industry. *Clinical Biomechanics, 13*, 561–573.

Padula, R., Comper, M., Sparer, E., & Dennerlein, J. (2017). Job rotation designed to prevent musculoskeletal disorders and control risk in manufacturing industries: A systematic review. *Applied Ergonomics, 58*, 386–397.

Palmgren, A. (1924). Die Lebebsdaue rvon Kugellagern. *Zeitschrift des Vereines Deutscher Ingenieure (ZVDI), 68*, 339–341.

Philippidis, T., & Passipoularidis, V. (2007). Residual strength after fatigue in composites: Theory vs. experiment. *International Journal of Fatigue, 29*, 2104–2116.

Potvin, J., Ciriello, V., Snook, S., Maynard, W., & Brogmus, G. (2021). The liberty mutual manual materials handling (LM-MMH) equations. *Ergonomics, 64*, 955–970. https://doi.org/10.1080/00140139.2021.1891297

Roylance, D. (2020. *Fatigue*. Retrieved from https://ocw.mit.edu/courses/materials-science-and-engineering/3-11-mechanics-of-materials-fall-1999/modules/MIT3_11F99_fatigue.pdf

Rucker, N., & Moore, J. (2002). Predictive validity of the strain index in manufacturing facilities. *Applied Occupational and Environmental Hygiene, 12*, 63–73.

Schechtman, H., & Bader, D. (1997). In vitro fatigue of human tendons. *Journal of Biomechanics, 30*, 829–835.

Schechtman, H., & Bader, D. (2002). Fatigue damage of human tendons. *Journal of Biomechanics, 35*, 347–353.

Sesek, R. (1999). Evaluation and refinement of ergonomic survey tools to evaluate worker risk of cumulative trauma disorders (dissertation).

Shepherd, J., & Screen, H. (2013). Fatigue loading of tendon. *International Journal of Experimental Pathology, 94*, 260–270.

Shepherd, J. H., Legerlotz, K., Demirci, T., Klemt, C., Riley, G., & Screen, H. (2014). Functionally distinct tendon fascicles exhibit different creep and stress relaxation behaviour. *Proceedings of the Institution of Mechanical Engineers. Part H, Journal of Engineering in Medicine, 228*, 49–59.

Shirazi-Adl, A., El-Rich, M., Pop, D. G., & Parnianpour, M. (2005). Spinal muscle forces, internal loads and stability in standing under various postures and loads—application of kinematics-based algorithm. *European Spine Journal, 14*, 381–392.

Smith, D., Chen, X., Xu, B., McIntosh, T., Gennarelli, T., & Meaney, D. (1997). Characterization of diffuse axonal pathology and selective hippocampal damage following inertial brain trauma in the pig. *Journal of Neuropathology and Experimental Neurology, 56*, 822–834.

Snook, S. (1978). The design of manual handling tasks. *Ergonomics, 21*, 963–985.

Snook, S., Campanelli, R., & Hart, J. (1978). A study of three preventive approaches to low back injury. *Journal of Occupational Medicine, 20*, 478–481.

Snook, S., & Ciriello, V. (1991). The design of manual handling tasks: Revised tables of maximum acceptable weights and forces. *Ergonomics, 34*, 1197–1213.

Solomonow, M., Baratta, R., Banks, A., Freudenberger, C., & Zhou, B. (2003). Flexion–relaxation response to static lumbar flexion in males and females. *Clinical Biomechanics, 18*, 273–279.

Stein, T., Alvarez, V., & & McKee, A. (2015). Concussion in chronic traumatic encephalopathy. *Current Pain and Headache Reports, (*10*)*, 19, 47.

Stephens, R., Fatemi, A., Stephens, R., & Fuchs, H. (2001). *Metal fatigue in engineering* (2nd ed.). New York: Wiley.

Sun, H., Andarawis-Puri, N., Li, Y., Fung, D., Lee, J., Wang, V., . . . Flatow, E. L. (2010). Cycle-dependent matric remodeling gene expression response in fatigue-loaded rat patellar tendons. *Journal of Orthopaedic Research, 28*, 1380–1386.

Thornton, G. M., Schwab, T., & Oxland, T. (2007). Cyclic loading causes faster rupture and strain rate than static loading in medial collateral ligament at high stress. *Clinical Biomechanics, 22*, 932–940.

Wang, J. (2006). Mechanobiology of tendon. *Journal of Biomechanics, 39*, 1563–1582.

Ward, W., Santi, P., Duvall, A., & Turner, C. (1981). Total energy and critical intensity concepts in noise damage. *The Annals of Otology, Rhinology, and Laryngology, 90*, 584–590.

Waters, T., Lu, M., & Occhipinti, E. (2007). New procedure for assessing sequential manual lifting jobs using the revised Niosh lifting equation. *Ergonomics, 50*, 1761–1770.

Waters, T., Occhipinti, E., Colombini, D., Alvarez-Casado, E., & Fox, R. (2016). Variable lifting index (VLI): A new method for evaluating variable lifting tasks. *Human Factors, 58*, 695–711.

Waters, T., Putz-Anderson, V., & Garg, A. (1994). *Applications manual for the revised NIOSH lifting equation*. Cincinnati, OH: DHHS (NIOSH) Publication Number 94–110.

Waters, T., Putz-Anderson, V., Garg, A., & Fine, L. (1993). Revised NIOSH equation for the design and evaluation of manual lifting tasks. *Ergonomics, 36*, 749–776.

Wikipedia (2010. *Vibration fatigue*. Retrieved from https://en.wikipedia.org/wiki/Vibration_fatigue

Wilke, H., Neef, P., Caimi, M., Hoogland, T., & Claes, L. (1999). New in vivo measurements of pressures in the intervertebral disc in daily life. *Spine, 24*, 755–762.

Wright, J., Carroll, L., Sham, T.-L., Lybeck, N., & Wright, R. (2016). Determination of the creep–fatigue interaction diagram for alloy 617. In *Proceedings of the ASME 2016 Pressure Vessels and Piping Conference (PVP2016), July 17–21, 2016* (pp. 10). Vancouver, BC: American Society of Mechanical Engineers, Vancouver.

Yingling, V., Callaghan, J., & McGill, S. (1997). Dynamic loading affects the mechanical properties and failure sites of lumbar spines. *Clinical Biomechanics, 12*, 301–305.

Zelik, K., Nurse, C., Schall, M., Jr., Sesek, R., Marino, M., & Gallagher, S. (2021). An ergonomic assessment tool for evaluating the effect of back exoskeletons on injury risk. *Applied Ergonomics, 99*, 103619.

Zitnay, J., Jung, G., Lin, A., Qin, Z., Li, Y., Yu, M., . . . Weiss, J. (2020). Accumulation of collagen molecular unfolding is the mechanism of cyclic fatigue damage and failure in coll. *Science Advances, 6*, 1–10.

9

Fundamentals of Fatigue Failure Analysis

Introduction

On Sunday, May 8, 1842, a celebration was held in honor of King Louis Phillipe I in the gardens of Versailles outside Paris, France. Late in the afternoon, as the festivities were drawing to a close, over 750 people boarded a train at the Versailles railway station for the short trip back to Paris. Regrettably, as the train was traveling between Bellevue and Meudon, an axle on the lead locomotive fractured, causing the engine to derail. The derailment led to a scattering of the firebox contents from the lead steam engine and when the trailing locomotive crashed into the first and the trailing carriages traveled over the resulting flames a large conflagration ensued. This accident caused a still undetermined (but large) death toll variously estimated to have been between 52 and 220 (Wikipedia, 2020). The large mortality figure was certainly due, in part, to the prevailing practice at the time of locking passengers inside their compartments during train trips. It was the first rail accident in France and was the worst rail disaster the world had experienced up to that point.

In the investigation that followed, a mechanical engineer named William John Macquorn Rankine (1820–1872) examined the broken axle to identify the cause of failure. His analysis led him to conclude that repeated submaximal cyclic stresses on the axle led to crack development in areas where stresses in the structure were concentrated and that the length of these cracks increased as the result of continuing repeated stress (Lahrman, 2016). Unfortunately, these exceptional insights were ignored by other engineers for quite some time, who persisted in believing that the application of stress led to recrystallization of the metal, resulting in failure of the axle. Adherence to the latter (incorrect) hypothesis unfortunately prevented progress in the area for quite some time, until engineers like William Fairburn (1789–1874) demonstrated the process of fatigue failure in flexural tests of large wrought and cast-iron girders (Lahrman, 2016).

Confirmation of this theory led to the development of a body of knowledge that has greatly increased our understanding of how and why materials fail when exposed to repetitive stress. Several advances ensued in the years that followed. Work by August Wöhler (1819–1914) led to a systematic approach of testing fatigue in materials and the development of the stress versus life (*S–N*) curve. Wöhler also was the first person to point out that it is the *range* of stress experienced by a material (not the maximum stress) that is the critical factor in fatigue damage development. Other important contributions were made by Gerber (Gerber, 1874) and John Goodman (Goodman, 1930) in the development of models describing the influence of mean stresses in the fatigue process. In 1924, A. Palmgren developed a linear cumulative damage model for materials that experienced variable amplitude loading (Palmgren, 1924). This work was the basis of a linear

Musculoskeletal Disorders: The Fatigue Failure Mechanism, First Edition. Sean Gallagher and Mary F. Barbe.

fatigue damage criterion developed by Miner in 1945, which is now known as the Palmgren-Miner linear damage rule, a measure used extensively in fatigue design (Miner, 1945). Other important developments were the application of the statistical distribution developed by Waloddi Weibull (1887–1979), allowing for probability-based fatigue life testing and analysis, and the rainflow counting technique of Matsuishi and Endo (1968) that allows continuous variable loading regimens to be broken into stress reversals and subsequently analyzed to estimate cumulative damage development.

As the brief history given earlier describes, the study of material fatigue has a history spanning over 175 years. While the study of fatigue initiated in metals, subsequent research has indicated that the same process is observed in all materials, including those making up the musculoskeletal system, as discussed in Chapter 7. As it happens, many of the techniques and relationships uncovered over the centuries appear highly relevant to the development of musculoskeletal disorders (MSDs). In fact, some of the techniques developed over the years provide ready solutions to some daunting challenges faced by musculoskeletal researchers. Other techniques and knowledge may also prove useful as our understanding of the MSD process progresses. The purpose of this chapter is to describe what is known so far about damage development in materials exposed to repeated stress, especially information that would appear useful with respect to evaluating damage development that may result from exposure to repetitive stress by musculoskeletal tissues.

Fatigue Terminology

The word fatigue comes from the Latin word 'fatigare' which means "to weary" or "to tire out." It is clear that things can "tire out" in many ways because fatigue has been used to describe a variety of phenomena. When the term "fatigue" is mentioned in the context of the musculoskeletal system, the usual connotation is physiological fatigue associated with exercise or heavy exertion. This is the feeling of tiredness or exhaustion often related to physical exertion that results in a deterioration in performance, ion imbalances in the muscle, and the buildup of lactic acid (Wan, Qin, Wang, Sun, & Liu, 2017). Fatigue has also been used to describe a decline in cognitive function (i.e., mental fatigue), a condition associated with prolonged cognitive activity, for example (Tran, Craig, Craig, Chai, & Nguyen, 2020).

However, we will not be focusing on physiological or mental fatigue in this book. Instead, we will be using the term to describe the "tiring out" and failure of the molecular bonds that bind the material together as the result of exposure to repeated stress. Material fatigue is the result of repeated loading and unloading cycles (or creep) at stresses below the ultimate stress of the material. This cyclic loading will eventually lead to an initial microfailure in the material, which sets the stage for a progressive expansion of damage and deterioration of the material properties. Complete failure of musculoskeletal tissues is relatively rare but it does occur. For example, frank ruptures of the Achilles tendon and bone fractures are a few examples of complete failure of musculoskeletal tissues that can result from material fatigue. However, musculoskeletal tissues do not have to exhibit complete material failure to result in significant pain, dysfunction, and disability. Even partial damage can result in significant detriments to the individual so afflicted.

As discussed in Chapter 7, multiple lines of evidence indicate that fatigue failure is experienced by musculoskeletal tissues. It would therefore make sense that we use our knowledge of the process of fatigue failure to our advantage when trying to minimize injury development in musculoskeletal tissues. We are still learning about fatigue failure; however, due to its long history, a great deal is known. The remaining parts of this chapter will introduce important fundamentals of fatigue failure theory and will present techniques of particular interest that may be quite helpful in our understanding of the cumulative damage development in musculoskeletal tissues.

Figure 9.1 provides examples of different types of cyclic loading and measures of stress that are important in characterizing sinusoidal constant amplitude stress cycles. Algebraic expressions are provided below in Equation 9.1 for S_a (alternating stress); S_m (mean stress); ΔS (stress range), S_{max} = maximum stress, S_{min} = minimum stress:

$$S_a = \frac{\Delta S}{2} = \frac{S_{\max} - S_{\min}}{2} \tag{9.1}$$

$$S_m = \frac{S_{\max} + S_{\min}}{2}$$

$$S_{\max} = S_m + S_a$$

$$S_{\min} = S_m - S_a$$

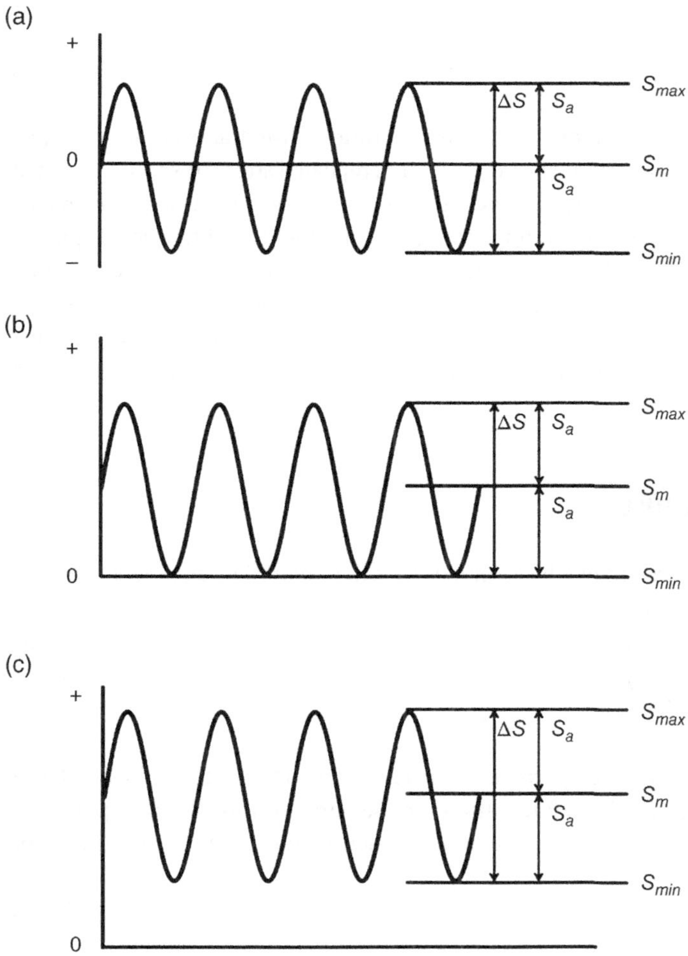

Figure 9.1 Cyclic loading regimens: (a) completely reversed cyclic loading; (b) repeated stress; (c) fluctuating stress. Note: S_a = alternating stress; S_m = mean stress; ΔS = stress range; S_{max} = maximum stress; S_{min} = minimum stress. Plus (+) = tensile load, minus (–) = compressive load.

Figure 9.1a represents *fully reversed loading* which has a mean stress of 0, and cycles from compression (negative) to tension (positive) with equivalent peak stresses in each direction. This is a common loading mode for many materials; however, it seems to be a relatively rare loading regimen in musculoskeletal tissues. Figure 9.1b shows loading termed *repeated or unidirectional loading*. In this type of loading, stress cycles start from a minimum of zero to some positive or negative value (positive in our example). Note that in this case the mean stress is no longer zero but has a positive value halfway between zero and the peak stress of the cycle. This type of loading would be similar to what tendons might experience, starting at close to zero stress when relaxed, and experiencing tensile stress with muscle contraction. Figure 9.1c illustrates a loading pattern known as *fluctuating stress*. This pattern never experiences zero stress, but cycles while always staying either above zero as in this case (illustrating constant tension), or below zero (constant compression). An example of this type of loading in the musculoskeletal system would be loads on the spine when lifting. When standing the spine would have a compressive load resulting from the weight of the upper body acting on the spine (estimated at 500 N for an average man), but when lifting an object (a 20-pound box, for example), the compressive load might cycle to 2,000 N and return to 500 N when the lift is completed.

Another commonly used relationship is called the *stress ratio:*

$$R = \frac{S_{\text{min}}}{S_{\text{max}}} \tag{9.2}$$

Values of R can be used to describe some of the loading conditions listed above. For example, $R = -1$ represents fully reversed loading, while $R = 0$ represents repeated stress. It should be noted that while the preceding equations are usually expressed in terms of stress, several surrogate measures can replace stress in these equations, including strain, load, moment, and torque (Stephens, Fatemi, Stephens, & Fuchs, 2001). It should also be noted that while loading cycles are well defined in Figure 9.1, variable amplitude loading is quite common in musculoskeletal tissues. When variable amplitude loading is experienced, cycles may become less easily identifiable, and we must identify *stress reversals* to evaluate cyclic loading effects. A procedure to do so will be described later in this Chapter.

Mechanisms of Fatigue Failure

It has long been recognized that there are two basic modes by which materials experience failure. These are through (a) a one-time application of high magnitude stress (at or beyond the so-called "ultimate stress" [US] of the material) or (b) repeated sub-maximal stress applications (Peterson, 1950). The American Society for Testing and Materials (ASTM) has defined the latter failure mode (fatigue failure) as under:

> . . .the process of progressive localized permanent structural change occurring in a material subjected to conditions that produce fluctuating stresses and strains at some point (or points) and that may culminate in cracks or complete fracture after a sufficient number of fluctuations
>
> (ASTM, 2000).

Failure of materials often appears to be sudden and without warning; however, this is due to the insidious nature of the failure mechanism, which might have been underway for a considerable period prior to failure (Stephens et al., 2001). Furthermore, the fatigue failure process is characterized by damage that starts locally and then spreads as repetitive stress continues. Eventually, the damage developed can be great enough to lead to a significant failure or even a complete fracture (or rupture) of the material.

However, while this definition is largely applicable to most materials, certain aspects may not be as applicable to musculoskeletal tissues. For example, the ASTM definition given earlier characterizes fatigue damage as permanent in nature. This is not necessarily the case for musculoskeletal tissues. For example, tissues such as muscle and bone can experience damage due to repeated applications of stress but can rely on the body's healing capacity to repair the damaged tissue. In fact, the repaired muscle tissue can be superior in strength than it was prior to damage. Unfortunately, not all musculoskeletal tissues are able to repair themselves quite so well. In many cases, the repair of musculoskeletal structures (such as a tendon) requires extended periods of time and while healed to an extent, these structures are not replaced with material that is equivalent to the original quality.

In standard monolithic materials such as metals, the fatigue failure process is known to initiate on the surface of the material in an area where stress is concentrated. Stress concentrations are often the result of a change in the geometric shape of a material. For example, the presence of a notch or hole in the material (or even a scratch or groove on the surface) can lead to significant stress concentrations that may eventually lead to crack nucleation. There are two main phases of crack growth. The first phase of crack growth typically occurs along the plane of maximum shear loading. Eventually, this phase ends and a new phase begins where the crack growth occurs in the plane of maximum tensile stress (Figure 9.2). However, under complex loading (i.e., torsional or multiaxial), macroscopic crack growth in the shear plane may be seen.

However, musculoskeletal tissues are not traditional engineering materials (metals or plastics) but instead behave as a specialized composite material. Composites tend to demonstrate a slightly different type of fatigue damage development process. Fatigue damage development in composite materials tends to be characterized by multiple damage modes, such as crazing and cracking of the matrix, fiber or matrix decohesion, fiber fracture, delamination, void growth, and multidirectional

Figure 9.2 Process of fatigue failure in a material, starting from surface nucleation to crack propagation and failure (Stage I and Stage II).

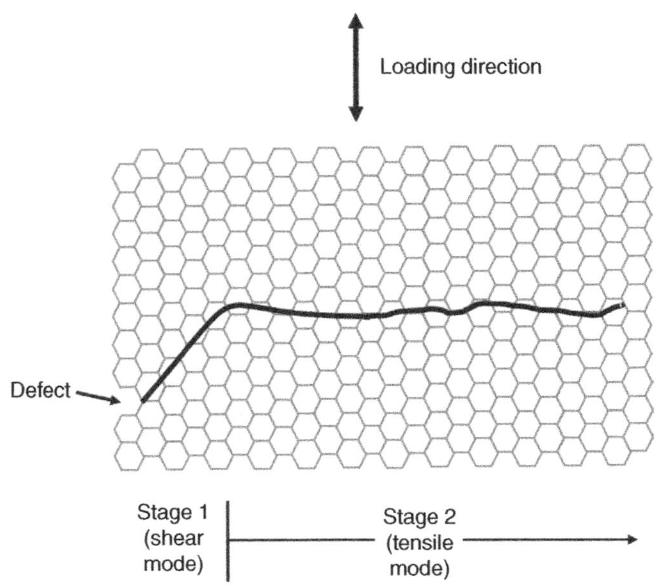

cracking (Mao & Mahadevan, 2002). These types of damage behaviors have been demonstrated in tendon in response to fatigue loading *in vivo* (Andarawis-Puri, Flatow, & Soslowski, 2015). Such damage modes can develop relatively early in the fatigue life of composites. Compared to traditional engineering materials, the processes of crack nucleation and propagation are more complex in composite materials. Even in equivalent loading scenarios, cracks may initiate in different locations and act in different directions in composites. Furthermore, damage in composite materials begins to accumulate more quickly (initially) than in monolithic materials such as metals but often progresses at a slower rate in the middle of the damage accumulation process (Mao & Mahadevan, 2002).

Musculoskeletal tissues are typically subjected to a wide range of loading conditions. These can be rather straightforward and highly repetitive activities (such as walking or running), or they can be highly variable and complex activities (such as performing multiple tasks with wide-ranging demands in an occupational setting). Interspersed with repetitive cyclic loading, there may also be situations in which a constant load is experienced by musculoskeletal structures, leading to a phenomenon known as *creep fatigue*. This type of loading would be experienced when standing still, in which the weight of the upper body places a constant static compressive stress on the lumbar spine, or when exerting a constant grip pressure on an item (such as a drill) for a substantial period of time. Obviously, musculoskeletal tissues can experience both cyclic and creep loading, each of which can cause stress and damage to musculoskeletal tissues.

Fortunately, techniques have been developed to ascertain the amount of damage developed in materials in both simple and complex loading situations. It is clear that many of the techniques used in assessing damage accumulation in inert materials (such as metals and plastics) are highly applicable to the development of damage in musculoskeletal materials; however, there are some differences in response. This chapter will describe techniques derived from fatigue failure theory that can be utilized to assess the risk associated with injury to musculoskeletal tissues under a variety of loading conditions.

The process of fatigue failure in a material begins with nucleation of a small micro-failure in the material incurring the stress, usually on or near the surface, near an internal or surface flaw, or an area of stress concentration (Roylance, 2020). The area surrounding the initial micro-failure experiences a subsequent increase in stress concentration at the site of damage, and with repeated loadings, the area of damage starts to expand. At moderate load levels, the rate of growth tends to be slow at this early stage and may be difficult to detect (Stephens et al. 2001). With continued load exposure, a new phase of damage propagation will ensue. In this secondary phase of growth, the area of damage increases in a stable manner—subcritical with respect to the integrity of the involved structure. However, eventually, a damage threshold is surpassed (critical in light of prevailing loading conditions) where rapid and unstable damage accumulation occurs, eventually compromising structural integrity.

The Stress-Life (*S*–*N*) Curve

The relationship between applied stress and the number of cycles to failure in a material is exponential in nature and is typically described in an *S–N diagram*. This S-N diagram describes how the number of cycles to failure (*N*) varies with respect to constant cyclic stress (*S*). An example *S–N* diagram is provided in Figure 9.3. As can be seen in this figure, higher levels of loading will result in failure in fewer cycles and lower levels of loading will endure for an exponentially larger number of cycles. In fact, millions of cycles may be necessary to create failure in low load situations,

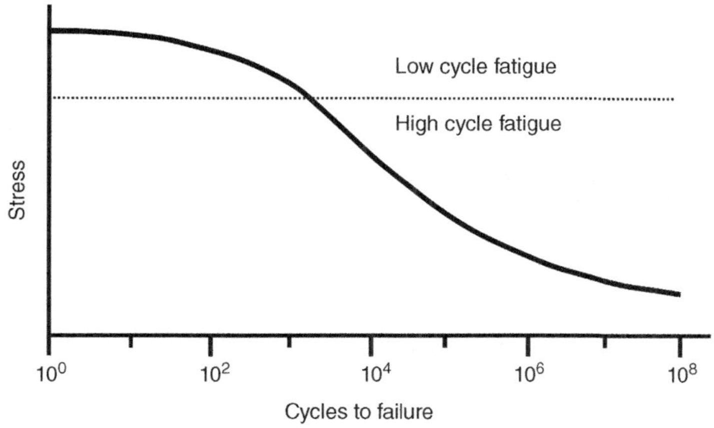

Figure 9.3 Stress-life (*S–N*) curve. Low-cycle fatigue (characterized by repeated plastic deformation), High-Cycle fatigue (characterized by repeated elastic deformation).

and for many engineering materials like steel, there exists a fatigue (or endurance) limit—usually around 30% of the material's US—where failure will not occur no matter the number of cycles experienced in fully-reversed loading conditions (Ashby, Shercliff, & Cebon, 2010).

Note that the curve is divided into two parts: low cycle fatigue (LCF) and high cycle fatigue (HCF). These portions of the curve are differentiated by the type of deformation experienced by the subject material at these different stress levels. LCF is characterized by repeated plastic deformation; whereas, in the HCF region material deformation is elastic in nature. When repeated plastic deformation is experienced, materials will fail rather quickly (i.e., in a low number of cycles). Life estimation in the LCF region is often obtained using a strain-based approach (Stephens et al., 2001). However, deformation in the elastic range can be tolerated for a large number of cycles, and fatigue life estimates often employ a stress-life approach, through the use of the *S–N* curve.

When a material has been fatigue-tested at multiple levels of stress (as in the Schechtman Bader data shown in Chapter 6), an *S–N* curve is drawn through the median life observed for each stress level tested. This provides a line that estimates equal probabilities of survival and failure at each stress level. The following represents several important terms that are defined for such a curve drawn in such a manner (American Society for Testing and Materials (ASTM), 2000):

Fatigue Life (N_f): the number of cycles of stress or strain of a specified character that a given specimen can sustain before failure of a specified nature is experienced.

Fatigue Strength (S_{Nf}): the estimated value of the stress at failure for exactly N_f cycles, as determined by an *S–N* diagram.

Fatigue Limit (S_f): the limiting value of the median fatigue strength as N_f gets very large.

Depending on the stress magnitude, a material experiencing fatigue failure may spend different amounts of time in the damage propagation phase. At high-stress magnitudes, crack nucleation occurs relatively early in the process, and a proportionately larger amount of time will be spent in the damage growth phase prior to final failure. At lower stress levels, greater time is spent in the nucleation of damage (microfailure), and proportionately less time is spent in damage growth below failure (Figure 9.4).

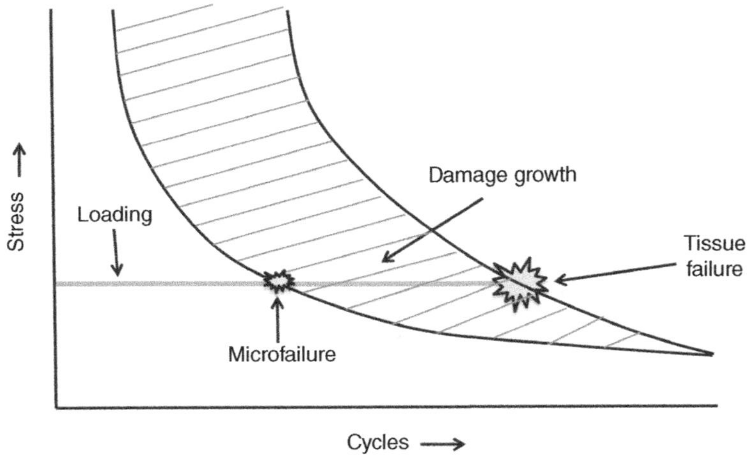

Figure 9.4 Difference in the proportion of time spent in damage nucleation, growth, and failure dependent on stress level.

Plastic Strain Fatigue Life Estimation Methods

Another method that is often used to estimate the fatigue life of a material is the strain-based approach (ε-N). Strain-based methods appear particularly well-suited to the estimation of fatigue life in low-cycle fatigue (fatigue that occurs in less than 10,000 cycles), although plastic strain methods can be used in high-cycle fatigue. Under these conditions materials often experience plastic strain (as opposed to elastic strain) which leads to more rapid deterioration of the material.

Two methods are commonly used to estimate plastic strain fatigue life. One is the Morrow Energy Model, which estimates fatigue life based on the strain energy density, which can be obtained from the inner area of a hysteresis loop (Morrow, 1965). The other is the Coffin–Manson model (life vs. plastic strain range), which uses the width of hysteresis loops to estimate the number of cycles needed to produce failure (Tavernelli & Coffin, 1962).

As indicated above, both strain-based life estimation methods derive information from *hysteresis loops*, which are plots of the stress and strain characteristic of viscoelastic materials in which the unloading curve does not follow the same path as the loading curve. The deviation of these paths is representative of the strain energy that is lost between loading and unloading resulting from the internal friction in the material. During this process, energy is lost in the form of heat.

Figure 9.5 shows a hysteresis loop that identifies important characteristics associated with the strain-life methods. Note in particular the different paths taken during the loading portion of the curve as opposed to the unloading portion. These different loading paths provide important information that can be used to estimate the fatigue life of the material, as discussed in more detail below.

Morrow Energy Model

The Morrow Energy model uses the plastic strain energy density to estimate the fatigue life of a material, represented by the area inside the hysteresis loop. The physical interpretation of this measure is the energy associated with the distortion of material that results from the change in the shape of the material during the loading and unloading processes. This relationship has been shown to provide good estimates of fatigue failure in metallic materials as well as in

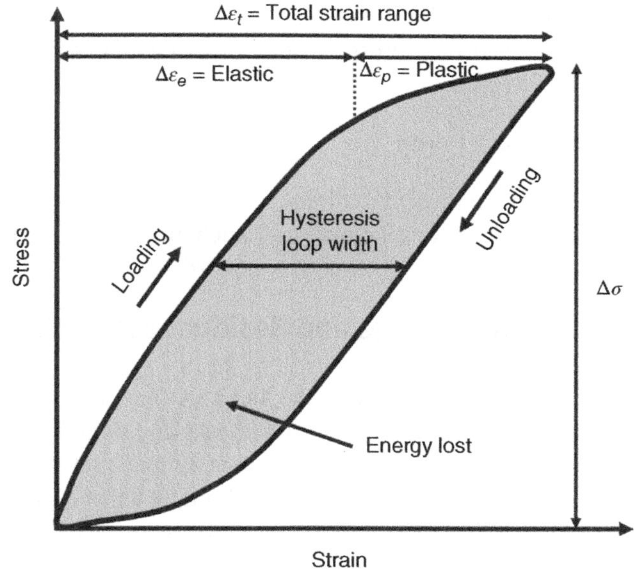

Figure 9.5 Hysteresis loop.

polymers (Kanchanomai & Mutoh, 2004). The following equation (9.3) is used to quantify this relationship:

$$N_f^m \times W_p = C \tag{9.3}$$

where N_f represents fatigue life, m represents the fatigue exponent, W_p denotes the plastic strain energy density, and C denotes the material ductility coefficient. A modified version of this model has been developed to account for the effect of experimental frequency:

$$\left(N_f \times \upsilon^{k-1}\right)^m \times W_p = C \tag{9.4}$$

where υ and k represent the frequency and frequency exponent, respectively. The application of this model has been shown to predict fatigue life well in bioinspired materials (Panadero, Vikingsson, Gomez Ribelles, Sencadas, & Lanceros-Mendez, 2013). In this study, the fatigue life of a trabecular scaffold made of poly-ε-caprolactone was well described by this model. Interestingly, it was found that the number of cycles increased up to fivefold with water-infused specimens due to the incompressibility of water (Panadero et al., 2013).

The Coffin–Manson Model

The Coffin–Manson model establishes a relationship between the plastic strain range (represented by the width of a hysteresis loop) and the fatigue life of a material. The plastic strain range can also be obtained by subtracting the elastic strain range from the total strain range (Kanchanomai & Mutoh, 2004). The relationship between the plastic strain range and the number of cycles to failure is described by the following equation:

$$\left(N_f\right)^\alpha \times \Delta\varepsilon_p = \theta \tag{9.5}$$

where N_f represents fatigue life, α is the fatigue ductility exponent, and θ is the fatigue ductility coefficient. Low cycle fatigue appears to be well-estimated using this equation for many common materials. As with the Morrow Energy model, a modified version of the Coffin–Manson model has been developed to address variable experimental frequencies, as represented in the following equation:

$$\left(N_f \times \upsilon^{k-1}\right)^{\alpha} \times \Delta\varepsilon_p = \theta \tag{9.6}$$

where υ and k represent the frequency and frequency exponent, respectively, as derived from the fatigue life-frequency relationship (Kanchanomai & Mutoh, 2004).

Cumulative Damage and Residual Strength Models

It has long been recognized in the literature that MSDs are the result of an accumulation of damage resulting from exposure of musculoskeletal tissues to repeated stress (Armstrong et al., 1993; NRC-IOM, 2001; National Institute for Occupational Safety and Health (NIOSH), 1981). Several authors in the field have developed methods of assessing cumulative loading (Callaghan, Salewytsch, & Andrews, 2001; Jager, 2000; Kumar, 1990; Marras, Ferguson, Lavender, Splittstoesser, & Yang, 2014; Norman, et al., 1998). Most of these studies have relied on rectangular integration methods or the calculation of area under the loading curve. While several of these methods have shown significant relationships with MSD outcomes, there are several limitations associated with these approaches. For example, certain factors known to be of critical importance in the development of cumulative damage in materials are not addressed by these models, such as the importance of the stress range in the development of cumulative damage. Previous approaches often do not capture the importance of the exponential increase in the effect of repetition in cumulative damage development with an increase in stress. There is no process in these methods to estimate the residual strength of materials, and so forth. Finally, they do not have an underlying mechanism that provides insight into how and why injuries are occurring, and how the area under the curve relates to such a mechanism.

A major benefit provided by fatigue failure theory is that damage accumulation in materials has been examined extensively (Post, Case, & Lesko, 2008) and several validated methods of estimating the amount of cumulative damage incurred by material exist, even when loading conditions are variable and complex. This section will examine some of the techniques to assess the damage accumulation models that may be helpful in understanding the risk imposed on musculoskeletal tissues. There have been two primary modeling approaches used when estimating failure of materials due to variable amplitude loading: damage accumulation models and models to assess the residual strength of materials (Post et al., 2008).

Musculoskeletal tissues typically experience variable loading conditions ("spectrum loading", to use the fatigue failure jargon) during daily living or in occupational settings or athletic pursuits. While the S–N curve can provide an estimate of the number of cycles needed to cause tissue failure for at a single level of repeated stress, other techniques are necessary to assess the cumulative damage development of materials when service histories have a complex array of loading situations involving different levels of stress and repetitions at these levels of stress. The earliest and still the most used cumulative damage model for such situations is the Palmgren-Miner model.

The Palmgren-Miner model is a linear cumulative damage estimate of fatigue life due to spectrum loading, as proposed by Palmgren (Palmgren, 1924) and Miner (Miner, 1945). This rule is represented by the following equation:

$$D = \Sigma \frac{n_i}{N_i} = \frac{n_1}{N_{f1}} + \frac{n_2}{N_{f2}} + \cdots = 1 \tag{9.7}$$

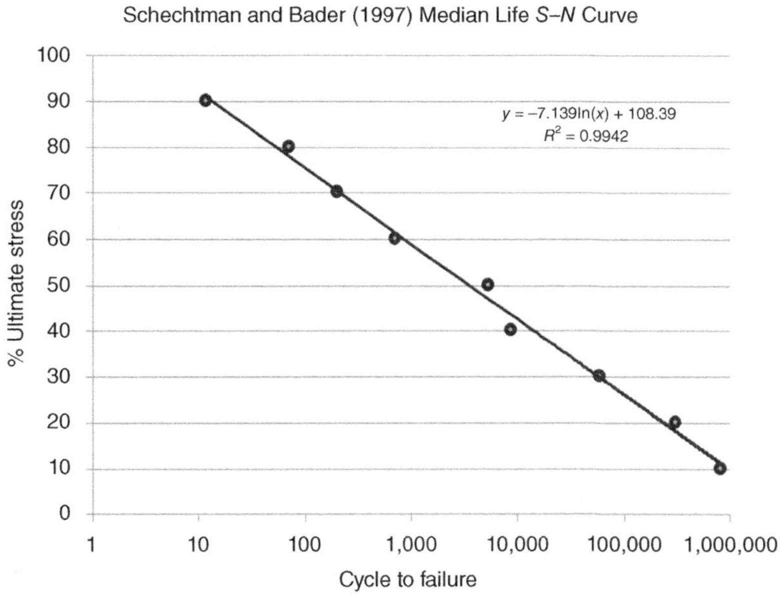

Figure 9.6 Median life data for extensor digitorum longus tendon. Modified from Schechtman, H., & Bader, D. (1997). In vitro fatigue of human tendons. *Journal of Biomechanics*, *30*, 829–835.

where the damage D is a constant (usually 1.0, though this can vary), n_i . . . represents the number of exposure cycles experienced at stress levels where N_{fi} . . . cycles would result in failure. When the right-hand sum is equal to the constant value, the material would be expected to begin the process of fatigue failure.

A rudimentary example of the Palmgren-Miner technique is provided below. In this illustration, the need to examine both force and repetition in combination should become apparent. Suppose that a tendon is repeatedly stressed for 250 cycles at 40% of ultimate tensile stress, 500 cycles at 30% ultimate tensile stress, and 2,000 cycles at 20% ultimate tensile stress (UTS). Let us also assume that the cycles to failure for 60, 50, and 40% UTS are 8,700, 60,000, and 315,000 cycles, respectively (Figure 9.6). The Palmgren-Miner model estimates the cumulative damage (*D*) by summing the quotients of the number of cycles experienced at each stress level divided by their respective cycles to failure, as seen in Equation 9.8 below:

$$D = \frac{250}{9{,}700} + \frac{500}{60{,}000} + \frac{2{,}000}{315{,}000} \cong 0.043 \qquad (9.8)$$

From this analysis, we would expect the cumulative damage experienced by the tissue to be approximately 4.3% of its fatigue life. Additional analysis can be performed to determine the *percentage* of damage associated with the repeated stress at each stress level, as shown in Table 9.1.

The table above demonstrates that approximately two-thirds of the total damage in the preceding scenario is due to the 250 cycles performed at the 40% UTS level. Repeated stress at the other two levels combined (despite many more repetitions) accounts for only about a third of the total. These results demonstrate the huge impact that stress magnitude plays on the effect of repetition. In fact, this data suggests that even though 8 times *greater* cycles are experienced at 20 versus 40%, this higher cycle count results in four and a half times *less* damage accumulation in the tissues. This is a critical insight in terms of understanding the vastly different impact of repetition at different stress levels in the development of tissue damage. This example clearly demonstrates why

Table 9.1 Determination of the Percentage of Total Damage for Scenario Above

Stress level	Damage per stress level	Percentage of total damage
40% UTS	250/8,700 = 0.029	0.029/0.43 = 66.2%
30% UTS	500/60,000 = 0.008	0.008/0.43 = 19.2%
20% UTS	2,000/315,000 = 0.006	0.006/0.43 = 14.6%

the effect of repetition should not be considered in isolation (or examined simply as the main effect) while evaluating the effects of force and repetition. Repetition's role in damage to tissues can only be truly understood when evaluated in combination with stress magnitude.

The Palmgren-Miner rule often provides a useful approximation of the accumulation of fatigue damage in a material; however, it must be understood that it is only an approximation. Numerous factors can influence the development of fatigue failure and these factors can influence the fatigue failure process in a manner not captured by the simple linear relationship expressed above. One factor that can affect fatigue life is the sequence of loading experienced by a material. Such loading sequence effects usually occur in either early or late stages of the fatigue process and can have a significant effect on fatigue life in certain materials, often as the result of *residual stresses* (stresses remaining in a material due to prior loading events). Such factors are not taken into account by the Palmgren-Miner rule though they can potentially have large influences on fatigue life (Roylance, 2020).

However, loading sequence effects can either extend or reduce the fatigue life of a material, and in many cases complex loading histories (as would be common with musculoskeletal tissues) may have sequence effects that cancel each other out, or result in effects that are highly erratic and unpredictable (Stephens et al., 2001). There are still no specific guidelines as to when one should take load sequence effects into account. Despite these limitations, the Palmgren-Miner rule remains the single most commonly used method by engineers in fatigue prediction for reliability design analysis (Post et al., 2008; Roylance, 2020).

Another approach to fatigue estimation, apart from the cumulative damage modeling approach discussed earlier, is using residual strength models. In these models, the failure criterion is described in terms of the residual strength of the material (S_r) and the maximum applied stress (σ_p) such that:

$$S_r(n) \le \sigma_p(n) \rightarrow Failure \tag{9.9}$$

Thus, the residual strength available within the material to withstand a load is calculated and if the load experienced [$S_r(n)$] is greater than the residual strength [$\sigma_p(n)$], the material would be predicted to fail. Residual strength in these models is treated as a monotonically decreasing function, as opposed to the monotonically increasing cumulative damage function of the Palmgren-Miner rule. The argument in favor of such models is that material damage is evaluated in terms of a specific physical quantity that can be measured and, for some materials, quantified at various points during their fatigue life (Post et al., 2008).

An early example of the use of a residual strength approach in composite materials that generally perform well is that of Broutman and Sahu (Broutman & Satu, 1972). This model assumes a linear decrease in residual strength and requires the same data as used by the Palmgren-Miner model, specifically an S–N curve providing an estimate of the fatigue life (N_i) for each level of stress application. The Broutman and Satu (1972) model is provided below:

$$S_r = S_u - \sum_i (S_u - \sigma_p)\frac{n_i}{N_i} \tag{9.10}$$

Table 9.2 Calculation of Residual Strength

S_u (MPa)	σ_p (MPa)	n_i	N_i	$(S_u - \sigma_p)\frac{n_i}{N_i}$ (Mpa)	% total reduction in S_r
100	20	2,000	315,000	0.508	18.0
100	30	500	60,000	0.583	20.7
100	40	250	8,700	1.724	61.3
			Total	2.815	100.0

where S_r is the predicted residual strength of the material, S_u is the material's original ultimate strength, σ_p is the maximum applied stress during a fatigue cycle, n_i is the number of cycles applied at a given stress level, and N_i is the estimated number of cycles to failure (from the *S–N* curve) at that stress level. Therefore, the model estimates what the *new* maximum load is that the material can withstand after a period of fatigue loading.

For clarity, we will calculate the residual strength of a tendon using the same data used in our example of variable loading with the Palmgren-Miner rule above. Table 9.2 illustrates the calculations necessary to estimate the residual strength of the tendon given the same variable loading regimen.

Thus, the reduction in residual strength (S_r) due to this variable loading sequence would be estimated at 2.815 MPa. Since the original strength (S_u) was 100 MPa, the predicted residual strength would be 97.185 MPa, compared to the original 100 MPa. As with the Palmgren-Miner rule calculations, we can calculate the percentage decrease in residual strength associated with each of the three fatigue loading conditions. As can be seen, the 250 cycles at 40 MPa was responsible for 61.2% of the decrease in residual strength, with the other two conditions contributing approximately 20% apiece.

Effects of Mean Stress on Fatigue Life

Many engineering materials experience fully reversed loaded (alternating compressive and tensile stress reversals) during their service life; however, it appears that this circumstance is less prevalent in musculoskeletal tissues. Instead, the latter tend to experience repeated stress or fluctuating stress (see Figure 9.1). In such cases, the mean stress experienced by the material will be non-zero and may have a significant influence on fatigue life. The presence of a moderate to high mean stress level during loading can also lead to a phenomenon known as *cyclic creep*, which may result in additional decreases in fatigue life, and add to the overall deformation experienced by the material (Bazant & Panula, 1979). As we prepare to calculate the fatigue life of musculoskeletal tissues encountering variable amplitude loading, we need to introduce techniques that take into account the impact of the mean stress on fatigue life.

Despite the fact that musculoskeletal tissues rarely experience fully reversed loading, this loading condition plays an important role in the analysis of conditions having variable amplitude loading conditions with nonzero mean stresses (common to musculoskeletal tissues). Essentially the fully reversed loading condition serves as the standard loading condition, and variable loading conditions and loading with nonzero mean stresses are corrected for and placed in the context of fully reversed loading, as we shall see.

Nonzero mean stresses (be they tensile or compressive) can significantly influence the fatigue life of a material. In general, tensile mean stresses have a detrimental effect on the number of cycles to failure, while compressive mean stresses can have a beneficial effect on fatigue life for many materials. The process of correcting for the effects of non-zero mean stresses involves the use of equations developed for the task by a number of authors. The most popular of these is the modified Goodman equation (Goodman, 1930) and is shown below:

$$\frac{S_a}{S_{Nf}} + \frac{S_m}{S_u} = 1 \qquad (9.11)$$

where S_a represents the stress amplitude, S_{Nf} is the fatigue strength (the stress expected to cause failure in N_f cycles), S_m is the mean stress, and S_u is the ultimate stress that can be borne by the material. The modified Goodman equation is sometimes criticized for being excessively conservative in its estimates of the fatigue life of the material at hand. Another equation, similar in formulation, but resulting in less conservative estimates of fatigue life is the Gerber equation (Gerber, 1874), shown below:

$$\frac{S_a}{S_{Nf}} + \left(\frac{S_m}{S_u}\right)^2 = 1 \qquad (9.12)$$

While the modified Goodman equation results in a straight line, the Gerber equation results in an arc (Figure 9.7). Actual experimental data on fatigue life tend to reside between these two lines. When used to design for the so-called "infinite life", every point on the modified Goodman line (or Gerber curve) corresponds to failure in 10^6 cycles. Thus, combinations of stress amplitude and mean stress that resides beneath the Goodman line or Gerber curve would be said to have "infinite" life and points above the curves would have "finite" life.

However, while infinite life design is one procedure that the Goodman and Gerber equations are often used for, another (perhaps more common) use is to correct for mean stresses associated with variable amplitude loading tasks. Due to the fact that musculoskeletal tissues commonly experience variable amplitude loading, this equation is a very useful tool for researchers interested in determining the cumulative damage associated with such loading.

Let us examine how these equations are used to perform mean stress corrections on loading curves having non-zero tensile stress. This loading situation is very common to musculoskeletal tissues such as ligaments and tendons, which tend not to experience axial compressive forces, but range from near zero stress at rest to some positive amount of tensile stress. Consider the loading curve illustrated in Figure 9.8.

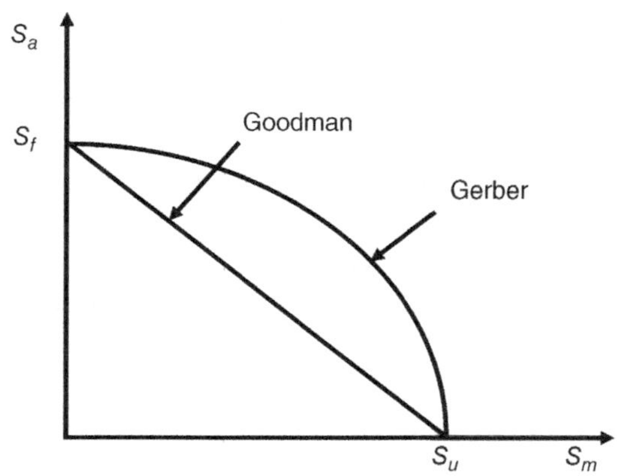

Figure 9.7 Goodman and Gerber estimates of constant fatigue life given the stress amplitude and mean stress experienced by a material. In design for infinite life, these curves are constructed such that they correspond to 10^6 cycles. However, these estimates can be adjusted to represent fatigue lives for any number of cycles (*Note.* see text for abbreviations).

Figure 9.8 Hypothetical tendon loading with a stress amplitude (S_a) of 15 MPa and a mean stress (S_m) of 15 MPa.

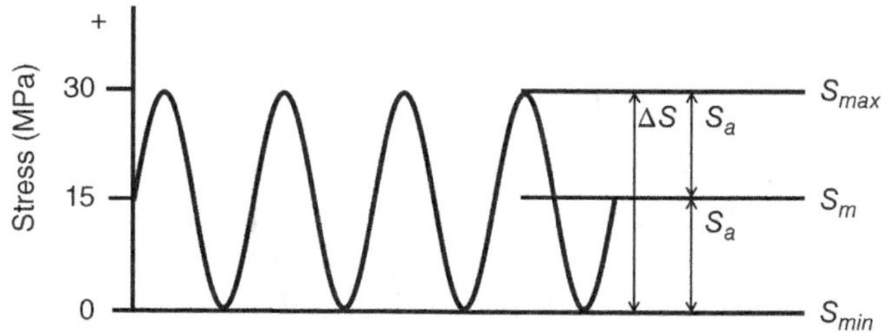

A mean correction of this loading condition is performed so that these (and potentially other) conditions can be brought into a standard loading condition so that comparisons can be made between loading histories having a variety of mean stresses and stress magnitudes. In fatigue failure analysis the standard loading condition is fully reversed loading ($R = -1$). The problem is to take the non-zero mean stress and transform it into its stress equivalent in the context of the fully reversed loading condition. In doing so, the original loading history and the transformed (fully reversed) loading history would be expected to have the same number of cycles to failure. The way that means stress is corrected in fully reversed loading is by increasing the stress amplitude of the fully reversed version so that it matches the impact of the tensile mean stress in the original. Let us use the modified Goodman equation to perform a mean correction for the data in Figure 9.8 above. Once again, the Goodman equation is:

$$\frac{S_a}{S_{Nf}} + \frac{S_m}{S_u} = 1 \tag{9.13}$$

We will assume that the ultimate stress of the tendon is 100 MPa (Schechtman & Bader, 1997). We know that the mean stress for the loading history above is 15 MPa, thus we can determine the relationship between the amplitude of the fully reversed stress given the stress amplitude and mean stress of the original.

$$\frac{S_a}{S_{Nf}} + \frac{15\,\text{MPa}}{100\,\text{MPa}} = 1$$

Thus,

$$S_{Nf} = 1.18 S_a \tag{9.14}$$

This tells us that the fully reversed fatigue strength stress amplitude should equal 1.18 times the original stress amplitude or 17.65 MPa. The fully reversed loading condition (equivalent in cycles to failure compared to the nonzero mean stress shown in Figure 9.8) is shown in Figure 9.9.

Cycle Counting in Variable Amplitude Stress Exposures

Musculoskeletal loading patterns in occupational settings tend to exhibit substantial variability (Mathiassen 2006; Mathiassen, Möller, & Forsman, 2003). Fortunately, several techniques exist to evaluate highly variable loading patterns in the context of a fatigue failure process. One of the issues that has faced musculoskeletal researchers over the years is how to count repetitions in complex variable amplitude exposures. This issue is becoming even more relevant with the advent

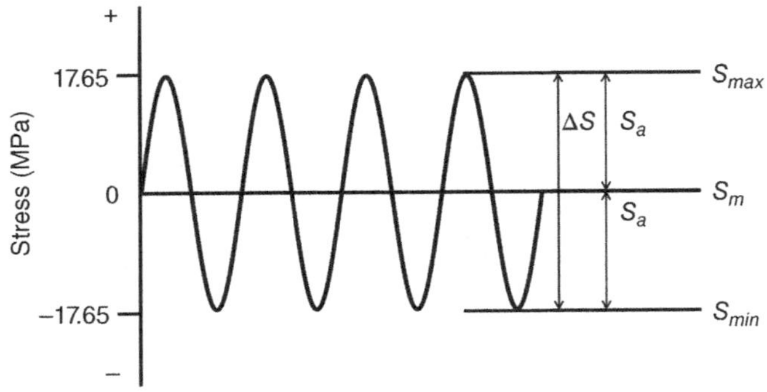

Figure 9.9 The equivalent fully reversed load history to the nonzero mean stress history shown in Figure 9.8, based on the modified Goodman equation. Goodman, J. (1930). *Mechanics applied to engineering* (Vol. 1). London: Longmans Green and Co.

of methods allowing researchers to obtain data on stressful exposures on a continuous basis. Small and easy-to-wear inertial measurement units are now able to obtain kinematic data that can be used to estimate measures such as the moment about the L5-S1 joint on a continuous basis. The question is how do we analyze the highly variable loads experienced by the lumbar spine in a manner that allows us to understand the cumulative impact of this loading on the spine.

Fortunately, this issue has been studied extensively by experts in the fatigue failure domain, and several validated methods have been developed that allow estimation of fatigue life resulting from continuous measures of variable amplitude repeated stress. The objective of these methods is to take these variable load amplitude histories and break down the curve in a manner that the data can then be used by a cumulative damage or residual strength model to estimate the cumulative damage experienced by the material in question.

It has been determined that the best counting methods (those that correlate best with experimental results) have certain attributes in common. First, they count cycles from the lowest valley to the highest peak, and then, they count other cycles in a manner that maximizes the ranges that are counted (Stephens et al., 2001). Every part of the curve must be accounted for and must be counted once and only once. Also, the best counting methods count smaller stress ranges (down to a predetermined threshold) once and only once. Many such methods have been developed, but we will describe the technique known as *rainflow analysis* (Matsuishi & Endo, 1968), which is generally acknowledged to be the best technique for variable amplitude cycle counting. The term "rainflow" refers to the fact that this technique identifies maximum stress ranges using a technique that, if the loading curve is turned 90°, would look as though rain was flowing down a series of pagoda roofs.

As an example of this technique, imagine a mono-task job in which repeated tensile stress of varying magnitude is experienced by a worker. The cycle time is 30 s, and the continuous measurement of stress is shown in Figure 9.10a. Figure 9.10b presents the rainflow counting procedure. Figure 9.10c provides the cycle breakdown resulting from the rainflow procedure.

Because identification of cycles is difficult in variable amplitude loading, rainflow analysis evaluates the so-called *stress reversals*. A stress reversal is simply a point at which stress reaches a local maximum or minimum, and then reverses to go in the opposite direction. Once the stress reversals in the loading history have been identified, they can be formed into cycle equivalents and the results used in cumulative damage or residual strength models to ascertain the degree of damage expected to occur as the result of the loading history.

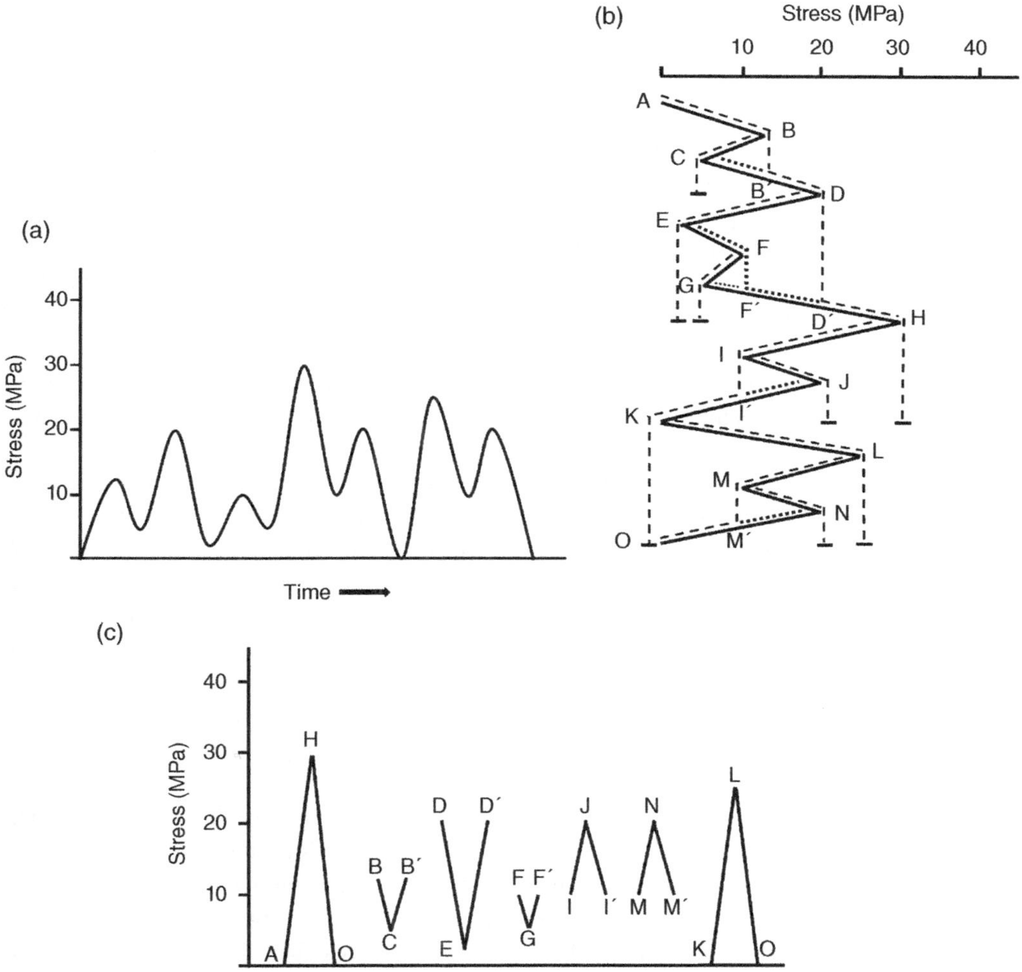

Figure 9.10 (a) Tendon stress history for 30-s work task; (b) Rainflow algorithm to identify stress reversals; (c) Complete cycles resulting from rainflow analysis.

The algorithm used for rainflow counting starts with the arrangement of the loading history so that either the lowest valley or the highest peak is the starting point. Assuming one starts at the lowest stress point (e.g., point A in Figure 9.10b), one would draw a line following the loading curve until one encounters a point that is *less than or equal to* the stress level at which one started for the first reversal. For example, in Figure 9.10b, We started at 0 MPa at point A and continued to point B at which point the line drops off the A–B "roof". At this point, the line passes point C but point C (5 MPa) is not equal to or lower than the stress at point A, so we keep going. The line keeps going down the C–D roof and falls past points E through G (none equal to or lower than point A) and the line falls again off of the G–H roof and passes points I and J until it finally arrives at point K which has a stress of 0 MPa, meeting our criterion for stopping. The total stress range of this first reversal (A–H) is 30 MPa.

For negative to positive reversals, we draw our line until we encounter a point that is *greater than or equal to* the point at which we started. Staring at point B (12.5 MPa) and the following stress in the negative direction we drop off the B–C roof and come upon point D. Point D (20 MPa) has higher stress than where we started and so we stop. The first negative to positive reversal ranges from 12.5 to 5 MPa for a stress range of 7.5 MPa.

One might have noticed that with the A-H reversal, that certain regions of the ascending stress curves were not originally accounted for (such as a portion of the C–D segment). This segment (and others similar to it) are picked up later in the count. For example, you can see that there is a short segment C–B′ that picks up the small segment left out of the original A–H reversal. This process is continued until all parts of the loading curve have been accounted for. Thus, every part of the curve is counted once and only once. By rearranging the loading history so that we start with the lowest or highest loading point, we ensure that the counted reversals always pair up into full cycles of equal magnitude, as seen in Figure 9.10c.

The results of the rainflow analysis can now be analyzed using techniques such as those developed by Goodman (Goodman, 1930) and Gerber (Gerber, 1874). If we assume this worker performs this task every 30 s for a total of 7.5 hr during the workday, the cumulative damage estimates would be as shown in Table 9.3.

The preceding analysis uses the Schechtman and Bader data of *in vitro* tendon fatigue to estimate the cumulative damage development for this example (Schechtman & Bader, 1997). As can be seen, the total estimated cumulative damage experienced in a workday is approximately 3.5% of that necessary to initiate a fatigue failure process. Note also the percentage damage is associated with the various cycles. One can observe that two cycles (A–H–O and K–L–O) account for approximately two-thirds of the total damage. If these tasks could be modified to reduce stress, cumulative damage (and injury risk) could be substantially reduced. Note also the correspondence between the stress range of the cycles and the percentage cumulative damage experienced by the tendons in this example. As identified by Wohler in the 1800s, the stress range represents a critical driver of fatigue damage in materials.

Several other cycle counting methods have been developed including the Range-Pair method, Racetrack Counting, the Level Crossing Method, and the Peak Counting Method; however, Rainflow Analysis has demonstrated strong correlations with experimental data and remains the most popular of the cycle counting methods (Stephens et al., 2001). Having techniques that break down and analyze variable amplitude loading histories is a great benefit to musculoskeletal researchers, as musculoskeletal tissues experience precisely that variety of loading. The ability to

Table 9.3 Estimates of Cumulative Damage from Rainflow Analysis, Assuming the Load History in Figure 9.10 is Repeated 900 Times During a Workday

Cycle	Stress amplitude (MPa)	Mean stress (MPa)	Fully reversed equivalent stress (MPa)	N_f	n	n/N_f
A–H–O	15	15	17.65	64,832	900	0.0134
B–C–B′	3.75	8.75	9.09	459,728	900	0.0020
D–E–D′	8.75	11.25	9.86	196,679	900	0.0046
F–G–F′	2.25	7.5	2.43	566,629	900	0.0016
I–J–I′	5	15	5.88	346,620	900	0.0026
M–N–M′	5	15	5.88	346,620	900	0.0026
K–L–O	12.5	12.5	14.29	104,698	900	0.0086
		Totals			6,300	0.0354

Table 9.4 A Representation of a Hypothesized Tendon Loading History Broken Into Bins Comprised of Combinations of Stress Range and Mean Stress for Subsequent Analysis

	Mean stress (MPa)								
Stress range (MPa)	**2.5**	**5**	**7.5**	**10**	**12.5**	**15**	**17.5**	**20**	**22.5**
5	564	126	47	32	17	14	8	5	
10		317	118	78	52	13	4	2	1
15			298	135	78	31	9	5	3
20				232	64	22	6	8	6
25					133	43	8		
30						57	11	6	5
35							13		
40								8	
45									4

have a technique that provides a consensus method for counting cycles and assessing the effects of stress in complex loading situations will become even more important as techniques allowing real-time exposure of musculoskeletal stresses in the workplace (or in athletic endeavors), as estimates of cumulative damage and injury risk would quickly.

For large-scale data collection, it may be helpful as a data reduction method to place data representing combinations of stress range and mean stress in "bins" such as those shown in Table 9.4. These bins can provide a basis to analyze spectrum loading (a loading history comprised of non-uniform or variable amplitude, fatigue). Such data could be analyzed using the Goodman or Gerber equations (Gerber, 1874; Goodman, 1930), or other cumulative damage models. Figure 9.11 shows a graphical method of displaying the results of a separate spectrum loading history.

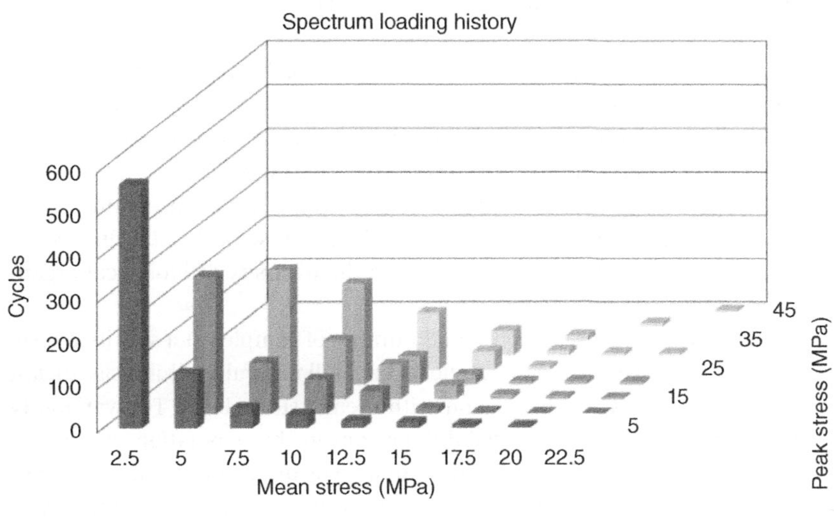

Figure 9.11 Graphical depiction of the results of a spectrum loading history.

Weibull Analysis of Fatigue Life

Wallodi Weibull (1887–1979), a Swedish engineer and mathematician, was the developer of a statistical distribution of great importance to the analysis of material failure. He was involved in the study of metallurgical failures and reported that the normal distribution did not accurately reflect the true distribution of failures observed in fatigue testing. This realization was the impetus for the desire to develop a distribution that was flexible and able to describe a wide variety of distributions, including the normal and exponential distributions, in a distribution dependent on the estimation of two (or three) parameters. In fitting this distribution to empirical data on fatigue life, many important aspects regarding the distribution of failures can be described, including the failure probability (or conversely the reliability) of a material at a certain stress level and cycle count, the rate of failure, and the material's characteristic life.

The Weibull analysis offers many advantages in understanding the fatigue failure process in a material. For example, the distribution has been shown to provide reasonably accurate estimates of the fatigue characteristics of a material with only a handful of data points. The Weibull distribution assumes the failure rate to be a power equation of time:

$$\lambda(t) = a t^b \tag{9.15}$$

where a and b represent different constants. The failure rate is often expressed using the following equation for the sake of convenience:

$$\lambda(t) = \frac{\beta}{\theta}\left(\frac{t}{\theta}\right)^{\beta-1} \tag{9.16}$$

where β is the shape parameter or the slope of the Weibull plot, θ is the scale parameter or "characteristic life" of Weibull. The slope of the line derived from the Weibull analysis provides information regarding the physical nature of the damage (slopes >1 suggest an accelerating damage process, while slopes <1 suggest a decelerating rate of damage with many early failures perhaps as the result of material defects). A slope equal to 1 is indicative of a constant damage rate. In situations where data points adhere closely to the line, a single failure mode is indicated; however, if the plot of points shows significant deviation from the fitted line, this may be an indication that mixed modes of failure are involved.

Even when identical fatigue testing is performed on seemingly identical metal specimens, a very large variation in fatigue life is usually observed (Johnson, 1964). Reasons for this wide scatter may be due to many factors, including inherent variability of the molecular makeup of material itself, variations in the geometry of the specimen, and variations associated with the testing protocol (e.g., machine calibration or specimen alignment). In some cases, the effect of the prior loading history of the specimen being tested might be an influence. When musculoskeletal tissues are involved, significant additional variability in fatigue life due to the diversity of biological organisms would also be expected.

Fatigue testing usually involves testing a relatively small number of samples at a specified level of stress or multiple levels of stress. Results of such fatigue testing will naturally exhibit significant variability in fatigue life both between stress levels and within each stress level. The variability observed in testing provides an estimate of the variability present in the population of possible specimens that might be tested. Examining this variability can help us understand what the population distribution of fatigue life looks like and can provide us with information regarding how many cycles specimens might last at different levels of reliability. For example, if we wanted to

Table 9.5 Fatigue Life Data for Human Extensor Digitorum Longus Tendons and Associated Median Ranks

Failure rank	Cycles	Median rank
1	74,876	0.067
2	112,724	0.163
3	173,579	0.260
4	260,411	0.356
5	313,313	0.452
6	314,788	0.548
7	354,398	0.644
8	467,923	0.740
9	707,333	0.837
10	770,594	0.933

Modified from Schechtman, H., & Bader, D. (1997). In vitro fatigue of human tendons. *Journal of Biomechanics, 30*, 829–835.

design for 90% reliability of a material, how many cycles would the sample data suggest us to design for at a given level of stress?

Let us examine the results of a sample of fatigue testing on the human extensor digitorum longus tendon at 20% of the estimated ultimate tensile stress (Schechtman & Bader, 1997). The failure data consist of 10 EDL tendon specimens and have been arranged in ascending order of cycles to failure (Table 9.5). Note the large variability in cycles to failure in this table, with the highest value being over 10 times the value of the lowest. The median rank for each specimen is provided. Median rank is calculated by taking (Failure Rank-0.3)/(Total # Failures+0.4).

From these data, we can obtain variables needed for a regression allowing us to develop a Weibull plot, as shown in Table 9.6. To get a measure of the failure probability of the material we need to obtain the double log of the quantity one divided by 1 minus the median rank. The other variable requires taking a log of either some measure of time or loading cycles. Since our data are obtained in terms of cycles, we will take the log of the cycles to failure for each specimen (Table 9.6). If one regresses the double natural log of 1 over 1-Median Rank against the natural log of the cycles, regression parameters allowing calculation of the Weibull parameters alpha and beta is possible, along with a Weibull plot which helps to understand the distribution.

Results of the regression equation provide coefficients for the regression intercept (−19.0520) and the beta weight for the slope of the regression (1.47566). from these results, the Weibull parameters can be obtained. The shape parameter of the Weibull distribution is obtained directly from the regression slope. Thus, the shape parameter is 1.47566. Shape parameter value of >1 indicates a failure rate that is increasing with time, also considered a "wearing out" process. The *characteristic life* (the number of cycles at which 63.2% of specimens would be predicted to fail) is calculated as follows:

$$Characteristic\ Life = e^{\left(\frac{-intercept}{slope}\right)} = e^{\left(\frac{-(-19.0520)}{1.47566}\right)} \cong 404{,}672 \text{ cycles} \quad (9.17)$$

Table 9.6 Initial Data Required for Regression to Determine Weibull Plot and Parameters

ln(ln(1/(1 − Median Rank)))	ln(Cycles)
−2.664	8.038
−1.723	9.425
−1.202	10.640
−0.822	10.819
−0.509	11.060
−0.230	11.281
0.033	11.548
0.299	11.678
0.594	11.734
0.993	11.896

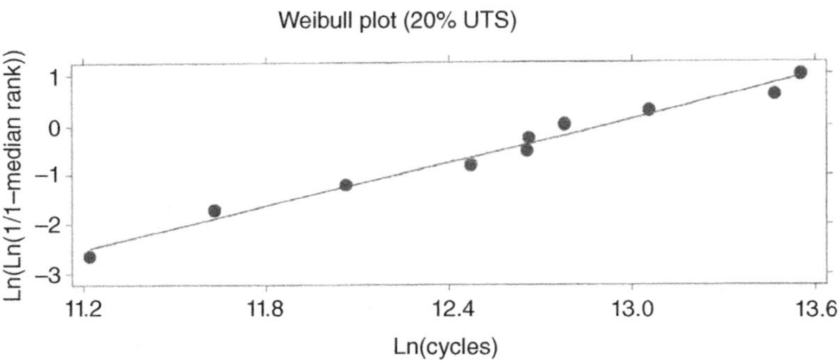

Figure 9.12 Weibull plot for the EDL tendon fatigue loaded at 20% UTS.

Figure 9.12 provides the Weibull plot for this data set. The data suggest that the line fits these data well with an adjusted $R^2 = 0.98$. If significant deviations from the line were present, it might indicate that different failure modes were at work.

The estimated probability of failure (or conversely the reliability) at any particular number of cycles can be estimated, given the shape and scale parameters of the Weibull distribution. The two-parameter Weibull cumulative distribution function is shown below in equation (9.18):

$$F(x,\alpha,\beta) = 1 - e^{-\left(\frac{x}{\beta}\right)^{\alpha}} \tag{9.18}$$

where x represents the number of cycles for which a failure probability is desired, α represent the Weibull shape parameter, and β equals the characteristic life. As an example, to obtain the failure probability associated with the lowest cycle value observed (74,876) for the 20% UTS fatigue test, the following calculation would be performed:

$$F(74{,}876, 1.48, 404{,}686) = 1 - e^{-\left(\frac{74{,}876}{404{,}686}\right)^{1.48}} = 0.079 \tag{9.19}$$

Table 9.7 Failure Probabilities and Reliability for EDL Tendons as a Function of the Number of Cycles Experienced at 20% UTS

Cycles	Failure probability	Reliability
74,876	0.0790	0.9210
112,724	0.1400	0.8600
173,579	0.2485	0.7515
260,411	0.4059	0.5941
313,313	0.4958	0.5042
314,788	0.4982	0.5018
354,398	0.5603	0.4397
467,923	0.7105	0.2895
707,333	0.8982	0.1018
770,594	0.9253	0.0747

Thus, 7.9% of tendons would be expected to fail in 74,876 cycles at 20% UTS. Reliability is the complement of the failure probability:

$$Reliability = e^{-\left(\frac{x}{\beta}\right)^{\alpha}} = e^{-\left(\frac{74,876}{404,686}\right)^{1.48}} = 0.921 \quad (9.20)$$

Reliability represents the proportion of tendons that would be expected to survive 74,876 cycles when loaded at 20% UTS, in this case, 92.1%. A similar type of Weibull analysis calculations can be performed for other cycles to failure to get a picture of the probabilities of tendon failure (or tendon reliability) over a wide range of cycles (Table 9.7).

The number of cycles to failure expected at specified levels of reliability can also be calculated. The following equation (9.21) can be utilized for this analysis:

$$F(x,\theta,\beta) = x * \left(-LN(\theta)\right)^{\frac{1}{\beta}} \quad (9.21)$$

where x denotes the characteristic life, theta equals the desired level of reliability, and beta equals the characteristic life. To assess the estimated number of cycles at a reliability of 0.01, the following calculation can be made:

$$F(404,686, 0.01, 1.48) = 404,686 * \left(-LN(0.01)\right)^{\frac{1}{1.48}} = 1,135,683 \quad (9.22)$$

Table 9.8 provides estimated cycles to failure for tendons at various levels of reliability.

Creep Loading and Creep-Fatigue

Up until this point, we have focused on the effects of fatigue damage due to cyclic loading, as this is expected to be the predominant method of damage to materials (musculoskeletal and otherwise). However, musculoskeletal tissues also experience creep loading every day, often in combination with cyclic loading. Creep loading is caused by a constant (non-varying or static) stress

Table 9.8 Estimated Cycles to Failure for Various Levels of Reliability for Tendons Stressed at 20% UTS

Reliability	Cycles
0.01	1,135,693
0.1	710,982
0.25	504,622
0.5	315,913
0.75	174,389
0.9	88,464
0.99	18,082

being imposed on the material. Both methods of loading can lead to material deformation and damage.

A simple illustration of the interaction between creep and cyclic loading in occupational workers is given below.

A male worker in a manual bag palletizing operation is simply standing at his workstation, waiting for delivery of the materials that he will soon have to palletize. Assuming that he is an average size male, his lumbar spine will be subjected to a constant compressive load of approximately 500 N. This constant load will lead to a constant slow creep deformation of the materials making up his spine, due to the viscoelastic nature of the spine's constituent parts. If experienced for a sufficiently long time, the creep load alone may lead to the development of damage in spinal structures.

Imagine now that the bagged materials are being delivered to the workstation and the worker must now lift the materials onto a pallet. The spine will now be subjected to repetitive loading characterized by substantial variation in compressive loading on the lumbar spine, perhaps cycling from 500 to 3,000 N. In general, cyclic fatigue will lead to damage development much more rapidly than exposure to creep stress. However, it is clear that both methods of stress exposure can lead to the development of damage given sufficient repetitions (or time). The question is: Can we estimate the effects of the combination of creep and fatigue loading, a situation that surely happens with musculoskeletal tissues?

Fortunately, a recommended procedure has been established for assessing the damage accumulation associated with a cyclic creep load. According to the Code of the American Society of Mechanical Engineers, the combination of creep and cyclic loading should be evaluated by summing the damage fractions of both cyclic and creep loading (Wright et al., 2016). The equation below describes how to evaluate the interaction of creep and fatigue loading:

$$\sum_j \left(\frac{n}{N_d}\right)_j + \sum_k \left(\frac{\Delta t}{T_d}\right)_k \tag{9.23}$$

where n represents the number of cycles experienced and N denotes the number that will lead to failure for a particular loading condition; Δt and T_d represent the specific creep loading time for a given task and the time that would lead to failure at that creep loading level, respectively. The left-hand term might be recognized as the Palmgren-Miner rule that is commonly used to assess cyclic damage for highly variable cyclic loading conditions, as discussed in detail above. The right-hand term denotes a "time fraction" for determining the damage associated with creep loading. This time fraction represents the amount of creep time experienced divided by the creep time required to lead to tissue damage at a particular level of static loading.

Using this model, we can evaluate the combined effects of creep and fatigue loading, assuming we have information regarding the responses to both types of loading from a given material. Fortunately, there are a couple of studies in the musculoskeletal literature that have examined both creep and fatigue loading on biological tissues that allow for such an evaluation (Thornton et al., 2007). The analysis that follows employs the dataset provided by Thornton et al. (2007), analyze the creep-fatigue interaction on rabbit medial collateral ligaments.

The data used for this evaluation is obtained from a study of ligament fatigue and creep damage performed by Thornton et al. (2007). In this study, 47 medial collateral ligaments (MCLs) from 37 female rabbits were used to assess the number of cycles to failure (rupture) at 15, 30, and 60% Ultimate Tensile Strength (UTS), and the time necessary to cause rupture for Creep (static) loading at the same percentages of UTS. Cyclic loading tests were performed at 1 Hz, and creep tests involved continuous loading at the assigned load magnitude. The authors provided the following regression equations that provided the best fits for cycles/time to rupture for fatigue and creep loading results (note that the data for a creep at 15% UTS resulted in only one creep failure, thus these data were not used in the development of the creep equation):

$$T_{fatigue} = 2.06 * 10^{6}\left(\frac{\sigma_0}{\sigma_{UTS}}\right)^{-3.72} \tag{9.24}$$

$$T_{creep} = 1.54 * 10^{4}\left(\frac{\sigma_0}{\sigma_{UTS}}\right)^{-1.78} \tag{9.25}$$

Based on these relationships, estimates of the combined effects of creep and fatigue loading can be made. Such estimates can help to understand the impact of the duty cycle on cumulative damage development in musculoskeletal tissues when a combination of cyclic and creep loading is experienced. The following section provides estimates of the effects of the duty cycle when cyclic and creep loading are combined.

Based on the equations given earlier, we can estimate the individual contributions associated with creep and fatigue loading at various percentages of UTS and duty cycle. For the purposes of the calculations below, we calculate the effect of one cycle of fatigue loading (damage per cycle) by taking the hours of cyclic fatigue that would be predicted for a specific %UTS from Thornton et al.'s (2007) data, multiplying it by 3,600 (the number of loading cycles per hour), and then dividing 1 by the calculated cycles to failure. Similarly, for creep loading, we took the number of hours to creep rupture, multiplied this value by 3,600, and divided 1 by the calculated seconds to rupture to obtain the amount of damage associated with 1 s of creep loading for each specific %UTS. Table 9.9 provides data of fatigue failure damage per cycle and creep damage per second for 30–60% of ultimate tensile strength.

With this data, we can evaluate the combination of cyclic and creep for a given load history. Consider the load history illustrated in Figure 9.13. This load history contains four cycles (to different percentages of UTS) combined with four different static creep loads ranging from 1–4 s in length.

To calculate the total cumulative damage associated with this load history, we would sum the cumulative damage associated with each of the four cycles and then add the additional damage associated with the creep loading portion. The cyclic loading portion would be as represented in equation 9.26:

$$Cyclic\ CD = 0.00012288 + 0.00055533 + 0.00004214 + 0.00028184 = 0.00100219 \tag{9.26}$$

Table 9.9 Fatigue Damage Per Cycle and Creep Damage Per Second at Various Percentages of Ultimate Tensile Strength

Percent ultimate tensile stress	Fatigue damage per cycle	Creep damage per second
30% UTS	0.00004214	0.0000077
40% UTS	0.00012288	0.0000128
50% UTS	0.00028184	0.0000191
60% UTS	0.00055533	0.0000264

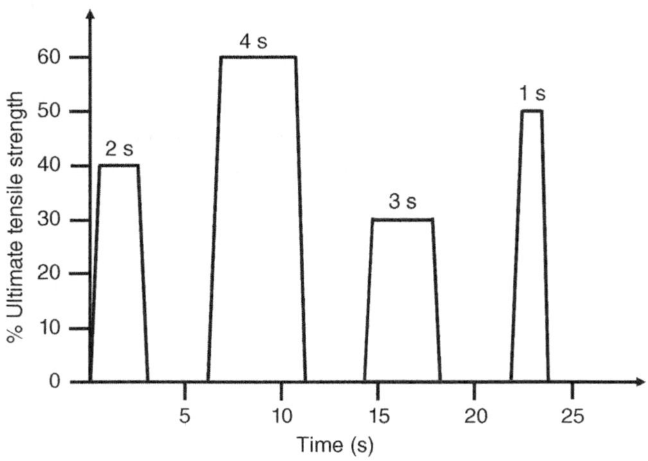

Figure 9.13 Example of a load history containing four loading cycles combined with 4 lengths of creep loading.

The creep loading portion would involve taking the appropriate creep damage per second (for each given load) and multiplying it by the number of seconds the creep was experienced.

$$Creep\ CD = 0.0000128 * 2 + 0.0000264 * 4 + 0.0000077 * 3 + 0.0000191 * 1 = 0.0001734 \quad (9.27)$$

The total cumulative damage associated with both types of loading would be the sum of these sums:

$$Total\ CD = 0.00100219 + 0.0001734 = 0.00117559 \quad (9.28)$$

From this dataset, we can also determine the proportion of the cumulative damage associated with the cyclic portion and the creep portion of loading.

$$Proportion\ of\ Total\ CD\ from\ Cyclic\ Loading = \frac{0.00100219}{0.00117559} = 0.85 \quad (9.29)$$

$$Proportion\ of\ Total\ CD\ from\ Creep\ Loading = \frac{0.0001734}{0.00117559} = 0.15 \quad (9.30)$$

Thus, we can conclude that 85% of the cumulative damage was due to cyclic loading while 15% was the result of the creep portion.

There is a shortage of studies examining the effects of both creep and fatigue in biological tissues. In fact, the two studies that we are aware of have used either wallaby tail tendons (Wang et al., 1995) or Burgunder rabbit medial collateral ligaments (Thornton et al., 2007). We are aware of no such studies that used human tissues. While tendons and ligaments are similar throughout the animal kingdom, it would be helpful to have data regarding creep and fatigue responses on specific human tendons to evaluate whether significant differences exist.

Limitations of this analysis include the use of rabbit medial collateral ligaments as a basis for predicting creep-fatigue interaction and a limited number of specimens per loading level. In spite of these limitations, we believe that this analysis gives a reasonable picture of the effects of creep-fatigue interaction on cumulative damage development.

Summary

Musculoskeletal tissues are physical materials, and it would be surprising if they did not respond to the application of repeated stress in the same manner as all other physical materials. The process starts with an initial insult at a location of high stress in the material, and with repeated loading, a progression of damage starts to accumulate in that now weakened area. Eventually, the damage can become significant enough to lead to damage that results in material dysfunction and pain. This chapter has provided an overview of certain fatigue failure analysis methods that have particular relevance to the development of musculoskeletal disorders. However, this chapter only scratches the surface with respect to the analytical methods that have been developed in the fatigue failure realm, many others of which may be relevant to MSD development as well. A vast amount of fatigue failure research has been focused on the materials humans use to build things, but surprisingly little has been devoted to fatigue of the structures of which humans are made. One reason is certainly the difficulty presented by having these structures largely hidden from view (and therefore difficult to measure) in the living state. Another reason is the added complexity presented by the dynamic biological environment in which these structures exist, particularly the fact that these viscoelastic tissues not only incur damage but also have a self-healing capacity. It is proper time that we increase research devoted to the scrutiny of the workings of this complex system more closely. The benefits derived from our improved understanding of the operation of this complex biomechanical system would be immense indeed.

Bibliography

American Society for Testing and Materials (ASTM) (2000). *Annual book of ASTM standards, metals test methods and analytical procedures* (Vol. 03.01). Conshohocken, PA: ASTM.

Andarawis-Puri, A., Flatow, E., & Soslowski, L. (2015). Tendon basic science: Development, repair, regeneration, and healing. *Journal of Orthopaedic Research*, *33*, 780–784.

Armstrong, T., Buckle, P., Fine, L., Hagberg, M., Jonsson, B., Kilbom, A., . . . Viikari-Juntura, E. (1993). A conceptual model for work-related neck and upper-limb musculoskeletal disorders. *Scandinavian Journal of Work, Environment & Health*, *19*, 73–84.

Ashby, M., Shercliff, H., & Cebon, D. (2010). *Materials: Engineering, Science, Processing and Design* (2nd ed.). Oxford, UK: Elsevier Butterworth-Heinemann.

Bazant, Z., & Panula, L. (1979). Practical prediction of time-dependent deformations of concrete. Part VI: Cyclic creep, nonlinearity and statistical scatter. *Materials and Structure*, *12*, 175–183.

Broutman, L., & Satu, S. (1972). A new theory to predict cumulative fatigue damage in fiberglass reinforced plastics. In *Composite materials: testing and design (second conference) ASTEM STP 497* (pp. 178–188). American Society for Tesing and Materials.

Callaghan, J., Salewytsch, A., & Andrews, D. (2001). An evaluation of predictive methods for estimating cumulative spinal loading. *Ergonomics, 44*, 825–837.

Gerber, W. (1874). Bestimmung der zulossigenin eisen construcionen. *Zeitschrift Bayer Architekten Ingenieure Vereines, 6*, 101–110.

Goodman, J. (1930). *Mechanics applied to engineering* (Vol. 1). London: Longmans Green and Co.

Jager, M. J. (2000). Evaluation and assessment of lumbar load during total shifts for occupational manual materials handling jobs within the Dortmund lumbar load study– DOLLY. *International Journal of Industrial Ergonomics, 25*, 553–571.

Johnson, L. (1964). *The statistical treatment of fatigue experiments*. Amsterdam: Elsevier Publishing Company.

Kanchanomai, C., & Mutoh, Y. (2004). Low-cycle fatigue prediction model for pb-free solder 96.5Sn-3.5Ag. *Journal of Electronic Materials, 33*, 329–333.

Kumar, S. (1990). Cumulative load as a risk factor for back pain. *Spine, 15*, 1311–1316.

Lahrman, D. (2016). A brief history of fatigue failure analysis, damage tolerance, and remediation. *Metal Finishing News*. Retrieved from https://www.lsptechnologies.com/resources/a-brief-history-of-fatigue-failure-analysis-damage-tolerance-and-remediation

Mao, H., & Mahadevan, S. (2002). Fatigue damage modelling of composite materials. *Composite Structures, 58*, 405–410.

Marras, W., Ferguson, S., Lavender, S., Splittstoesser, R., & Yang, G. (2014). Cumulative spine loading and clinically meaningful declines in low-Back function. *Human Factors, 56*, 29–43.

Mathiassen, S. (2006). Diversity and variation in biomechanical exposure: What is it, and why would we like to know? *Applied Ergonomics, 37*, 419–427.

Mathiassen, S. E., Möller, T., & Forsman, M. (2003). Variability in mechanical exposure within and between individuals performing a highly constrained industrial work task. *Ergonomics, 46*, 800–824.

Matsuishi, M., & Endo, T. (1968). Fatigue of metals subjected to varying stress. In *Paper presented to the Japanese Society of Mechanical Engineers*. Fukuoka, Japan: Japanese Society of Mechanical Engineers.

Miner, M. A. (1945). Cumulative damage in fatigue. *Journal of Applied Mechanics, 16*, A159–A164.

Morrow, J. (1965). Cyclic plastic strain energy and fatigue of metals. In B. Lazan (Ed.), *Internal friction, damping, and cyclic plasticity* (pp. 45–87). West Conshohocken, PA: ASTM International.

Nash, J. C. (1966). *Fatigue of self-healing structure: A generalized theory of fatigue failure*. New York: American Society of Mechanical Engineers.

National Institute for Occupational Safety and Health (NIOSH) (1981). *Work practices guide for manual lifting*. Cincinnati: National Institute for Occupational Safety and Health.

Norman, R., Wells, R., Neumann, P., Frank, J., Shannon, H., & Kerr, M. (1998). A comparison of peak vs cumulative physical work exposure risk factors for the reporting of low back pain in the automotive industry. *Clinical Biomechanics, 13*, 561–573.

NRC-IOM, N. R.-I (2001). *Musculoskeletal disorders and the workplace: Low Back and upper extremities*. Washington, DC: The National Academies Press.

Palmgren, A. (1924). Die Lebebsdaue rvon Kugellagern. *Zeitschrift des Vereines deutscher Ingenieure, 68*, 339–341.

Panadero, J., Vikingsson, L., Gomez Ribelles, J. L., Sencadas, V., & Lanceros-Mendez, S. (2013). Fatigue prediction in fibrin poly-ε-caprolactone macroporous scaffolds. *Journal of the Mechanical Behavior of Biomedical Materials, 28*, 55–61.

Peterson, R. (1950). Discussion of a century ago concerning the nature of fatigue, and review of some of the recent researches concerning the mechanism of fatigue. *ASTM Bulletin, 164*, 50.

Post, N., Case, S., & Lesko, J. (2008). Modeling the variable amplitude fatigue of composite materials. *International Journal of Fatigue, 30*, 2064–2086.

Roylance, D. (2020). Fatigue. Retrieved from https://ocw.mit.edu/courses/materials-science-and-engineering/3-11-mechanics-of-materials-fall-1999/modules/MIT3_11F99_fatigue.pdf

Schechtman, H., & Bader, D. (1997). In vitro fatigue of human tendons. *Journal of Biomechanics, 30*, 829–835.

Stephens, R., Fatemi, A., Stephens, R., & Fuchs, H. (2001). *Metal fatigue in engineering* (2nd ed.). New York, NY: Wiley.

Tavernelli, J., & Coffin, J. L. (1962). Experimental support for generalized equation predicting low cycle fatigue. *Transactions of the ASME. Journal of Basic Engineering, 84*, 533.

Thornton, G., Schwab, T., & Oxland, T. R. (2007). Cyclic loading causes faster rupture and strain rate than static loading in medial collateral ligament at high stress. *Clinical Biomechanics, 22*, 932–940.

Tran, Y., Craig, A., Craig, R., Chai, R., & Nguyen, H. (2020). The influence of mental fatigue on brain activity: Evidence from a systematic review with meta-analyses. *Psychophysiology, 57*, e13554.

Wan, J., Qin, Z., Wang, P., Sun, Y., & Liu, X. (2017). Muscle fatigue: General understanding and treatment. *Experimental & Molecular Medicine, 49*, e384.

Wang, X., Ker, R., & Alexander, R. (1995). Fatigue rupture of wallaby tail tendons. *The Journal of Experimental Biology, 198*, 847–852.

Wikipedia. (2020). Retrieved from Versailles Rail Accident: https://en.wikipedia.org/wiki/Versailles_rail_accident

Wright, J., Carroll, L., Sham, T.-L., Lybeck, N., & Wright, R. (2016). Determination of the creep-fatigue interaction diagram for alloy 617. In *Proceedings of the ASME 2016 Pressure Vessels and Piping Conference (PVP2016)* (pp. 10). Vancouver, BC: EPRI 2016 Creep Fatigue Workshop In Collaboration with ASME PVP.

10

Fatigue Failure in a Biological Environment

Introduction

The traditional domain of fatigue failure analysis has been in the analysis of the fatigue life of engineering materials such as metals, plastics, and composite materials. Failure of materials, such as those contained in airplanes, bridges, buildings, and other structures has resulted in the loss of many lives, causing countless injuries and involving considerable financial cost. There are many known modes of failure for these materials, but one study has estimated that 50–90% of all mechanical failures are the result of fatigue or repetitive loading (Stephens, Fatemi, Stephens, & Fuchs, 2001). Even when examining fatigue in such inert materials, there is a complex interaction of factors that will influence the development of failure including load, time, temperature, corrosion, structural (and microstructural) aspects, the geometry of the material involved, and so on. The interaction of such factors can result in widely varying fatigue lives even in seemingly identical parts.

As complicated as the fatigue failure process can be in inert materials when one adds dynamic biological materials to the mix, an entirely new dimension of complexity is introduced. The musculoskeletal system, like other systems in the human body, seeks to maintain *homeostasis*. Homeostasis is defined as "any self-regulating process by which biological systems tend to maintain stability while adjusting to conditions that are optimal for survival" (Britannica, 2020). Multiple systems have been developed in musculoskeletal tissues to help maintain homeostasis. As already discussed in Chapter 3 and again being discussed in detail later in this chapter, the biological tissues that make up our musculoskeletal system possess mechanoreceptors that are highly responsive to the stress imposed upon them; these tissues will invoke specific physiological reactions in accordance with the magnitude and frequency of that stress.

Another unique feature of biological tissues is, of course, is their capacity to self-heal, which will be discussed more in Chapter 11. The healing response is triggered in response to an insult to a tissue, with the magnitude of the physiological response varying according to the degree of tissue injury experienced (Carp, Barbe, Winter, Amin, & Barr, 2007), the involved tissue(s) (see Chapter 11), and the time necessary for healing in the involved tissue(s) (Ekstrand, Askling, Magnusson, & Mithoefer, 2013). All musculoskeletal tissues exhibit some manner of healing capacity, although the characteristics of the healing response and the extent to which the tissues can successfully be healed vary widely (see Chapter 11). In general, tissues with greater blood flow (e.g., muscle and bone) and greater numbers or accessibility of active progenitor/stem cells, tend to heal more fully and quickly; whereas tissues with poor blood flow and fewer stem cells (e.g.,

Musculoskeletal Disorders: The Fatigue Failure Mechanism, First Edition. Sean Gallagher and Mary F. Barbe.

tendons, ligaments, and cartilage) take much longer to heal, and the quality of the repair is generally inferior (Sharma & Maffulli, 2005).

A Model of Fatigue Failure in Self-Healing Materials

In biological systems, both tissue damage and tissue repair processes are continually in progress. The key to the prevention of MSDs is in trying to ensure that the amount of damage accrued in tissues does not exceed the capacity of the repair mechanisms to heal. However, tissue damage can develop relatively rapidly, while the repair process is a complex and time-consuming process that can take several weeks, months, or years. Even when the repair process is complete, many types of tissues (such as tendons, ligaments, and cartilage) never regain their original strength and/or tissue quality. Thus, preventing or minimizing the degree of damage is critical to the maintenance of tissue homeostasis.

Nash (1966) put forth a generalized model of fatigue failure for self-healing biological materials, which can be expressed as follows:

$$D(t) = D_D(t) + D_A(t) + D_S(t) - H(t) \tag{10.1}$$

where $D(t)$ represents total tissue damage over a time frame, $D_D(t)$ denotes the damage occurred due to disease, $D_A(t)$ is damage due to aging, $D_s(t)$ is damage due to imposed stresses on tissues, and $H(t)$ represents healing over the time frame of interest. If one is considering a time frame when disease is not present and when the effect of aging is not significant, this equation can be simplified as per equation (10.2):

$$D(t) = D_S(t) - H(t) \tag{10.2}$$

where $D(t)$ represents total tissue damage over a time frame, $D_s(t)$ is damage due to imposed stresses on tissues, and $H(t)$ represents healing over the time frame of interest (Nash, 1966). The term $D_s(t)$ can be determined using the Palmgren-Miner rule, as described earlier. To do this, one would have to know or estimate the ultimate strength (US) of the tissue in question and need to be able to quantify the stress experienced by the tissue. One would then simply have to know the healing rate of the stressed tissue over time to quantify the total amount of cumulative damage accrual in the tissue.

Healing of tissues requires periods of unloading (rest) and some controlled loading so that damage accumulation can cease, so that repair mechanisms can have the time necessary to heal the tissue, and so that that matrix cells can realign in the direction of the typical forces on the tissues. But how much rest is needed? The model described earlier would suggest that the amount of rest necessary for healing would have to be related to the type of tissue damaged and the amount of damage incurred in some (as yet undetermined) manner. It might be possible, however, to examine the relationship of cumulative tissue loads (developed using fatigue failure techniques) with the amount of rest available to determine whether certain ratios of cumulative loading to rest result in lower MSD rates, while others lead to increased risk. Poorly vascularized tissues would be expected to be more susceptible to fatigue loading compared to highly vascularized tissues, due to the reduced availability of the biochemical and nutritional elements required for healing.

Deterioration of musculoskeletal function is among the most universal and demoralizing manifestations of the aging process. Human beings experience musculoskeletal loading every day of their lives (more than 100 years in some cases), and the sum of the loads experienced by musculoskeletal tissues over a lifetime must be quite impressive. The unremitting nature of loading on musculoskeletal tissues (through creep and fatigue) and the consequent accumulation of damage, clearly takes a substantial toll over time.

Degeneration of musculoskeletal tissues is a complex process that involves the degradation of many physiological processes, but mechanical fatigue of tissues also seems to play an important role. Key to the influence of the degenerative process is the fact that several tissues associated with MSDs (e.g., tendons, ligaments, and cartilage) do not heal quickly and when damage occurs they never regain their original strength. Continued loading of a damaged and weakened structure may result in a vicious cycle leading to tissue deterioration. For instance, damage in a structure will affect its ultimate strength, thereby reducing the repetitive loading that the structure will be able to withstand in the future. Other effects of a damaged structure may be that increased loading will be transferred to a secondary restraint, which may, in turn, experience damage due to repeated stress.

Responses of Inert Versus Biological Materials to Stress

As mentioned earlier, there are substantial differences in stress response when comparing inert materials with musculoskeletal tissues. The response of inert materials to stress application follows a general pattern in which escalating stress and repetition result in increased damage development (Stephens et al., 2001). However, evidence suggests a more complex response to the application of repeated stress in musculoskeletal tissues. On one hand, the right amount of high stress properly applied can convey significant health benefits and help maintain (or improve) musculoskeletal health. This is why exercises (such as weightlifting) can be beneficial for musculoskeletal health. On the other hand, if the stress applied to tissues is either insufficient or excessive, musculoskeletal tissues can experience a loss of homeostasis, leading to atrophy or the development of cumulative damage (Andarawis-Puri & Flatow, 2011; Barbe et al., 2013; LeBlanc, Spector, Evans, & Sibonga, 2007; Sun et al., 2010).

An example of the differential responses of inert versus biological tissues to applied stress can be seen in the lack of stress being applied to each type of material. For example, if a prolonged lack of stress is experienced by an inert material (such as a piece of metal or plastic), there will virtually be no impact on its material properties. However, when a prolonged lack of stress is experienced by musculoskeletal materials, the result may be tissue atrophy. The most extreme example of this phenomenon is the rapid loss of musculoskeletal tissue experienced by the astronauts who experience prolonged periods of weightlessness during space flights. When exposed to the lack of stress in a microgravity environment, the body responds quickly by resorbing both bone and muscle tissues (LeBlanc et al., 2007). For example, losses in bone mineral density experienced by 14 International Space Station Crew members per month in microgravity ranged from an average of ~1% in the lumbar spine to 2.7% in the femoral neck (Lang et al., 2004). These losses occur despite exercise programs put in place to mitigate bone loss during space flight (LeBlanc et al., 2007). Bone losses in astronauts are primarily observed in the load-bearing bones of the lower extremity and the spinal column, with relatively little bone loss observed in the upper extremities (Amin, 2010). Studies indicate that the loss of bone does not seem to be associated with a decrease in bone formation activity, as bone formation markers such as osteocalcin appear not to be affected significantly (Smith et al., 1999). Rather the loss appears to be due to accelerated resorption of bone, as indicated by the bone resorption marker n-telopeptide (NTX) (Smith et al., 1998, 1999). In an environment where stress reduction on bone is less severe (and often used as an analog to space flight), prolonged bed rest leads to changes in bone markers like those observed in space flight, though the response is predictably not as extreme (LeBlanc et al., 2007).

The reduced stress environment of space flight makes a significant impact on muscles because of the reduced need for muscular contraction to support the body or locomote (NASA, 2021). When exposed to microgravity, muscles quickly develop atrophy. Studies have indicated up to a

20% decrease in muscle mass during spaceflights that last only 5–11 days (NASA, 2021). Muscle volume loss in 16 Mir space station crew members completing 4–6-month flights was approximately 15% in the muscles of the back and legs (LeBlanc, Lin, Shackelford, Sinitsyn, & Evans, 2000). According to this study, the loss of muscle tends to be concentrated in the same anatomical region as bone loss, supporting numerous findings that state that these musculoskeletal tissues are both mechanically and functionally interrelated (Kaji, 2014). One can surely appreciate that the reduced forces required of muscle in this environment would lead to decreased bone loading; therefore, to bone resorption according to Wolff's law. However, given the small numbers of subjects and the variable responses in bone and muscle loss observed in individuals, the precise relationship remains poorly understood.

The catabolic processes resulting from the reduced stress on musculoskeletal tissues in spaceflight can occur with rapidity. However, as is the case in recovery from tissue damage caused by repeated stress, the road to recovery from this "reduced stress" catabolic event is considerably longer than the time required to produce the bone loss. In fact, complete recovery of bone loss accrued from an extended duration space flight can take 1–3 years (LeBlanc et al., 2007). Bone resorption in astronauts appears to return to normal levels a couple of days after return to Earth (and the resultant increase in stress), while the bone formation rate is like that observed pre-flight upon landing. However, bone formation increases significantly after a couple of weeks of walking (LeBlanc et al., 2007).

It is quite clear that with the reduced stress experienced by musculoskeletal tissues in microgravity a threshold is crossed that invokes a change in the normal metabolism of the affected tissues. At some point, the body seems to make the decision that the decreased level of imposed stress no longer warrants the maintenance of tissue that now appears superfluous. Exactly what this threshold is, and how and why it is crossed remains unclear. However, what this finding clearly demonstrates is that musculoskeletal tissues *need* a certain amount of stress to maintain structural integrity and proper function.

The beneficial effects of stress include situations in which high stress is experienced for a limited number of loading cycles (Sun et al., 2010). This type of activity is, of course, the type that weightlifters perform in which they lift weights close to their maximum capacity with limited repetitions (three sets of 10 repetitions, for example). Such strength training activities have been demonstrated to provide substantial physiologic benefits such as increased metabolism and improved cardiac function and can provide substantial benefits to musculoskeletal tissues as well. These benefits include increased bone mass and strength, improved muscle strength and function, increased toughness of tendons and ligaments, and better joint function. Muscles may exhibit an increase in their physiological-cross sectional area, largely the result of hypertrophy of muscle fibers (Ahtiainen, Pakarinen, Alen, Kraemer, & Häkkinen, 2003). Tendons have been shown to demonstrate an increase in stiffness with exercise in both animal and human studies (Kubo, Kaneshia, & Fukunaga, 2001; Woo, Gomez, Amiel, Ritter, Gelberman, & Akeson, 1981). This increased stiffness may be due in part to the increased number and diameter of collagen fibrils observed in tendons after resistance training (Kongsgaard, Aagaard, Kjaer, & Magnusson, 2005; Michna & Hartmann, 1989).

However, while it is apparent that a limited number of high-stress exertions can have beneficial effects, it is just as clear that excessive exposure to high-stress results in the development of damage (Sun et al., 2010; Wu et al., 2013), which can occur in multiple musculoskeletal tissues. Thus, the response of the organism to the imposition of high stress appears highly dependent on the cycles experienced. A compelling example of this relationship can be found in a study of the application of high stress (with two different levels of repetition) to patellar tendons in an *in vivo* rat model (Sun et al., 2010). These authors demonstrated that when 100 cycles of loading were imposed (at about 50% of the tendon strength), a repair/remodeling process was observed consistent with tendon hypertrophy (an anabolic or "tissue building" response). However, when 7,200 cycles were applied at the same loading magnitude, a catabolic (tissue breakdown) response was observed. In the high cycle condition, microstructural fatigue damage accumulation of the tendon was observed, reminiscent of that observed in tendinopathy (Andarawis-Puri & Flatow, 2011). This indicates the presence of another stress-related threshold in musculoskeletal tissues that demonstrates a cycle-dependent differential response to stress. It would appear that with a low number of high-stress cycles (and presumably limited amounts of damage), the organism can muster processes designed to preserve and even improve tissue loading characteristics. However, after a certain number of high-stress cycles, the response transitions to one in which cumulative damage accumulation takes place. The cycle threshold of the transition between anabolic and catabolic responses is undoubtedly influenced by the level of stress applied, with fewer cycles to the transition in higher stress exertions and an increasingly greater number of cycles as applied stress decreases.

Healing of Damaged Tissues

Of all the differences between inert and biological materials, probably the most significant difference is the ability of biological tissues to self-heal. When an inert (non-self-healing) material experiences fatigue damage, the lack of a healing process means that the damage that has propagated will not be repaired (if left on its own) and continued exposure to repeated stress can only lead in one direction: further damage accumulation and ultimately failure. Biological organisms, on the other hand, have the valuable (or one might say essential) ability to repair damaged tissue, as discussed in more detail in Chapter 11.

Musculoskeletal tissues typically enjoy a baseline rate of turnover (or replacement) of materials. For example, the turnover rate in bone results in the replacement of about 10% of the skeleton every year (Wikipedia Contributors, 2021). The turnover of collagen in tendons has variously been estimated at ~1–2% per day (Miller et al., 2005; Schechtman & Bader, 1997), with higher values observed post-exercise. In addition to baseline material replacement rates, when an injury occurs to a tissue, a healing process is invoked. Such a healing process occurs in both plants and animals and both exhibit similar characteristics (Cremaldi & Bhushan, 2018).

Healing is a complex process, which occurs in several overlapping phases (Gouin & Kiecolt-Glaser, 2011) as shown in Chapter 11 for individual tissues. After an acute trauma, the process starts with an inflammatory response, involving vasoconstriction in the damaged region and the development of a fibrin clot to reduce blood loss in the area. The damaged area is subsequently infiltrated by inflammatory cells, fibroblasts, and granulation tissues. Some of these cells attract phagocytes and other specialized cells to the site. Others will become involved with the proliferation of repair materials that will be used in the process of tissue regeneration and capillary regrowth. The final phases, tissue remodeling and maturation, then occur taking a significant period of time, perhaps weeks, months, or years (dependent on numerous factors, such as the tissue type and size of the insult). As a cascading and integrated process, the ultimate quality of the repair is dependent on many factors, including the success of the initial stages (Gouin & Kiecolt-Glaser, 2011).

It seems there must be a fundamental relationship between the rate of damage development in a material and the rate at which the body can heal that damage. A study on fatigue damage and healing of rat cortical bones provides some insight into the development of fatigue damage and the healing response of the damage accrued (Wu et al., 2013). In this study, the right ulna and radius bones of 40 Sprague–Dawley rats were subjected to repeated stress using a four-point bending task, with 10,000 cycles being delivered once every alternate day for 2 weeks. The load had a magnitude of 0.058 N/g and the loading frequency was 4 Hz. The rats were randomly assigned to four groups and were sacrificed at 1, 2, 3, or 4 weeks into the microcrack repair process.

Fatigue microdamage was observed in all loaded ulnae in the region between force-bearing points 1–2 and points 3–4, primarily in the form of microcracks. The microcrack length and density were observed in each of the four groups. Microcracks were healed 2–3 weeks after application of the fatigue loading. Figure 10.1 provides data on the crack length resulting from fatigue damage, and the healing of microcracks from this study (Wu et al., 2013). Diffuse microcrack damage was repaired via damage-targeted remodeling that stimulated osteoclast resorptive activity, while linear microcracks were repaired by osteocyte-activated resorption. Diffuse damage may not provoke the latter healing method due to a lack of focal injury-induced apoptotic response (Herman, Cardoso, Majeska, Jepsen, & Schaffler, 2010).

Figure 10.2 provides a simple model of this relationship. In this model, we will talk in terms of the *kinetics* of damage development and healing. Kinetics in this sense refers to the rates at which these reactions in the material take place. If the damage kinetics are lower than the healing kinetics, we would expect a restorative repair in the musculoskeletal tissue. However, if damage kinetics exceed the healing kinetics, the damage accumulates in the tissue and this accumulation will continue as long as repeated stress is experienced. Damage kinetics are primarily the result of repeated stress experienced by the tissues and the resultant process of fatigue failure. The higher the rate of cumulative damage, the greater the risk that damage may exceed

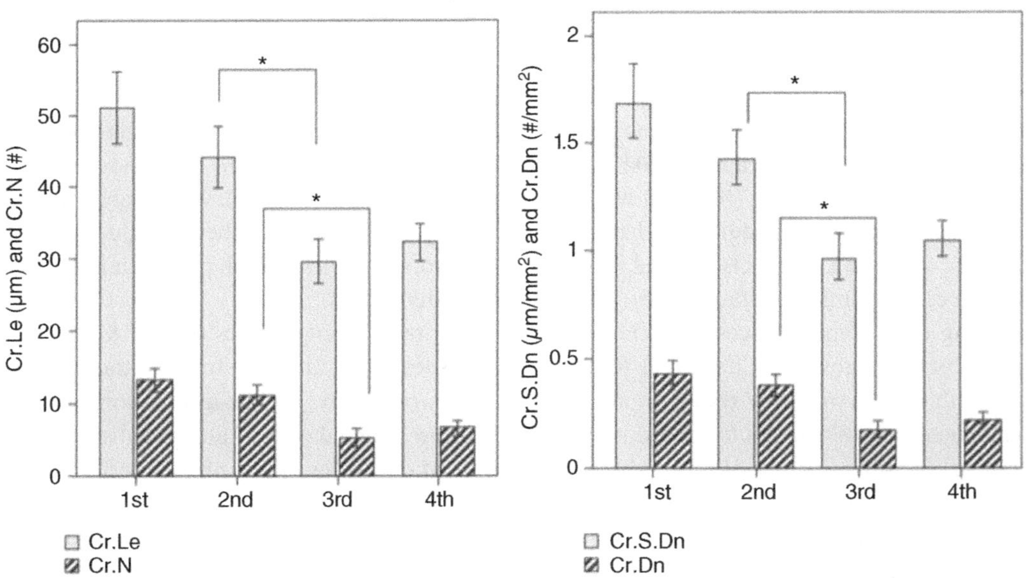

Figure 10.1 Data on fatigue microcrack damage to bone and subsequent healing of microcrack damage. Microcrack length (Cr. Le) and the average number of cracks (Cr. N) are shown on the left for rats euthanized 1, 2, 3, and 4 weeks post-fatigue damage. The crack surface density (Cr.S.Dn) and crack density (Cr.Dn) for groups euthanized after 1–4 weeks are shown on the right. Wu, B., Zhang, C., Chen, B., Zhang, L., Dai, R., Wu, X.,... Liao, E. (2013). Self-repair of rat corical bone microdamage after fatigue loading in vivo. *International Journal of Endocrinology*, 8, 321074, Open Access.

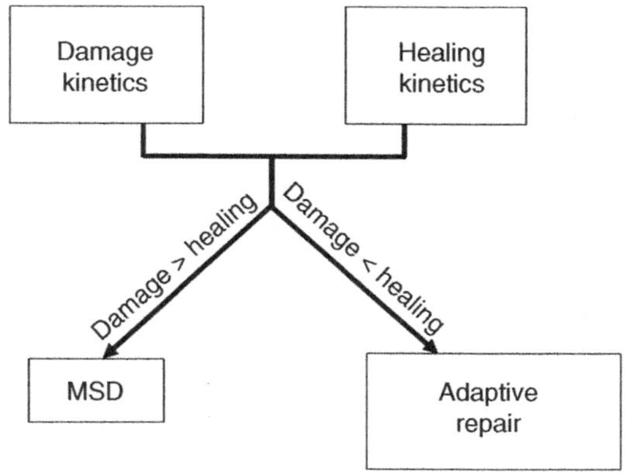

Figure 10.2 Simple model of the interplay between the kinetics of damage and healing.

the rate of healing. Healing kinetics can be influenced by several factors. For example, healing kinetics can be positively impacted by factors such as sleep quality, rest breaks, and exercise (Guo & DiPietro, 2010). On the other hand, factors such as aging, obesity, and certain disease states (such as diabetes) can negatively impact healing rates (Godbout & Glaser, 2006; Guo & DiPietro, 2010; Gouin & Kiecolt-Glaser, 2011). Obviously, lower rates of fatigue damage along with higher rates of healing kinetics are the most desirable condition and would more likely lead to adaptive repair of the damage incurred. However, all too often, the damage kinetics may exceed healing capacity, potentially leading to accumulating damage in the tissues and the development of MSDs.

Because the processes of damage development and healing are generally hidden from view (much occurs at the microscopic level), the damage/repair relationship in biological tissues is not easily measured. As a result, remains to be understood and many important questions need to be answered. For example, a common finding when performing fatigue failure tests of musculoskeletal tissues *ex vivo* is that the number of cycles to failure (even at lower levels of stress) is much lower than the materials have been shown to last during a lifetime (Brinckmann, 1988; Schechtman & Bader, 1997; Thornton & Bailey, 2013). Certainly, healing would be expected to confer some benefit in this regard, but how much? Another question is—to what degree is rest helpful to the healing process (rest being defined as the absence of loading)?

There would seem to be four main options as to how musculoskeletal tissues manage to last so much longer than demonstrated during *ex vivo* tests: (a) the loads experienced by tissues *in vivo* are in reality much lower than our models estimate, (b) tissue strength *in vivo* is much greater than *ex vivo*, (c) the body's healing process can greatly extend the fatigue life of musculoskeletal tissues, or (d) some combination of the previously mentioned factors. There is not much in the way of evidence that the first two options are in fact the case. On the other hand, the self-healing process would appear to be the major difference between *ex vivo* and *in vivo* states (Ker, 2002). While these questions cannot directly be answered with our current knowledge of these relationships in the biological setting, there is some indirect evidence that the presence of remodeling and healing processes in a material incurring damage from repeated stress can substantially increase the fatigue life of a material. This evidence comes, interestingly enough, from a field that has mimicked the biological self-healing process, but it applies such a process to standard (formerly inert) materials such as polymers and metals. As described in the following section, this research is being performed in the new and rapidly expanding field of self-healing materials (Aissa, Therriault, Haddad, & Jamroz, 2012; Wool, 2008).

Self-Healing in Engineered Materials

Self-healing materials have only recently become recognized as a defined field of study, with the first international conference on the topic held in 2007 (Wikipedia, 2020). Though the field as a discipline is nascent (developed primarily during the twenty-first century), a remarkable first known use of self-healing materials stems from ancient times (Wikipedia, 2020). Specifically, the Romans developed a type of lime mortar that possessed self-healing characteristics. They developed a specific composite material that, when mixed with the lime in the mortar, developed crystals that would grow in the mortar in areas where cracks would develop. The evolving crystal development during this process helped bind the mortar mixture and countered the development of fatigue crack development. Some of the structures in which this self-healing mortar was used include the Pantheon and the Colosseum, structures still standing after 1,900 years (Wikipedia, 2020). Remarkably, examination of non-biological self-healing materials and inhibition of fatigue damage provides some interesting insights that appear quite relevant to the process in biological tissues. A particular benefit of examining engineered self-healing materials is that careful control can be exercised in experiments studying the effects of healing kinetics versus damage kinetics, so that the roles of damage and healing can be better understood (Maiti, Shankar, Geubelle, & Kieffer, 2006).

An example of how modern materials achieve a self-healing capacity in a polymer material is as follows. A microencapsulated self-healing agent is embedded in the substance of the polymer, as is a catalyst of this agent. When the polymer is subjected to fatigue loading, a crack is nucleated and it starts to propagate through the material. The microcapsules containing the healing agent are ruptured as a result of the crack growth and enter the crack plane through capillary action. The healing agent makes contact with the embedded catalyst and begins the process of polymerization of the healing agent (see Figure 10.3). This polymer fills the crack resulting in a slowing or a complete arrest of the crack growth (Jones et al., 2007).

Several studies that have examined fatigue failure of biological tissues *ex vivo* have indicated that unlike materials such as steel (Stephens et al., 2001), a lack of an endurance limit is observed in these tissues (Huber et al., 2016; Schechtman & Bader, 1997; Thornton & Bailey, 2013). Typically, testing on tissues such as tendons and ligaments suggests that at low levels of loading, these tissues will last in the low millions of cycles. However, during life, the service history of these materials may be tens or hundreds of millions of cycles, well above the predicted life *by ex vivo* tests. For example, it has been estimated that an average American may walk approximately 5,000 steps/day (Bassett Jr., Wyatt, Thompson, Peters, & Hill, 2010). If one maintains that average daily and attains 80 years of age that would equate to approximately 146 million steps taken in a lifetime. However, *ex vivo* testing of tendons indicates that even at a fairly low loading level (say 20% UTS), this would be hundreds of times greater than the number of cycles required to develop macroscopic damage to the tendon. The prime candidate for potential fatigue life extension is the body's healing process (Ker, 2002; Nash, 1966; Schechtman & Bader, 1997).

The effectiveness of the healing response in these self-healing materials is dependent upon two primary factors: (a) the kinetics of the mechanical loading and (b) the kinetics of the healing response (Jones et al., 2007). The kinetics of fatigue crack growth is dependent on the stress ratio ($R = K_{min}/K_{max}$), the frequency of loading (f), and the maximum applied stress intensity factor. If R and F remain constant, $K_{max} - K_{min}$ (sometimes denoted as ΔK) will control the growth rate. Higher values of this variable will increase the rate of cumulative damage as defined by the Paris power law (Stephens et al., 2001):

$$\frac{da}{dN} = C\left(\Delta K\right)^{n} \tag{10.3}$$

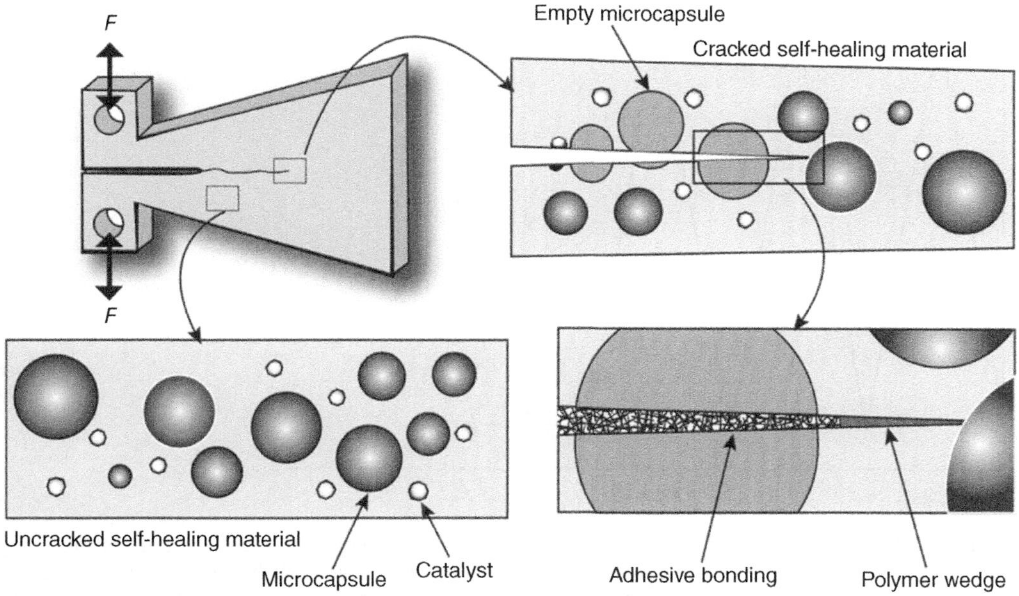

Figure 10.3 Material healing process in an engineered polymer. Adapted from Jones, A., Rule, J., Moore, J., Sottos, N., & White, S. (2007). Life extension of self-healing polymers with rapidly growing fatigue cracks. *Journal of the Royal Society, Interface*, 4, 395–403.

Where n denotes the slope of the line and a is the coefficient found by extending the straight line to $\Delta K = 1\,\mathrm{MPa\,m}^{1/2}$. Note that if $K_{min} = 0$, K_{max} alone can represent the stress intensity factor.

During fatigue loading of an engineered self-healing material, it is not unusual to have the mechanical damage accruing at the same time that a healing process is occurring (the same probably happens in our tissues as well). These studies demonstrate that a key to the effectiveness of the self-healing system is the rate at which the healing process occurs in relation to the mechanical kinetics of the loading. This becomes critical, particularly when the fatigue mechanics are high. Figure 10.4 provides an illustration of the stress intensity factor.

The fatigue life extension ratio is given by Eq. (10.4):

$$\lambda = \frac{N_{healed} - N_{control}}{N_{control}} \tag{10.4}$$

Where N_{healed} represents the number of cycles to failure of a self-healing specimen, and $N_{control}$ is the number of cycles of the control (i.e., non-healing) specimen. It should be recognized that repairs performed early in the damage process would help prevent long-term damage.

When K_{max} approaches the quasistatic fracture toughness (K_{Ic}) of the material, an unstable fracture of the material will occur. The ratio of K_{max}/K_{Ic} provides a value for stress intensity that is a good measure of the mechanical kinetics of crack growth. At lower values of stress intensity (say $K_{max}/K_{Ic} = 0.45$) having slower material crack growth, the healing kinetics may be effective at reducing or even arresting the rate of crack growth (and have a reasonable fatigue life extension ratio) even if the deployment of the healing agent is not excessively rapid. However, as the stress intensity increases (say to 0.68), a slowly deploying healing agent will be much less effective in

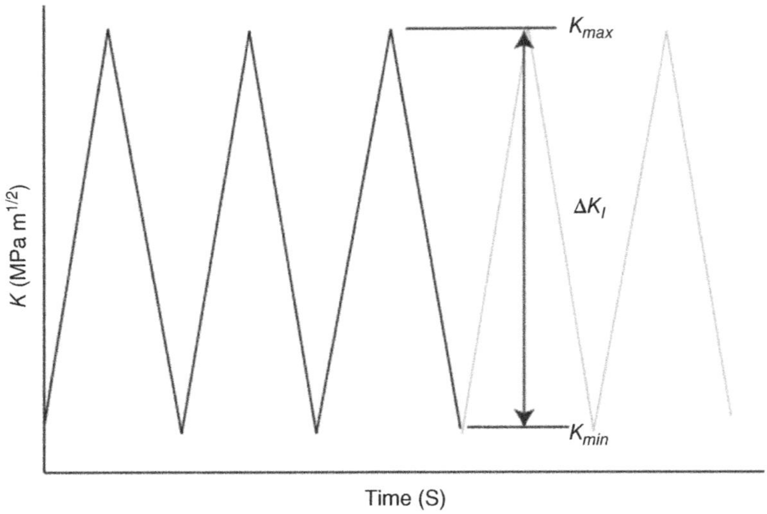

Figure 10.4 Stress Intensity Factor (K) associated with a loading regimen. K_{max} and K_{min} represent the maximum and minimum values of stress intensity in the loading history, and ΔK_I the stress intensity range. Jones, A., Rule, J., Moore, J., Sottos, N., & White, S. (2007). Life extension of self-healing polymers with rapidly growing fatigue cracks. *Journal of the Royal Society, Interface*, 4, 395–403.

extending fatigue life. However, a healing agent with faster healing kinetics may be able to significantly extend or arrest the crack growth development.

Figure 10.5 presents the results of a study conducted by Jones et al. (2007) involving three healing agents (C, D, and E) with C possessing the slowest healing kinetics and E having the fastest. Fatigue tests were all performed at $K_{max} = 0.676\,\text{MPa}\sqrt{m}$. When compared against the neat control condition (A), the life-extension ratio afforded by the healing agents C, D, and E were 16.8, 25.1, and 31.9, respectively. When comparing the number of cycles achieved, the control condition (A) exhibited a fatigue life of ~86,400 cycles, while healing agent E exhibited a fatigue life of approximately 2,815,000 cycles (32 times more cycles than the control condition having no healing agent). This finding indicates that the presence of a healing agent (particularly one with fast healing kinetics) has the potential to vastly increase the fatigue life of a material. Figure 10.6 demonstrates that a threshold exists regarding the level of damage kinetics and damage accumulation at a constant healing rate. In this example, a loading level K_{max} of $0.50\,\text{MPa}\,\text{m}^{1/2}$ in the presence of a high healing rate will lead to no damage accumulation. However, when the loading is increased to K_{max} of $0.676\,\text{MPa}\,\text{m}^{1/2}$ the healing rate is not sufficient to prevent damage accumulation.

When the mechanical kinetics of crack growth is high and poses a challenge to the speed with which the healing agent can deploy, it will decrease the ability of the healing agent to inhibit crack propagation. In such a case introduction of rest periods was shown to extend the fatigue life of the material (Jones et al., 2007). Figure 10.7 illustrates an example where a polymer is subjected to fast mechanical kinetics ($K_{max} = 0.801$). Without the introduction of rest periods, the healing agent cannot achieve significant life extension in the material. However, the introduction of rest periods can lead to significant life extension. In this case, the rest periods were 10–12 hr in length. This rest period allows time for the healing agent to both reduce the continued propagation of the crack and also allows time for the healing agent to continue to set up.

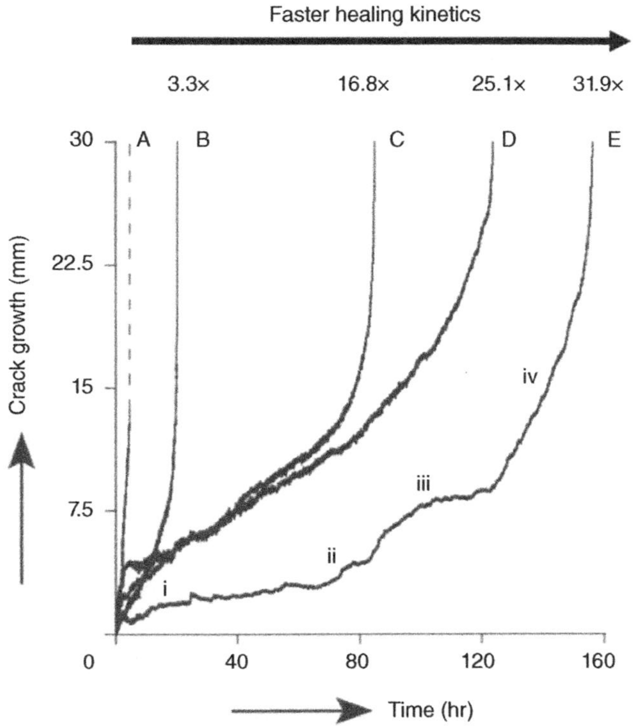

Figure 10.5 Fatigue life for healing agents with different healing kinetics (lines C, D, and E) vs. two controls (A, B). Jones, A., Rule, J., Moore, J., Sottos, N., & White, S. (2007). Life extension of self-healing polymers with rapidly growing fatigue cracks. *Journal of the Royal Society, Interface*, 4, 395–403.

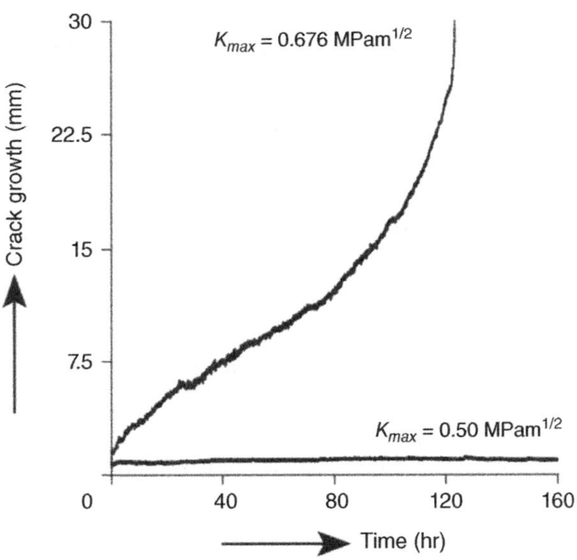

Figure 10.6 Fatigue crack growth at a high material healing rate for two different levels of loading. Fatigue cracks can be totally arrested at $K_{max} = 0.50\,\text{MPa}\,\text{m}^{1/2}$, but when exposed to a higher stress intensity ($K_{max} = 0.676\,\text{MPa}\,\text{m}^{1/2}$) fatigue crack growth will occur. Jones, A., Rule, J., Moore, J., Sottos, N., & White, S. (2007). Life extension of self-healing polymers with rapidly growing fatigue cracks. *Journal of the Royal Society, Interface*, 4, 395–403.

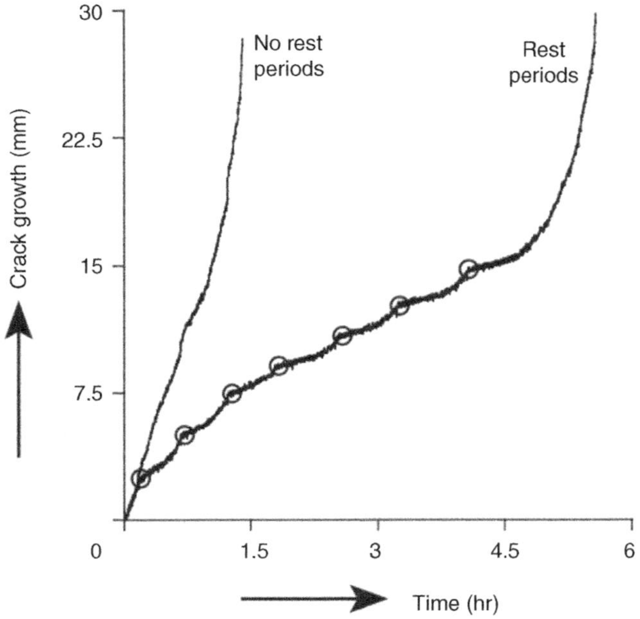

Figure 10.7 Introduction of rest periods can extend the fatigue life of a material subjected to high mechanical kinetics (K_{max} = 0.801 MPa m$^{1/2}$). In this case, rest periods of 10 hr increase fatigue life more than threefold. If an additional rest period was introduced, the fatigue life would increase proportionally. Jones, A., Rule, J., Moore, J., Sottos, N., & White, S. (2007). Life extension of self-healing polymers with rapidly growing fatigue cracks. *Journal of the Royal Society, Interface*, 4, 395–403.

The information given earlier regarding the ability of self-healing materials to repair or significantly increase fatigue life may provide some insights into certain aspects of the healing process of musculoskeletal tissues. While there are limitations regarding such a comparison, certain findings seem to comport with what is known about the healing process in the body. For example:

1) It appears that the presence of a self-healing process can significantly extend fatigue life in materials.
2) The self-healing capacity of musculoskeletal tissues may help to explain the higher fatigue life observed for musculoskeletal tissues during life than that observed during *ex vivo* material testing.
3) The extent to which the healing process can be successful in this endeavor is going to be a function of the interplay between mechanical damage kinetics and the healing kinetics of the tissues involved.
4) The introduction of rest periods may be beneficial to healing for two reasons. First, they provide a respite to the fatigue loading experienced by the material. Second, they permit time to let the healing process consolidate gains and to continue unimpeded.
5) The gain in fatigue life associated with the introduction of rest periods increases in proportion to the frequency of the rest periods provided.

Factors Influencing Healing Kinetics

As we have discussed already, to maintain musculoskeletal health a balance must be maintained between the damage kinetics imposed on a tissue and the healing kinetics. If the damage accrued exceeds the healing capacity, the tissue will enter a catabolic (tissue breakdown) state. There are several factors, including psychological stress and several personal characteristics (such as age, sex, and obesity) that are known to have detrimental effects on the healing process (Guo & DiPietro, 2010). The following subsections will discuss the potential influence of these factors on the healing process.

Psychological (Psychosocial) Stress

An association between psychosocial stress at the workplace and the incidence of MSDs has been reported in numerous studies over the past few decades (e.g., Bongers, De Winter, Kompier, & Hildebrandt, 1993; Bongers, Kremer, & ter Laak, 2002; Westman, Linton, Öhrvik, Wahlén, & Leppert, 2008). Several hypotheses have been put forth as to why the association between psychosocial stresses and MSDs is so prevalent (Deeney & O'Sullivan, 2009). These include the biopsychosocial model of job stress (Engel, 1977), the hyperventilation theory (Schleifer, Ley, & Spalding, 2002), the migraine theory (Knardahl, 2002), the muscle spindle theory (Johansson & Sojka, 1991), the nitric oxide/oxygen ratio hypothesis (Eriksen, 2004), and the Cinderella hypothesis (Hagg, 1991).

Commonly cited MSD risk factors associated with psychosocial stress include high work demands, job control, monotonous work, and the degree of social support a worker has in the workplace (Davis & Heaney, 2000; Deeney & O'Sullivan, 2009). Job demands include work that is performed under time pressure, work pressure and that has low workload variability (NIOSH, 1997). High job demands have been associated with increased risk of neck and shoulder complaints in several studies (Bernard, Sauter, Fine, Petersen, & Hales, 1994; Smith, Mihashi, Adachi, Koga, & IshitakeT., 2006; Van Den Heuvel, Van Der Beek, Blatter, Hoogendoorn, & Bongers, 2005). Job control is generally defined as the degree of influence a worker exercises over different aspects of his job such as scheduling and job performance. The lack of job control has been associated with increased MSD symptoms in the upper extremities in several studies (Bernard et al., 1994; Hales et al., 1994; Lagerström, Wenemark, Hagberg, & Hjelm, 1995). Jobs that are associated with tedium and which possess little variety are considered monotonous work. Several studies have demonstrated a relationship between monotonous work and MSDs, including those on the neck and shoulder (Harkness, Macfarlane, Nahit, Silman, & Mcbeth, 2003; Johansson et al., 1993; Ryan & Bampton, 1988). Finally, the lack of *social support* (generally defined as how an individual draws support from interpersonal interactions) has been shown to be associated with neck and shoulder MSDs (Aasa, Barnekow-Bergkvist, Angquist, & Brulin, 2005) and back pain (Skov, Borg, & Orhede, 1996). However, social support is not as consistently associated with MSD risk as some of the other psychosocial factors (Burdorf, Van Riel, & Brand, 1997; Engstrom, Johansson, Jonsson, & Medbo, 1995).

While associations between psychosocial factors and MSDs have been plentiful, specific mechanisms by which psychological stresses result in the development of MSDs are scant. However, the damage and healing model described earlier may provide a possible mechanism by which psychosocial stress may directly impact the development of MSDs. Specifically, psychological stress is known to negatively impact the healing of tissues via a well-established mechanism. This mechanism involves the secretion of glucocorticoids and catecholamines that inhibit the healing response and that reduce sleep time and quality (also known to negatively impact healing). Psychological stress is also associated with certain unhealthy behaviors (e.g., smoking and drinking) that can also reduce the effectiveness of healing.

Psychological stress has been shown in many studies to significantly inhibit the healing response of tissues (Godbout & Glaser, 2006). This has been reported in both animal and human studies. For example, one study demonstrated that students facing examination stress during the academic year demonstrated a 40% increase in the time it took to heal a 3.5 mm biopsy punch wound on the hard palate compared to an identical wound placed on the contralateral side during a period of

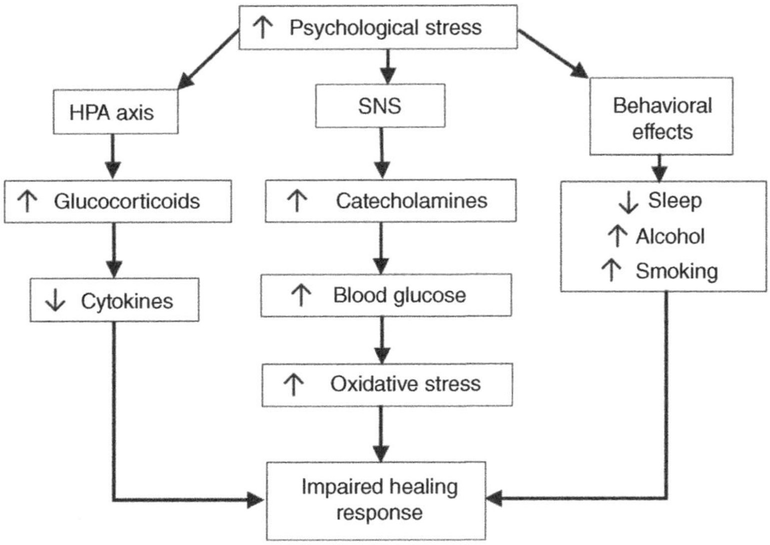

Figure 10.8 Mechanisms associated with the impaired healing response resulting from psychological stress (*Note.* SNS = sympathetic nervous system; HPA = hypothalamic–pituitary–adrenal). From Gallagher, S., & Barbe, M. (2021). The impaired healing hypothesis: A mechanism by which psychosocial stress and personal characteristics increase MSD risk? *Ergonomics*, 8, 1–14. https://doi.org/10.1080/00140139.2021.1974103.

vacation (Marucha, Kiecolt-Glaser, & Favagehi, 1998). All 11 subjects demonstrated a slowed healing response under stress and averaged a 3-day increase in the time to heal. A possible immunological mechanism was exhibited as the production of IL-1 (beta) mRNA was shown to decline by 68%. In another study, caregivers operating in stressful situations have demonstrated a similar reduced healing response (Kiecolt-Glaser, Marucha, Malarkey, Mercado, & Glaser, 1995). Compared with controls, stressed caregivers experienced wound healing averaging 9 days longer (48 vs. 39 days). Similarly, individuals living in hostile marital relationships showed a 60% decrease in the rate of wound healing, which was associated with a reduction in IL-1 (beta), IL-6, and TNF-alpha levels at the wound site (Kiecolt-Glaser et al., 2005).

The delay in healing resulting from stress is partly attributable to the hypothalamus–pituitary–adrenal (HPA) axis secretion of glucocorticoid (GC) hormones. A significant impact of GC compounds is the decreased proliferation and differentiation of immune cells, along with a decrease in gene transcription, and reduced cell adhesion activity vital in the immune healing response (Sternberg, 2006). One potent GC (cortisol) acts as a strong anti-inflammatory agent that counters the immune responses involved in the initial phase of healing (Guo & DiPietro, 2010). In this manner, psychological stress can impair the initiation of a normal healing response, resulting in a significant delay in the healing process. Figure 10.8 illustrates some of the pathways by which psychological stress can lead to impaired wound healing.

Effects of Personal Characteristics on Wound Healing

Age

Unsurprisingly, individuals of increased age may have a wound healing response that takes a significantly longer time than that of individuals of a younger age. However, while the wound healing process takes longer, in healthy aged individuals, the quality of healing is not necessarily impaired

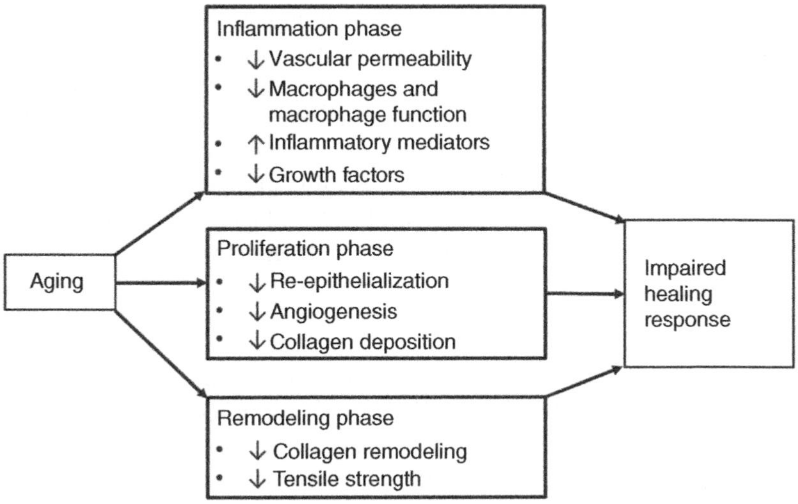

Figure 10.9 Effect of aging on the healing process. Gallagher, S., & Barbe, M. (2021). The impaired healing hypothesis: A mechanism by which psychosocial stress and personal characteristics increase MSD risk? *Ergonomics*, 8, 1–14. https://doi.org/10.1080/00140139.2021.1974103.

(Gosain & DiPietro, 2004). The extended wound healing time appears to be associated with a delayed inflammatory response. For example, some of the altered wound healing activity includes reduced macrophage activity, delayed T-cell infiltration, and changes in chemokine production (Swift, Burns, Gray, & DiPietro, 2001). In fact, each phase of the healing response appears to be affected by age-related changes (Guo & DiPietro, 2010). Some of these changes include delayed macrophage arrival and function, increased cytokine secretion, decreased presence of growth factors, slower collagen deposition, and remodeling. At the end of the process, decreased wound strength will often result (Gosain & DiPietro, 2004). Figure 10.9 illustrates factors associated with aging that can lead to decreased healing rates.

Obesity

Health issues associated with obesity are numerous and include increased risk of type II diabetes, heart disease, high blood pressure, stroke, sleep apnea, and significant respiratory problems. In addition to these health problems, obese individuals demonstrate an impaired wound healing capability, as well as an increased number of complications during the wound healing process (Guo & DiPietro, 2010). Complications may include skin wound infections (common in surgical incision sites in obese individuals), wounds that burst open due to increased tension at the wound site, pressure ulcers, and venous ulcers (Wilson & Clark, 2004). Many of these problems stem from a decrease in blood perfusion and ischemia present in adipose tissue. The same tension that causes a wound to experience *dehiscence* (bursting open) may also contribute to reduced perfusion at the wound site, leading to decreased delivery of oxygen and biochemical compounds necessary to heal the wound (Anaya & Dellinger, 2006; Wilson & Clark, 2004).

Type II Diabetes is strongly associated with obesity and can negatively impact both the development of musculoskeletal disorders as well as the healing kinetics to a greater degree (Brem & Tomic-Canic, 2007; Lin et al., 2017). Hypoxia is often observed in diabetic wounds and can prolong the injury healing time of wounds by increasing the levels of oxygen radicals in diabetics (Guo &

DiPietro, 2010). A decrease in the amount of angiogenesis is also commonly observed in diabetics (Brem & Tomic-Canic, 2007). The neuropathy attendant to diabetes may also increase wound healing times (Guo & DiPietro, 2010). Tendinopathy, tendon ruptures, and impaired tendon healing are all more prevalent among people with diabetes (Maffulli, Longo, Maffulli, Khanna, & Denaro, 2011). High blood glucose levels appear to inhibit the proliferation of tendon-derived stem cells and increase the rate of cell apoptosis (Lin et al., 2017). The healing of tendons appears to be significantly delayed in a hyperglycemic environment (Lin et al., 2017). Figure 10.10 shows some of the factors that lead to impaired wound healing in diabetics (Guo & DiPietro, 2010).

Sex

The rate of collagen synthesis is a critical factor in the healing of musculoskeletal tissues. Research over the past two decades has demonstrated that a sex difference exists with respect to the rate of collagen synthesis between males and females, with decreased collagen synthesis in the latter (Kjaer et al., 2009). Females have a lower rate of basal collagen synthesis compared to males, and also demonstrate a decreased collagen synthesis rate compared to males after exposure to exercise (Miller et al., 2006a, 2006b). This decreased collagen synthesis rate has been linked with estrogen levels, as varying levels of estradiol have been associated with a diminished rate of collagen synthesis in females (Hansen et al., 2008). These findings are supported by *ex vivo* studies in which it has been found that estradiol receptors are present in ligaments (Sciore, Frank, & Hart, 1998), and the finding that the very presence of estradiol itself can inhibit collagen synthesis in ligaments and tendons (Liu et al., 1996; Yu, Panossian, Hatch, Liu, & Finerman, 2001). The influence of estradiol levels on collagen synthesis may not be direct but may be the result of the effect that estradiol has on circulating insulin-like growth factor (IGF-I), a substance directly related to the rate of collagen synthesis (Kjaer et al., 2009)

Relationship of Damage Versus Healing Kinetics

Figure 10.11 shows the model of the relationship between damage development in musculoskeletal tissues and the healing response. This model is considered at the level of the individual rather than the population. To maintain homeostasis of the tissues, the damage

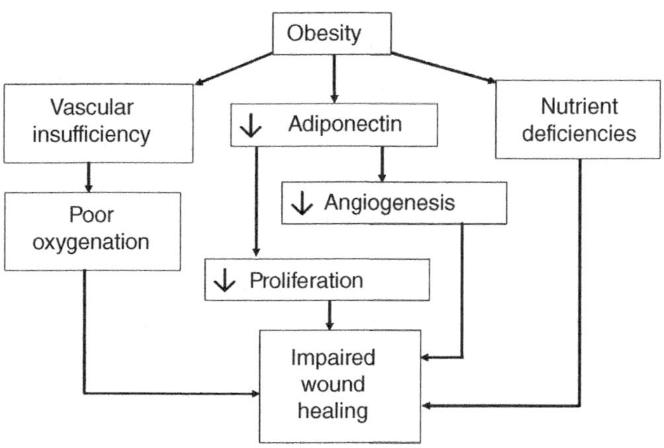

Figure 10.10 Effects of obesity on healing. Gallagher, S., & Barbe, M. (2021). The impaired healing hypothesis: A mechanism by which psychosocial stress and personal characteristics increase MSD risk? *Ergonomics*, 8, 1–14. https://doi.org/10.1080/00140139.2021.1974103.

accumulation must be less than or equal to the capacity of the system to heal. In such cases, the tissue can perform a restorative repair. However, if the rate of damage development exceeds the repair capacity, homeostasis cannot be sustained and the tissue can accrue cumulative damage. The latter imbalance can obviously happen in different ways. One way is that the damage accumulation is greater than the healing capacity as mentioned previously. Here repeated physical stress (in relation to the tissues' ultimate strength) will dominate the relationship. It may be noted that some studies have indicated that psychosocial stress may increase the magnitude of muscle contraction or stress experienced (Davis & Marras, 2003), and such additional stress may be a portion of the repeated stress variable in the upper left-hand corner of the figure.

The other way in which an unwanted imbalance between damage and healing kinetics can be experienced is that the healing kinetics is negatively impacted by certain variables. As illustrated in Figure 10.11, certain personal characteristics and/or the presence of psychological stress could have a negative impact on healing process. As discussed earlier, psychological (or psychosocial) stress has been shown to negatively impact the healing process through several pathways, including glucocorticoid and catecholamine release and disruption of sleep. Increasing age and obesity may also have a deleterious impact on healing capacity. Any factors that negatively impact healing capacity may lead to a situation where the fatigue life of the loaded tissue may be reduced, resulting in the development of damage and ultimately an MSD.

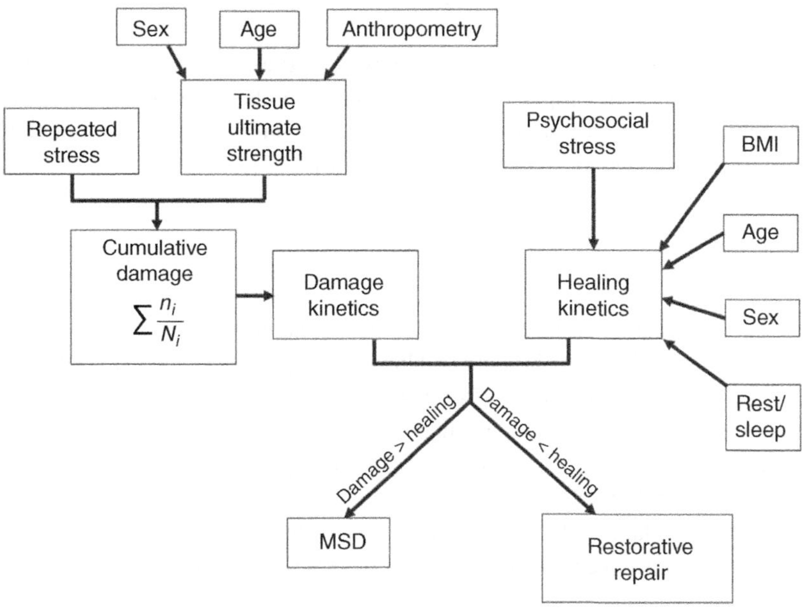

Figure 10.11 An individual-level model of the relationship of damage versus healing kinetics and selected MSD risk factors. Note: $\Sigma \frac{n_i}{N_i}$ represents cumulative damage as calculated via the Palmgren-Miner rule. Gallagher, S., & Barbe, M. (2021). The impaired healing hypothesis: A mechanism by which psychosocial stress and personal characteristics increase MSD risk? *Ergonomics*, 8, 1–14. https://doi.org/10.1080/00140139.2021.1974103, Miner, M. A. (1945). Cumulative damage in fatigue. *Journal of Applied Mechanics*, 16, A159–A164, and Palmgren, A. (1924). Die Lebebsdaue rvon Kugellagern. *Zeitschrift des Vereines deutscher Ingenieure*, 68, 339–341.

Summary

Musculoskeletal tissues are dynamic structures residing in a complex biological system. These tissues are highly responsive to stress and will react in accordance with changes in the stress environment. If the stress on the tissues undergoes a long decrease, musculoskeletal tissues will atrophy. On the other hand, a moderate number of high-stress exertions can lead to an anabolic response in the tissues, leading to stronger and more resilient tissues. However, when exposed to sufficient repeated stress, musculoskeletal tissues (like all materials) will experience fatigue failure. This has been demonstrated in both *ex vivo* and *in vivo* studies. Fortunately, the biological setting provides remodeling and healing processes that can replace old cells with new ones and can affect repairs when damage occurs, as discussed further in Chapter 11. These remodeling and repair capacities would be expected to provide a substantial extension of the fatigue life of tissues. Studies using engineered self-healing materials indicate that having a process to repair material damage can indeed increase fatigue life substantially compared to an inert material, up to 32 times greater fatigue life in one experiment. The fact that minor damage can be repaired at an early stage of the fatigue process is particularly helpful in reducing the development of more significant damage.

Being situated in a biological environment brings other influences into play that can impact musculoskeletal health. For example, the presence of psychological stress has been shown to impair the effectiveness of the body's healing process. Other factors that negatively impact healing include obesity, aging, and being female. All these factors have been associated with increased MSD prevalence and incidence. Their negative impact on the healing process may significantly reduce the fatigue life of tissues, a finding demonstrated in studies of engineered self-healing materials.

Clearly, the multiple systems that support musculoskeletal tissues in the biological environment add great complexity to understanding the fatigue life of these tissues. A clearer understanding of the interaction between damage accumulation and healing is needed and represents one of the most important research issues in the field of musculoskeletal health.

Bibliography

Aasa, U., Barnekow-Bergkvist, M., Angquist, K. A., & Brulin, C. (2005). Relationships between work-related factors and disorders in the neck-shoulder and low-back region among female and male ambulance personnel. *Journal of Occupational Health*, *47*, 481–489.

Ahtiainen, J., Pakarinen, A., Alen, M., Kraemer, W. J., & Häkkinen, K. (2003). Muscle hypertrophy, hormonal adaptations and strength development during strength training in strength-trained and untrained men. *European Journal of Applied Physiology*, *89*, 555–563.

Aissa, B., Therriault, D., Haddad, E., & Jamroz, W. (2012). Self-healing materials systems: Overview of major approaches and recent developed technologies. *Advances in Materials Science and Engineering*, *17*, 854203.

Amin, S. (2010). Mechanical factors and bone health: Effects of weightlessness and neurologic injury. *Current Rheumatology Reports*, *12*, 170–176.

Anaya, D., & Dellinger, E. (2006). The obese surgical patient: A susceptible host for infection. *Surgical Infections*, *7*, 473–480.

Andarawis-Puri, N., & Flatow, E. (2011). Tendon fatigue in response to mechanical loading. *Journal of Musculoskeletal and Neuronal Interactions*, *11*, 106–114.

Barbe, M., Gallagher, S., Massicotte, V., Tytell, M., Popoff, S., & Barr-Gillespie, A. (2013). The interaction of force and repetition on musculoskeletal and neural tissue responses and sensorimotor behavior in a rat model of work-related musculoskeletal disorders. *BMC Musculoskeletal Disorders, 14*, 303.

Bassett, D., Jr., Wyatt, H., Thompson, H., Peters, J., & Hill, J. (2010). Pedometer-measured physical activity and health Behaviors in U.S. adults. *Medicine & Science in Sports & Exercise, 42*, 1819–1811.

Bernard, B., Sauter, S., Fine, L., Petersen, M., & Hales, T. (1994). Job task and psychosocial risk factors for work-related muscu-loskeletal disorders among newspaper employees. *Scandinavian Journal of Work, Environment and Health, 20*, 417–426.

Bongers, P., De Winter, C., Kompier, M., & Hildebrandt, V. (1993). Psychosocial factor at work and musculoskeletal disease. *Scandinavian Journal of Work, Environment and Health, 19*, 297–312.

Bongers, P., Kremer, A., & ter Laak, J. (2002). Are psychosocial factors, risk factors for symptoms and signs of the shoulder, elbow, or hand/wrist? A review of the epidemiological literature. *American Journal of Industrial Medicine, 41*, 315–342.

Brem, H., & Tomic-Canic, M. (2007). Cellular and molecular basis of wound healing in diabetes. *The Journal of Clinical Investigation, 117*, 1219–1222.

Brinckmann, P. B. (1988). Fatigue fracture of human lumbar vertebrae. *Clinical Biomechanics, 3*(Suppl. 1), S1–S23.

Britannica, T. E. (2020). *Homeostasis*. Retrieved from Encyclopedia Britannica: https://www.britannica.com/science/homeostasis

Burdorf, A., Van Riel, M., & Brand, T. (1997). Physical load as a risk factor for musculoskeletal complaints among tank terminal workers. *American Industrial Hygiene Association Journal, 58*, 489–497.

Carp, S., Barbe, M., Winter, K., Amin, M., & Barr, A. (2007). Inflammatory biomarkers increase with severity of upper-extremity overuse disorders. *Clinical Science (London, England), 112*, 305–314.

Cremaldi, J., & Bhushan, B. (2018). Bioinspired self-healing materials: Lessons from nature. *Beilstein Journal of Nanotechnology, 9*, 907–935.

Davis, K., & Heaney, C. (2000). The relationship between psychosocial work characteristics and low back pain: Underlying methodological issues. *Clinical Biomechanics, 15*, 389–406.

Davis, K., & Marras, W. (2003). Partitioning the contributing role of biomechanical, psychosocial, and individual risk factors in the development of spine loads. *The Spine Journal, 3*, 331–338.

Deeney, C., & O'Sullivan, L. (2009). Work related psychosocial risks and musculoskeletal disorders: Potential risk factors, causation and evaluation methods. *Work, 34*, 239–248.

Dictionary.com (2021). *Homeostasis*. Retrieved from http://Dictionary.com: https://www.dictionary.com/browse/homeostasis?s=t

Ekstrand, J., Askling, C., Magnusson, H., & Mithoefer, K. (2013). Return to play after thigh muscle injury in elite football players: Implementation and validation of the Munich muscle injury classification. *British Journal of Sports Medicine, 47*, 769–774.

Engel, G. (1977). The need for a new medical model: A challenge for biomedicine. *Science, 196*, 129–136.

Engstrom, T., Johansson, J., Jonsson, D., & Medbo, L. (1995). Empirical evaluation of the reformed assembly work at the Volvo Uddevalla plant: Psychosocial effects and performance. *International Journal of Industrial Ergonomics, 16*, 293–308.

Eriksen, W. (2004). Linking work factors to neck myalgia: The nitric oxide/oxygen ratio hypothesis. *Medical Hypotheses, 62*, 721–726.

Gallagher, S., & Barbe, M. (2021). The impaired healing hypothesis: A mechanism by which psychosocial stress and personal characteristics increase MSD risk? *Ergonomics, 8*, 1–14. https://doi.org/10.1080/00140139.2021.1974103

Godbout, J., & Glaser, R. (2006). Stress-induced immune dysregulation: Implications for wound healing, infectious disease and cancer. *Journal of Neuroimmune Pharmacology, 1*, 421–427.

Gosain, A., & DiPietro, L. (2004). Aging and wound healing. *World Journal of Surgery, 28*, 321–326.

Gouin, J.-P., & Kiecolt-Glaser, J. (2011). The impact of psychological stress on wound healing: Methods and mechanisms. *Immunology and Allergy Clinics of North America, 31*, 81–93.

Guo, S., & DiPietro, L. (2010). Factors affecting wound healing. *Journal of Dental Research, 89*, 219–229.

Hagg, G. (1991). Static work loads and occupational myalgia – A new explanation model. *Electromyographical Kinesiology*, 141–144.

Hales, T., Sauter, S., Peterson, M., Fine, L., Putz-Anderson, V., Schleifer, L., . . . Bernard, B. (1994). Musculoskeletal disorders among visual display terminal users in a telecommunications company. *Ergonomics, 37*, 1603–1621.

Hansen, M., Miller, B., Holm, L. D., Petersen, S., Skovgaard, D., Frystyk, J., . . . Langberg, H. (2008). Effect of administration of oral contraceptives in vivo on collagen synthesis in tendon and muscle connective tissue in young women. *Journal of Applied Physiology, 586*, 3005–3016.

Harkness, E., Macfarlane, G., Nahit, E., Silman, A., & Mcbeth, J. (2003). Mechanical and psychosocial factors predict new onset shoulder pain: A prospective cohort study of newly employed workers. *Journal of Occupational and Environmental Medicine, 60*, 1603–1621.

Herman, B., Cardoso, L., Majeska, R., Jepsen, K., & Schaffler, M. (2010). Activation of bone remodeling after fatigue: Differential response to linear microcracks and diffuse damage. *Bone, 47*, 766–772.

Huber, G., Nagel, K., Skrzypiec, D., Klein, A., Püschel, K., & Morlock, M. (2016). A description of spinal fatigue strength. *Journal of Biomechanics, 49*, 875–880.

Johansson, H., & Sojka, P. (1991). Pathophysiological mechanisms involved in genesis and spread of muscular tension in occupational muscle pain and in chronic musculoskeletal pain syndromes: A hypothesis. *Medical Hypotheses, 35*, 196–203.

Johansson, J., Kadefors, R., Rubenowitz, S., Klingenstierna, U., Lindstrom, I., Engstrom, T., & Johansson, M. (1993). Musculoskeletal symptoms, ergonomic aspects and psychosocial factors in two different truck assembly concepts. *International Journal of Industrial Ergonomics, 12*, 35–48.

Jones, A., Rule, J., Moore, J., Sottos, N., & White, S. (2007). Life extension of self-healing polymers with rapidly growing fatigue cracks. *Journal of the Royal Society, Interface, 4*, 395–403.

Kaji, H. (2014). Interaction between muscle and bone. *Journal of Bone Metabolism, 21*, 29.

Ker, R. (2002). The implications of the adaptable fatigure quality of tendons for their construction, repair, and function. *Comparative Biochemistry and Physiology (part A), 133*, 987–1000.

Kiecolt-Glaser, J., Loving, T., Stowell, J., Malarkey, W., Lemeshow, S., Dickinson, S., & Glaser, R. (2005). Hostile marital interactions, proinflammatory cytokine production, and wound healing. *Archives of General Psychiatry, 62*, 1377–1384.

Kiecolt-Glaser, J., Marucha, P., Malarkey, W., Mercado, A., & Glaser, R. (1995). Slowing of wound healing by psychological stress. *Lancet, 346*, 1194–1196.

Kjaer, M., Langberg, K., Heinemeier, M., Bayer, M., Hansen, M., . . . Magnusson, S. (2009). From mechanical loading to collagen synthesis, strucural changes and function in human tendon. *Scandinavian Journal of Medicine and Science in Sport, 19*, 500–510.

Knardahl, S. (2002). Psychophysiological mechanisms of pain in computer work: The blood vessel-nociceptor interaction hypothesis. *Work and Stress, 16*, 179–189.

Kongsgaard, M., Aagaard, P., Kjaer, M., & Magnusson, S. P. (2005). Structural Achilles tendon properties in athletes subjected to different exercise modes and in Achilles tendon rupture patients. *Journal of Applied Physiology, 99*, 1965–1971.

Kubo, K., Kaneshia, H., & Fukunaga, T. (2001). Effects of different duration isometric contractions on tendon elasticity in human quadriceps muscles. *The Journal of Physiology, 536*, 649–655.

Lagerström, M., Wenemark, M., Hagberg, M., & Hjelm, E. (1995). Occupational and individual factors related to musculoskeletal symptoms in five body regions among Swedish nursing personnel. *International Archives of Occupational and Environmental Health*, *68*, 27–35.

Lang, T., LeBlanc, A., Evans, H., Lu, Y., Genant, H., & Yu, A. (2004). Cortical and trabecular bone mineral loss from the spine and hip in long-duration spaceflight. *Journal of Bone and Mineral Research*, *19*, 1006–1012.

LeBlanc, A., Lin, C., Shackelford, L., Sinitsyn, V., Evans, H., Belichenko, O., . . . Feeback, D. (2000). Muscle volume, MRI relaxation times (T2), and body composition after spaceflight. *Journal of Applied Physiology*, *89*, 2158–2164.

LeBlanc, A., Spector, E., Evans, H., & Sibonga, J. (2007). Skeletal responses to space flight and the bed rest analog: A review. *Journal of Musculoskeletal and Neuronal Interaction*, *7*, 33–47.

Lin, Y., Li, Y., Rui, Y., Dai, G., Shi, L., Xu, H., . . . Teng, G. (2017). The effects of high glucose on tendon-derived stem cells: Implications of the pathogenesis of diabetic tendon disorders. *Oncotarget*, *8*, 17518–17528.

Liu, S., Shaikh, R., Panossian, V., Yang, R., Nelson, S., Soleiman, N., . . . Lane, J. (1996). Primary immunolocalization of estrogen and progesterone target cells in the human anterior cruciate ligament. *Journal of Orthopaedic Research*, *14*, 526–533.

Maffulli, N., Longo, U., Maffulli, G., Khanna, A., & Denaro, V. (2011). Achilles tendon ruptures in diabetic patients. *Archives of Orthopaedic and Trauma Surgery*, *131*, 33–38.

Maiti, S., Shankar, C., Geubelle, P., & Kieffer, J. (2006). Continuum and molecular-level Modeling of fatigue crack retardation in self-healing polymers. *ASME Journal of Engineering and Materials Technology*, *128*, 595–602.

Mangine, G., Hoffman, J., Gonzalez, A., Townsend, J., Wells, A., Jajtner, A., . . . Stout, J. (2015). The effect of training volume and intensity on improvements in muscular strength and size in resistance-trained men. *Physiological Reports*, *3*, e12472.

Marucha, P., Kiecolt-Glaser, J., & Favagehi, M. (1998). Mucosal wound healing is impaired by examination stress. *Psychosomatic Medicine*, *60*, 362–365.

Michna, H., & Hartmann, G. (1989). Adaptation of tendon collagen to exercise. *International Orthopaedics*, *13*, 161–165.

Miller, B., Hansen, M., Olesen, J., Flyvbjerg, A., Schwarz, P., Babraj, J., . . . Kjær, M. (2006a). No effect of menstrual cycle on myofibrillar and connective tissue synthesis in contracting skeletal muscle. *The American Journal of Physiology*, *290*, E163–E168.

Miller, B., Hansen, M., Olesen, J., Schwarz, P., Babraj, J., Smith, K., . . . Kjær, M. (2006b). Tendon collagensynthesis at rest and after exercise in women. *Journal of Applied Physiology*, *102*, 542–547.

Miller, B., Olesen, J., Hansen, M., Døssing, S., Crameri, R., Welling, R., . . . Rennie, M. (2005). Coordinated collagen and muscle protein synthesis in human patella tendon and quadriceps muscle after exercise. *The Journal of Physiology*, *567*(Pt 3), 1021–1033.

Miner, M. A. (1945). Cumulative damage in fatigue. *Journal of Applied Mechanics*, *16*, A159–A164.

NASA. (2021). Muscle atrophy. Retrieved from NASA Information: https://www.nasa.gov/pdf/64249main_ffs_factsheets_hbp_atrophy.pdf

Nash, J. C. (1966). *Fatigue of self-healing structure: A generalized theory of fatigue failure*. New York, NY: American Society of Mechanical Engineers.

NIOSH (1997). *Musculoskeletal disorders and workplace factors*. Cincinnati, OH: National Institute for Occupational Safety and Health.

Palmgren, A. (1924). Die Lebebsdaue rvon Kugellagern. *Zeitschrift des Vereines deutscher Ingenieure*, *68*, 339–341.

Paris, P., Gomez, M., & Anderson, W. (1961). A rational analytic theory of fatigue. *Trends in Engineering*, *13*, 9.

Punnett, L., Pruss-Ustun, A., Nelson, D., Fingerhut, M., Leigh, J., Tak, S., & Phillips, S. (2005). Estimating the global burden of low back pain attributable to combined occupational exposures. *American Journal of Industrial Medicine, 48*, 459–469.

Ryan, G., & Bampton, M. (1988). Comparison of data process operators with and without upper limb symptoms. *Community Health Studies, 12*, 63–68.

Schechtman, H., & Bader, D. (1997). In vitro fatigue of human tendons. *Journal of Biomechanics*, 829–835.

Schleifer, L., Ley, R., & Spalding, T. (2002). A hyperventilation theory of job stress and musculoskeletal disorders. *American Journal of Industrial Medicine, 41*, 420–432.

Sciore, P., Frank, C., & Hart, D. (1998). Identification of sex hormone receptors in human and rabbit ligaments of the knee by reverse transcription-polymerase chain reaction: Evidence that receptors are present in tissue from both male and female subjects. *Journal of Orthopaedic Research, 16*, 604–610.

Sharma, P., & Maffulli, N. (2005). Tendon injury and tendinopathy: Healing and repair. *Journal of Bone and Joint Surgery (American), 87*, 187–202.

Singh, S., Young, A., & McNaught, C. (2017). The physiology of wound healing. *Surgery (Oxford), 35*, 473–477.

Skov, T., Borg, V., & Orhede, E. (1996). Psychosocial and physical risk factors for musculoskeletal disorders of the neck, shoulders, and lower back in sales people. *Occupational and Environmental Medicine, 53*, 351–356.

Smith, D., Mihashi, M., Adachi, Y., Koga, H., & IshitakeT. (2006). A detailed analysis of musculoskeletal disorder risk factors among Japanese nurses. *Journal of Safety Research, 37*, 195–200.

Smith, S., Nillen, J., LeBlanc, A., Lipton, A., Demers, L., Lane, H., & Leach, C. (1998). Collagen cross-link excretion during space flight and bed rest. *Journal of Clinical Endocrinology and Metabolism, 83*, 3584–3591.

Smith, S., Wastney, M., Morukov, B., Larina, I., Nyquist, L., Abrams, S., . . . Lane, H. (1999). Calcium metabolism before, during, and after a 3-mo space-flight: Kinetic and biochemical changes. *American Journal of Physiology, 277*, R1–R10.

Stephens, R., Fatemi, A., Stephens, R., & Fuchs, H. (2001). *Metal fatigue in engineering* (2nd ed.). New York, NY: Wiley.

Sternberg, E. (2006). Neural regulation of innate immunity: A coordinated nonspecific host response to pathogens. *Nature Reviews Immunology, 6*, 318–328.

Sun, H., Andarawis-Puri, N., Li, Y., Fung, D., Lee, J., Wang, V., . . . Flatow, E. L. (2010). Cycle-dependent matric remodeling gene expression response in fatigue-loaded rat patellar tendons. *Journal of Orthopaedic Research, 28*, 1380–1386.

Swift, M., Burns, A., Gray, K., & DiPietro, L. (2001). Age-related alterations in the inflammatory response to dermal injury. *The Journal of Investigative Dermatology, 117*, 1027–1035.

Thornton, G., & Bailey, S. (2013). Healing ligaments have shorter lifetime and greater strain rate during fatigue than creep at functional stresses. *Journal of Biomechanical Engineering, 135*, 1713–1721.

Toy, L. (2005). How much do we understand about the effects of ageing on healing? *Journal of Wound Care, 14*, 472.

Van Den Heuvel, S., Van Der Beek, A., Blatter, B., Hoogendoorn, W., & Bongers, P. (2005). Psychosocial work characteristics in relation to neck and upper limb symptoms. *Pain, 114*, 47–53.

Westman, A., Linton, A., Öhrvik, J., Wahlén, P., & Leppert, J. (2008). Do psychosocial factors predict disability and health at a 3-year follow-up for patients with non-acute musculoskeletal pain? A validation of the Örebro musculoskeletal pain screening questionnaire. *European Journal of Pain, 12*, 641–649.

Wikipedia (2020). *Self-healing materials*. Retrieved from https://en.wikipedia.org/wiki/Self-healing_material

Wikipedia Contributors (2021. *Wikipedia, the free encyclopedia*. Retrieved from Bone remodeling: https://en.wikipedia.org/w/index.php?title=Bone_remodeling&oldid=1021128734

Wilson, J., & Clark, J. (2004). Obesity: Impediment to postsurgical wound healing. *Advances in Skin & Wound Care*, *17*, 426–435.

Woo, S., Gomez, M., Amiel, D., Ritter, M. A., Gelberman, R. H., & Akeson, W. H. (1981). The effects of exercise on the biomechanical and biochemical properties of swine digital flexor tendons. *Biomechanical Engineering*, *103*, 51–56.

Wool, R. (2008). Self-healing material: A review. *Soft Matter*, *4*, 400–418.

Wu, B., Zhang, C., Chen, B., Zhang, L., Dai, R., Wu, X., . . . Liao, E. (2013). Self-repair of rat corical bone microdamage after fatigue loading in vivo. *International Journal of Endocrinology*, *8*, 321074.

Yu, W., Panossian, V., Hatch, J., Liu, S., & Finerman, G. (2001). Combined effects of estrogen and progesterone on the anterior cruciate ligament. *Clinical Orthopaedics*, *21*, 268–281.

11

Injury and Self-Repair of Musculoskeletal Tissues

Introduction

Injuries in musculoskeletal and neural tissues can occur via a variety of mechanisms ranging from direct lacerations or mechanical deformation (e.g., contusions, compressions, or strains) to indirect causes (e.g., ischemia and neurological damage), and/or the accumulation of degenerative changes and therefore fatigue damage, due to repeated overuse, aging, or repeated sports injuries. A complex series of molecular, vascular, and cellular responses are initiated the moment a tissue is injured. The first responses after injury are the establishment of hemostasis and then inflammation to clear the damaged cells. For example, injuries from mechanical deformations generate a sterile inflammatory response (lacking viral or bacterial exposure) that is essential for the clearance of damaged and necrotic cells and tissues (Barbe, Hilliard, Fisher, et al., 2020; Toumi, F'Guyer, & Best, 2006; Wang, 2018). If viruses or bacteria have entered the tissues, the purpose of the immune response is also to encapsulate and fight such infection also. Acute inflammatory responses can be amplified as needed by activating soluble mediators and immune cell infiltration. The wound healing phases of hemostasis and acute inflammation are followed by proliferation, remodeling, and maturation (which can overlap) in an attempt to restore normal tissue architecture and function after an injury (Figure 11.1).

Injury-Induced Inflammation

Acute Inflammation—Primary and Secondary Responses

Under normal conditions, an acute inflammatory response is initiated to clear damaged cells and tissues. This response is characterized by a quick accumulation of fluid and plasma components and an influx of neutrophils into the affected tissue. The cardinal

clinical signs of inflammation are heat (calor), redness (rubor), swelling (edema), and pain (dolor) (as shown in the upper zone of Figure 11.2). With very localized musculoskeletal and neural tissue injury, signs, such as redness, swelling, or heat are often difficult to detect. However, pain is a good indication of even discrete underlying injury, since pain occurs due to increased pressure on nerves caused by edema.

Factors released by the injured cells participate in their own clearance or repair. The first signals released from damaged and necrotic cells are damage-associated molecular pattern molecules (DAMPS; Table 11.1), such as IL-1α, a key inflammatory cytokine produced by the damaged cells.

Musculoskeletal Disorders: The Fatigue Failure Mechanism, First Edition. Sean Gallagher and Mary F. Barbe.

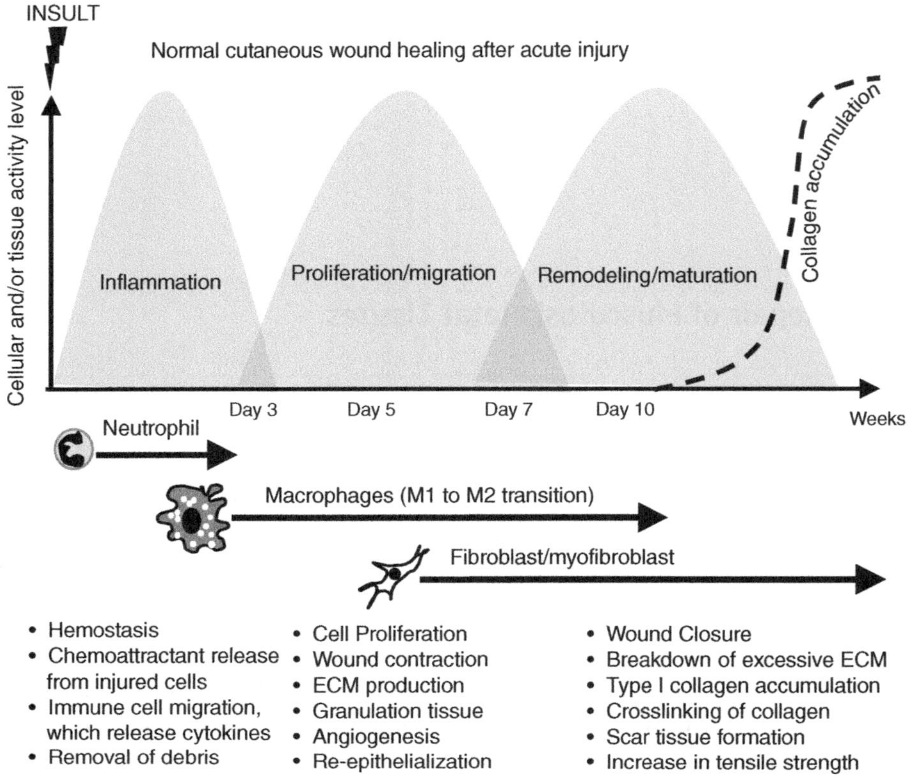

Figure 11.1 Relative time course of inflammatory cell, fibroblast recruitment, and healing of skin wounds. A typical skin wound heals by means of three overlapping phases of tissue repair (inflammation, proliferation/migration, and remodeling/maturation). In the inflammatory phase, injured cells release chemoattractant molecules that induce immune cells to migrate to the wound site (chemotaxis) to protect the injured cells against microbes, or in the case of a sterile injury to clear damaged cells and tissues. In the proliferation and migration phase, fibroblasts are transformed into myofibroblasts by bioactive substances derived from macrophages. These transformed cells contribute to the formation of granulation tissue and wound contraction. In the remodeling and maturation phase, new matrix components are deposited and crosslinked, and proteolytic enzymes break down excessive extracellular matrix, although scarring in the form of collagen accumulation can occur. Abbreviations: ECM = extracellular matrix; M1 = pro-inflammatory macrophages; M2 = anti-inflammatory/repair related macrophages. Modified from Mori, R., Tanaka, K., & Shimokawa, I. (2018). Identification and functional analysis of inflammation-related miRNAs in skin wound repair. *Development, Growth & Differentiation*, 60(6), 306–315. https://doi.org/10.1111/dgd.12542. http://Wiley.com.

Also, extracellular matrix (ECM) polysaccharide Hyaluronan (HA) is rapidly catabolized by hyaluronidases, resulting in fragmentary, low-molecular-weight HA that promotes inflammation. On the resolution of inflammation, both the amount and size of HA return to basal levels. Regarding their function, DAMPs are chemotactic for neutrophils, similar to several other chemokines (chemotactic cytokines) produced by neighboring cells after DAMP exposure (Wang, 2018). Chemotaxis refers to the migration of cells into the interstitial space. In this case, the infiltrating cells are immune cells.

Interestingly, the early infiltrating platelets, neutrophils, and mast cells play crucial roles in the process of vasodilation (necessary to recruit additional immune cells) by their production and release of a variety of biochemical mediators involved in this process (Figure 11.2; Table 11.1). The

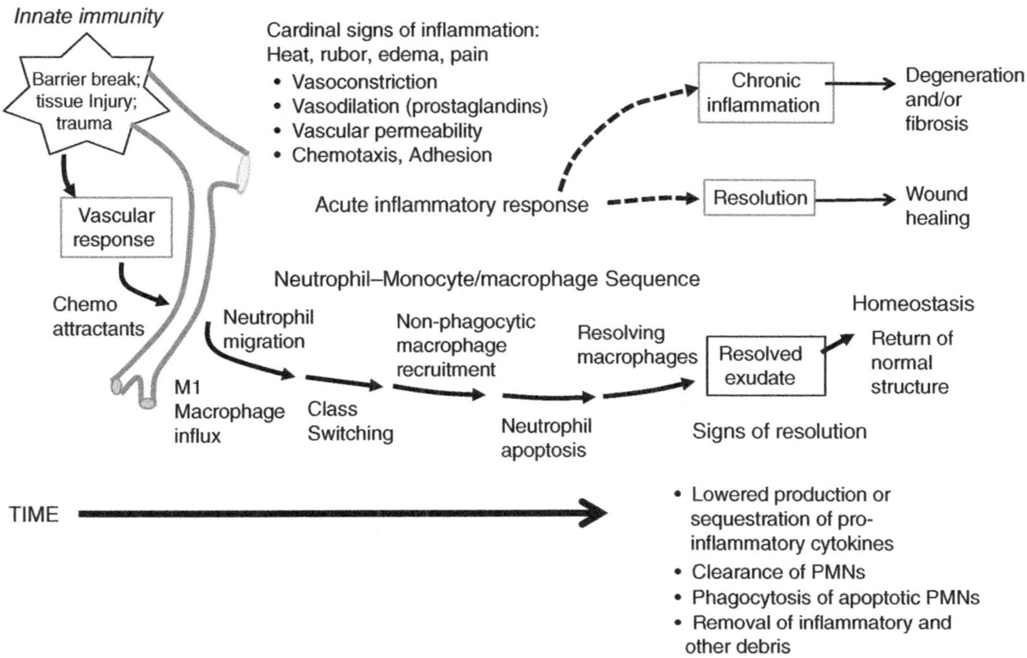

Figure 11.2 Time-course of the initiation and resolution of acute inflammation generated by an acute injury. Abbreviations: M1 macrophages = pro-inflammatory macrophages; PMNs = polymorphonuclear immune cells. Modified from Serhan, C. N. (2017). Treating inflammation and infection in the 21st century: New hints from decoding resolution mediators and mechanisms. *The FASEB Journal*, 31(4), 1273–1288. https://doi.org/10.1096/fj.201601222R.

mediators include histamine, prostaglandins, bradykinin, serotonin, and cytokines (including TNFα and IL-1). Note, the type of infiltrating immune cells depends on the type of stimulus (i.e., injury, infectious, or allergic) and the specific molecules and inflammatory mediators released by the injured cells and tissues.

Platelets are the first repair components to appear after an injury (Eisinger, Patzelt, & Langer, 2018). They are anuclear, cytoplasmic fragments derived from megakaryocytes. Their primary function is to initiate the coagulation cascade and form the fibrin plug that fills the tissue gap, a process called hemostasis. Platelets are activated within seconds of an endothelial lesion and they release a variety of growth factors and cytokines upon contact with collagen and other ECM components. For example, they release PDGF, which initiates the clearance and healing cascade by being chemotactic to neutrophils and monocytes/macrophages and inducing fibroblast proliferation needed for tissue repair, respectively. Platelets also release pro-inflammatory cytokines, including interleukin-1 (IL-1α and IL-1β), IL-6, TNFα, and transforming growth factor-beta (TGFβ). As shown in Tables 11.1 and 11.2, these cytokines are either key mediators of inflammation, tissue healing, or of both these processes; they mediate tissue healing if also involved in inducing collagen and fibronectin production by fibroblasts (Table 11.1).

After a sterile muscle injury, neutrophils (typically short-lived phagocytes) invade within 2 hr of injury (McCracken & Allen, 2014; Wang, 2018) (Figure 11.2). Functionally, neutrophils adopt three possible strategies: (a) removal of cellular debris by phagocytosis, an activity shared with macrophages that are also attracted by the chemotactic factors released by neutrophils and injured cells; (b) release of growth and pro-angiogenic factors; (c) resolution of inflammation (Wang, 2018).

Table 11.1 Examples of Mediators of Inflammation

DAMPS (damage-associated molecular pattern molecules)—endogenous danger molecules released from damaged cells (alarmins and pathogen-associated molecular patterns [PAMPs])

- HMGB1 (DNA binding high mobility group box 1)—chemoattractant and activator of granulocytes
- Hyaluronan (HA) fragments—Extracellular matrix HA rapidly catabolized by hyaluronidases, resulting in fragmentary, low-molecular-weight HA.
- Cytokines
    - Interleukin (IL-1) α—chemotactic for neutrophils and macrophages (i.e., inflammatory); fibrogenic
    - IL-33—immune system modulator; augments inflammatory "storm"

Pro-inflammatory cytokines

- IL-1α—see earlier
- IL-1β—produced and released primarily by macrophages and nonimmune cells (fibroblasts and endothelial cells) during cell injury and inflammation; chemotactic for immune cells. Can stimulate connective tissue growth factor (CCN2/CTGF) production.
- IFNγ (Interferon-gamma)—pleiotropic, can promote macrophage activation, though it is anti-proliferative and pro-apoptotic also.
- PDGF (platelet-derived growth factor)—chemotactic to neutrophils and macrophages; induces fibroblast proliferation for tissue repair.
- TNFα (Tumor necrosis factor-alpha)—produced by macrophages during acute inflammation; chemotactic for immune cells; responsible for several signaling events that lead to necrosis or apoptosis (i.e., cytotoxicity).

Other chemical mediators released during acute inflammation

- Bradykinin—activates signaling pathways resulting in increased vascular permeability, vasodilation, hypotension, pain, fever; produced by platelets, neutrophils, mast cells.
- CGRP (calcitonin gene-related peptide)—a neurotransmitter, a modulator of pain perception
- Histamine—involved in vasodilation, enhancement of vascular permeability, mediation of acute inflammation; produced by platelets, neutrophils, mast cells, and
- MMPs—matrix metalloproteinases, proteolytic enzymes that break down extracellular matrix (ECM) proteins
- Prostaglandins—lipid autacoids derived from arachidonic acid; involved in vasodilation; produced by platelets, neutrophils, mast cells, and other immune cells.
- RNS (Reactive Nitrogen Species)—perform a similar function as ROS do.
- ROS (Reactive Oxygen Species)—highly reactive free radicals that are cytotoxic effectors.
- Serotonin—increases vascular permeability; it is produced by platelets, neutrophils, mast cells.
- SP (Substance P)—a neurotransmitter; a modulator of pain perception; vasodilator; can increase collagen production
- VEGF (vascular endothelial growth factor)—stimulates angiogenesis

Table 11.2 Examples of Mediators of Tissue Repair (Including Fibrotic Repair)

Anti-inflammatory cytokines

- IL-10—potent anti-inflammatory cytokine that suppresses TNFα and IL-1 production.
- IL-13—suppresses the production of pro-inflammatory cytokines by macrophages; it is pro-fibrotic also.
- IL-4—IL-13 homolog; inhibits the production of pro-inflammatory cytokines and chemokines.

Growth factors and modulators

- CCN2/CTGF (cell communication network factor 2/connective tissue growth factor)—a matricellular protein that regulates cell adhesion, migration, and survival; a downstream mediator of TGFβ and induces collagen production by fibroblasts.
- EGF (epidermal growth factor)—stimulates the proliferation of different cell types, including fibroblasts and epithelial cells.
- IL-13—see earlier
- PDGF—induces fibroblast proliferation for tissue repair.
- TGFβ—a highly pleiotropic cytokine that plays an important role in wound healing, angiogenesis, immunoregulation; anti-inflammatory; induces collagen production by fibroblasts.
- VEGF—influences the rate of wound closure/re-epithelialization, angiogenesis, granulation tissue formation during the proliferative phase.

Glucocorticoids

- Any group of corticosteroids (e.g., hydrocortisone) involved in the metabolism of carbohydrates, proteins, and fats; anti-inflammatory.

The latter process occurs when neutrophils become apoptotic and are phagocytosed by macrophages (Figure 11.2); phagocytosis is a process that initiates a feed-forward pro-resolution program characterized by the release of tissue-repair related cytokines (e.g., TGFβ) and potent anti-inflammatory cytokines(e.g., IL-10). Thereafter, neutrophils undergo rapid decline and are replaced by macrophages (Tidball & Villalta, 2010; Tidball & Wehling-Henricks, 2015; Wang, Wehling-Henricks, Samengo, & Tidball, 2015; Welc et al., 2020).

Monocyte-derived macrophages are polarized into M1 (pro-inflammatory) and M2 (anti-inflammatory and repair) phenotypes (Hu et al., 2012; Tidball & Wehling-Henricks, 2015) (Figure 11.3). Many M1 macrophages are bone-marrow-derived phagocytes that are recruited to damaged muscles by chemotactic and adhesion molecules, as well as pro-inflammatory cytokines released by injured cells (Wynn & Vannella, 2016). M1 macrophages are activated by the pro-inflammatory cytokines (including IFNγ and TNFα), an activation that leads to their increased production of additional inflammatory cytokines (Roszer, 2015). An influx of M1 macrophages is required for proper clearance of injury-induced debris (Lech & Anders, 2013; Mann et al., 2011; Yang & Hu, 2018). The resident type of macrophages is normally quiescent. However, these resident macrophages can also proliferate and alter their phenotype to phagocytic in nature in response to released pro-inflammatory cytokines (Wynn & Vannella, 2016). Note, there are many heterogeneous populations of immune cells, including macrophages, that fulfill tissue-specific and niche-specific functions. These functions range from dedicated homeostatic functions (e.g., clearance of cellular debris, play central roles in tissue immune surveillance, response to infection, and the resolution of inflammation.

This complex acute phase response occurs not only at the site of localized injury in order to recruit immune cells, but can also spread to adjacent tissue. Secondary damage can occur in tissues surrounding the original injury site via continued phagocytosis and their release of cytotoxic effectors, including ROS and RNS, respectfully, and proteolytic enzymes (matrix metalloproteinases,

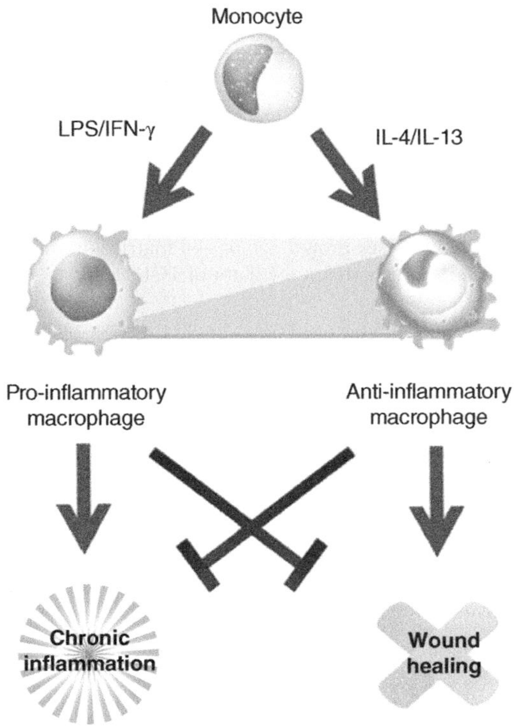

Figure 11.3 M1 (pro-inflammatory) versus M2 (anti-inflammatory) macrophage phenotypes paradigm. Both types of macrophages represent opposite ends of a continuum of intermediate phenotypes and are produced after monocyte stimulation with lipopolysaccharide (LPS), interferon-gamma (IFN-γ), and other pro-inflammatory cytokines in M1 macrophages, or interleukin (IL) 4 or 13 in M2 macrophages. The characteristic M1 profile is beneficial for pathogens and tumor elimination yet is detrimental if persistent and for wound healing. The M2 profile improves chronic inflammatory diseases and regeneration, yet continued presence is also associated with fibrosis. From Funes, S. C., Rios, M., Escobar-Vera, J., & Kalergis, A. M. (2018). Implications of macrophage polarization in autoimmunity. *Immunology*, 154(2), 186–195. https://doi.org/10.1111/imm.12910.

MMPs) that break down ECM proteins. Interestingly, while experimental depletion of neutrophil numbers or blocking their function reduces this collateral damage, such actions also reduce muscle repair and regeneration (Teixeira et al., 2003; Toumi et al., 2006). Similarly, experimental depletion of macrophages early after injury diminishes the inflammatory response, as expected, but also decreases wound debridement, tissue repair, and regeneration (Duffield et al., 2005; Zhang et al., 2012). Acute inflammation can also become systemic in order to amplify or depress the widespread activation of immune defense pathways.

Termination of the Acute Phase Response

Acute inflammatory responses are usually terminated by specific inhibitors and are followed by regenerative processes to restore normal tissue architecture and function. After acute inflammation, the next essential step for muscle regeneration and repair is a transition from a pro-inflammatory milieu to an anti-inflammatory one (Yang & Hu, 2018). Table 11.2 lists and defines several key mediators of tissue repair. In muscles, for example, increases in anti-inflammatory cytokines (IL-10 and IL-13), inhibit most pro-inflammatory responses (Dagdeviren et al., 2016) and stimulate an increase in repair-related M2 macrophages. Functional subtypes of M2 macrophages include M2a, M2b, and M2c. M2a subtypes are anti-inflammatory macrophages that promote wound healing or fibrosis in response to the cytokines IL-4 and IL-13 (Figure 11.3). M2b macrophages are activated in response to immune complexes and lipopolysaccharide, while M2c are deactivated macrophages that respond to IL-10, TGFβ1, and glucocorticoids to produce additional repair-related mediators, such as more IL-10 and TGFβ1 (Arango Duque & Descoteaux, 2014; Lech & Anders, 2013).

Under certain conditions, the ability to clear injured tissues is impaired (e.g., with diabetes or aging). Additionally, depending on other superimposed processes in the involved tissues, acute inflammatory responses can stimulate either further injury, chronic inflammation, or healing responses (including tissue adaptation, repair, or resorption). For example, an acute local inflammation may become chronic, or injury-repair cycles too persistent to allow for complete resolution of inflammation, each leading to persistent inflammation.

Wound Healing–Physiological Versus Pathological

Three primary outcomes are possible after tissue injury: (a) complete resolution with the total restoration of normal tissue structure; (b) repair with scar formation of varying degrees, depending on the level of injury; (c) chronic inflammation accompanied by degeneration, and no resolution of the inflammation or repair. Complete restoration is the regeneration or recreation of the tissue to a state in which it may even be in a better form or condition than it was before the injury. Repair is the process of mending tissue after damage. The mended area may not return to its pre-injury structure but may heal with a collagenous scar (i.e., a fibrotic scar or fibrosis) that fills the damaged tissue region. Repair of biological tissues can be accomplished through the processes of inflammation and remodeling, as long as the damage does not exceed the ability of tissues to repair. The lack of resolution of acute inflammatory responses leads to chronic inflammation, which is characterized by the prolonged presence of pro-inflammatory M1 macrophages and other immune cells (Figure 11.3). This can occur as the result of repeated tissue injury in which there is not enough time for the resolution of acute inflammatory responses and tissue repair. Persistent neutrophil and macrophage activities can also amplify a local injury by their enhanced production of pro-inflammatory cytokines. The pro-inflammatory cytokines produced by M1 macrophages and injured cells can escalate secondary tissue injuries since they are cytotoxic at high concentrations, particularly in the case of high levels of TNFα (Lech & Anders, 2013). Additionally, as systemic levels of pro-inflammatory cytokines elevate with chronic inflammation, inflammatory responses can be stimulated at distance sites far from the initial injury site. This increase in systemic inflammation can act as a co-morbidity for heart disease, diabetes, and rheumatoid arthritis, and vice versa, with concurrent presence of these inflammatory disorders enhancing injury-induced musculoskeletal inflammatory responses (Carp, Barr, & Barbe, 2008; Gallagher & Barbe, 2021).

Physiological Wound Healing

As shown in Figure 11.1, physiological wound healing after skin injury involves distinct phases that develop in an orderly but overlapping manner: hemostasis/acute inflammation, proliferation, and remodeling/maturation, with the objective being restorative repair. The first phase was discussed in Section "Injury-Induced Inflammation." The second phase of wound healing, the proliferative phase, is characterized by the migration of fibroblasts and stem/progenitor cells into the injury site, which proliferates to fill in the wound site. This phase is also called the granulation tissue formation phase because microscopically the wound site appears to be filled with many small immune cells and proliferating fibroblasts. The primary function of fibroblasts and related fibroblastic cells is to produce a new extracellular matrix. The first collagen subtype produced is collagen type III. This collagen subtype is unorganized fibrillar collagen that consists of only one collagen alpha chain, in contrast to most other collagens, and a weaker thinner fibril than collagen type I. Therefore, one main purpose of the next phase of repair and healing, the remodeling/maturation phase, is the gradual replacement of collagen III with the thicker, well-aligned network of collagen I fibrils that become cross-linked during this last phase, further enhancing strength. Fibroblasts realign along the axis of force through the tissue during remodeling. However, some tissues do not recover fully to their original structure and strength due to poor vascularization, persistent inflammation, or excessive fibrosis/scar formation, as discussed next.

Pathological Healing

Pathological injury can result from persistent injury, chronic cyclical inflammation, disrupted vascular supply and vascular function, excessive proliferation and activity of fibroblastic cells, conversion of fibroblasts into contractile type myofibroblasts, and increased production of fibrogenic mediators and therefore fibrotic tissue. In further detail, repeated injury and damage cycles, as depicted in Figure 11.4, give tissues little chance to complete the healing process, and persistent inflammation results in a chronic release of inflammatory mediators. Some of these mediators, such as TNFα, are cytotoxic at high levels, worsening cellular damage at or around the injury site, thus worsening tissue tolerance to loading, a key feature of fatigue failure as described in Figure 11.4.

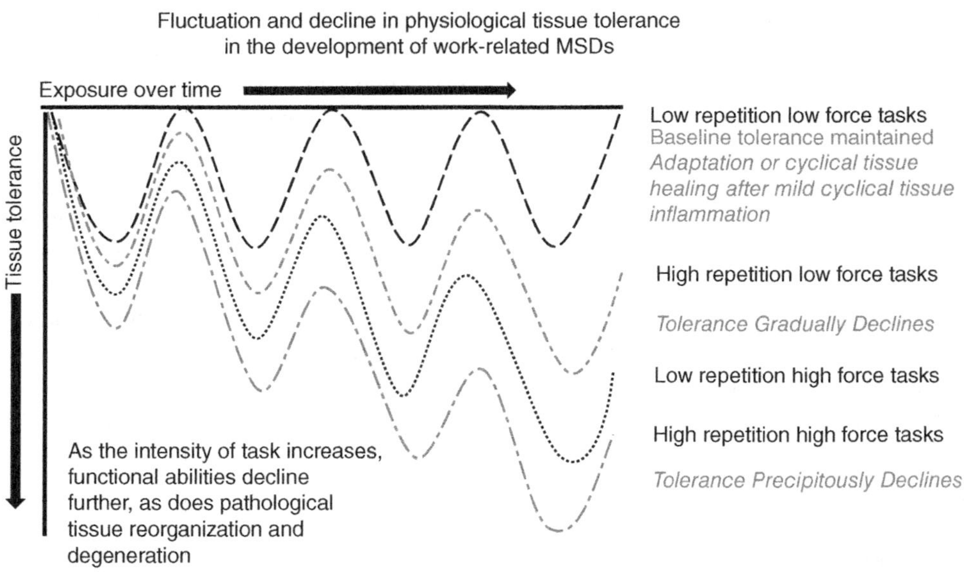

Figure 11.4 A model depicting the long-term effects of repeated tissue inflammation on tissue tolerance consistent with a fatigue failure theory of MSD development. In cases where the tissue exposure level remains below a critical threshold (upper curve), repeated bouts of inflammation are successful in resolving tissue disruption and restoring normal tissue tolerance through healing. When tissue exposure exceeds a critical threshold, incomplete tissue healing may result in a subsequent reduction in tissue tolerance (lower curves). Depending on the degree of exertion, this decline in tissue tolerance may be gradual or precipitous (as in the high repetition high force group). In addition to the overall decline in tissue tolerance, inflammatory episodes will result in transient periods of even lower tissue tolerance, resulting in fluctuations in tissue tolerance, as depicted. The modification of tissue exposure levels during these transient tissue tolerance minima may have an important impact on the maximization of tissue tolerance. Modified from Barr, A. E., & Barbe, M. F. (2004). Inflammation reduces physiological tissue tolerance in the development of work-related musculoskeletal disorders. *Journal of Electromyography and Kinesiology*, 14(1), 77–85. https://doi.org/10.1016/j.jelekin.2003.09.008.

Repeated injury and damage cycles in many tissue types are also associated with marked increases in non-contractile tissue (primarily collagen) (Barr & Barbe, 2002; Kjaer, 2004). For example, several of the inflammation-related cytokines listed in Tables 11.1 and 11.2 are also pro-fibrogenic, such as IL-1β and IL-13. Persistent release of such cytokines can cause excessive proliferation and activity of fibroblastic cells and production of fibrogenic growth factors, such as TGFβ1 and CCN2/CTGF (Barbe et al., 2020a, 2020b; Barbe, Harris, et al., 2021; Frara et al., 2021). Substance P, a nociceptor neuropeptide that is released by activated pain fibers after injury, acute or repeated, has also been shown to increase collagen production by tenocytes and fibroblastic cells (Fisher et al., 2015; Frara et al., 2018) leading to neurogenic driven fibrosis. Additionally, fibrogenic processes are perpetuated by the extended activity or prolonged presence of M2 macrophages that actively produce collagen precursors and factors that stimulate fibroblasts, such as TGFβ1 (Krzyszczyk, Schloss, Palmer, & Berthiaume, 2018; Tidball & Villalta, 2010; Tidball & Wehling-Henricks, 2015; Wang et al., 2015). An increased level of Substance P in the environment can also enhance TGFβ1 production. This is a key point since increased TGFβ1 induces fibroblasts to differentiate into myofibroblasts, key collagen-producing cells types in the ECMs of many soft tissues (Kjaer, 2004; Kjaer et al., 2009). Myofibroblasts have high levels of alpha-smooth muscle actin (which increases their contractile activity) and high levels of PDGF (an inflammatory modulator and pro-fibrogenic mediator, Tables 11.1 and 11.2) (Contreras, Rebolledo, Oyarzun, Olguin, & Brandan, 2016). The contractile activity of myofibroblasts is important during physiological wound healing; however, they are also heavy producers of collagen and contribute to tissue fibrosis with prolonged activation (Barr & Barbe, 2002; Kjaer, 2004). The result of a pathological remodeling phase is often excessive fibrosis (scar formation) in the tissues, which reduces tissue pliability and function.

Other factors can also negatively affect wound healing, including disrupted vascular supply that can lead to local tissue ischemia and necrosis. Invading neutrophils and macrophages lead to secondary tissue damage in nearby healthy tissue through phagocytosis, free radical damage, and tissue catabolism. Persistent tissue inflammatory responses can elevate circulating levels of pro-inflammatory cytokines that can induce recruitment of leukocytes into widespread tissues areas, leading to a pathological enhancement of bone resorption, cartilage degradation, and more due to enhanced systemic inflammation. Nerves innervating peripheral tissues also play a role in all phases of the healing response. These nerves include autonomic efferent, nociceptive afferent, and perivascular terminals of noradrenergic and cholinergic fibers. Overactivation of such endings can lead to a dysregulation of vascular function, enhanced pain, and poor wound healing. The patient's overall health must also be considered, such as malnutrition, infection, physiological and even psychological stress. For example, the presence of metabolic disorders, such as diabetes, can directly reduce the success of wound healing. We will discuss various contributions of overall health to healing further in Chapter 12.

Unique Injury and Healing Mechanisms and Capacity in Specific Musculoskeletal and Neural Tissues

Tendons

Tendon injury

Tendon injuries are relatively common, especially in people who play sports (30–50%) (Florit et al., 2019), with occupational tasks (Fedorczyk et al., 2010; Gao et al., 2013; Smith et al., 2020), and other repeated stressors that induce fatigue failure in the tendon tissues (Kjaer, 2004; Kjaer et al., 2009). Most tendon injuries occur near joints, such as the shoulder, elbow, knee, and ankle. A common tendon injury is a strain, which is damage to a tendon or muscle to which it connects, or enthesis damage if the injury is where the tendon attaches to the bone. Acute trauma from falling or suddenly twisting a tendon can cause a strain. Inactive people may be more vulnerable to such strains, especially if they suddenly become active or experience muscle weakness because of inactivity. Although acute trauma can occur, tendon injuries are mostly the result of an accumulation of degenerative changes, due to overuse, repeated sports injuries and stress, or aging. In other words, tendon injuries are usually the result of many tiny tears or gradual wear and tear (i.e., fatigue). Such accumulation weakens the tendon over time and can result in ruptures, which most commonly affect the Achilles, biceps, knee, and quadriceps tendons.

Signs and symptoms of tendinopathies can vary, although they are most often characterized by load-related pain and loss of function. An inflamed or irritated tendon can become swollen and warm to the touch due to blood vessel damage that leads to hemorrhage and edema. Injured tendons are very painful due to damage of sensory nerve endings in epitenon and peritenon connective tissues, and later on, due to the ingrowth of these nerve endings from exterior regions of the tendon into the injured tendon interior (the tendon proper). Tendon injuries can lead to stiffness and loss of strength in the affected tendon. Also, crepitus (a "grating" sound or sensation when moving or palpating a tendon) may develop that is indicative of a roughening of the tendon surface and inner lining of a tendon sheath, or the development of granulation or bony material in a tendon (the lateral known as heterotopic ossification of tendon regions).

Injury-induced tendon inflammation—Acute versus chronic/persistent

Although quite controversial in the past, an acceptance of inflammation in the etiology of tendinopathies represents the most striking shift in the field in the last decade. With the use of modern molecular methods and improved cell phenotyping markers, it is now known that a variety of immune cells infiltrate tendons early after injury and that a failure to resolve inflammatory responses is linked to tendinopathies accompanied by chronic pain. Tendon biopsies collected from patients with tendon pain show increased inflammatory processes, including interferon signaling. In contrast, tendon biopsies collected from patients with tendinopathy without pain show the presence of M2-type macrophages that are anti-inflammatory and pro-repair. How inflammation fits into the larger picture of the progression of tendinopathies remains less clear. Known features of the phases of healing after acute tendon injuries are summarized in Figure 11.5 (depicted as solid shapes). This figure also depicts the effects of repeated injury cycles on these phases of healing (as dashed lines). The main difference is that the inflammatory and proliferative phases are extended temporally, a prolongation that contributes to cumulative degenerative and fibrotic changes within the tendon proper or its sheaths. Key changes occurring with tendinopathies are also summarized in Figure 11.7.

Inflammatory responses increase within 1 day of tendon injury and subside quickly or may last for 6 weeks or more weeks, depending on the extent of the injury and superimposed biological responses and factors. This inflammatory phase is key for minimizing or eliminating additional damage and the removal of damaged and necrotic cells. It begins by a release of danger signals from injured or stressed cells, including heat shock proteins (cell stress-related proteins), DAMPS, like HMGB1 and IL-33 (see Table 11.1), and inflammatory cytokines. HMGB1 elevates in response to mechanical overload and initiates the progression of tendinopathy in mouse models. There is also increased production of inflammatory and chemotactic cytokines, increased vascular permeability and immune cell infiltrate (Figure 11.5). These immune cells release inflammatory mediators that recruit additional immune cells and fibroblast infiltration. An increase in VEGF stimulates the ingrowth of small blood vessels into the injured tendon site (i.e., angiogenesis), bringing even more immune cells and

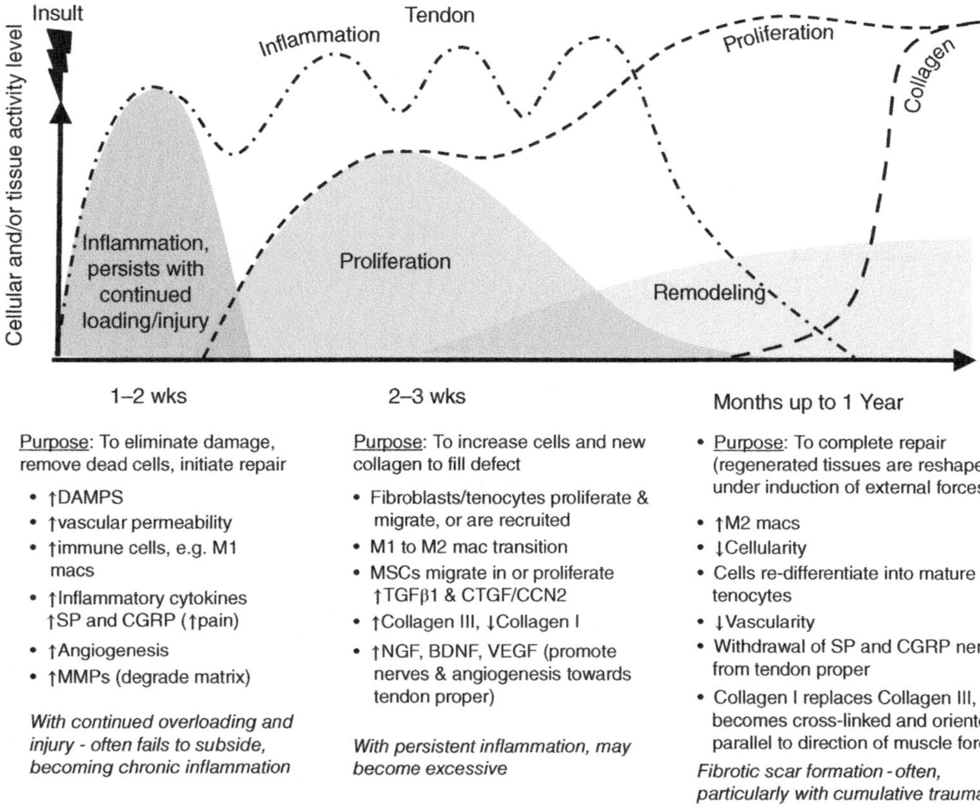

Figure 11.5 A summary of the inflammation, proliferation, and remodeling phases after tendon injury, their time frames, and several major events occurring during each phase. The acute phases of inflammation, proliferation, and remodeling (solid shapes) are extended temporally by repeated injury cycles (depicted as dashed lines). BDNF = Brain-derived growth factor; M1 and M2 = macrophage subtypes; NGF = nerve growth factor. Other abbreviations as defined in Tables 11.1 and 11.2. Modified from Mori, R., Tanaka, K., & Shimokawa, I. (2018). Identification and functional analysis of inflammation-related miRNAs in skin wound repair. *Development, Growth & Differentiation*, 60(6), 306–315. https://doi.org/10.1111/dgd.12542. http://Wiley.com.

mesenchymal stem cells into the tendon proper. There is an early ingrowth of nerve endings from the paratendon and proximal myotendinous junctions into the injured zone of the tendon proper, and an ingrowth of pain-related sensory nerve endings [e.g., sensory endings that are immunopositive for Substance P and calcitonin gene-related peptide (CGRP)] that accompany small blood vessels. Such ingrowth enhances pain symptoms, vasodilation, and further immune cell infiltration. Macrophages and tendon fibroblasts upregulate their production and activate proteinases, such as matrix metalloproteinases (MMPs) that degrade the damaged ECM (Figures 11.5 and 11.6). This point signals the onset of the proliferative phase (Figure 11.5), with increased release of Substance P and CGRP enhancing anabolism. In addition to enhancing the proliferation of several cell types including tenocytes, Substance P stimulates collagen stimulation by tenocytes both independently and through TGFβ1 signaling mechanisms (Frara et al., 2021). Also, HMGB1 and IL-33 are molecular switches that signal a switch from the production of mature collagen (type I) to immature collagen (type III). Thus, inflammation is an important driver of tendon healing.

Yet, the inflammatory phase does not always subside and apoptotic cells may fail to be cleared (which weakens a tendon's biomechanical properties). Continued mechanical loading of tendons

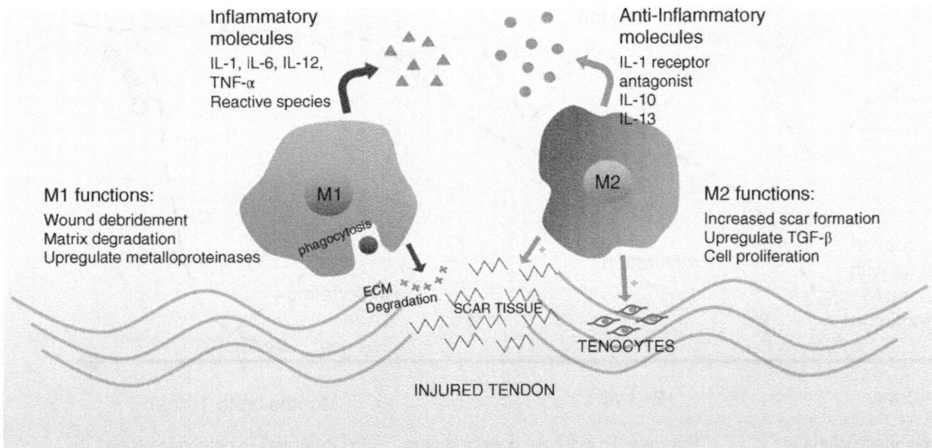

Figure 11.6 A comparison of the function of M1 and M2 macrophage phenotypes in the healing tendon. IL = interleukin; TGF-β = transforming growth factor-beta; TNFα = tumor necrosis factor-alpha. From Sunwoo et al. (2020); http://Wiley.com. https://doi.org/10.1002/jor.24667.

at high repetition or high force loads is associated with persistent or cyclical inflammatory responses (Fedorczyk et al., 2010; Gao et al., 2013), increased Substance P production by tenocytes, fibroblastic cells, and nerve endings in tendons (Frara et al., 2018) (which increases pain and fibrotic tendon changes), increased MMP production and activation (which enhances tissue degradation), and the switch from pro-inflammatory M1 type macrophages to pro-repair M2 type macrophages, as shown in Figure 11.6, does not occur (Barbe, Harris, et al., 2021). While one can postulate that a repeated injury cycle is propagating the inflammatory phase, several mechanosensitive ion channels and other proteins (such as Piezo channels, transient receptor potential channels, and integrins) are activated by mechanical movement of a cell, including in macrophages (Yang & Plotnikov, 2021). Mechanical activation of the mechanosensitive proteins in macrophages can trigger a wide range of intracellular signaling pathways including pathways that enhance their migration. Mechanosensitive proteins in macrophages, fibroblasts, and myofibroblast can also activate signaling pathways that synergize with chemical signaling pathways mediated by pro-inflammatory cytokines and growth factors, thereby linking inflammatory and mechanosensitive signaling pathways (Yang & Plotnikov, 2021). This link may be one of the biochemical means by which continued fatigue loading can lead to fatigue failure (specifically, in this case, the perpetuation of inflammatory responses that can weaken cells and tissues further).

Capacity and extent of tendon self-repair

The inflammatory phase in tendons, discussed earlier, is an important driver of the proliferative phase, which is followed by a remodeling phase that takes up to 1 year to complete (Figure 11.5) (Sharma & Maffulli, 2005; Woo et al., 1999). Cellular proliferation is the key characteristic, although the cells are from multiple sources. Intrinsic tenocytes increase in number and fibroblasts proliferate and migrate from the epitenon and endotenon into the tendon defect. Stromal fibroblasts are also recruited and proliferate in response to inflammatory cytokines (e.g., IL-1α). These fibroblasts often upregulate their alpha-smooth muscle actin production, thus becoming contractile type myofibroblasts, that can aid closure of the defect. M1 macrophages transition into repair type (M2) macrophages, and additional M2 macrophages gradually arrive via the additional tendon blood vessels to start the healing process and up-regulation of anti-inflammatory cytokines (e.g., IL-10) and repair type growth factors (e.g., TGFβ; Figure 11.6).

A heterogeneous group of mesenchymal stem cells also migrate in or proliferate from within the tendon. Considering the low regenerative ability of adult tendons, it may seem odd to discuss the presence of progenitor cells in tendons. Their regenerative abilities are quite strong in fetal and neonatal tendons but are considerably weaker in adult tendons. In adult tendons, there are resident preexisting progenitor cells that expand and differentiate after tendon transection to contribute to the healed scar tissue (Scx+ and S100beta4+ cells). There are progenitor populations in the paratendon (alpha-smooth muscle actin expressing cells that migrate to bridge defects, and that differentiate into Scx + tenocytes) and in tendon sheaths (osteocalcin expressing cells that proliferate after partial tendon injuries in mice), and more. More investigation is warranted on these adult MSCs and how to stimulate their participation in tendon healing. It is clear currently is that there are missing or misregulated cues underlying the inability of tendon progenitor/stem cells to regenerate adult tendons.

The proliferative phase typically lasts only a few weeks and is further characterized by increased fibroblast numbers and collagen synthesis in response to increased TGFβ1 and CCN2/CTGF (defined in Table 11.2). There is increased deposition of immature type of tendon collagen (type III) at the tendon injury site, and transient downregulation of mature collagen type I. There may also be an increase in the deposition of components important in the repair of the extracellular matrix, such as proteoglycans (Wang, 2006; Wang & Komatsu, 2016). Tendon nerve endings also participate in the proliferative phase by increasing their production and release of VEGF and neural factors (including, nerve growth factor (NGF) and BDNF that promote the rapid expansion of the vascular network and nerves toward the tendon proper.

The next phase, the remodeling process in injured tendons, is initiated approximately 6 weeks after an acute injury/strain and lasts for up to 1 year after injury (Figure 11.5). This stage is sometimes divided into two separate parts, the first being the consolidation stage and the second being the maturation stage (Sharma & Maffulli, 2005). The consolidation stage represents the period during which repair tissues evolve from a cellular to a fibrous configuration and when the collagen fibrils become aligned in the direction of mechanical stress. The maturation process begins at about 10 weeks post-trauma and shows a slow change to a more "scar-like" tendon tissue that has greater stiffness and tensile strength than an undamaged tendon. In the case of tendons, a fibrotic scar often fills the damaged tissue gap. During remodeling, fibroblast cells in the tendons differentiate or redifferentiate into mature tenocytes, cellularity and vascularity typically decrease, there is a withdrawal of Substance P+ and CGRP+ nerve fibers from the tendon proper (reducing pain), and stronger collagen type I fibrils gradually replace the immature and weaker collagen type III fibrils in the tendon proper.

However, damaged tendons may never return to normal structural or biomechanical properties, even after long periods of recovery. Tendons exposed to cyclical loading develop degenerative changes pathologies, including microtears that show greater mean tear size and density in tendons experiencing repetitive stress loading, compared to tendons in unloaded limbs, congruent with fatigue failure theory (Nakama, King, Abrahamsson, & Rempel, 2005). The weaker and less organized collagen type II may not be replaced completely by collagen type I (Figure 11.7), decreasing the fatigue loading threshold (fatigue loading is explained in detail in Chapter 7). In brief, collagen fibrils are tightly aligned linearly in normal uninjured tendons, kinks develop in focal tendon regions after exposure to low-level fatigue loading, a greater number of kinked and separated collagen fibrils develop with exposure to moderate level fatigue loading, while tendons exposed to high levels of fatigue loading exhibit a severe disruption in fibril alignment, more fibril separations, thinning, and discontinuities (Fung et al., 2009) (Figure 11.7). A fibrovascular scar often persists at the prior injury site that has inferior biomechanical properties, compared to a healthy tendon. Surgery may be needed to excise remaining clumps of dead cells and fibrotic regions in order to induce tendon repair (Yang, Rothrauff, & Tuan, 2013). After a rupture, even with surgical repair, re-rupture often occurs due to incomplete tendon regeneration and an

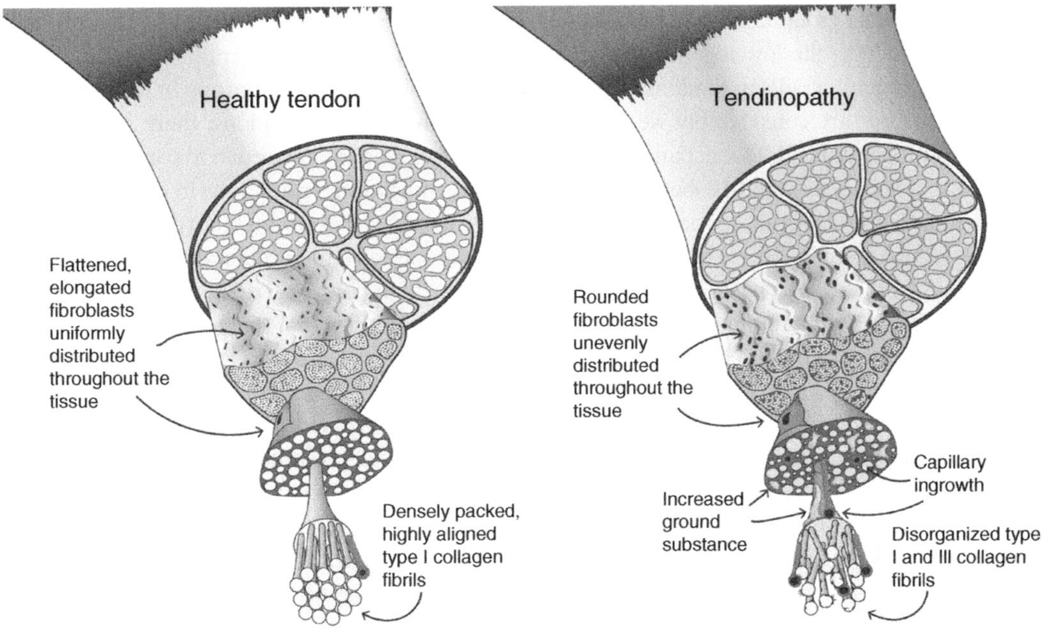

Figure 11.7 Graphical representation of the morphological features in a healthy tendon and a tendon with tendinopathy. From Mead, M. P., Gumucio, J. P., Awan, T. M., Mendias, C. L., & Sugg, K. B. (2018). Pathogenesis and management of tendinopathies in sports medicine. *Translational Sports Medicine*, 1(1), 5–13. https://doi.org/10.1002/tsm2.6. http://Wiley.com.

inability of the tendon tissues to regain pre-rupture strength. Additionally, the heterotopic bone may have formed within the tendon or at the site of a tendon-to-bone attachment (the enthesis), and osteoclasts may be attracted to this same region that engages in bone resorption, each impairing healing. One means by which osteoclasts gain access to tendon tissues is an excess of vessels that fail to withdraw from the tendon proper during the remodeling phase (Figure 11.7). Lastly, adhesions often form between the paratendon or tendon sheath and the tendon surface in fibrotic tendons (Smith et al., 2020), which may reduce a tendon's sliding function (Stecco et al., 2008).

Ligaments

Ligament injury

Ligament injuries are common in the ankle, knee, wrist, thumb, neck, or back. Several factors can increase the risk of injury, including repeated mechanical stress (fatigue), acute trauma (a fall, contusive blow, or other high impact events), twisting the ligament into an awkward position, tears (after a fall or high impact even) or weakness in the surrounding muscles due to a sedentary lifestyle. Ligament sprains can occur after a ligament overstretch or tear and can be temporary to long-lasting. Overstretch of a ligament (but with no tear) is designated as a mild sprain, partial tears are moderate sprains, while a complete tear of the ligament is considered as a severe sprain. The latter type of sprain leads to joint instability in the associated joint and often requires surgical treatment.

Signs and symptoms of a ligament tear include pain and tenderness or palpation, and perhaps also swelling and bruising. It may be difficult to move the associated joint due to a loss of joint stability. Movement is impaired when a ligament is torn, resulting in looseness in the joint or an inability to move the joint normally.

Table 11.3 Differences Observed Between Normal Ligament Tissue and Repaired (Scarred) Ligament Tissue

Normal ligament	Repaired ligament (scar tissue)
• Large collagen fibrils	• Smaller collagen fibrils
• Low cell and matrix turnover	• High cell and matrix turnover
• Well-aligned collagen	• Disorganized collagen
• Densely packed collagen	• Flaws between fibers
• High matrix-cell ratio	• Lower matrix-cell ratio
• Low cell density	• Higher cell density
• Mature collagen crosslinks	• Immature collagen crosslinks
• Type I collagen	• More collagen III
• Small proteoglycans	• Larger proteoglycans
• Rare cell division	• More cell division

Adapted from Hauser, R. A., & Dolan, E. E. (2011). Ligament injury and healing: An overview of current clinical concepts. *Journal of Prolotherapy*, 3(4), 836–846.

Capacity and extent of ligament self-repair

The healing of ligament follows the same process as all soft tissues in the body that consists of the same three overlapping phases as shown in Figures 11.1 and 11.5: inflammation, proliferation, and remodeling. During the inflammation phase, which lasts about 48–72 hr after an acute ligament injury, blood collects at the site of injury and platelet cells are deposited which interact with ligament matrix components to change shape and initiate clot formation. The proliferation phase involves the action of numerous growth factors that attract immune cells to the injury to both clean up damaged tissue and begin deposition of new tissue to rebuild the ligament matrix. The newly deposited repair material resembles scar tissue and contains more blood vessels, fat cells, and inflammatory cells than in normal ligament tissue (Hauser & Dolan, 2011). During the remodeling phase, the scar tissue gradually achieves some improvement in material characteristics (becoming more akin to the original tissue). However, even the fully remodeled tissue never attains the quality of normal ligament in terms of appearance or function. Table 11.3 provides a comparison of the characteristics of normal ligament tissue versus a repaired (scar) ligament.

As with tendons, ligaments are poorly vascularized tissues. This inhibits the healing process and makes it more likely that fatigue damage will exceed the ability of the tissue to heal. Steroid injections and NSAIDs have been used to reduce ligament pain and inflammation, although these treatments may inhibit healing perhaps by inhibiting tissue clearance during the inflammatory phase.

Skeletal Muscle

Muscle injury

There are several types of acute muscle injuries, including contusions, elongation, strain, tears, and lacerations. Contusions occur after an impact on a muscle that compresses or even tears one or more myofibers. Elongation injuries occur when a muscle is stretched beyond its capacity, which also tears one or more myofibers. A muscle strain is caused by intense and rapid contractions of a muscle. If the contractions are too strong and are sufficiently repetitive, the muscle fibers may be unable to resist and may undergo fatigue damage. Muscle strains can be categorized into three grades based on the extent and degrees of myofiber tearing: Grade 1) mild muscle damage to individual muscle fibers (<5%), resulting in a minimal loss of strength and motion; Grade 2) more extensive damage with involvement of more muscle fibers, and Grade 3) complete rupture of a muscle.

A milder cellular or subcellular muscle injury may also occur, such as after repetitive or sustained contraction of the same muscle fibers, as described for tendon. In contrast, persistent repeated strains or activity at high force levels can result in higher levels of injury and chronic inflammation. Such repetitive or sustained contractions have been linked to impairment of calcium regulation in affected muscle fibers (Allen, Lamb, & Westerblad, 2008; Hadrevi et al., 2019; Ortenblad, Lunde, Levin, Andersen, & Pedersen, 2000). Disruption of calcium homeostasis can cause calcium overload due to leakage of calcium from the sarcoplasmic reticulum, impaired calcium uptake into the sarcoplasmic reticulum, or increased cell membrane Ca^{2+} influx (Gissel, 2005; Sogaard, 1995). These disturbances may activate intracellular Ca^{2+}-dependent proteins, such as calpains that lead to further cell damage by degrading intracellular proteins and cellular membranes and inducing nuclear DNA (Amici et al., 2017). This type of muscle cell damage can induce metabolic overload and a higher reliance on anaerobic processes leading to increased levels of lactate and pyruvate in the muscle, for example, changes associated with increased muscle pain (also termed *myalgia*) (Rosendal et al., 2004).

Signs and symptoms of muscle injuries include increased pain during muscle contractions and reduced muscle function. Palpation of the muscle results in localized pain, as does a movement that involves the injured muscle fibers. More severe injuries will result in loss of strength, the appearance of a hematoma, and occupationally, a depression or cavity at the location where muscle fibers have been torn.

Injury-induced muscle inflammation

Similar to most tissues, the process of muscle injury healing involves three main phases: (a) degeneration or inflammation; (b) regeneration; (c) remodeling (Figure 11.8). The inflammatory phase takes place during the first few days after injury, first with necrosis of the injured muscle fibers (partially due to lesions of the sarcolemma, and then a loss of calcium homeostasis, as discussed earlier. During this period, a hematoma may form at the injury site depending on the size and extent of the injury. Thereafter, the inflammatory process in muscle proceeds similarly as in cutaneous wound healing events shown in Figures 11.1 and 11.2. There is an infiltration of neutrophils to remove the necrosed muscle tissue and the secretion of pro-inflammatory molecules, including several cytokines and growth factors, from injured cells and infiltrating neutrophils. After a controlled acute strain injury, muscle fiber necrosis and inflammation are observed by 24 hr, significantly increased inflammation within 24 hr, followed by resolution of the inflammation by 7 days although an increase in collagenous tissues (fibrosis) may also be evident at this point (Butterfield, Best, & Merrick, 2006).

In contrast, persistent repeated strains or activity at high force levels result in repeated or cyclical bouts of inflammation. In one study, pro-inflammatory cytokines were examined in muscles and tendons collected from 4 groups: control rats, immediately after training for 5 weeks to learn the high repetition low force task (the point of the initial injury), and 18 and 24 weeks after performing this task for 2 hr/day, 3 days/week (Figure 11.9; Gao et al., 2013). The inflammatory cytokines showed cyclical changes across the weeks of training and task performance, with peaks after the initial training period, then resolution by 18 weeks despite the continued task performance, and then an increase again by 24 weeks, indicative of a cyclical inflammation that may further enhance tissue injuries. In this study by Gao et al. (2013), greater cytokine expression was observed in tendons than in muscles suggesting different response processes in these tissues.

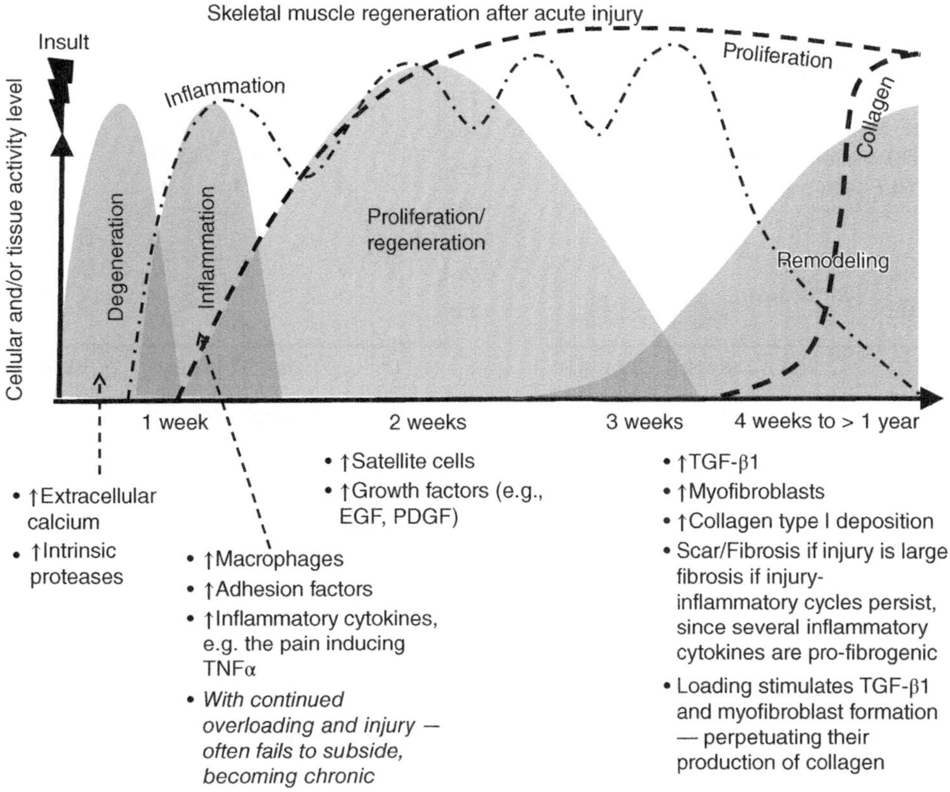

Figure 11.8 Phases and main events after muscle injury. The typical acute phases of inflammation, proliferation, and remodeling (solid shapes) are prolonged by repeated injury cycles (depicted as dashed lines). (Gharaibeh, Burhan & Chun-Lansinger, Yuri & Hagen, Tanya & Ingham, Sheila & Wright, Vonda & Fu, Freddie & Huard, Johnny. (2012). Biological approaches to improve skeletal muscle healing after injury and disease. Birth defects research. Part C, *Embryo Today: Reviews*, 96, 82-94. 10.1002/bdrc.21005.)

As described for tendons, two main phenotypes of macrophages infiltrate skeletal muscles. The pro-inflammatory M1 macrophages infiltrate first to assist with the removal of injured tissue. Pro-inflammatory processes, such as this macrophage influx, are required for proper muscle repair and clearance of injury-induced debris (Lech & Anders, 2013; Mann et al., 2011; Yang & Hu, 2018), while anti-inflammatory M2 macrophages arrive later to help attenuate the inflammatory response by producing IL-10 (Barbe, Harris, et al., 2021). Factors released by the M2 macrophages also promote the formation of myotubes (Dort, Fabre, Molina, & Dumont, 2019). Yet, several researchers have reported that M2a type macrophages have been shown to play important roles in fibrosis in lung, liver, skin, and muscle (Desguerre et al., 2009; Higashi-Kuwata et al., 2010; Hu et al., 2012; Murphy et al., 2010; Tidball & Villalta, 2010; Tidball & Wehling-Henricks, 2015; Wang et al., 2015), particularly in concert with persistent/chronic inflammation (Barbe, Harris, et al., 2021).

Capacity and extent of muscle self-repair

Skeletal muscle has a remarkable ability for self-repair after injury, partly due to its strong blood supply and robust numbers of progenitor/stem cells, a category that includes the satellite cells described in the following text. The regeneration of new muscle cells is initiated in the late phase

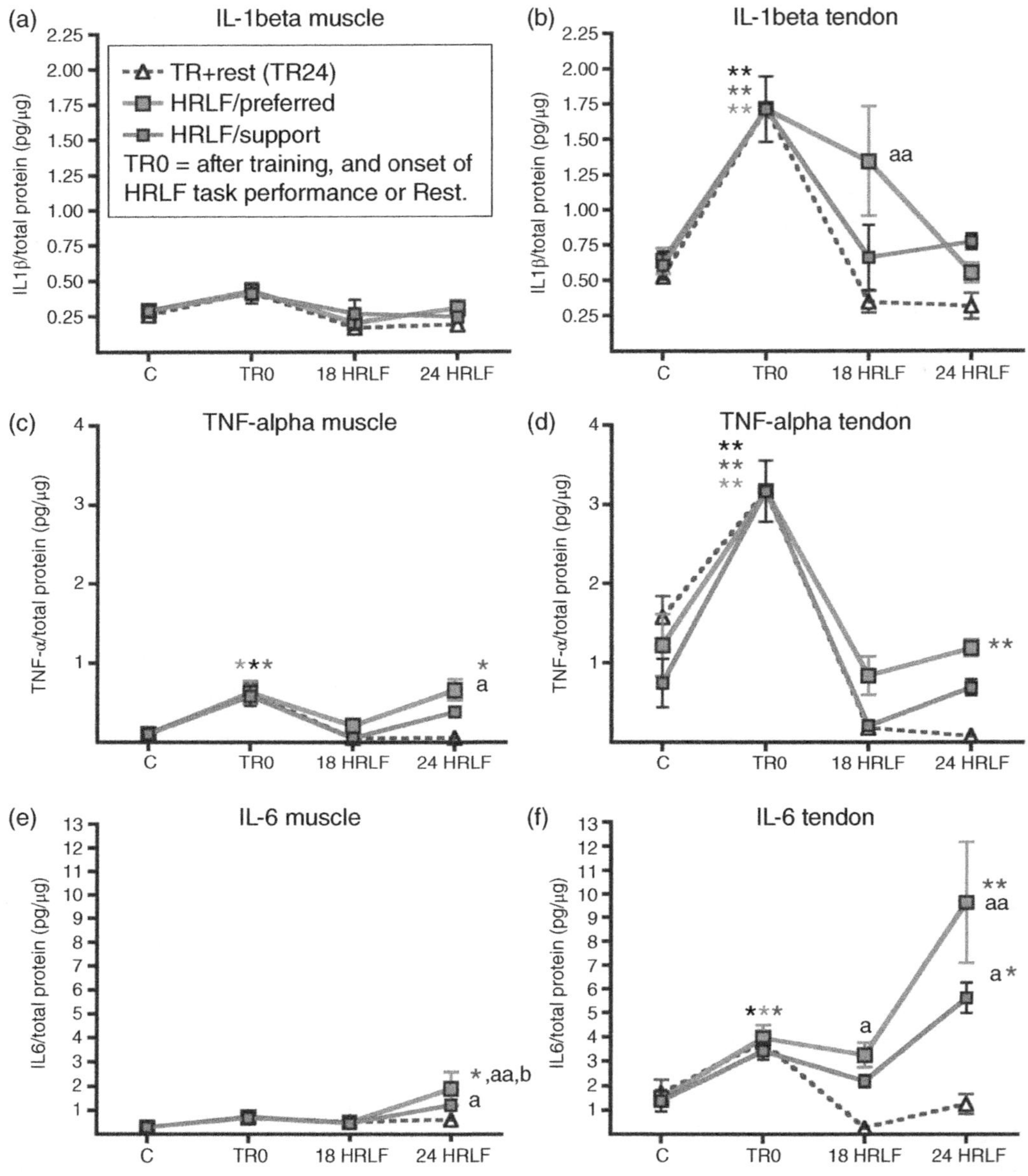

Figure 11.9 Persistent inflammation with continued task performance. Pro-inflammatory cytokines show cyclical increases in forelimb muscles and tendons of rats performing a repetitive high repetition low force (HRLF) task for 24 weeks Groups: control rats (C), trained only rats (TR0), TR + Rest (TR24; trained rats that rested for 24 weeks, dotted line), and high repetition low force (HRLF) rats that worked for 18 or 24 weeks. Preferred reach limbs (gray line) and contralateral support limb (black line) data are shown. *p, 0.05, **p, 0.01 and ***p, 0.001, compared to C; a:p, 0.05 and aa: p, 0.01, compared to TR + Rest; b:p, 0.05, compared to HRLF support limbs. Gao, H. G., Fisher, P. W., Lambi, A. G., Wade, C. K., Barr-Gillespie, A. E., Popoff, S. N., & Barbe, M. F. (2013). Increased serum and musculotendinous fibrogenic proteins following persistent low-grade inflammation in a rat model of long-term upper extremity overuse. *PLoS One*, 8(8), e71875. https://doi.org/10.1371/journal.pone.0071875./Public Library of Science/CC BY.

of the inflammatory process and can take up to 4 weeks, with peak regenerative activity occurring about 2 weeks after an acute injury although full regeneration can take up to months depending on the level of injury (Figure 11.8; Table 11.7). However, the tissue gap induced with volumetric muscle damage may never completely be filled with normal muscle tissue but with fibrotic or fatty tissue instead (Greising et al., 2017), indicating limitations in repair by even a tissue with strong regenerative properties.

The ability of a muscle to regenerate is governed by the interaction between satellite cells and their microenvironment. Satellite cells are a population of adult stem cells that are unipotent muscle precursor cells (Mukund & Subramaniam, 2020). These cells are necessary for repair since myofiber cells do not possess the ability to divide. Satellite cells typically reside between the basal lamina and sarcolemma in a quiescent state (i.e., their "niche"). This niche in which they are embedded is composed of acellular components including growth factors, ECM proteins, chemokines, MMPS, as well as fibroadipogenic progenitor cells (FAPs) (Judson, Low, Eisner, & Rossi, 2017). Beyond this niche, local interstitial cells, motor neurons, vascular and secreted factors can influence satellite cells. Injury disrupts this intrinsic and extrinsic environment, activating the satellite cells and stimulating their migration to areas with injured myofiber cells. Satellite cells proliferate during this phase, differentiate and form into myoblasts that develop into regenerated myofibers. Some satellite cells do not form myoblasts but instead reproduce to replenish the population of satellite cells to prepare for future repair needs (Mukund & Subramaniam, 2020). Bone marrow-derived cells are also thought to be involved in the replenishment of myoblasts (Yin, Price, & Rudnicki, 2013). Endothelial cells and fibroblasts also proliferate or infiltrate to replace injured vessels and muscle connective tissues. This replenishment is aided by many of the same growth and repair factors listed in Table 11.2, including PDGF and EGF. The density and efficacy of these progenitor/stem cells reduce with age (Almada & Wagers, 2016), a change that may contribute to the reduced healing and sarcopenia observed with aging.

Once the myoblasts have been replaced and are appropriately situated, they differentiate into myofibers, and the muscle remodeling process can proceed. During this phase, regeneration of myofibers continues along with the maturation of new myofibers (Mukund & Subramaniam, 2020). This phase also experiences an increase in revascularization of the injury site along with additional connective tissue repair. Revascularization is critical both for muscle regeneration and also to reduce the likelihood of fibrosis development. Muscle repair is complete when myofibers are regenerated and innervation of the newly repaired myofibers is established (Mukund & Subramaniam, 2020).

Muscle fibrosis can occur as the result of a severe injury or even smaller repeated injury and inflammation (Barbe et al., 2020b; Kjaer, 2004; Kjaer et al., 2009). Some of this results from the transformation of resident fibroblasts into myofibroblasts after injury. Myofibroblasts are stimulated by repair growth factors (particularly, TGFβ) to synthesize and release ECM components (such as fibrous collagens types I and II, and more). Additionally, the mesenchymal transition of fibroadipogenic progenitor cells occurs into activated fibroblast populations. Activation of myofibroblasts and fibroblastic cells leads to additional collagen deposition and an expansion of the muscle's extracellular matrix. Muscle fibrosis does not typically resolve completely, even after months of rest (Stauber, 2004; Stauber, Smith, Miller, & Stauber, 2000). Such fibrosis can lead to muscle stiffening (and sometimes a weaker muscle) since denser connective tissues contain a clear predominance of collagen fibers over ground substances and are less flexible than loose connective tissues (Binder-Markey, Broda, & Lieber, 2020; Mathewson et al., 2014).

Cartilage

Cartilage injury

Cartilage injuries are known as chondral injuries. Common mechanical mechanisms of primary cartilage injury include a single traumatic joint loading or direct blows to the joint, such as during sports injuries, a fall, or automobile accidents, as well as repeated compressive impact loading—each leading to fatigue failure of cells or matrix in the damaged site. Mechanical damage of articular cartilage, a type of hyaline cartilage, occurs most commonly in the knee, although the elbow, wrist, ankle, shoulder, and hip joints can also be affected. Elastic cartilage, fibrocartilage, and hyaline cartilage are also subject to damage from mechanical insult.

Symptoms of cartilage damage may be absent since cartilage is aneural (lacking in innervation in the cartilage proper). As a consequence, cartilage damage may propagate and progress considerably before detection (and thus intervention). Even moderate structural damage that is detectable radiographically may not correlate with patient reports of pain and dysfunction. When symptomatic, the pain is likely due to inflammatory processes in the surrounding joint tissues, such as synovial membrane or ligaments, or in subchondral bone tissues that are well innervated with pain signaling nerves (nociceptors). In such cases, the symptoms can include severe pain, inflammation and swelling, and often some degree of disability. If the injured cartilage is associated with a joint, the disability includes stiffness and limitations in the joint's range of motion.

Direct acute trauma results in localized abolishment of chondrocyte anabolic function and biomechanical changes in the extracellular matrix (detectable as early as 0–3 days post-injury) or chondrocyte death from apoptosis (detectable as early as 96 hr post-injury). Direct impacts, even low-energy impacts, may also initiate microcracks in the collagen network. Following initiation of microcracks, repetitive mechanical loads to cartilage during normal daily activities (including walking) may propagate these cracks within the extracellular collagenous matrix, thus spreading the injury into adjacent cartilage regions. Even small acute cartilage injuries can progress to larger cartilage lesions over time if left untreated, eventually leading to post-traumatic osteoarthritis (PTOA). Thus, in articular cartilage, likely due to its avascular, low progenitor/stem cells and therefore, low healing/repair characteristics, once a microcrack is initiated, a fatigue failure process commences.

In more detail, post-injury morphological changes in the cartilage include structural, cellular, and matrix damage (Table 11.4). Structural damage can range from mild changes (surface

Table 11.4 Types of Cartilage Damage and Subsequent Events

Primary: Direct acute trauma	• Loss of chondrocyte anabolic function, • Chondrocyte death from apoptosis, • Biochemical changes in extracellular matrix (e.g., increased inflammatory cytokines & glycosaminoglycans), • Weakened biomechanical properties, • Microcracks that propagate may lead to progressive cartilage damage, • Significantly increased risk of post-traumatic arthritis (PTA) and post-traumatic osteoarthritis (PTOA).
Secondary (indirect): Extra-cartilage soft tissue trauma (e.g., ligaments, menisci, synovial tissue)	• Damage to extra-cartilage soft tissue • Joint instability with increased abnormal loading, which leads to cartilage wear and tear • Increased release of inflammatory cytokines from inflamed soft tissues • Biochemical changes in extracellular matrix (see earlier) • Significantly increased risk of PTOA

irregularities) and breaking of collagen fibrils to moderate changes (loss of some rows of chondrocytes due to apoptosis, and moderate clustering, defined as multinucleate groups of chondrocytes), and then to substantial changes (a substantial loss of chondrocytes, chaotic structure, substantial cells clustering, and osteoclast invasion from subchondral bone) (Driban, Barr, Amin, Sitler, & Barbe, 2011). The most advanced stages of cartilage damage include cyst formation and subchondral bone lesions. Cellular indices of damage follow suit with the structural changes, ranging from small superficial clusters to substantial clustering, and eventually hypocellularity from cell death (Driban et al., 2011; Driban et al., 2020). The damage to the ECM is partially a result of increased production of inflammatory cytokines that are also cytotoxic, such as TNFα and TNFα receptors by the damaged chondrocytes. The chondrocytes also lose anabolic function and an increase in their apoptosis rate by 96 hr post-injury. Loss of chondrocyte function contributes to a loss of collagen type 2 (the main type of collagen in cartilage) and proteoglycans in the extracellular matrix, and significantly increased breakdown and release of glycosaminoglycans (GAGs, a type of proteoglycans) (D'Lima, Hashimoto, Chen, Colwell Jr., & Lotz, 2001). Interesting, decreased GAGs in articular cartilage are both a sign and a stimulator of further deterioration of load-bearing cartilage. In contrast, collagen I production may increase, changing the matrix from pliable hyaline cartilage to stiffer fibrocartilage. These changes when combined weaken the cartilage's biomechanical loading properties. Chondrocyte apoptosis and a lack of replenishment of the matrix by this cell type lead to a loss of cartilage thickness that is visible using radiological or MRI imaging as joint space narrowing.

Articular cartilage injuries may also occur indirectly (secondary cartilage injuries) after the injury of ligamentous or other structures within a joint, such as the synovial membranes, labrum in the shoulder, and anterior cruciate ligaments and menisci in the knee. These extra-cartilage soft tissue injuries lead first to joint instability that can then enhance degeneration of articular cartilage as a consequence of repetitive loading at abnormal angles and strains. Inflammatory mediators released from inflamed synovial tissues (such as the release of inflammatory cytokines during synovitis) can also enhance cartilage degeneration by inducing biochemical changes in the extracellular matrix of cartilage that weakens its biomechanical properties. Repetitive wear and tear, and even long periods of mechanical stress on the cartilage, can also lead to cartilage damage (Driban et al., 2011, 2020). For example, obese individuals are more likely to damage their knee over a 20-year period than a person of normal weight does, simply because the body and joints are under much higher degrees of physical stress.

Capacity and extent of articular cartilage self-repair

Unfortunately, once injured, articular cartilage has a very limited capacity to self-heal after damage, as shown in Figure 11.10 (Wei & Dai, 2021). Several contributing reasons are listed in Table 11.5. For example, unlike other types of tissues, cartilage is an avascular tissue that is nourished by diffusion, which requires movement of the joint. There are no blood vessels to promote migration or immediate-early repair responses provided by macrophages. Long periods of inactivity or immobility post-trauma decrease the diffusion of nutrients through the cartilage matrix (how this avascular tissue receives its nutrients). This increases the risk of damage to the cartilage and reduces the diffusion of nutrients, thereby exacerbating the already low anabolic state in damaged chondrocytes.

Like most tissues, cartilage contains resident populations of mesenchymal stem/progenitor cells (MSCPs), including cartilage-derived progenitor cells that can be found in both normal and injured

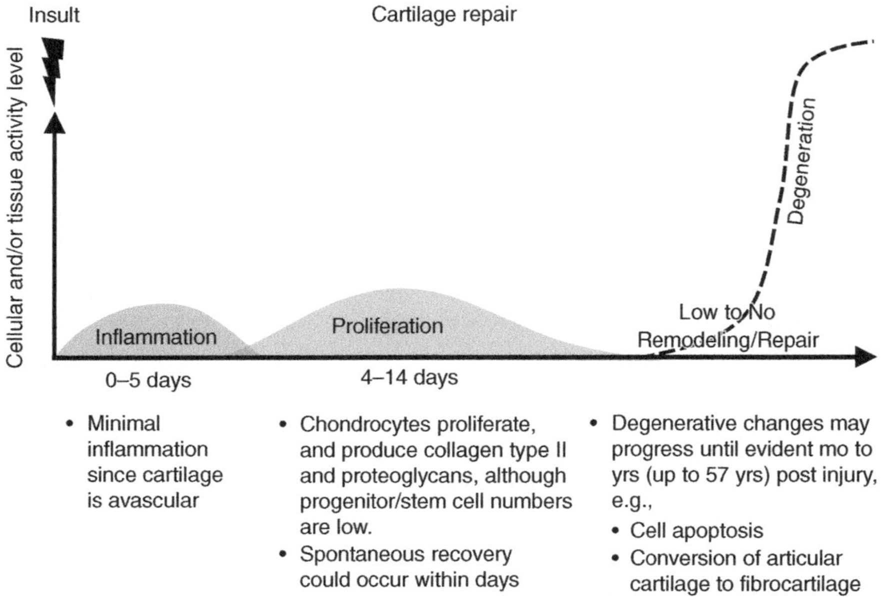

Figure 11.10 Phases of cartilage repair. The mechanisms underlying the degeneration are further explained in Figure 11.11.

Table 11.5 Limitations to Articular Cartilage Self-Repair

Avascular nature of cartilage	Limits infiltration of immune cells that clear damaged or necrosing cells (no early repair response).
	Limits influx of bone marrow-derived stem cells.
	Nutrients in synovial fluid required for repair and regeneration must rely on diffusion only, which is insufficient in deeper defects.
The low number of progenitor cells	Only a very small number of resident cartilage progenitor cells are present.
Weak recruitment signals	Signals that could stimulate chondrocytes of stem/progenitor cells to migrate to the injury site are weak or too limited.
Dense matrix	May hinder the migration of chondrocytes and cartilage progenitor cells.
Inhibitory nature of the matrix	Some matrix components, such as dermatan sulfate and other proteoglycans, can inhibit cell migration and adhesion, such as the migration of progenitor cells in synovial membranes.
Age >55 years	Reduced healing capacity due to increased cell senescence, reduced numbers of chondrocytes and stem/progenitor cells (which are low already), reduced chondrocyte proliferation and matrix synthesis.
Infection, inflammation, metabolic insufficiency	Interfere with repair and healing processes

cartilage. In a joint, there are also tissue-specific MSCPs in tissues surrounding the articular cartilage, including in synovium, synovial fluid, meniscus, fat pads, and perichondrium. Yet, the numbers of resident cartilage-derived progenitor cells in cartilage are quite low in number (Dowthwaite et al., 2004; Wei & Dai, 2021). The migration of MSCPs from surrounding joint tissues to the area of cartilage damage is restricted by the density of the extracellular matrix of cartilage, and some of the components of the matrix are inhibitory to cell migration (such as dermatan sulfate, a proteoglycan in hyaline cartilage). Although chondrocytes have been shown to produce endogenous recruitment signals for stem/progenitor cells (such as TGFβ, bone morphogenic factors, insulin-like growth factors, and fibroblast growth factors), their levels are too limited to recruit sufficient numbers of stem/progenitor cells for successful regeneration. Thus, intrinsic healing mechanisms are quite limited in cartilage.

If the cartilage damage is full thickness and extends to the subchondral bone, an extrinsic healing mechanism can help the healing process, due to blood seeping into the cartilage. This mechanism involves the development of a fibrin clot, which is later replaced by granulation tissue and fibrocartilage, which has different biomechanical properties and less gliding abilities than articular hyaline cartilage. Consequently, cartilage lesions represent a complex and challenging problem for surgeons and rehabilitation clinicians.

Capacity and extent of fibrocartilage self-repair

As with articular cartilage, the self-healing rate of fibrocartilage is slow and dependent upon the nature, size, and site of the injury. The periphery appears to heal more effectively, with the rate and extent of healing dependent on whether intrinsic or extrinsic healing mechanisms are operant, as noted earlier. A slower rate of healing appears to be superior to a faster rate of healing (Cole & Malek, 2004). The size of the defect also plays a major role in healing effectiveness. In a study performed on Shetland Ponies, small defects (3 mm) in menisci were not visible after 6 months; however, 9 and 15 mm defects were still apparent after that time frame (Convery, Akeson, & Keown, 1972).

Progression of cartilage degeneration after trauma

Figure 11.11 shows a slow progression from an initial cartilage injury to late-stage osteoarthritis that may be due to cumulative damage from fatigue loading, although perhaps also due to biochemical changes that contribute to slowly progressing apoptosis of chondrocytes (and their inability to replace themselves), induced even after a single high impact trauma (Driban et al., 2020). The latency time to late-stage osteoarthritis can be quite long. Late-stage post-traumatic osteoarthritis of the ankle, for example, may take up to 34 years, with a range of 6–57 years after the initial injury. This is because injury initiates a cascade of pathological processes in the cartilage, characterized most clearly by an active breakdown of the ECM of the articular cartilage, in particular collagen II and aggrecan. Early-stage osteoarthritis may spontaneously reverse itself, typically if the trauma is non-invasive (superficial layers only), or at the point of ADAMTS-mediated aggrecan degradation (ADAMTS is short for "a disintegrin and metalloproteinase with thrombospondin motifs"). However, late-stage osteoarthritis is at the point of no return when MMP3 mediated aggrecan and collagen type II degradation is evident typically in parallel with TGFβ activation. Additionally in the latter, chondrocytes have changed into a catabolic and hypertrophic phenotype, and/or a dedifferentiated phenotype or apoptotic state. This often occurs after damage in deeper layers of the cartilage or subchondral bone. An increase in inflammatory cytokines and mediators inhibits chondrocyte proliferation and the synthesis of extracellular matrix proteins. Overproduction of ROS results in further cell senescence or death. The subchondral bone becomes more permeable (particularly if the injury penetrates this layer) and osteogenic cytokines potentially leak into the cartilage (such as bone morphogenic proteins and TGFβ), changes that stimulate osteophyte formation.

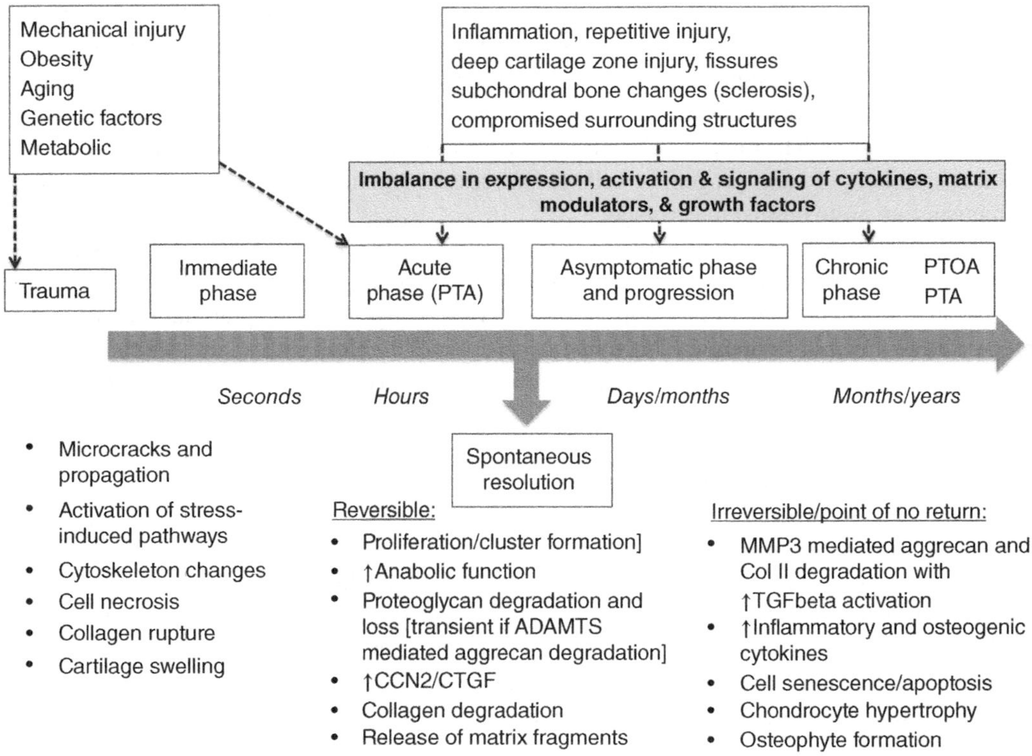

Figure 11.11 Primary initiating events of cartilage degeneration, contributors to early versus late osteoarthritis, main events occurring at each point. Abbreviations: ADAMTS = a disintegrin and metalloproteinase with thrombospondin motifs; CCN2/CTGF = cell communication network factor 2/ connective tissue growth factor; MMPs = matrix metalloproteinases; PTA = post-traumatic arthritis; PTOA = post-traumatic osteoarthritis; TGFβ = transforming growth factor-beta. Modified by Barbe from Punzi, L., Galozzi, P., Luisetto, R., Favero, M., Ramonda, R., Oliviero, F., & Scanu, A. (2016). Post-traumatic arthritis: Overview on pathogenic mechanisms and role of inflammation. *RMD Open*, 2(2), e000279. https://doi.org/10.1136/rmdopen-2016-000279.

Bone

Bone injury

Bone injuries vary from microdamage within the cortical or trabecular bone, contusions, fractures to full breaks. A bone contusion or bone bruise occurs after a small injury on the surface of a bone. They are fairly common and are most likely to occur in knees and heels. A bone bruise is typically the result of a direct hit to the bone (such as from a fall, accident, or direct hit to the bone) and includes symptoms of stiffness and swelling of a joint, difficulty using the injured joint, and tenderness and pain that lasts longer than a usual bruise. Depending on the injury, a nearby ligament may also be injured. They can last from a few days to a few months. In contrast, bone microdamage from fatigue failure can be divided into microfractures, diffuse bone damage, and linear microcracks (Figure 11.12) (Barbe et al., 2018; Robling & Turner, 2009; B. Wu, Zhang, et al., 2013; Z. Wu, Laneve, & Niebur, 2013). Such microdamage are tiny fractures in a bone caused when the force applied to a bone exceeds the strength of the bone, as also discussed in Chapter 7. This can be achieved through strenuous activities such as running, dance, military training, gymnastics, or repetitive overuse. Such microdamage has long been reported in different nonbiological,

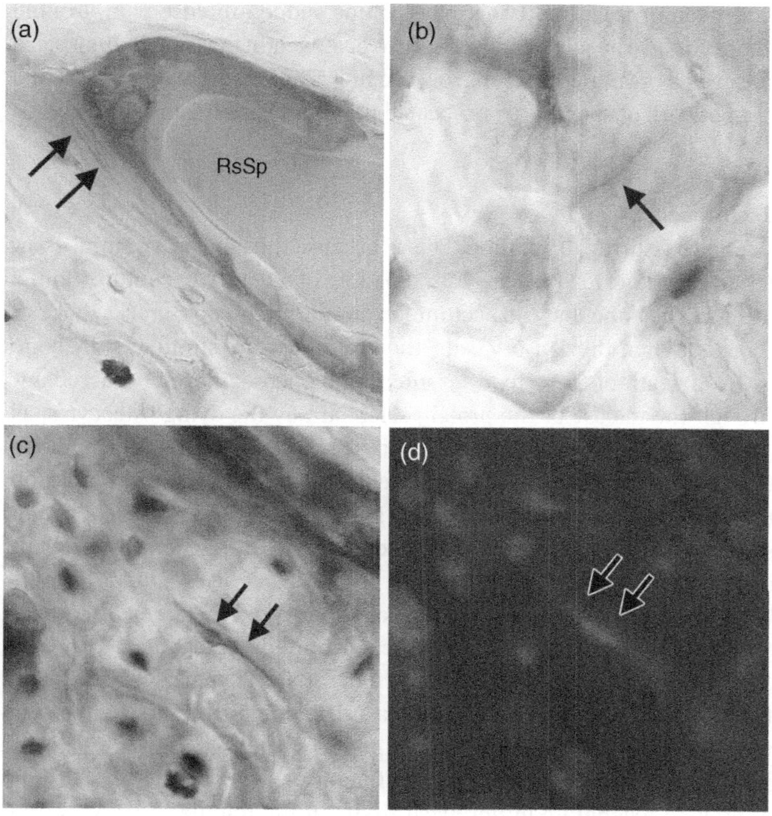

Figure 11.12 Examples of microcracks in forearm bone occurring as a consequence of prolonged reaching and grasping at high force and high repetition levels. (a) Small linear microcracks in trabeculae near an osteoclastic cutting resorptive space. (b–d) Microcracks in the outer region of cortical bone. (d) The same crack as panel C using orange fluorescence (for further verification). From Barbe, M. F., Massicotte, V. S., Assari, S., Monroy, M. A., Frara, N., Harris, M. Y., ... Popoff, S. N. (2018). Prolonged high force high repetition pulling induces osteocyte apoptosis and trabecular bone loss in distal radius, while low force high repetition pulling induces bone anabolism. *Bone, 110*, 267–283. doi:10.1016/j.bone.2018.02.014.

engineering materials as a result of fatigue and can signal imminent failure of the material. In a bone, as microcracks expand, they sever the connections between osteocytes located in the osteocytic canalicular network (see Chapter 3) by shearing their dendritic extensions. Microcracks disrupt osteocyte function and initiate their apoptosis (Dominguez & Agnew, 2019; B. Wu, Zhang, et al., 2013; Z. Wu, Laneve, & Niebur, 2013). A large number of microcracks reduce the quality of the bone and increase its risk for fracture (Dominguez & Agnew, 2019). Yet, their occurrence is important—the initiation and propagation of microdamage dissipate the energy of applied forces that would otherwise result in a larger catastrophic break of the entire bone (thereby, increasing bone toughness; refer to Chapter 7 for further explanation). Also, microcrack-induced osteocyte apoptosis releases chemical signals that activate osteoclastic bone remodeling in areas prone to microdamage (Barbe et al., 2018). In summary, microcracks serve an adaptive role.

A bone fracture, on the other hand, is a bone break that involves damage to a deeper area of bone. It commonly occurs because of car accidents, falls, or sports injuries, yet also as a result of low bone density and osteoporosis, which weaken the bones. There are many types of fractures, but the main categories are displaced, non-displaced, open, and closed fractures.

Signs and symptoms of a broken or fractured bone may include sudden intense pain, trouble using or moving the injured area or nearby joints, an inability to bear weight, a visibly out-of-place or misshapen limb or joint, as well as swelling, bruising, or bleeding. The intense pain persists due to the disruption of the dense network of sensory axons located in the periosteum and the trabecular bone compartment.

Capacity and extent of bone self-repair

Every bone is continuously renewed during its lifetime. This is because the bone is a natural composite tissue that is subjected to repetitive loading each day. Loading of a bone can rupture atomic bones and the crystal structures of the bone that can accumulate in submicroscopic cracks that can eventually become visible cracks. When the sensory cells, the osteocytes, are stimulated by bone loading, remodeling begins. Even death of the osteocytes after bone microdamage or macrodamage initiates remodeling through the release of the protein sclerostin by the dying osteocytes, as described previously by Barbe et al. (Barbe et al., 2018). As discussed in Chapter 3, during bone repair and remodeling, osteoclasts remove bone tissue and osteoblasts and rebuild it in a typically coupled manner. This, combined with a strong vascular supply and high numbers of mesenchymal stem/progenitor cells present within a bone, marrow provides bone with a generally excellent intrinsic capacity for repair and regeneration.

Microfractures, diffuse bone damage, and linear microcracks are repaired by targeted remodeling in both trabecular and cortical bones. Osteoclasts from the surrounding intact bone form cutting cones across the microfracture gap to reestablish the Haversian canals. Then osteoblasts follow to produce new bone that fills the defect, and when the osteoblasts become surrounded by the new matrix, they convert to osteocytes. If the microfractures and apoptotic osteocytes are not healed/replaced, increased bone porosity may result, enhancing bone fragility.

The goal of fracture healing is to regenerate mineralized tissue in the fracture healing to the point that mechanical strength is restored in the bone. After a fracture, the temporal steps of bone healing occur in three main phases (inflammation, repair, and remodeling) similar to other tissues. These steps can be further divided into six sub-steps: fracture, hematoma, inflammation, fibrovascular (also known as soft callus formation), bone formation (also known as hard callus formation), and remodeling. These phases are depicted more simply in Figure 11.13, and in more detail in Figure 11.14. In brief, after an injury or disruption of the bone or its surrounding periosteum, a hematoma is formed at the site of fracture or break that provides an immediate provisional matrix. At this point, platelet degranulation releases chemokines to recruit inflammatory cells to the region. The inflammatory phase induces the reparative stage characterized by mesenchymal cell expansion and migration from the periosteum and endosteum, and angiogenesis. A soft callus is formed that consists of fibrous tissue and unmineralized matrix and blood vessels. This granulation tissue then converts into a cartilaginous callus that later ossifies, via either endochondral or intramembranous ossification mechanisms. During the remodeling phase, osteoclasts resorb primary bone and the process of remodeling restores bone shape and structure. The periosteal bone callus is converted into the mature bone and any unnecessary callus is resorbed.

In more detail, fracture healing begins with hemostasis (hopefully, or there is a drop in survival rate) and then a hematoma spanning the area of disruption in the periosteum, bone itself, and marrow region (Figure 11.14b). This is followed by an inflammatory reaction in which a variety of immune cells invade the region to clear the damaged cells and tissues (including T and B cells, mast cells, macrophages, eosinophils if there is a bacterial or viral invasion, and neutrophils)

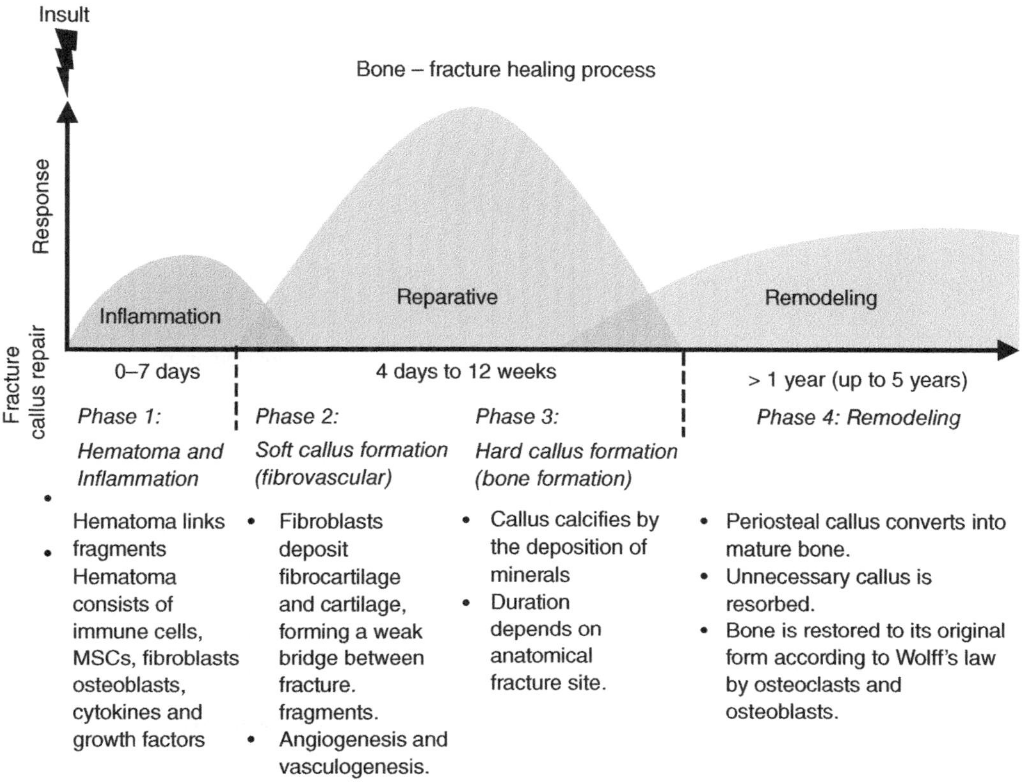

Figure 11.13 Phases of bone repair after a fracture.

(Figure 11.14c). They release cytokines that are either pro-inflammatory or growth factors, as well as complement factors, that will be chemotactic for mesenchymal stem/progenitor cells and endothelial cells, indicating the onset of the fibrovascular phase of soft callus formation (Figure 11.14d). During this phase, endothelial cells are involved in revascularization via angiogenesis (sprouting of nearby vessels) and de novo vasculogenesis that is important at this point since the tissues in the region of injury have lost their blood and therefore nutrient supply. Factors made and released during this phase include HIF-1alpha (hypoxia-inducible factor 1 alpha, a transcription factor that promotes angiogenesis and erythropoiesis), VEGF (also involved in angiogenesis), and MMPs (involved in tissue degradation to remove the hematoma). Deficiencies in angiogenesis result in delayed or insufficient fracture repair. Various factors are produced that aid the transition of mesenchymal progenitor/stem cells into osteoblasts, chondroblasts, fibroblasts, myocytes, or adipocytes (in other words, all of the cells needed to rebuild the periosteum, bone, entheses, myotendinous junctions, and marrow). During the next phase, the fibrocartilagenous soft callus is converted into a mineralized bony callus (Figures 11.13 and 11.14e). Endochondral and intramembranous ossification processes are involved at this point, based on if there is increased motion in the healing fracture site or a stabilized fracture, respectively. Lastly, remodeling occurs in a coupled osteoblast–osteoclast synthesis and lysis process in which immature woven bone is converted into mature lamellar bone (Figure 11.13f). This last step is the point in which the bone is remodeled based on its imposed forces.

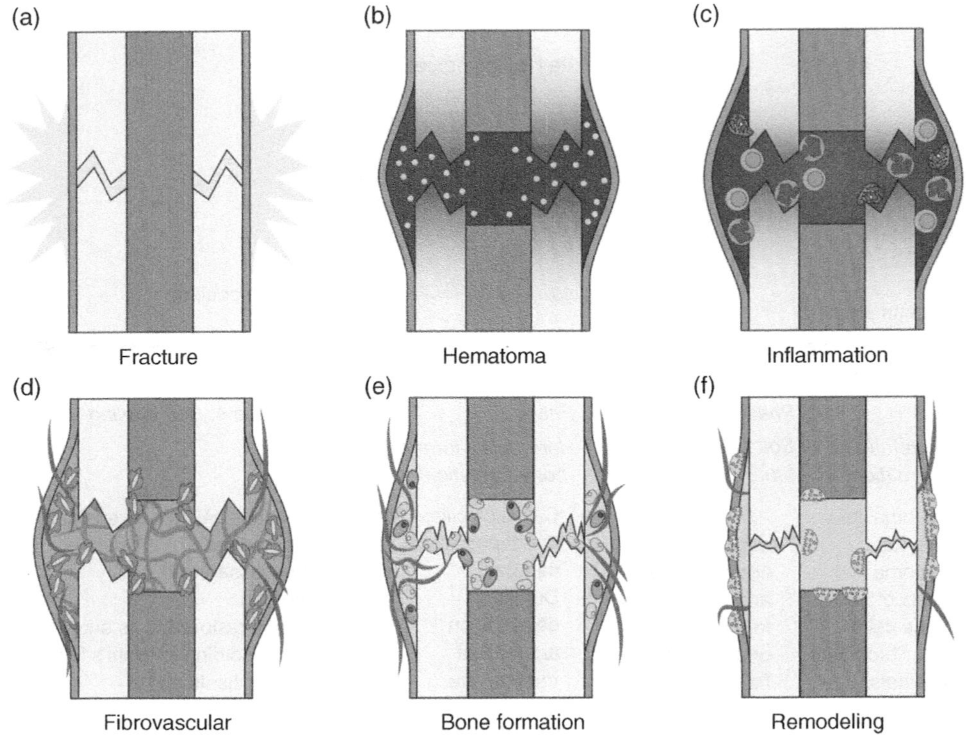

Figure 11.14 Fracture healing is a temporally defined process. (a) Fracture, showing disruption of the periosteum and bone, (b) Hematoma which serves as a provisional matrix (~0–3 days) post-fracture), (c) Inflammatory phase (~3–5 days), (d) Fibrovascular phase (soft callus formation with fibrous tissue, unmineralized matrix, and angiogenesis, ~2–3 weeks), (e) Hard callus formation/secondary bone formation (6–12 weeks), and (f) Remodeling and bone healing (up to 5 years for restoration to original form). From Bahney, C. S., Zondervan, R. L., Allison, P., Theologis, A., Ashley, J. W., Ahn, J., . . . Hankenson, K. D. (2019). Cellular biology of fracture healing. *Journal of Orthopaedic Research: Official Publication of the Orthopaedic Research Society*, 37(1), 35–50. https://doi.org/10.1002/jor.24170. Wiley.

The length of the healing process in bone is dependent on a number of factors (several of which are summarized in Table 11.6). Although a typical time frame is approximately 6–12 weeks, its original structure and full biomechanical strength may not be fully restored for up to 5 years after the initial bone break or fracture. Not surprisingly, smaller and simpler fractures will heal better than the more complex and involved fractures (such as comminuted or displaced fractures). Bones of the upper limb tend to heal more quickly than those of the lower limb because of less loading (Mirhadi, Ashwood, & Karagkevrekis, 2013). Trabecular bone tends to heal more quickly than compact bone, due to the larger area of bony contact and an increased number of bone cells present. Furthermore, bone healing depends not only on the magnitude and type of loading but also on the rate and frequency of cyclic loading. These parameters may improve the quality of the viscoelastic properties of the material constituents of bone (Epari, Duda, & Thompson, 2010; Xi et al., 2020). The rate of compressive loading on bone has also been found to enhance bone healing (Goodship, Cunningham, & Kenwright, 1998; Hente, Fuchtmeier, Schlegel, Ernstberger, & Perren, 2004). Lastly, while some studies show that bones adapt their strength and mass to keep the strain caused by physiological loads close to a set point (Frost, 1994), a Damage-Repair Theory better explains catabolic changes observed in overloaded trabecular

Table 11.6 Factors Modifying Bone Self-Repair, Growth, and Maintenance

Factors modifying the load applied to bone	Factors modifying the ability of bone to resist load or self-repair
• Biomechanical factors (including ground reaction force magnitude and rates, acceleration/shock, anthropometry and alignment, running-gait kinematics) • Training factors (including duration and frequency of training sessions, and running intensity/speed). • Muscle strength and endurance • Training surfaces and terrain • Shoes and inserts (orthoses and insoles) – can alter stability and kinematics • Physical activity history (if osteocytes have acclimated to a particular loading force, more force is needed to stimulate bone deposition).	• Deficiencies in revascularization (e.g., from aging, surgery, type II diabetes mellitus, smoking—delayed or insufficient fracture repair. • Aging—Decreased callus formation + inhibited angiogenesis, reduced VEGF and MMP9, fewer or senescent stem cells. • Chronic Inflammation (e.g., from rheumatoid arthritis, Crohn's disease)—Increased systemic inflammatory cytokines that increase osteoclastogenesis (and therefore bone resorption), or cause an imbalance in M1/M2 macrophages. • Medication use that influences bone (i.e., long-term nonsteroidal anti-inflammatory drug use or glucocorticoid use). • Diet and nutrition (including eating behaviors, and caloric, calcium, and vitamin D intake). • Physical activity history • Endocrine status and hormones (including the age of menarche and menstrual status) • Genetics or bone disease • Large deficits that are hard to repair

Modified from Warden, S.J., Davis, I. S., & Fredericson, M. (2014). Management and prevention of bone stress injuries in long-distance runners. *The Journal of Orthopaedic and Sports Physical Therapy, 44*(10), 749–765. doi: 10.2519/jospt.2014.5334. Epub 2014 Aug 7. PMID: 25103133.

and cortical bone and postulates that damage accumulates in the bone if the loading is so high that self-repair mechanisms cannot keep pace with the level of damage or overload-induced resorption (Li, Li, Zou, & Fok, 2011). At this point, osteopenia and osteoporosis (and fragility) become evident in the bone.

Bone repair and maintenance require innervation

Although a fairly new field and still under investigation, the somatosensory nervous system is generally believed to play a role in mediating the anabolic response of bone to physiological mechanical loading. Several studies have established that neurons communicate with cells in the bone microenvironment and regulate bone homeostasis (Elefteriou, 2018). Both the periosteum and trabecular bone compartments contain a dense network of TrkA (the high-affinity receptor for nerve growth factor)-positive sensory fibers that are responsive to mechanical stimuli (Takegahara et al., 2006). These sensory neurons sense and respond to mechanical stimuli. A study in mice investigating the role of sensory neurons during forelimb axial loading demonstrated their importance in potentiating the anabolic response to mechanical stimuli to achieve maximal load-induced bone formation (Tomlinson et al., 2017).

Sensory denervation with capsaicin treatment reduces neuropeptides levels in the sciatic nerve and hind leg long bones (e.g., Substance P and CGRP), and also leads to reduced tibial bone mineral density and strength. Similarly, peripheral nerve injury that also causes bone denervation leads to significant bone loss and increased fracture risk in the denervated bone. Evidence from fracture studies suggests a distinct role of Substance P in regulating the bone formation and resorption processes of fracture healing. The density of Substance P fibers changes temporally in areas of bone formation and bone resorption. Specifically, Substance P fibers that co-expressed the nerve growth marker GAP-43 have been shown to sprout into the fracture site on Day 3 post-fracture, and then remain in the periosteum until cortical bone bridging has occurred (day 21). The density of Substance P fibers remains increased until resorptive remodeling of the fracture callus is complete (day 35). On the other hand, although the general trend is that sensory innervation is supportive of bone health, aberrant overactivity of sensory neurons can increase pain and may also lead to pathological conditions, such as ossification of the soft tissue, due to the osteogenic properties of sensory neuropeptides (Burr & Allen, 2019). Yet, more information is needed on this topic, particularly as related to bone and joint pain.

Nerve

Nerve injury

Typical modes of peripheral nerve injury include compression, overstretching, contusion, and frank ruptures. Repeated compression and overstretching are the most common causes of nerve damage. Several other modes of nerve injury include crush, persistent inflammatory or immunological causes, chronic constriction injury (such as with the median nerve in the carpal tunnel or compression of a nerve root by a ruptured and prolapsed vertebral disc), and vascular disease.

Clinical signs of nerve damage include acute pain, chronic pain, loss of sensation and discrimination, declines in nerve conduction velocity, and motor dysfunction. Examples of motor dysfunction following nerve injury include muscle weakness, atrophy, or paralysis. Abnormal sensations, such as hyperalgesia (i.e., increased sensitivity to painful stimuli) and mechanical allodynia (i.e., increased sensitivity to typically non-noxious stimuli), may also develop. The latter symptoms are hallmarks of neuropathic pain discussed previously in Chapter 4.

With regard to the pain, both nerve injury as well as repeated or prolonged activation of nociceptors (sensory axons that convey pain information), can lead to altered gene expression within these neurons so that the density, distribution, and even expression type of ion channels on the neuronal membrane change. For example, repeated exposure to inflammatory mediators or nerve injury can lead to increased density of voltage-gated sodium and calcium channels on nociceptor terminals. This change results in a dramatic increase in abnormal action potentials and subsequent neuropathic pain (Gold & Gebhart, 2010; Yan et al., 2017). Both injury and inflammation can also induce spontaneous activity in the nerve axon itself and then enhanced or chronic pain (Bove et al., 2019). A large aggregation of various ion channels on the neuronal membrane can also contribute to spontaneous nerve activity.

Injury-induced nerve inflammation

Biochemical signs of mild-to-moderate peripheral nerve damage include increased production and release of a variety of mediators of inflammation, pain, and vasodilation. For example, IL-1, TNFα, IL-6, bradykinins, and other inflammatory mediators as listed in Table 11.1, are released by injured nerves. This "inflammatory soup" contributes to further inflammation by recruiting macrophages intraneurally. These inflammatory mediators enhance pain by sensitizing nociceptors through the activation of the neuron or by lowering the threshold for firing in the larger nerve trunk. Injured or sensitized nerve terminals increase their production and release of nociceptor-related neuropeptides, including Substance P, vasoactive intestinal peptide, and calcitonin gene-related protein (CGRP), each of which contributes to vasodilation and thus to immune cell infiltration, as well as further sensitization of nerve terminals. Schwann cells also increase their production of bradykinins, and thus vasodilation and inflammatory cell infiltration. Neural growth factors, such as nerve growth factor, when upregulated in cells and tissues surrounding nociceptor endings also drive gene expression of the nociceptor-related neuropeptides. This change may lead to a vicious cycle of inflammation and sensitization, as seen in chronic pain conditions.

Capacity and extent of peripheral nerve repair

More extensive nerve damage in which the axons are transected, extensively crushed, or ruptured induces a stereotyped neuronal degenerative response known as Wallerian degeneration ("Augustus Volney Waller (1816–1870), 1969"). General steps are listed in Figure 11.15 and diagramed in Figure 11.16. After nerve transection, there is an initial lag phase of 6–24 hr in a neuron's response to the axotomy. During this phase, there is a rapid short-term calcium ion wave (that aids in the sealing of nerve stump endings), a loss of axonal current, and the loss of axoplasmic flow of proteins from the cell body to distant axonal regions. The latter results in a depletion of several key proteins in the distal axonal stumps that are typically transported from the cell body down the axons. Depletion of one protein, nicotinamide adenine dinucleotide, leads to the loss of ATP, then an energy failure and an increase in ROS levels and calpain-mediated proteolysis of the axonal structural proteins. Depletion of another protein, a Wallerian degeneration inhibitor called nicotinamide mononucleotide adenylyltransferase 2, activates proteins that trigger axonal dieback (Coleman & Hoke, 2020).

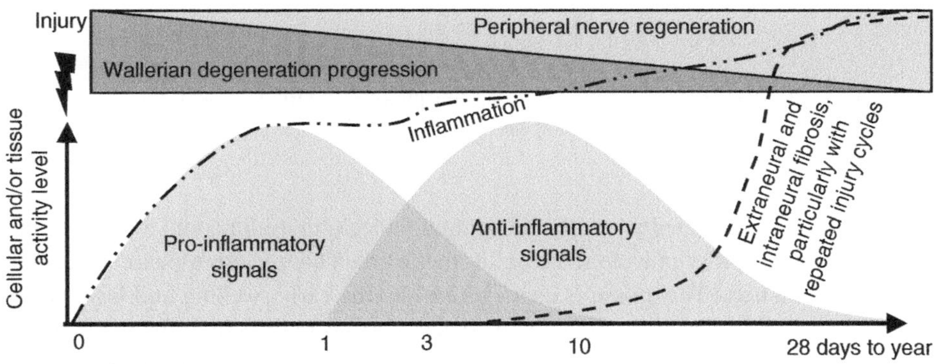

Acute phase:

- ↑Pro-inflammatory gene and cytokine release
- Schwann cell activation and myelin release
- Resident macrophage activation and M1 macrophage influx
- Axonal and myelin breakdown
- Rapid Wallerian degeneration
- Synthesis of growth-promoting proteins by neurons
- Neurotrophic factor release by Schwann cells

Chronic phase:

- Resolution of inflammation
- Macrophage efflux (exit) from nerve, or return to quiescence
- Injury-type dependent axonal regeneration
- Axon regrowth
- Axon remyelination by Schwann cells
- Intraneural and extraneural fibrosis may develop, if induction continues or dependent on level of injury

Figure 11.15 Main steps of Wallerian degeneration and nerve regeneration. The acute phases of inflammation, proliferation, and remodeling (solid shapes) are extended by repeated injury cycles (depicted as dashed lines). Figure modified from Siqueira Mietto, B., et al. (2015). Role of IL-10 in resolution of inflammation and functional recovery after peripheral nerve injury. *Journal of Neuroscience, 35*(50), 16431–16442. Article ID 251204. https://doi.org/10.1155/2015/251204.

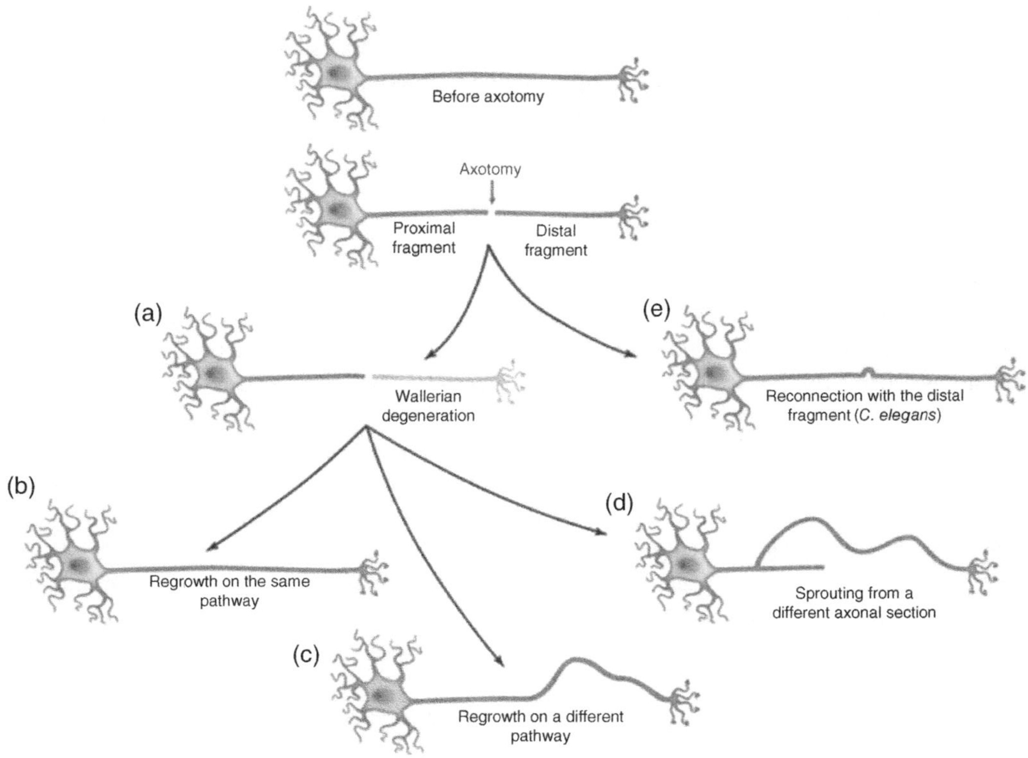

Figure 11.16 Main steps in the Wallerian degeneration. From Hilliard, M.A. (2009). Axonal degeneration and regeneration: a mechanistic tug-of-war. *Journal of Neurochemistry* 108(1), 23–32. https://doi.org/10.1111/j.1471-4159.2008.05754.x Wiley.

A second calcium ion wave is elicited when the mitochondria begin to dysfunction, a change that destabilizes the microtubules that provide structure to the axons. The execution phase of axonal degeneration then commences. This phase is characterized by the early swelling and beading of axons, followed by catastrophic fragmentation and die-back of axons to the site of the transection. This is accompanied by Schwann cell necrosis and myelin degradation. Simultaneous infiltration of macrophages and other phagocytes aids the loss of Schwann cells and axons by phagocytosing even partly injured cells in an effort to debride the injury site. Axonal degeneration can also occur by apoptosis and pruning mechanisms (a loss of local neurotrophic factors, such as nerve growth factor) (Gamage et al., 2017). This execution phase can last weeks to months and sometimes even years. If not reversed, the nerve's target atrophies due to a lack of neural input (Llobet Rosell & Neukomm, 2019), with the best-known example of this is muscle atrophy after long-term nerve damage.

Fortunately, the clearance of the aforementioned inhibitory debris in the injured peripheral nerve leads to an environment that supports axonal regrowth with weeks to months post-injury. The remaining Schwann cells (myelinating and non myelinating types) undergo extensive reprogramming post-injury in order to promote and guide axonal repair (Nocera & Jacob, 2020). Within weeks post injury, these cells transform into a repair phenotype with down-regulation of pro-myelinating genes and the *de novo* expression of regeneration genes. This reprogramming involves the upregulation of multiple transcription mechanisms that control and regulate repair (Moreau & Boucher, 2020). The repair type Schwann cells begin to proliferate, produce and secrete growth-related neurotrophins, extend long parallel processes, and align in tracts to guide future axonal regrowth (Moreau & Boucher, 2020). Axons in the proximal stump of the transected nerve begin to sprout and extend toward the target, guided by the new Schwann cells tracts. Thereafter, there is a redifferentiation of the Schwann cells into myelinating types that then remyelinate the newly regenerated axons, leading to a restoration of physiological function (Moreau & Boucher, 2020). Although this entire process may take months to years to reach completion, successful reinnervation of the target end-organ is possible in many circumstances.

However, nerve repair does not always result in a restorative repair, similar to several previously mentioned tissues. Chronic inflammation leads to the development of fibrotic tissue in extraneural and intraneural tissues (Barbe, Harris, et al., 2021; Bove, Harris, Zhao, & Barbe, 2016; Bove, Weissner, & Barbe, 2009). This can occur as a result of a persistent presence of inflammatory cytokines or profibrotic macrophages subtypes. Such nerve fibrosis can contribute to nerve compression and tethering to paraneural tissues, and thus further injury and inflammation, particularly if the fibrosed nerve lies within a constrained space, such as the median nerve within carpal tunnel (Clark et al., 2003; Clark, Al-Shatti, Barr, Amin, & Barbe, 2004).

The degree of functional recovery after peripheral nerve injury also depends on the extent to which the connective tissue investments of a nerve are disrupted at the injury site. A more extensive rupture requires significant fibroblastic repair of these connective tissue investments. A greater degree of fibrous stroma (i.e., nerve fibrosis) and a lower number of axons occur after inelastic and rupture injuries than with elastic or crush injuries (Yeoh, Warner, Eli, & Mahan, 2020). This appears to be the result of a higher incidence of misdirection of growing axons through the fibrosed region. Long-term loss of axons depletes the end organ of neurotrophic growth factors needed for homeostasis, leading to atrophy of the target end organ. For example, it is difficult to rescue atrophied muscles after long-term denervation due to loss of the motor end plates or the replacement of muscle fibers with non-contractile fatty or collagenous connective tissues (Barbe, Testa, et al., 2021; Fisher et al., 2015; Hodges & Danneels, 2019). Other tissues can be similarly negatively affected after long-term denervation (as discussed for bone in previous Section "Bone repair and maintenance requires innervation").

Effects of Continued Tissue Loading on the Healing Process

Mechanical parameters are known to be an important stimulus for tissue formation during healing; however, the transduction from mechanical stimuli to cellular activity is not completely understood (Ghiasi, Chen, Vaziri, Rodriguez, & Nazarian, 2017; Isaksson, 2012). Several authors have examined the mechanical loads favoring the growth of various tissues (Carter, Beaupre, Giori, & Helms, 1998; Claes & Heigele, 1999). According to a few authors, the mechanical environment that favors the growth of specific tissues is the same in which the tissue performs its normal function. For example, a bone forms best in a low stress-low strain environment, cartilage forms under a low strain, high compression environment, while connective tissues and fibrocartilage form in high strain regions.

Overexertion is an initiating and a propagating injury stimulus in MSDs, such as overuse injuries. The authors have speculated that the mechanisms leading to tissue repair may be hindered by the continued cycle of tissue trauma in repetitive motion injury (Barbe & Popoff, 2020; Gallagher & Schall Jr., 2017). Although cumulative loading of viscoelastic tissues in the short term may increase the likelihood that applied loads will result in tissue injury, it becomes an overexertion event that initiates a cyclical and perhaps persistent inflammatory response. Phagocytic cell infiltration, an increase in the number of free radicals, and induction of inflammatory cytokines by

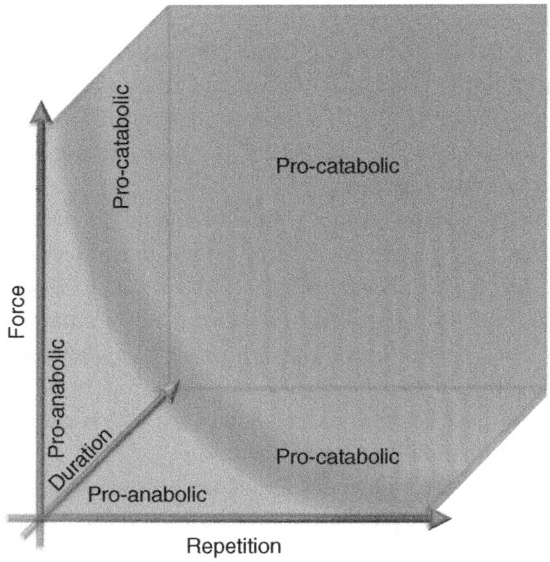

Figure 11.17 Schematic diagram demonstrating that interactions of force, repetition, and duration of tissue loading can elicit a pro-anabolic response up to a point at which the combination of these factors exceeds a threshold resulting in a net catabolic response due to tissue fatigue failure. The point at which the threshold is crossed varies from one individual to another, as do the factors that influence its location (including, age, gender, genetic background, metabolic disease, and presence of chronic inflammatory disorders). Modified from Barbe, M. F., & Popoff, S. N. (2020). Occupational activities: Factors that tip the balance from bone accrual to bone loss. *Exercise and Sport Sciences Reviews*, 48(2), 59–66. https://doi.org/10.1249/JES.0000000000000217. https://pubmed.ncbi.nlm.nih.gov/32004169.

persistent injury and inflammation can lead to tissue degeneration, such as tissue necrosis, pathological tissue reorganization, and subsequent biomechanical failure. Repeated bouts of injury, inflammation and fibrosis eventually contribute to decreasing tissue tolerance and increasing catabolism over time (Figure 11.17). At that point, lower levels of exertion lead to tissue damage that can further reduce tissue tolerance and functional performance.

Summary

Many *in vivo* injuries and disorders affect more than one part of the musculoskeletal system (e.g., tendons, ligaments, muscles, cartilages, bones and nerves) (NIOSH, 2011). Acute tissue injury results in micro- or macro-damage, followed by acute inflammatory cell infiltration, and usually, a rapid progression into healing. The healing rate after this acute injury is affected mainly by the extent of the injury and a tissue's individual vascular and progenitor/stem cell characteristics. Estimated healing times for individual tissues after acute injury are presented in Table 11.7. These are estimates only as further research is warranted to confirm these times in both individual and composite tissues.

Variations in healing time are likely to be affected by fatigue failure mechanisms with repeated stress and strain on the tissues during movement. The responses of tissues to repeated injury have similar underpinnings but they are exacerbated by repetitive stress and strain and repeated exposure to inflammatory cytokines, some of which are cytotoxic and some of which are pro-fibrogenic, each of which further weakens the tissues (Barr & Barbe, 2002; Kjaer, 2004). Thus, dependent on the type and extent of trauma, not only are tissues subject to microdamage from an acute event as summarized in Table 11.8, but this damage can be propagated by repeated loading and heightened by cytotoxic

Table 11.7 Estimated Healing Times After Acute Injury

Tissue	Time	Grade injury	Variation by grade injury
Skin	12 days–2 weeks		
Tendon	3 weeks to 1 year, depending on extent and type of injury	Tendinitis Tendinosis Laceration/rupture	3–7 weeks 1–6 months Months to 1 year
Ligament	3 days to 1 year, depending on the extent of the injury	Grade 1 Grade 2 Grade 3	0–3 days 3 weeks–6 months 5 weeks–1 year
Muscle	1 week–6 months, depending on the extent of the injury	Grade 1 Grade 2 Grade 3	1–4 weeks 3–12 weeks 1–6 months
Articular Cartilage	Spontaneous in days, or low to none		
Bone fracture	6 weeks–12 weeks to bony callus, but up to 5 years for full restoration		
Nerve	28 days–1 years		

Table 11.8 Effects of Repeated Fatigue Loading on Tissue Healing and Repair Processes

Tissue	Inflammation	Proliferation	Remodeling/maturation	Failure indices
Tendon	Prolonged, persistent, or cyclical	Higher cell density in tendon proper and thickened sheaths (fibroplasia)	Increased ground substance (i.e., fibrosis), excessive vascularization and nerve ending ingrowth, disorganized collagen fibrils with an overabundance of weaker type III.	Kinks that increase in density; tear propagation to rupture
Ligament	Needs more investigation	Higher cell density	Same as for tendon	Tear propagation to rupture
Muscle	Prolonged, persistent, or cyclical	Higher cell density between myofibers and thickened sheaths	The remarkable ability of self-repair, yet, often develops excessive collagen deposition between myofibers (i.e., fibrosis) with repeated loading	Tear propagation to rupture
Cartilage	Prolonged, but low since avascular	Insufficient for the replacement of damaged cells	Mostly degenerative	Microcrack propagation, cell apoptosis, and loss of matrix
Bone	Prolonged, persistent, or cyclical	If balanced, both osteoblasts and osteoclasts proliferate. If pathologically imbalanced, osteoclasts show higher density.	The remarkable ability of self-repair; yet, if osteoclasts show higher number and activity than osteoblasts, osteopenia to osteoporosis can result	Microcrack propagation
Nerve	Prolonged, persistent, or cyclical	Higher density of fibroblasts—intra- and extra-neural	Delayed regrowth and remyelination as long as inflammation persists	Demyelination to axonal dieback

mediators that further damage the tissues, increased macrophage produced and released proteases that degrade the tissues, and by the deposition of weaker matrix materials. Each makes tissues even more susceptible to damage with repeated loading—in strong support of a fatigue failure process.

Bibliography

Allen, D. G., Lamb, G. D., & Westerblad, H. (2008). Skeletal muscle fatigue: Cellular mechanisms. *Physiological Reviews*, *88*(1), 287–332.

Almada, A. E., & Wagers, A. J. (2016). Molecular circuitry of stem cell fate in skeletal muscle regeneration, ageing and disease. *Nature Reviews. Molecular Cell Biology*, *17*(5), 267–279. https://doi.org/10.1038/nrm.2016.7

Amici, D. R., Pinal-Fernandez, I., Mazala, D. A., Lloyd, T. E., Corse, A. M., Christopher-Stine, L., . . . Chin, E. R. (2017). Calcium dysregulation, functional calpainopathy, and endoplasmic reticulum stress in sporadic inclusion body myositis. *Acta Neuropathologica Communications*, *5*(1), 24. https://doi.org/10.1186/s40478-017-0427-7

Arango Duque, G., & Descoteaux, A. (2014). Macrophage cytokines: Involvement in immunity and infectious diseases. *Frontiers in Immunology*, *5*, 491. https://doi.org/10.3389/fimmu.2014.00491

Augustus Volney Waller (1816–1870) (1969). Wallerian degeneration. *JAMA*, *208*(13), 2469–2470. Retrieved from https://www.ncbi.nlm.nih.gov/pubmed/4891558

Bahney, C. S., Zondervan, R. L., Allison, P., Theologis, A., Ashley, J. W., Ahn, J., . . . Hankenson, K. D. (2019). Cellular biology of fracture healing. *Journal of Orthopaedic Research: Official Publication of the Orthopaedic Research Society*, *37*(1), 35–50. https://doi.org/10.1002/jor.24170

Barbe, M. F., Harris, M. Y., Cruz, G. E., Amin, M., Billett, N. M., Dorotan, J. T., . . . Bove, G. M. (2021). Key indicators of repetitive overuse-induced neuromuscular inflammation and fibrosis are prevented by manual therapy in a rat model. *BMC Musculoskeletal Disorders*, *22*(1), 417. https://doi.org/10.1186/s12891-021-04270-0

Barbe, M. F., Hilliard, B. A., Amin, M., Harris, M. Y., Hobson, L. J., Cruz, G. E., . . . Popoff, S. N. (2020a). Blocking CTGF/CCN2 reverses neural fibrosis and sensorimotor declines in a rat model of overuse-induced median mononeuropathy. *Journal of Orthopaedic Research: Official Publication of the Orthopaedic Research Society*, *38*(11), 2396–2408. https://doi.org/10.1002/jor.24709

Barbe, M. F., Hilliard, B. A., Amin, M., Harris, M. Y., Hobson, L. J., Cruz, G. E., & Popoff, S. N. (2020b). Blocking CTGF/CCN2 reduces established skeletal muscle fibrosis in a rat model of overuse injury. *The FASEB Journal*, *34*(5), 6554–6569. https://doi.org/10.1096/fj.202000240RR

Barbe, M. F., Hilliard, B. A., Fisher, P. W., White, A. R., Delany, S. P., Iannarone, V. J., . . . Popoff, S. N. (2020). Blocking substance P signaling reduces musculotendinous and dermal fibrosis and sensorimotor declines in a rat model of overuse injury. *Connective Tissue Research*, *61*(6), 604–619. https://doi.org/10.1080/03008207.2019.1653289

Barbe, M. F., Massicotte, V. S., Assari, S., Monroy, M. A., Frara, N., Harris, M. Y., . . . Popoff, S. N. (2018). Prolonged high force high repetition pulling induces osteocyte apoptosis and trabecular bone loss in distal radius, while low force high repetition pulling induces bone anabolism. *Bone*, *110*, 267–283. https://doi.org/10.1016/j.bone.2018.02.014

Barbe, M. F., & Popoff, S. N. (2020). Occupational activities: Factors that tip the balance from bone accrual to bone loss. *Exercise and Sport Sciences Reviews*, *48*(2), 59–66. https://doi.org/10.1249/JES.0000000000000217

Barbe, M. F., Testa, C. L., Cruz, G. E., Frara, N. A., Tiwari, E., Hobson, L. J., . . . Ruggieri, M. R., Sr. (2021). Nerve transfer for restoration of lower motor neuron-lesioned bladder function.

Part 2: Correlation between histological changes and nerve evoked contractions. *American Journal of Physiology. Regulatory, Integrative and Comparative Physiology*, *320*(6), R897–R915. https://doi.org/10.1152/ajpregu.00300.2020

Barr, A. E., & Barbe, M. F. (2002). Pathophysiological tissue changes associated with repetitive movement: A review of the evidence. *Physical Therapy*, *82*(2), 173–187. https://doi.org/10.1093/ptj/82.2.173

Barr, A. E., & Barbe, M. F. (2004). Inflammation reduces physiological tissue tolerance in the development of work-related musculoskeletal disorders. *Journal of Electromyography and Kinesiology*, *14*(1), 77–85. https://doi.org/10.1016/j.jelekin.2003.09.008

Binder-Markey, B. I., Broda, N. M., & Lieber, R. L. (2020). Intramuscular anatomy drives collagen content variation within and between muscles. *Frontiers in Physiology*, *11*, 293. https://doi.org/10.3389/fphys.2020.00293

Bove, G. M., Delany, S. P., Hobson, L., Cruz, G. E., Harris, M. Y., Amin, M., . . . Barbe, M. F. (2019). Manual therapy prevents onset of nociceptor activity, sensorimotor dysfunction, and neural fibrosis induced by a volitional repetitive task. *Pain*, *160*(3), 632–644. https://doi.org/10.1097/j.pain.0000000000001443

Bove, G. M., Harris, M. Y., Zhao, H., & Barbe, M. F. (2016). Manual therapy as an effective treatment for fibrosis in a rat model of upper extremity overuse injury. *Journal of the Neurological Sciences*, *361*, 168–180. https://doi.org/10.1016/j.jns.2015.12.029

Bove, G. M., Weissner, W., & Barbe, M. F. (2009). Long lasting recruitment of immune cells and altered epi-perineurial thickness in focal nerve inflammation induced by complete Freund's adjuvant. *Journal of Neuroimmunology*, *213*(1–2), 26–30. https://doi.org/10.1016/j.jneuroim.2009.06.005

Burr, D. B., & Allen, M. R. (2019). *Basic and applied bone biology* (2nd ed.). London: Elsevier/Academic Press.

Butterfield, T. A., Best, T. M., & Merrick, M. A. (2006). The dual roles of neutrophils and macrophages in inflammation: A critical balance between tissue damage and repair. *Journal of Athletic Training*, *41*(4), 457–465. Retrieved from https://www.ncbi.nlm.nih.gov/pubmed/17273473

Carp, S. J., Barr, A. E., & Barbe, M. F. (2008). Serum biomarkers as signals for risk and severity of work-related musculoskeletal injury. *Biomarkers in Medicine*, *2*(1), 67–79. https://doi.org/10.2217/17520363.2.1.67

Carter, D. R., Beaupre, G. S., Giori, N. J., & Helms, J. A. (1998). Mechanobiology of skeletal regeneration. *Clinical Orthopaedics and Related Research*, *355 Suppl*, S41–S55. https://doi.org/10.1097/00003086-199810001-00006

Claes, L. E., & Heigele, C. A. (1999). Magnitudes of local stress and strain along bony surfaces predict the course and type of fracture healing. *Journal of Biomechanics*, *32*(3), 255–266. https://doi.org/10.1016/s0021-9290(98)00153-5

Clark, B. D., Al-Shatti, T. A., Barr, A. E., Amin, M., & Barbe, M. F. (2004). Performance of a high-repetition, high-force task induces carpal tunnel syndrome in rats. *The Journal of Orthopaedic and Sports Physical Therapy*, *34*(5), 244–253. https://doi.org/10.2519/jospt.2004.34.5.244

Clark, B. D., Barr, A. E., Safadi, F. F., Beitman, L., Al-Shatti, T., Amin, M., . . . Barbe, M. F. (2003). Median nerve trauma in a rat model of work-related musculoskeletal disorder. *Journal of Neurotrauma*, *20*(7), 681–695. https://doi.org/10.1089/089771503322144590

Cole, B. J., & Malek, M. (2004). *Articular cartilage lesions: A practical guide to assessment and treatment.* New York, NY: Springer-Verlag.

Coleman, M. P., & Hoke, A. (2020). Programmed axon degeneration: From mouse to mechanism to medicine. *Nature Reviews Neuroscience*, *21*(4), 183–196. https://doi.org/10.1038/s41583-020-0269-3

Contreras, O., Rebolledo, D. L., Oyarzun, J. E., Olguin, H. C., & Brandan, E. (2016). Connective tissue cells expressing fibro/adipogenic progenitor markers increase under chronic damage: Relevance in fibroblast-myofibroblast differentiation and skeletal muscle fibrosis. *Cell and Tissue Research, 364*(3), 647–660. https://doi.org/10.1007/s00441-015-2343-0

Convery, F. R., Akeson, W. H., & Keown, G. H. (1972). The repair of large osteochondral defects. An experimental study in horses. *Clinical Orthopaedics and Related Research, 82*, 253–262. Retrieved from https://www.ncbi.nlm.nih.gov/pubmed/5011034

Dagdeviren, S., Jung, D. Y., Lee, E., Friedline, R. H., Noh, H. L., Kim, J. H., . . . Kim, J. K. (2016). Altered interleukin-10 Signaling in skeletal muscle regulates obesity-mediated inflammation and insulin resistance. *Molecular and Cellular Biology, 36*(23), 2956–2966. https://doi.org/10.1128/MCB.00181-16

Desguerre, I., Mayer, M., Leturcq, F., Barbet, J. P., Gherardi, R. K., & Christov, C. (2009). Endomysial fibrosis in Duchenne muscular dystrophy: A marker of poor outcome associated with macrophage alternative activation. *Journal of Neuropathology and Experimental Neurology, 68*(7), 762–773. https://doi.org/10.1097/NEN.0b013e3181aa31c2

D'Lima, D. D., Hashimoto, S., Chen, P. C., Colwell, C. W., Jr., & Lotz, M. K. (2001). Impact of mechanical trauma on matrix and cells. *Clinical Orthopaedics and Related Research, 391 Suppl*, S90–S99. https://doi.org/10.1097/00003086-200110001-00009

Dominguez, V. M., & Agnew, A. M. (2019). Microdamage as a bone quality component: Practical guidelines for the two-dimensional analysis of linear microcracks in human cortical bone. *JBMR Plus, 3*(6), e10203. https://doi.org/10.1002/jbm4.10203

Dort, J., Fabre, P., Molina, T., & Dumont, N. A. (2019). Macrophages are key regulators of stem cells during skeletal muscle regeneration and diseases. *Stem Cells International, 2019*, 4761427. https://doi.org/10.1155/2019/4761427

Dowthwaite, G. P., Bishop, J. C., Redman, S. N., Khan, I. M., Rooney, P., Evans, D. J., . . . Archer, C. W. (2004). The surface of articular cartilage contains a progenitor cell population. *Journal of Cell Science, 117*(Pt 6), 889–897. https://doi.org/10.1242/jcs.00912

Driban, J. B., Barr, A. E., Amin, M., Sitler, M. R., & Barbe, M. F. (2011). Joint inflammation and early degeneration induced by high-force reaching are attenuated by ibuprofen in an animal model of work-related musculoskeletal disorder. *Journal of Biomedicine & Biotechnology, 2011*, 691412. https://doi.org/10.1155/2011/691412

Driban, J. B., Harkey, M. S., Barbe, M. F., Ward, R. J., MacKay, J. W., Davis, J. E., . . . McAlindon, T. E. (2020). Risk factors and the natural history of accelerated knee osteoarthritis: A narrative review. *BMC Musculoskeletal Disorders, 21*(1), 332. https://doi.org/10.1186/s12891-020-03367-2

Duffield, J. S., Forbes, S. J., Constandinou, C. M., Clay, S., Partolina, M., Vuthoori, S., . . . Iredale, J. P. (2005). Selective depletion of macrophages reveals distinct, opposing roles during liver injury and repair. *The Journal of Clinical Investigation, 115*(1), 56–65. https://doi.org/10.1172/JCI22675

Eisinger, F., Patzelt, J., & Langer, H. F. (2018). The platelet response to tissue injury. *Frontiers in Medicine (Lausanne), 5*, 317. https://doi.org/10.3389/fmed.2018.00317

Elefteriou, F. (2018). Impact of the autonomic nervous system on the skeleton. *Physiological Reviews, 98*(3), 1083–1112. https://doi.org/10.1152/physrev.00014.2017

Epari, D. R., Duda, G. N., & Thompson, M. S. (2010). Mechanobiology of bone healing and regeneration: in vivo models. *Proceedings of the Institution of Mechanical Engineers. Part H, 224*(12), 1543–1553. https://doi.org/10.1243/09544119JEIM808

Fedorczyk, J. M., Barr, A. E., Rani, S., Gao, H. G., Amin, M., Amin, S., . . . Barbe, M. F. (2010). Exposure-dependent increases in IL-1beta, substance P, CTGF, and tendinosis in flexor digitorum tendons with upper extremity repetitive strain injury. *Journal of Orthopaedic Research: Official Publication of the Orthopaedic Research Society*, *28*(3), 298–307. https://doi.org/10.1002/jor.20984

Fisher, P. W., Zhao, Y., Rico, M. C., Massicotte, V. S., Wade, C. K., Litvin, J., . . . Barbe, M. F. (2015). Increased CCN2, substance P and tissue fibrosis are associated with sensorimotor declines in a rat model of repetitive overuse injury. *Journal of Cell Communications and Signaling*, *9*(1), 37–54. https://doi.org/10.1007/s12079-015-0263-0

Florit, D., Pedret, C., Casals, M., Malliaras, P., Sugimoto, D., & Rodas, G. (2019). Incidence of tendinopathy in team sports in a multidisciplinary sports Club over 8 seasons. *Journal of Sports Science and Medicine*, *18*(4), 780–788. Retrieved from https://www.ncbi.nlm.nih.gov/pubmed/31827363

Frara, N., Fisher, P. W., Zhao, Y., Tarr, J. T., Amin, M., Popoff, S. N., & Barbe, M. F. (2018). Substance P increases CCN2 dependent on TGF-beta yet collagen type I via TGF-beta1 dependent and independent pathways in tenocytes. *Connective Tissue Research*, *59*(1), 30–44. https://doi.org/10.1080/03008207.2017.1297809

Frara, N., Giaddui, D., Braverman, A. S., Porreca, D. S., Brown, J. M., Mazzei, M., . . . Ruggieri, M. R., Sr. (2021). Nerve transfer for restoration of lower motor neuron-lesioned bladder function. Part 1: Attenuation of purinergic bladder smooth muscle contractions. *American Journal of Physiology. Regulatory, Integrative and Comparative Physiology*, *320*(6), R885–R896. https://doi.org/10.1152/ajpregu.00299.2020

Frost, H. M. (1994). Wolff's law and bone's structural adaptations to mechanical usage: An overview for clinicians. *The Angle Orthodontist*, *64*(3), 175–188. https://doi.org/10.1043/0003-3219(1994)064<0175:WLABSA>2.0.CO;2

Funes, S. C., Rios, M., Escobar-Vera, J., & Kalergis, A. M. (2018). Implications of macrophage polarization in autoimmunity. *Immunology*, *154*(2), 186–195. https://doi.org/10.1111/imm.12910

Fung, D. T., Wang, V. M., Laudier, D. M., Shine, J. H., Basta-Pljakic, J., Jepsen, K. J., . . . Flatow, E. L. (2009). Subrupture tendon fatigue damage. *Journal of Orthopaedic Research: Official Publication of the Orthopaedic Research Society*, *27*(2), 264–273. https://doi.org/10.1002/jor.20722

Gallagher, S., & Barbe, M. F. (2021). The impaired healing hypothesis: A mechanism by which psychosocial stress and personal characteristics increase MSD risk? *Ergonomics*, 1–14. https://doi.org/10.1080/00140139.2021.1974103

Gallagher, S., & Schall, M. C., Jr. (2017). Musculoskeletal disorders as a fatigue failure process: Evidence, implications and research needs. *Ergonomics*, *60*(2), 255–269. https://doi.org/10.1080/00140139.2016.1208848

Gamage, K. K., Cheng, I., Park, R. E., Karim, M. S., Edamura, K., Hughes, C., . . . Deppmann, C. D. (2017). Death receptor 6 promotes Wallerian degeneration in peripheral axons. *Current Biology*, *27*(6), 890–896. https://doi.org/10.1016/j.cub.2017.01.062

Gao, H. G., Fisher, P. W., Lambi, A. G., Wade, C. K., Barr-Gillespie, A. E., Popoff, S. N., & Barbe, M. F. (2013). Increased serum and musculotendinous fibrogenic proteins following persistent low-grade inflammation in a rat model of long-term upper extremity overuse. *PLoS One*, *8*(8), e71875. https://doi.org/10.1371/journal.pone.0071875

Gharaibeh, B., Chun-Lansinger, Y., Hagen, T., Ingham, S., Wright, V., Fu, F., & Huard, J. (2012). Biological approaches to improve skeletal muscle healing after injury and disease. Birth defects research. *Part C, Embryo Today: Reviews*, *96*, 82–94. https://doi.org/10.1002/bdrc.21005

Ghiasi, M. S., Chen, J., Vaziri, A., Rodriguez, E. K., & Nazarian, A. (2017). Bone fracture healing in mechanobiological modeling: A review of principles and methods. *Bone Reports*, *6*, 87–100. https://doi.org/10.1016/j.bonr.2017.03.002

Gissel, H. (2005). The role of Ca^{2+} in muscle cell damage. *Annals of the New York Academy of Sciences, 1066*, 166–180.

Gold, M. S., & Gebhart, G. F. (2010). Nociceptor sensitization in pain pathogenesis. *Nature Medicine, 16*(11), 1248–1257. https://doi.org/10.1038/nm.2235

Goodship, A. E., Cunningham, J. L., & Kenwright, J. (1998). Strain rate and timing of stimulation in mechanical modulation of fracture healing. *Clinical Orthopaedics and Related Research, 335 Suppl*, S105–S115. https://doi.org/10.1097/00003086-199810001-00012

Greising, S. M., Rivera, J. C., Goldman, S. M., Watts, A., Aguilar, C. A., & Corona, B. T. (2017). Unwavering pathobiology of volumetric muscle loss injury. *Scientific Reports, 7*(1), 13179. https://doi.org/10.1038/s41598-017-13306-2

Hadrevi, J., Barbe, M. F., Ortenblad, N., Frandsen, U., Boyle, E., Lazar, S., . . . Sogaard, K. (2019). Calcium fluxes in work-related muscle disorder: Implications from a rat model. *BioMed Research International, 2019*, 5040818. https://doi.org/10.1155/2019/5040818

Hauser, R. A., & Dolan, E. E. (2011). Ligament injury and healing: An overview of current clinical concepts. *Journal of Prolotherapy, 3*(4), 836–846.

Hente, R., Fuchtmeier, B., Schlegel, U., Ernstberger, A., & Perren, S. M. (2004). The influence of cyclic compression and distraction on the healing of experimental tibial fractures. *Journal of Orthopaedic Research: Official Publication of the Orthopaedic Research Society, 22*(4), 709–715. https://doi.org/10.1016/j.orthres.2003.11.007

Higashi-Kuwata, N., Jinnin, M., Makino, T., Fukushima, S., Inoue, Y., Muchemwa, F. C., . . . Ihn, H. (2010). Characterization of monocyte/macrophage subsets in the skin and peripheral blood derived from patients with systemic sclerosis. *Arthritis Research & Therapy, 12*(4), R128. https://doi.org/10.1186/ar3066

Hilliard, M. A. (2009). Axonal degeneration and regeneration: a mechanistic tug-of-war. *Journal of Neurochemistry, 108*(1), 23–32.

Hodges, P. W., & Danneels, L. (2019). Changes in structure and function of the Back muscles in Low Back pain: Different time points, observations, and mechanisms. *The Journal of Orthopaedic and Sports Physical Therapy, 49*(6), 464–476. https://doi.org/10.2519/jospt.2019.8827

Hu, W., Jiang, Z., Zhang, Y., Liu, Q., Fan, J., Luo, N., . . . Yu, X. (2012). Characterization of infiltrating macrophages in high glucose-induced peritoneal fibrosis in rats. *Molecular Medicine Reports, 6*(1), 93–99. https://doi.org/10.3892/mmr.2012.890

Isaksson, H. (2012). Recent advances in mechanobiological modeling of bone regeneration. *Mechanics Research Communications*, 22–31.

Judson, R. N., Low, M., Eisner, C., & Rossi, F. M. (2017). Isolation, culture, and differentiation of fibro/Adipogenic progenitors (FAPs) from skeletal muscle. *Methods in Molecular Biology, 1668*, 93–103. https://doi.org/10.1007/978-1-4939-7283-8_7

Kjaer, M. (2004). Role of extracellular matrix in adaptation of tendon and skeletal muscle to mechanical loading. *Physiological Reviews, 84*(2), 649–698. https://doi.org/10.1152/physrev.00031.2003

Kjaer, M., Langberg, H., Heinemeier, K., Bayer, M. L., Hansen, M., Holm, L., . . . Magnusson, S. P. (2009). From mechanical loading to collagen synthesis, structural changes and function in human tendon. *Scandinavian Journal of Medicine & Science in Sports, 19*(4), 500–510. https://doi.org/10.1111/j.1600-0838.2009.00986.x

Krzyszczyk, P., Schloss, R., Palmer, A., & Berthiaume, F. (2018). The role of macrophages in acute and chronic wound healing and interventions to promote pro-wound healing phenotypes. *Frontiers in Physiology, 9*, 419. https://doi.org/10.3389/fphys.2018.00419

Lech, M., & Anders, H. J. (2013). Macrophages and fibrosis: How resident and infiltrating mononuclear phagocytes orchestrate all phases of tissue injury and repair. *Biochimica et Biophysica Acta*, *1832*(7), 989–997. https://doi.org/10.1016/j.bbadis.2012.12.001

Li, H., Li, J., Zou, Z., & Fok, A. S. (2011). Fracture simulation of restored teeth using a continuum damage mechanics failure model. *Dental Materials*, *27*(7), e125–e133. https://doi.org/10.1016/j.dental.2011.03.006

Llobet Rosell, A., & Neukomm, L. J. (2019). Axon death signalling in Wallerian degeneration among species and in disease. *Open Biology*, *9*(8), 190118. https://doi.org/10.1098/rsob.190118

Mann, C. J., Perdiguero, E., Kharraz, Y., Aguilar, S., Pessina, P., Serrano, A. L., & Munoz-Canoves, P. (2011). Aberrant repair and fibrosis development in skeletal muscle. *Skeletal Muscle*, *1*(1), 21. https://doi.org/10.1186/2044-5040-1-21

Mathewson, M. A., Chambers, H. G., Girard, P. J., Tenenhaus, M., Schwartz, A. K., & Lieber, R. L. (2014). Stiff muscle fibers in calf muscles of patients with cerebral palsy lead to high passive muscle stiffness. *Journal of Orthopaedic Research: Official Publication of the Orthopaedic Research Society*, *32*(12), 1667–1674. https://doi.org/10.1002/jor.22719

McCracken, J. M., & Allen, L. A. (2014). Regulation of human neutrophil apoptosis and lifespan in health and disease. *Journal of Cell Death*, *7*, 15–23. https://doi.org/10.4137/JCD.S11038

Mead, M. P., Gumucio, J. P., Awan, T. M., Mendias, C. L., & Sugg, K. B. (2018). Pathogenesis and management of tendinopathies in sports medicine. *Translational Sports Medicine*, *1*(1), 5–13. https://doi.org/10.1002/tsm2.6

Mirhadi, S., Ashwood, N., & Karagkevrekis, B. (2013). Factors influencing fracture healing. *Trauma*, *15*(2), 1–16.

Moreau, N., & Boucher, Y. (2020). Hedging against neuropathic pain: Role of hedgehog Signaling in pathological nerve healing. *International Journal of Molecular Sciences*, *21*(23). https://doi.org/10.3390/ijms21239115

Mori, R., Tanaka, K., & Shimokawa, I. (2018). Identification and functional analysis of inflammation-related miRNAs in skin wound repair. *Development, Growth & Differentiation*, *60*(6), 306–315. https://doi.org/10.1111/dgd.12542

Mukund, K., & Subramaniam, S. (2020). Skeletal muscle: A review of molecular structure and function, in health and disease. *Wiley Interdisciplinary Reviews. Systems Biology and Medicine*, *12*(1), e1462. https://doi.org/10.1002/wsbm.1462

Murphy, B. S., Bush, H. M., Sundareshan, V., Davis, C., Hagadone, J., Cory, T. J., . . . Feola, D. J. (2010). Characterization of macrophage activation states in patients with cystic fibrosis. *Journal of Cystic Fibrosis*, *9*(5), 314–322. https://doi.org/10.1016/j.jcf.2010.04.006

Nakama, L. H., King, K. B., Abrahamsson, S., & Rempel, D. M. (2005). Evidence of tendon microtears due to cyclical loading in an in vivo tendinopathy model. *Journal of Orthopaedic Research: Official Publication of the Orthopaedic Research Society*, *23*(5), 1199–1205. https://doi.org/10.1016/j.orthres.2005.03.006

NIOSH. (2011). *National Manufacturing Agenda—June 2010*. http://www.cdc.gov/niosh/nora/comment/agendas/manuf (23 October 2011). Retrieved from http://www.cdc.gov/niosh/nora/comment/agendas/manuf

Nocera, G., & Jacob, C. (2020). Mechanisms of Schwann cell plasticity involved in peripheral nerve repair after injury. *Cellular and Molecular Life Sciences*, *77*(20), 3977–3989. https://doi.org/10.1007/s00018-020-03516-9

Ortenblad, N., Lunde, P. K., Levin, K., Andersen, J. L., & Pedersen, P. K. (2000). Enhanced sarcoplasmic reticulum ca(2+) release following intermittent sprint training. *American Journal of*

Physiology. Regulatory, Integrative and Comparative Physiology, 279(1), R152–R160. https://doi.org/10.1152/ajpregu.2000.279.1.R152

Punzi, L., Galozzi, P., Luisetto, R., Favero, M., Ramonda, R., Oliviero, F., & Scanu, A. (2016). Post-traumatic arthritis: Overview on pathogenic mechanisms and role of inflammation. *RMD Open, 2*(2), e000279. https://doi.org/10.1136/rmdopen-2016-000279

Robling, A. G., & Turner, C. H. (2009). Mechanical signaling for bone modeling and remodeling. *Critical Reviews in Eukaryotic Gene Expression, 19*(4), 319–338. https://doi.org/10.1615/critreveukargeneexpr.v19.i4.50

Rosendal, L., Larsson, B., Kristiansen, J., Peolsson, M., Sogaard, K., Kjaer, M., . . . Gerdle, B. (2004). Increase in muscle nociceptive substances and anaerobic metabolism in patients with trapezius myalgia: Microdialysis in rest and during exercise. *Pain, 112*(3), 324–334. https://doi.org/10.1016/j.pain.2004.09.017

Roszer, T. (2015). Understanding the mysterious M2 macrophage through activation markers and effector mechanisms. *Mediators of Inflammation, 2015*, 816460. https://doi.org/10.1155/2015/816460

Serhan, C. N. (2017). Treating inflammation and infection in the 21st century: New hints from decoding resolution mediators and mechanisms. *The FASEB Journal, 31*(4), 1273–1288. https://doi.org/10.1096/fj.201601222R

Sharma, P., & Maffulli, N. (2005). Tendon injury and tendinopathy: Healing and repair. *The Journal of Bone and Joint Surgery* American Volume, *87*(1), 187–202. https://doi.org/10.2106/JBJS.D.01850

Siqueira Mietto, B., et al. (2015). Role of IL-10 in Resolution of Inflammation and Functional Recovery after Peripheral Nerve Injury. *Journal of Neuroscience,* ***35***(50), 16431–16442.

Smith, T. T. G., Barr-Gillespie, A. E., Klyne, D. M., Harris, M. Y., Amin, M., Paul, R. W., . . . Barbe, M. F. (2020). Forced treadmill running reduces systemic inflammation yet worsens upper limb discomfort in a rat model of work-related musculoskeletal disorders. *BMC Musculoskeletal Disorders, 21*(1), 57. https://doi.org/10.1186/s12891-020-3085-z

Sogaard, K. (1995). Motor unit recruitment pattern during low-level static and dynamic contractions. *Muscle & Nerve, 18*(3), 292–300. https://doi.org/10.1002/mus.880180305

Stauber, W. T. (2004). Factors involved in strain-induced injury in skeletal muscles and outcomes of prolonged exposures. *Journal of Electromyography and Kinesiology, 14*(1), 61–70. https://doi.org/10.1016/j.jelekin.2003.09.010

Stauber, W. T., Smith, C. A., Miller, G. R., & Stauber, F. D. (2000). Recovery from 6 weeks of repeated strain injury to rat soleus muscles. *Muscle & Nerve, 23*(12), 1819–1825. Retrieved from http://www.ncbi.nlm.nih.gov/pubmed/11102904

Stecco, C., Porzionato, A., Lancerotto, L., Stecco, A., Macchi, V., Day, J. A., & De Caro, R. (2008). Histological study of the deep fasciae of the limbs. *Journal of Bodywork and Movement Therapies, 12*(3), 225–230. https://doi.org/10.1016/j.jbmt.2008.04.041

Sunwoo, J.Y., Eliasberg, C.D., Carballo, C.B., & Rodeo, S.A. (2020). The role of the macrophage in tendinopathy and tendon healing. *Journal of Orthopaedic Research, 38*(8),1666–1675. https://doi.org/10.1002/jor.24667.

Takegahara, N., Takamatsu, H., Toyofuku, T., Tsujimura, T., Okuno, T., Yukawa, K., . . . Kikutani, H. (2006). Plexin-A1 and its interaction with DAP12 in immune responses and bone homeostasis. *Nature Cell Biology, 8*(6), 615–622. https://doi.org/10.1038/ncb1416

Teixeira, C. F., Zamuner, S. R., Zuliani, J. P., Fernandes, C. M., Cruz-Hofling, M. A., Fernandes, I., . . . Gutierrez, J. M. (2003). Neutrophils do not contribute to local tissue damage, but play a key role in skeletal muscle regeneration, in mice injected with Bothrops asper snake venom. *Muscle & Nerve, 28*(4), 449–459. https://doi.org/10.1002/mus.10453

Tidball, J. G., & Villalta, S. A. (2010). Regulatory interactions between muscle and the immune system during muscle regeneration. *American Journal of Physiology. Regulatory, Integrative and Comparative Physiology*, *298*(5), R1173–R1187. https://doi.org/10.1152/ajpregu.00735.2009

Tidball, J. G., & Wehling-Henricks, M. (2015). Shifts in macrophage cytokine production drive muscle fibrosis. *Nature Medicine*, *21*(7), 665–666. https://doi.org/10.1038/nm.3896

Tomlinson, R. E., Li, Z., Li, Z., Minichiello, L., Riddle, R. C., Venkatesan, A., & Clemens, T. L. (2017). NGF-TrkA signaling in sensory nerves is required for skeletal adaptation to mechanical loads in mice. *Proceedings of the National Academy of Sciences of the United States of America*, *114*(18), E3632–E3641. https://doi.org/10.1073/pnas.1701054114

Toumi, H., F'Guyer, S., & Best, T. M. (2006). The role of neutrophils in injury and repair following muscle stretch. *Journal of Anatomy*, *208*(4), 459–470. https://doi.org/10.1111/j.1469-7580.2006.00543.x

Wang, J. (2018). Neutrophils in tissue injury and repair. *Cell and Tissue Research*, *371*(3), 531–539. https://doi.org/10.1007/s00441-017-2785-7

Wang, J. H. (2006). Mechanobiology of tendon. *Journal of Biomechanics*, *39*(9), 1563–1582. https://doi.org/10.1016/j.jbiomech.2005.05.011

Wang, J. H., & Komatsu, I. (2016). Tendon stem cells: Mechanobiology and development of tendinopathy. *Advances in Experimental Medicine and Biology*, *920*, 53–62. https://doi.org/10.1007/978-3-319-33943-6_5

Wang, Y., Wehling-Henricks, M., Samengo, G., & Tidball, J. G. (2015). Increases of M2a macrophages and fibrosis in aging muscle are influenced by bone marrow aging and negatively regulated by muscle-derived nitric oxide. *Aging Cell*, *14*(4), 678–688. https://doi.org/10.1111/acel.12350

Warden SJ, Davis IS, Fredericson M. Management and prevention of bone stress injuries in long-distance runners. *The Journal of Orthopaedic and Sports Physical Therapy* 2014 Oct;44(10):749–65. doi: https://doi.org/10.2519/jospt.2014.5334. Epub 2014 Aug 7. PMID: 25103133.

Wei, W., & Dai, H. (2021). Articular cartilage and osteochondral tissue engineering techniques: Recent advances and challenges. *Bioactive Materials*, *6*(12), 4830–4855. https://doi.org/10.1016/j.bioactmat.2021.05.011

Welc, S. S., Wehling-Henricks, M., Antoun, J., Ha, T. T., Tous, I., & Tidball, J. G. (2020). Differential effects of myeloid cell PPARdelta and IL-10 in regulating macrophage recruitment, phenotype, and regeneration following acute muscle injury. *Journal of Immunology*, *205*(6), 1664–1677. https://doi.org/10.4049/jimmunol.2000247

Woo, S. L., Hildebrand, K., Watanabe, N., Fenwick, J. A., Papageorgiou, C. D., & Wang, J. H. (1999). Tissue engineering of ligament and tendon healing. *Clinical Orthopaedics and Related Research*, *367 Suppl*, S312–S323. https://doi.org/10.1097/00003086-199910001-00030

Wu, B., Zhang, C., Chen, B., Zhang, L., Dai, R., Wu, X., . . . Liao, E. (2013). Self-repair of rat cortical bone microdamage after fatigue loading in vivo. *International Journal of Endocrinology*, *2013*, 321074. https://doi.org/10.1155/2013/321074

Wu, Z., Laneve, A. J., & Niebur, G. L. (2013). in vivo microdamage is an indicator of susceptibility to initiation and propagation of microdamage in human femoral trabecular bone. *Bone*, *55*(1), 208–215. https://doi.org/10.1016/j.bone.2013.02.019

Wynn, T. A., & Vannella, K. M. (2016). Macrophages in tissue repair, regeneration, and fibrosis. *Immunity*, *44*(3), 450–462. https://doi.org/10.1016/j.immuni.2016.02.015

Xi, L., Song, Y., Wu, W., Qu, Z., Wen, J., Liao, B., . . . Fang, D. (2020). Investigation of bone matrix composition, architecture and mechanical properties reflect structure-function relationship of cortical bone in glucocorticoid induced osteoporosis. *Bone*, *136*, 115334. https://doi.org/10.1016/j.bone.2020.115334

Yan, Y. Y., Li, C. Y., Zhou, L., Ao, L. Y., Fang, W. R., & Li, Y. M. (2017). Research progress of mechanisms and drug therapy for neuropathic pain. *Life Sciences*, *190*, 68–77. https://doi.org/10.1016/j.lfs.2017.09.033

Yang, G., Rothrauff, B. B., & Tuan, R. S. (2013). Tendon and ligament regeneration and repair: Clinical relevance and developmental paradigm. *Birth Defects Research. Part C, Embryo Today*, *99*(3), 203–222. https://doi.org/10.1002/bdrc.21041

Yang, S., & Plotnikov, S. V. (2021). Mechanosensitive regulation of fibrosis. *Cell*, *10*(5), 994. https://doi.org/10.3390/cells10050994

Yang, W., & Hu, P. (2018). Skeletal muscle regeneration is modulated by inflammation. *Journal of Orthopaedic Translation*, *13*, 25–32. https://doi.org/10.1016/j.jot.2018.01.002

Yeoh, S., Warner, W. S., Eli, I., & Mahan, M. A. (2020). Rapid-stretch injury to peripheral nerves: Comparison of injury models. *Journal of Neurosurgery*, 1–11. https://doi.org/10.3171/2020.5.JNS193448

Yin, H., Price, F., & Rudnicki, M. A. (2013). Satellite cells and the muscle stem cell niche. *Physiological Reviews*, *93*(1), 23–67. https://doi.org/10.1152/physrev.00043.2011

Zhang, M. Z., Yao, B., Yang, S., Jiang, L., Wang, S., Fan, X., . . . Harris, R. C. (2012). CSF-1 signaling mediates recovery from acute kidney injury. *The Journal of Clinical Investigation*, *122*(12), 4519–4532. https://doi.org/10.1172/JCI60363

12

Personal Characteristics and MSD Risk

Introduction

Among the many significant challenges faced in controlling the incidence of MSDs, one of the most substantial is the remarkable variability observed with respect to the personal characteristics of specific individuals. Biological variation is an important aspect of life and has many benefits. Through this powerful process, intricate interconnecting biological systems have been developed, and inbuilt redundancies established to maximize an individual's ability to resist injury and other undesirable consequences (West, 2014). However, along with these benefits, biological diversity creates noteworthy challenges in trying to develop methods by which to protect individuals from developing MSDs.

In this chapter, we will examine the influences of various personal characteristics with respect to the development of MSDs. Three primary personal characteristics, specifically those of age, sex, and anthropometry, will be focused on in the current chapter. Each of these factors can significantly influence the development of fatigue damage in musculoskeletal tissues and may also have a considerable impact on the remodeling and healing processes. In addition, we will discuss certain disease states that influence the expression of MSDs.

Biological Variability

Our efforts to reduce MSD risk in workers are greatly complicated by the biological variability exhibited by humans (across numerous dimensions). Different sources of variability are present and include factors involving both interindividual variability and intraindividual variability. Interindividual variability may include a host of factors including genetic variation (sex, anthropometric differences, etc.) or environmental factors that influence the characteristics of musculoskeletal tissues. These can lead, for example, to significant differences in the size and strength of tissues, resulting in tissues that have a wide range of ultimate strength and/or systems that may have significant variability in terms of tissue remodeling and healing capacities. Intraindividual factors may include differences in the same individual over time and may include aging effects, dietary changes, changes in sleep patterns and quality, and changes in the effectiveness of the healing process, all of which may affect the health status of the musculoskeletal tissues. All of these factors may have substantial impacts on an individual's rate of fatigue damage accrual thereby affecting their risk of MSD development.

Musculoskeletal Disorders: The Fatigue Failure Mechanism, First Edition. Sean Gallagher and Mary F. Barbe.

Age

Effects of Aging on the Musculoskeletal System

Deterioration of musculoskeletal system function is among the most universal and demoralizing manifestations of the aging process. Human beings experience musculoskeletal loading every day of their lives (for more than 100 years of age in some cases), and the sum of the loading experienced by musculoskeletal tissues over a lifetime must be quite impressive. The unremitting nature of loading on the musculoskeletal system and the consequent accumulation of damage in musculoskeletal tissues clearly can take a substantial toll as one ages.

The process of degeneration of musculoskeletal tissues is complex and involves the degradation of many physiological processes, but mechanical fatigue of tissues undoubtedly is an important factor. Key to the influence of the degeneration process is that several tissues associated with MSDs (e.g., tendons, ligaments, and cartilage) do not heal well and when damage occurs they may never regain their original strength after repair (Knight, Nigam, & Hore, 2017). Persistent loading of a damaged and weakened structure will result in a vicious cycle leading to continued tissue degeneration. For instance, damage in a structure will decrease its ultimate strength and reduce the amount of repeated stress that the structure would be able to endure in future loading events. Other effects of a damaged structure may be that a portion of the load may be transferred to a secondary restraint, which may, in turn, experience fatigue-related damage.

Aging is associated with several progressive and degenerative changes that significantly influence the function of different components of the musculoskeletal system. These changes are associated with a weakening of system components, making them susceptible to further damage and injury (Knight et al., 2017). Over time, these changes can lead to frailty and may lead to an increased risk of fractures, tendinosis, and other adverse outcomes. The following sections discuss some of the changes that occur in musculoskeletal system components during the aging process.

Muscle

A muscle typically attains its maximum strength in an individual's 20s and 30s and experience a modest decline during the next two decades (40s and 50s). Declines in strength accelerate after the age of 60 years and are associated with a decrease in muscle mass and speed of contractions (Choi, 2016). Muscles experience a loss of force-producing capacity primarily due to the loss of type II (fast-twitch) muscle fibers, in a process known as senile sarcopenia. Sarcopenia is thought to be due, in part, to a process of denervation of motor neuron fibers and degradation of the neuromuscular junction itself. As a result of these changes, the muscle becomes weakly stimulated, which may lead to atrophy (Power & Dalton, 2013; Stokinger, Maxwell, Shapiro, deCabo, & Valdez, 2017). Though type II fibers are significantly affected by this process, type I fibers remain relatively unaffected (Bougea et al., 2016), and may even show evidence of increased metabolic enzymes (Murgia et al., 2017). In addition, muscles become more prone to injury and are slower to repair with advancing age. The latter is likely due to the decreased number of progenitor (satellite) cells and cellular senescence (Bougea et al., 2016). Table 12.1 provides a summary of age-related changes that occur in skeletal muscles.

Tendon/Ligament

Several degenerative changes in the tendon are seen with age, with the first signs becoming apparent as early as the third decade (Kannus, Paavola, & Józsa, 2005). Such changes may be observed in both collagen and noncollagenous matrix components of the tendon, as well as in the

Table 12.1 Summary of Age-Related Changes in a Skeletal Muscle

• Reduction in protein synthesis • Reduction in size and number of muscle fibers (esp., lower limbs) • Reduced satellite and stem cells • Reduced muscle growth • Reduced repair capacity • Replacement of muscle fibers by non-contractile fibrous tissue	• Reduced motor neurons and degraded neuromuscular junctions • Increased fat deposition • Reduction in the number of mitochondria • Less-efficient metabolism (type II) • Reduced blood flow to major muscle groups

Knight, J., Nigam, Y., & Hore, N. (2017). Anatomy and physiology of ageing 10: The musculoskeletal system. *Nursing Times*, 113, 60–63.

vasculature of the structure. Of the biomechanical changes associated with the aging of tendons, decreased tensile strength is the most dramatic (Kannus et al., 1992). A notable finding in the aged tendons is the increase in advanced glycation end-product (AGE) crosslinks that would be expected to increase modulus and strength; however, excessive cross-linking instead appears to have a negative impact on different biomechanical factors such as ultimate strength, ultimate strain, and the modulus of elasticity (Kannus et al., 2005). It is thought that the decrease in strength may be due in large part to an overall reduction in collagen in the tendon (Tuite, Renstrom, & O'Brien, 1997).

The effect of aging in tendons (and other tissues) is partly the result of damage incurred due to physical loading experienced in the course of a lifetime. Such loading can lead to significant changes in tendon architecture such as those evidenced in tendinopathy (Arya & Kulig, 2010; Longo et al., 2008), including disoriented collagen fibers, fiber thinning and kinking, which significantly alter biomechanical properties. Such degenerative changes result in a decrease in the tensile strength of tendons and a reduced modulus (Lavagnino & Arnoczky, 2005).

Degenerative vascular and mechanobiological changes are also observed in tendons with growing age (McCarthy & Hannafin, 2013). For example, overall blood flow is found to decrease and there is a decrease in the number of capillaries per unit area (Funakoshi et al., 2010; Josza & Kannus, 1997; Rudzki et al., 2008). These include degeneration of the tenocytes and collagen fibers, lipid accumulation, and calcium deposits (Kannus et al., 2005). There are also considerable changes witnessed in the ability of tendons to adapt to mechanical loading through mechanotransduction (McCarthy & Hannafin, 2013). In addition, an increase in degradative enzyme production has been postulated to affect tendon homeostasis with age. Research has demonstrated that matrix metalloproteinase-1 (MMP-1) is associated with tendinosis (Fu et al., 2002) and that increases in MMP-1 production are associated with decreases in tensile strength and modulus responses in tendons (Lavagnino & Arnoczky, 2005).

As detailed in Chapter 3, ligaments are similar to tendons in that their primary function is to resist tensile loads. Both have a similar structure though ligaments contain a higher proportion of elastin fibers, thereby providing joint support while allowing some flexibility in joint movement. The biomechanical characteristics of ligaments have also been shown to be affected by the aging process (McCarthy & Hannafin, 2013). Woo and colleagues documented a progressive deterioration in the biomechanical properties of the femur-ACL-tibia complex with increasing age, including decreased ultimate strength, stiffness, and energy absorption (Woo, Hollis, Adams, Lyon, Takai, 1991). These data correlate well with other data demonstrating a decrease in ultimate strength and modulus in the ACL with age (Noyes & Grood, 1976).

Bone

Bone is also more susceptible to damage (e.g., fracture) as an individual ages (Boskey & Coleman, 2010). Elderly individuals have been estimated to experience a 10-fold increase in risk compared to younger individuals with similar bone mineral density (BMD) (Kanis, 2002). Studies that have examined fractures during extreme old age have found that the fracture risk in those > 85 years is up to 15 times greater than in individuals aged 60–65 years (Melton, 1996; Yates, Karasik, Beck, Cupples, & Kiel, 2007)

Different bone components must maintain a dynamic balance in which resistance to fracture is weighed against the mass added to the skeleton (Boskey & Coleman, 2010). Bones require both stiffness and strength to withstand the large loads they experience as well as toughness to absorb the energy from impacts. The strength of bone is determined by the amount as well as distribution of mineral content (or density) (Ammann & Rizzoli, 2003). During the aging process, the amount of minerals present in bone varies considerably. Bone mass achieves 90% of its peak value by the age of 20 years and continues to increase until about the age of 30 years (Knight et al., 2017; National Institutes of Health, 2021). However, by the time an individual approaches middle age, bone density starts to decline. This loss of bone material is of particular concern for women due to the decrease in estrogen levels observed with aging, which becomes particularly evident post-menopause. Studies have shown that women may lose up to two times the bone mass per year compared to men (Daly et al., 2013). Bone loss in both sexes continues into old age, with bone mass levels at 80 years of age reduced to nearly half the peak values that were attained in young adulthood (Lau & Adachi, 2011). The loss of strength that results from this process makes bone increasingly susceptible to fatigue damage (O'Brien, Brennan, Kennedy, & Lee, 2005).

As per the typical fatigue failure process, bone exposed to repeated stress will experience microcracks which initiate at the sub-micron level, which if not repaired will propagate, ultimately leading to a failure (O'Brien et al., 2005). The number of microcracks observed in bone, as well as their density and lengths, increases exponentially with advancing age in humans (Schaffler, Choi, & Milgrom, 1995; Vashishth, 2007). It is likely that the combination of both increased susceptibility to damage with age, as well as the decreased capacity to repair damage as described in detail in Chapter 11, both lead to increased fatigue damage accumulation and may contribute to the reduced strength and toughness of both cortical and trabecular bone (Boskey & Coleman, 2010; Currey, Brear, & Zioupos, 1996; Currey, Brear, & Zioupos, 1997; Hirano, Turner, Forwood, Johnston, & Burr, 2000).

Cartilage

Like all musculoskeletal structures, cartilage plays a unique role in bearing the biomechanical loads imposed upon it during joint movement. As an example, articular cartilage must distribute compressive stress and withstand the shear stresses experienced as a result of joint motion (Poole, 2005). As discussed in Chapter 3, the extracellular matrix (ECM) plays a key role in the biomechanical responses of articular cartilage to loading (Lotz & Loeser, 2012). During normal homeostasis of cartilage, the ECM responds to mechanical stress appropriately and prevents the development of structural or cellular damage.

Damage to articular cartilage increases with aging and along with it, the risk of osteoarthritis (OA). OA is the most prevalent joint disease and aging remains a predominant risk factor in the development of this disease (Zhang & Jordan, 2010). In individuals aged ≤45 years with other predisposing factors, OA is rare (Hashimoto, Ochs, Komiya, & Lotz, 1998). However, advancing age is not a guarantee of the development of OA (Lotz & Loeser, 2012). Instead, it is the physical exposure experienced during the passage of time interacting with aging-related material changes that appear to lead to the initiation and propagation of this disease (Lotz & Loeser, 2012). This pattern is aligned with the notion expressed previously that the effects of aging on musculoskeletal tissues may be viewed as a consequence of an imbalance between stressors that damage tissue and the systems that repair or protect against such damage (Kirkwood, 2005).

The aging process leads to changes in both the volume and makeup of the ECM, which, in turn, affects the cartilage's ability to withstand imposed biomechanical loading (Maroudas, 1990). Among these changes are an increased protein breakdown in cartilage and synovial fluid, causing changes in the makeup of the ECM (Dean, Martel-Pelletier, Pelletier, Howell, & Woessner, 1989), and an increased proportion of degraded collagen molecules (Bank et al., 1997). Another significant change is the formation of advanced glycation end-products (AGEs) which leads to increased cross-linking of collagen molecules. This results in biomechanical changes such as increased stiffness in cartilage which increases susceptibility to damage resulting from repeated stress (Bank, Bayliss, Lafeber, Maroudas, & Tekoppele, 1998; Chen et al. 2002).

The superficial zone of articular cartilage experiences the most significant loading and is, therefore, the most susceptible site to injury (Caramés et al., 2012; Dean et al., 1989). This is the site of the earliest changes in cartilage structure with fibrillation and the appearance of superficial defects. These defects represent the result of a systemic breakdown in the response of cartilage to repetitive loading (Armstrong & Mow, 1982).

Aging Summary

At birth, individuals possess a fresh set of musculoskeletal tissues that are normally unblemished. During the first two to three decades of life, these tissues grow and strengthen to the maximum they will attain in life. Thereafter, there begins a steady decline in the strength and function of tissues. Muscles start to experience a loss of type I muscle fibers (sarcopenia); tendons and ligaments become more rigid and brittle; bone density begins to decrease; the proteoglycans in cartilage degrade, thereby making joints less resilient and susceptible to damage. The loss in strength and function of the musculoskeletal tissues appears to be the result of a progressive loss of tissue homeostasis because of a combination of accumulating damage, decreased repair capacity, and the application of inferior repair materials. A vicious cycle is experienced in which fatigue damage weakens tissues, the repair is unable to bring the tissue back to its original strength, and the weakened tissue, in turn, becomes more susceptible to damage when exposed to subsequent repeated loading.

The generalized decline of musculoskeletal tissue strength that occurs with age will have notable impacts on the development of fatigue damage in musculoskeletal tissues. The weakening that occurs in these tissues is due to several factors, including prior damage, suboptimal healing of prior injuries, declines in the healing capacity, decreased function of systems supporting the musculoskeletal system, sarcopenia, and many others. Table 12.2 provides an example of this phenomenon. Using data from a study on the fatigue failure of tendons performed by Schechtman and Bader (1997), Table 12.2 illustrates how the decreased ultimate tensile strength with age affects the repeated loading that would be necessary to lead to damage. Let us assume an occupational task is performed that requires a tendon to be loaded to 200 N. With a young healthy tendon, the ultimate strength might be 800 N. At this level of loading (25% of ultimate strength), the tendon would be expected to fail in approximately 150,000 cycles. At this level of loading, assuming that when you reach a value of 1.0 to fail, each cycle of this task would be expected to experience 0.000007 of the way to failure. However, if (with age) the tendon ultimate strength decreased to 570 N, the 200 N load would now represent approximately 35% of the ultimate strength of the tendon. At this level of loading, the expected cycles to failure would be approximately 30,000 cycles. This indicates that

Table 12.2 Example of the Effect of a 200 N Load on a Young Tendon Versus an Older Tendon

	Tendon ultimate strength (US)	% US of the 200 N load	Cycles to failure	Damage per cycle
Young tendon	800 N	25%	150,000	0.000007
Old tendon	570 N	35%	30,000	0.000033

each cycle would represent 0.000033 of the way to failure, approximately five times the damage per cycle compared to that in the young tendon. Obviously, the damage will accrue much more quickly with the older tendon, leading to greater injury risk which would potentially reduce the ultimate strength of the tendon even further.

When considering the increased musculoskeletal injury risk of older individuals, one clear supposition may be made that one reason why aged individuals experience increased risk is that tissue degradation that occurs with aging leads to weaker tissues (reduced ultimate strength) and that these weaker tissues are at increased risk of injury when exposed to repetitive loading. The weaker tissues are likely the result of both damages that have accrued due to repeated loading, and the decrease in the capacity of the healing system to repair these tissues. It should be mentioned, however, that while the general trends discussed earlier are clear, there can be substantial differences in the effects on an individual basis. There are several actions that can be taken that may improve overall musculoskeletal health with age. These actions are discussed in Chapter 15.

Sex

Epidemiological, experimental, and clinical evidence suggest that there are significant sex differences in the expression of musculoskeletal pain (Rollman & Lautenbacher, 2001). Evidence exists to suggest that women have a higher incidence of certain musculoskeletal disorders and report pain at a higher rate than their male counterparts (Rollman & Lautenbacher, 2001; Treaster & Burr, 2004; Wijnhoven, de Vet, & Picavet, 2006). Some studies have indicated that the sex differences diminish when confounding factors such as work exposure are included in the analysis (Punnett & Herbert, 2000); however, controlling these and other confounding factors does not always eliminate the finding of increased risk among females, especially for upper extremity MSDs (Treaster & Burr, 2004).

The reasons for this sex difference in MSD reporting are likely multifactorial and may include factors such as differences in body size, muscle strength and makeup, the strength of various musculoskeletal tissues, differences in the biological responses to mechanical loads, differences in cardiovascular endurance, increased pain sensitivity, and perhaps a differential response to psychosocial stressors (Rollman & Lautenbacher, 2001). Cultural factors may also play a role with respect to sex differences in reporting discomfort or pain. For example, men may be less apt to report pain of a certain level; however, the same pain may be more culturally acceptable for women to report. Further, some women may be exposed to significant MSD exposure due to housework, childcare, and other tasks performed in the home setting (Alexanderson, Sydsjo, Hensing, Sydsjo, & Carsternsen, 1996).

The sections that follow examine the differences between males and females with respect to various tissues of the musculoskeletal system. As will be seen, there are several anatomical, biomechanical, psychological, and biological differences between males and females that affect both the capabilities of the musculoskeletal system and the likelihood of experiencing injuries.

Effects of Sex on the Musculoskeletal System Components

Muscle

One well-established difference between males and females is that absolute muscle strength is greater (on average) in males than in females (Miller, MacDougall, Tarnopolsky, & Sale, 1993). In general, the difference in strength appears to be more pronounced in the muscles of the upper limb compared to lower limbs (Chen, Liu, & Yu, 2012), which may be due to the lower proportion of lean tissue in the upper body of women. This difference appears to be primarily the result of larger overall fiber areas in male muscles compared to females (Miller et al., 1993). There does not appear to be a difference between males and females in the strength per cross-sectional area of muscle, number of motor units, or ability to activate motor units. Men, however, exhibit greater muscle mass that is the result of testosterone-induced muscular hypertrophy (Haizlip, Harrison, & Leinwand, 2015).

The strength difference between men and women may have ramifications beyond strength capacity. For example, it should be noted that the mechanical properties of the tendon appear to be associated with the strength capacity of the muscle to which it is attached (Muraoka, Muramatsu, Fukunaga, & Kanehisa, 2005). Given the strength differences between genders, it would follow that the mechanical properties of the tendon will be decreased (on average) in females as opposed to males. The decreased tendon mechanical properties of females (on average) would mean that for a given load application, the average female would be at a higher level of their tendon capacity compared to the average male. This would suggest that the average female tendon would experience more rapid fatigue failure at a given load compared to the average man based on the principles of fatigue failure theory. The same would hold true when considering the level of muscle capacity that males and females would be working at for a given load application. Due to the decreased strength capacity of females, it would be expected that increased muscle damage would be expected in female muscle tissue.

Tendon/ligament

It is clear that women have a higher probability of injury to tendons and ligaments compared to men performing similar activities (Bijur et al., 1997; Jones, Bovee, Harris III, & Cowan, 1993; Magnusson et al., 2007). For example, the incidence of anterior cruciate ligament injuries in women is up to six times greater than in men engaged in similar activities (Hewett, Myer, & Ford, 2001). There appear to be several reasons that may be responsible for this result. For example, studies have shown that the mechanical properties of tendons show significant differences between men and women. Tests of male and female tendon collagen fascicles biopsied during anterior cruciate ligament reconstruction elective surgery (fascicles sampled from the anterior portion of the patellar tendon) demonstrated that the ultimate stress attained was significantly higher for men as opposed to women, as was the elastic modulus (Magnusson et al., 2007).

In addition to the decreased mechanical strength of tendons and ligaments observed in women, there are differences in the metabolism of these tissues between the sexes. Women's tendons exhibit a lessened hypertrophic response to training regimens, a lower collagen synthesis rate after exercise, and a decrease in the overall rate of collagen synthesis compared to male tendons (Magnusson et al., 2007). The latter is believed to be the result of the action of estradiol (a hormone mediating estrogen activity), which has been shown to have an inhibiting influence on collagen formation (Liu, Al-shaikh, Panossian, Finerman, & Lane, 1997; Yu, Panossian, Hatch, Liu, & Finerman, 2001). In response to exercise, women do not exhibit the degree of increased collagen synthesis as observed in men (Magnusson et al., 2007; Miller et al., 2005). The decreased collagen synthesis rate observed in women may explain the lack of tendon hypertrophy in women in response to exercise compared to the hypertrophic response in exercising men (Magnusson et al., 2007).

The increased susceptibility of tendon and ligament injury in women may be the result of several sex-specific differences, both in the mechanical strength of these structures and hormonal differences that affect collagen synthesis. The decreased ultimate stress of tendon fascicles in women as opposed to men suggests that women exposed to equivalent repeated stress would be expected to experience more rapid fatigue damage than men. Injury risk may be further exacerbated by the reduced collagen synthesis rate and because women do not experience hypertrophy after exercise regimens. Men do experience hypertrophy with exercise which results in an increase the cross-sectional area in the tendon, reducing stress for a given load application. Thus, several gender-specific mechanical and hormonal responses are apparent in tendons and ligaments, the combination of which would suggest increased injury susceptibility in women, a finding confirmed in epidemiological studies.

Bone

Stress fractures are among the most common bone disorders and can be a source of considerable disability depending on the location of the injury (Wentz, Liu, Haymes, & Ilich, 2011). These injuries are believed to result from exposure of bone to repeated stress, leading to micro-trauma that accrues if bone damage accumulates at a rate greater than the rate of bone healing (Pepper, Akuthota, & McCarty, 2006). Stress fractures vary according to activity, but the highest rates of stress fractures are generally reported in female runners (Jones, Thacker, Gilchrist, Kimsey, & Sosin, 2002). A recent systematic review of sex/gender differences in stress fractures in the military and athletic populations recently concluded that females in both populations exhibited increased fracture incidence compared to males. In military populations, the incidence of males and females was 3% and 9.2%, respectively, and in the athletic populations, the incidence was 6.5% and 9.7%, respectively (Wentz et al., 2011). Common sites of stress fracture were found in the tibia, metatarsals, femur, calcaneus, and pelvis (females only).

As discussed in Chapter 6, the strength of bone is primarily a function of bone mineral content or BMD. There is a significant difference observed between women and men in the structure, strength, and metabolism of bone. Most of these differences during growth are the result of a difference in the size of bones of women compared to men as opposed to a difference in volumetric bone mineral density (Seeman, 2001). During aging, men and women lose similar amounts of bone by endosteal resorption; however, men have less bone loss from the periosteum thus men experience an overall smaller net bone loss. In addition, the loss of trabecular bone is qualitatively different in women compared to men. In women, trabecular bone loss involves complete loss of trabecular elements; while in men the loss of bone does not result in a complete loss but thinning of trabecular structures (Seeman, 2001). The difference in bone strength between the sexes becomes greater because of the decrease in estrogen, a hormone in women that protects bones, which declines sharply when women reach menopause. This can cause significant bone loss and explains why the chance of developing osteoporosis increases after women reach menopause.

The net result of the decrease in bone is that women's bones (on average) are weaker than those of men, largely because of the size differences in the bone between males and females, which

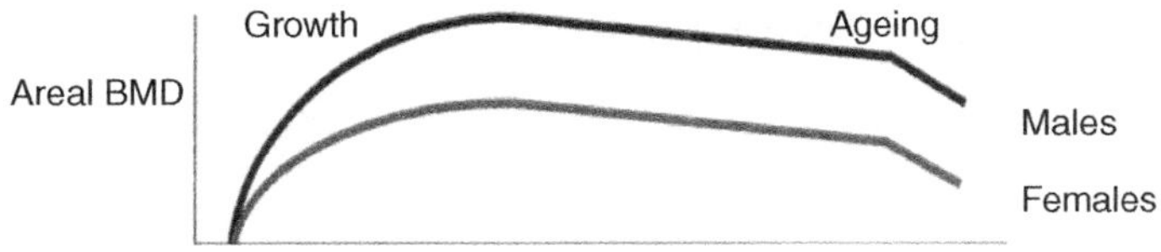

Figure 12.1 Differences in areal bone mineral density in males and females throughout life. Seeman, E. (2001). Sexual dimorphism in skeletal size, density, and strength. *The Journal of Clinical Endocrinology & Metabolism*, 86, 4576–4584.

become accentuated due to hormonal changes later in life. The weaker bone in females suggests increased susceptibility to damage accumulation due to fatigue failure when exposed to repeated stress. Figure 12.1 illustrates the difference in areal bone mineral density for males and females according to age.

Cartilage

Osteoarthritis (OA) is the most common and disabling disorder resulting from the breakdown of cartilage, affecting approximately 15% of the population (Guccione et al., 1994). This disorder tends to occur more frequently in lower extremity joints, such as the hip and the knee, with knee OA a lifetime prevalence of 40% in men and 47% in women (Johnson & Hunter, 2014). According to a meta-analysis of OA prevalence and incidence, females exhibit a higher prevalence and severity of OA overall and experience higher rates of hand, foot, and knee OA than men (Srikanth et al., 2005). Furthermore, women tend to show more severe radiographic evidence of OA than men, which may be increased further after menopause (Srikanth et al., 2005). The increased incidence of OA post-menopause indicates a possible role of estrogen in the process which may unmask OA symptoms by enhancing pain sensitivity (Johnson & Hunter, 2014).

Some of the gender disparity in OA incidence may be due to factors such as a decreased volume of knee cartilage compared to men, as well as decreased bone strength (Hanna et al., 2009; Johnson & Hunter, 2014). A study of gender differences in cartilage loss prior to the onset of OA reported that the average loss of total tibial cartilage was significantly greater in women than in men. Furthermore, this study found a predilection for increased progression of tibiofemoral cartilage defects in females (Hanna et al., 2009). Similarly, women were found to have a greater average percentage loss of cartilage volume loss in the patella (Hanna et al., 2009). These findings suggest that the greater incidence of OA in women may be due, at least in part, to differences in cartilage health prior to the onset of clinical symptoms (Hanna et al., 2009).

Recently, the Osteoarthritis Research Society International (OARSI) introduced a novel method of grading and staging the histopathology of articular cartilage damage progression (Pritzker et al., 2006). As shown in Figure 12.2, the grade establishes the progression of OA damage and is a measure of the severity of the osteoarthritic process. The stage is the horizontal extent of cartilage involvement, and the score represents the combined assessment of grade and stage (Pritzker et al., 2006). The grades and stages exhibit a classic fatigue failure damage progression, starting with the nucleation of small areas of fibrillation on the cartilage surface (Grade 1). Grade 2 exhibits propagation of the original fibrillation leading to the development of discontinuity on the surface. Grade 3 is associated with the development of vertical fissures (continued crack propagation) that extend into the midzone and eventually the deep zone. Further damage propagation is observed in the form of erosion in Grade 4. This is associated with cartilage matrix loss, first in the superficial zone and subsequently in deeper layers (termed "excavation"). Grade 5 is labeled as "denudation" and represents a complete loss of cartilage, leaving the articular surface as bone or mineralized

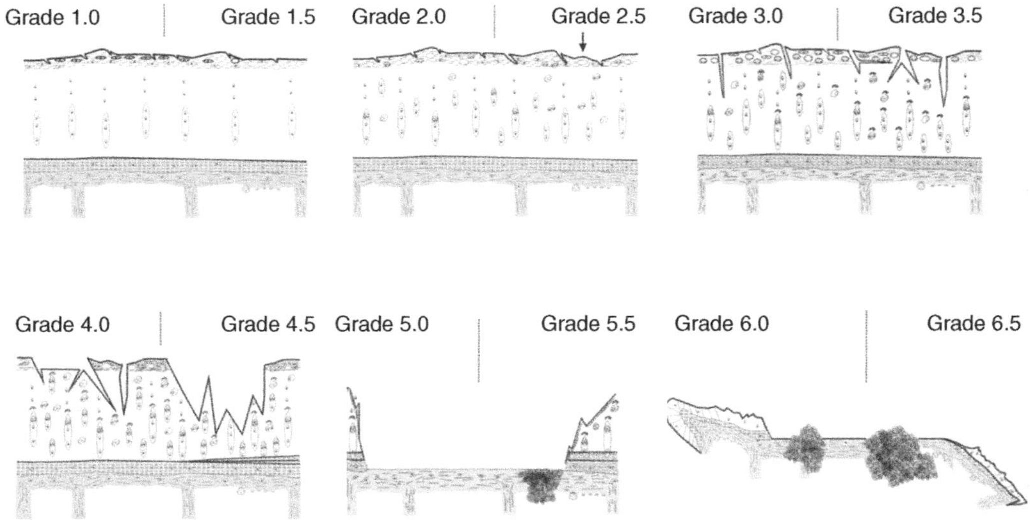

Figure 12.2 Grading of osteoporosis damage accumulation. See text for grade details. Pritzker, K., Gay, S., Jimenez, S., Ostergaard, K., Pelletier, J., Revell, P., . . . Van den Berg, W. (2006). Osteoarthritis cartilage histopathology: Grading and staging. *Osteoarthritis and Cartilage*, 14, 13–29./With permission of Elsevier.

cartilage. Grade 6 is classified as "deformation" and involves the more significant deformation of the articular surface involving some fibrocartilage growth and osteophyte formation (Pritzker et al., 2006).

The greater cartilage loss experienced in women prior to the onset of clinical symptoms suggests a weakening of articular joints making them more susceptible to the development of fatigue damage due to repeated loading (Hanna et al., 2009). This may help to explain the increased prevalence and incidence of OA in women, as well as the increased severity of prevalent OA observed in those of the female gender (Srikanth et al., 2005). Other potential gender-related differences factors related to OA incidence may include factors such as bone strength, alignment, ligament laxity, pregnancy, and changes due to menopause and neuromuscular strength (Johnson & Hunter, 2014). It should be noted that sex/gender differences in OA are particularly prominent in the knee and hip joints, but are less prominent in the hands (Srikanth et al., 2005).

Summary of Sex Differences in MSD Expression

As indicated by the preceding sections, studies examining the role of sex on a variety MSDs have generally found that females have a higher risk of MSDs than males for most disorders. There are several potential factors leading to this result. Such factors include the size and mechanical strength of musculoskeletal system components, differences in biological processes between men and women that affect musculoskeletal tissue health, potential differences in pain sensitivity and reporting, differential responses to psychosocial stress, and numerous other factors.

The examination of sex influence on the structure and function of musculoskeletal tissues provides evidence of significant differences in both mechanical characteristics and biological responses. Many of these sex/gender differences would be expected to substantially increase the risk of fatigue failure in females. Mechanically, females tend to exhibit smaller tissues with decreased mechanical strength (on average) compared to males and experience increased tissue loss with age (for example, in cartilage and bone) that would result in exacerbated fatigue failure risk.

While there is overlap between female and male populations in muscular strength, on average males demonstrate increased strength compared to females. This means that if an average man and an average woman perform a task requiring equivalent muscle force, the female would be likely be working at a higher percentage of maximum muscle strength compared to the male, perhaps leading to earlier muscle fatigue or injury. Female tendons and ligaments appear to exhibit significantly lower strength compared to male tendons and do not exhibit hypertrophy after exercise as male tendons do, which indicates an adaptive response for males to reduce future stress, a response generally absent in females (Magnusson et al., 2007). Females exhibit decreased bone strength compared to males (on average) and experience increased bone loss late in life. However, it should be noted that some studies have indicated that sex differences sometimes disappear when controlling for certain other variables, for example, workload (Punnett & Herbert, 2000).

Body Size and Composition

Among the many individual features that exhibit biological variability, body size is among the characteristics that is most pronounced. Body size and shape have varied systematically in humans over the years, influenced by factors such as genetics, nutrition, climate, diet, disease, geography, and technological sophistication (Ruff, 2002). Variability in body size and composition is substantial across many dimensions. According to a sampling of worldwide populations mean body mass can vary by 50% or more within sexes (Ruff, 1994). Variation in breadth measures is approximately 25%, somewhat larger than the variation observed for height (approximately 10%). Of course, the two factors discussed in previous sections (age and sex) may exert influences on both body size and composition. In general terms, the differences in body size in humans are likely to be the result of a combination of genetic influences and the developmental milieu (including factors such as diet and disease) (Ruff, 2002).

It is apparent that variability of body size and composition can both have significant effects on musculoskeletal performance and MSD risk. For example, the physical strength capacity of an individual has been found to be highly associated with the amount of lean body mass possibly leading to differential risk in the development of musculoskeletal disorders (Chen, Nelson, Zhao, Cui, & Johnston, 2013; Myers, Gebhardt, Crump, & Fleishman, 1983; Teves, Wright, & Vogel, 1985). Thus, individuals who have lower lean body mass (for which there may be many causes) would be expected to have decreased strength capacity and are likely to be operating at a higher percentage of strength capacity when performing a given task compared to an individual with higher lean body mass. This is likely to increase the risk of injury for the former as opposed to the latter.

Another aspect of body composition that has taken on increased importance in recent years is that of obesity. The disturbing rise of obesity (notably in the United States) is an emergent health crisis, involving many health-related concerns. Data from 2015 to 2016 indicated that nearly 40% of American adults were obese (compared to 34% in 2007–2008) (Hales, Fryar, Carroll, Freedman, & Ogden, 2018). The prevalence of severe obesity during the same period also rose from 5.7% to 7.7%. Obesity is typically determined using Body Mass Index (BMI). BMI is calculated using the height and weight of an individual according to the following formula:

$$BMI = \frac{m}{h^2}$$

where m is the body mass in kilograms and h denotes the height in meters. Table 12.3 provides the standard categorization of BMI values according to weight status.

Table 12.3 BMI Values and Corresponding Weight Categories

BMI	Weight status
Below 18.5	Underweight
18.5–24.9	Normal
25–29.9	Overweight
Over 30	Obese

Obesity carries with it numerous adverse systemic health effects, including increased risk of diabetes, cardiovascular disease, and hypertension. However, as will be seen later, obesity places significant burdens on the musculoskeletal system as well (both biomechanical and physiological). This section will discuss the impacts of body size and body composition on the capabilities of the musculoskeletal system, as well as the effects of these factors on the risk of MSDs.

Impact of Body Size and Composition on Muscle

Changes in muscle strength are associated with changes in muscle mass, muscle quality, and increases in adiposity (Hiol, von Hurst, Conlon, Mugridge, & Beck, 2021). Several studies have indicated that muscle mass is positively correlated with muscle strength (Beliaeff, Bouchard, Hautier, Brochu, & Dionne, 2008; Hiol, von Hurst, Conlon, Mugridge, & Beck, 2021). This would suggest that the loss of muscle mass with age might be of particular concern in older adults. However, obesity may impact the relationship between muscle mass and strength. It has been found that the relationship between muscle mass and strength is significant in non-obese individuals; however, this relationship disappears in individuals classified as obese. This may be due to an increase in intramuscular lipid content in obese individuals, which is believed to decrease strength, and lead to increased inflammation, functional deficits, and insulin insensitivity (Goodpaster et al., 1985).

Impact of Body Size and Composition on Tendons/Ligaments

Obesity has also been associated with several negative impacts that may enhance the risk of tendon disorders. For example, a systematic review of the effect of obesity on tendon disorders found that individuals with high rates of adiposity exhibit increased tendon pathologies, pain, and rupture compared to controls (Gaida, Ashe, Bass, & Cook, 2009). Tendons responsible for bearing significant loads, such as the Achilles and patellar, seem to be commonly affected (Abate, Schiavone, Di Carlo, & Salini, 2012; Klein, Weil, Weil, & Fleischer, 2013; Malliaras, Cook, & Kent, 2007). However, relationships with adiposity are also seen in tendons with lesser load-bearing responsibilities (Rechardt et al., 2010).

There are several possible reasons for the emergence of these relationships. For example, there are certainly reasons to believe that increased mechanical loading may play a role in the increased tendon disorders incidence in individuals with elevated BMI (Gaida, Ashe, Bass, & Cook, 2009). Obesity will cause heavier loads to be borne by load-bearing tendons and ligaments, such as the Achilles and patellar tendons. Increased loads will lead to a decrease in the expected fatigue life of the tendons so stressed. While tendons may try to adapt to the increased loads, there may be a limit to the adaptations that can be made to counter large increases in loading.

Another hypothesis suggests that increased adiposity leads to changes in the structure of the tendon resulting from the presence of bioactive substances (adipokines) that can lead to significant changes to tendon architecture and function (Abate et al., 2012). Several studies have shown an increased prevalence of tendon abnormalities with higher abdominal adipose tissue (Malliaras et al., 2007). Adipose tissue has been recognized as a significant endocrine organ, which secretes several bioactive peptides and hormones that can potentially modify tendon structure due to the development of a chronic low-grade inflammatory state (Abate, Schiavone, Di Carlo, & Salini, 2012). These factors can lead to degeneration of the tendon and an impaired healing response, both of which may lead to heightened injury risk.

Of course, it would not be surprising if the biomechanical and systemic responses to increased adiposity worked in tandem to increase the incidence of tendon injuries. Obesity serves to create a deleterious biochemical environment for the tendons and ligaments, which can lead to, increased tendon degeneration and impaired healing. At the same time, these tendons may experience increased loading due to the augmented weight-bearing responsibilities, the combination of which could clearly lead to an accelerated fatigue failure process in affected tendons.

Impact of Body Size and Composition on Bone

There is a substantial body of evidence that body size and composition have substantial impacts on measures of bone mass and density (Reid, 2002). For example, BMD shows a positive correlation with body weight (Felson, Zhang, Hannan, & Anderson, 1993). This relationship holds across sex and age and is true for virtually every portion of the skeleton. The effect of body weight on BMD appears stronger than that of age in many studies and may represent an important risk factor for osteoporosis (Reid, 2002). In addition, fractures appear to be strongly associated with body composition. In a study examining differences between those experiencing hip fractures compared to the normal group, those experiencing hip fractures were 3.5 kg lighter on average (Hassager & Christiansen, 1989), a finding replicated by others (Aloia et al., 1985; Kleerekoper et al., 1989).

The amount of soft tissue also appears to have an important influence on the process of bone turnover. Weight loss has been shown to significantly increase the rate of bone resorption by up to 50% (Hyldstrup, Andersen, McNair, Breum, & Transbol, 1993; Ricci et al., 2001). There appears to be a difference in effect between lean soft tissues mass versus fat soft tissue mass on bone. Lean tissue can provide benefits to bone, not only by the load carried by the skeleton by these tissues but also through the stress loading of bone resulting from muscle contraction (Reid, 2002). Fat mass also contributes to the load borne by the skeleton and is associated with increases in bone density, particularly in older women (Pluijm et al., 2001).

Impact of Body Size and Composition on Cartilage

Studies examining body composition measures such as fat-free mass (FFM) and fat mass (FM) in the body can have differential effects on tibial cartilage volume in individuals not experiencing clinical knee osteoarthritis (OA) (Wang et al., 2007). Specifically, FFM was positively correlated with tibial cartilage volume while FM was associated with adverse effects on cartilage, including a decreased tibial cartilage volume, and was associated with an increased number of cartilage defects (Wang et al., 2007). A reduction in muscle mass (a portion of FFM) has been associated with a decrease in both medial and lateral tibial cartilage across a 2-year period in people without OA. Therefore, an increased muscle mass appears to be protective against the loss of cartilage (Hudelmaier et al., 2003). This suggests that cartilage, like other musculoskeletal materials, is sensitive to the stress experienced and adapts accordingly. Decreased muscle mass would lead to decreased stress and a loss of cartilage volume as one ages. However, increased muscle mass may also be important in stabilizing the knee joint during dynamic activities which may also play a role in cartilage health.

Obesity is another body composition factor that is significantly associated with the development of knee OA (Felson, Anderson, Naimark, Walker, & Meenan, 1988). Several measures associated with obesity, including FM, BMI, and waist circumference have been positively correlated with the prevalence of OA (Abbate et al., 2006). In this study, increased BMI was associated with the increased prevalence and severity of cartilage defects. These cartilage defects have been shown to be predictive of future cartilage loss (Wang et al., 2007), strongly suggestive of the presence of a fatigue failure process.

Fatigue Failure Implications Regarding Personal Characteristics

Differences in personal characteristics (age, sex, and anthropometry) can have a profound effect on the rate at which individuals incur cumulative damage when exposed to repeated stress. Much of this effect may be due to a key precept of fatigue failure theory: the effect of an imposed stress is a function of the ultimate stress (US) of the exposed tissue. It is important to recognize that everyone's tissue ultimate stress will be unique, and variability between individuals will likely be immense. This means that if exposed to the same load and rate of repetition, different tissue strengths will lead to vastly different rates of damage development. Of course, everyone's unique tissue strength profile will be influenced by the factors discussed in this chapter (among others).

The understanding that individuals will experience different rates of damage accrual to identical loading conditions raises some interesting philosophical issues. For example, a common tactic of industry is to place younger, stronger individuals to work on jobs with greater physical demands. From a fatigue failure perspective, it must be said that such an approach makes some sense. For example, if a lifting task incurs a spinal compressive load of 2 kN and an older worker doing the job has a spine US of 4 kN (i.e., spinal load is 50% of his ultimate strength), it is likely that significant damage to spinal tissues will eventually accrue. Based on *ex vivo* studies carried on spinal motion segment strength, the characteristic life at this level of loading would be approximately 2000 cycles. However, if a younger worker with an 8 kN spine US is brought in to do the job, spinal damage would be expected to develop much more slowly. Based on the same *ex vivo* studies, the characteristic life at this level of loading (i.e., 25% of ultimate strength) would be estimated at approximately 47,000 cycles. Thus, the worker with the stronger spinal column would be expected to lift the equivalent load 45,000 cycles more than the worker with the weaker spine before reaching his or her characteristic life.

Of course, design according to individual tolerances is not the most effective method of reducing risk. In our earlier example, it would be better if the task compressive load on the spine were reduced to 1 kN, benefitting all workers. Further, it should be realized that even individuals with high tissue strength can be overloaded and develop cumulative damage. We are certainly not at the point where individualized safe load limits can be implemented with assurity. However, if MSDs are the result of a fatigue failure process, individualized "safe loads" may someday be possible and may make sense as one method of helping to control MSDs.

Relatedly, a common approach has been to design jobs such that 75% of females and 90% of males have the capability to perform a job, and should be protective of workers. However, it bears consideration when designing with such a criterion that greater risk (relatively speaking) will be borne by individuals with weaker tissues (and more risk will be experienced by women as compared to men), while individuals with higher tissue strengths will be increasingly protected. The latter individuals may be able to operate safely at a somewhat higher absolute level of loading than this population-based design criteria would suggest.

The wide ranges of tissue strengths noted earlier have significant implications for MSD prevention efforts. For example, it would make sense that as tissue strength declines with age, a commensurate decrease in repetitive loads on these tissues should be experienced. Ideally, repetitive loads for aging workers would be "stepped down" throughout their working life to accommodate for decreases in tissue tolerance. Similarly, sensitivity to the effects of gender on tissue strength should be considered in determining acceptable occupational loads. It is simply a fact of life that, on average, males will have stronger tissues than females. These differences can be substantial. According to data from Jager and Luttmann, the average female spine strength is 4,900 N while the average male spine strength is 6,625 N, a 26% difference (Jager & Luttmann, 1991). If exposed to a repetitive spinal load of equivalent magnitude, the damage will clearly accrue much more quickly in the female spine.

As a final point, it should be noted that we have focused in this chapter on physical personal characteristics, and their influence on risk. However, it should be noted that there are several personal characteristics that may also affect the risk that is outside of the physical domain. Specifically, there may be differences in physiological and/or psychological variables that may influence injury risk. These factors (and their relationship to MSD risk) are discussed in other chapters, including Chapters 10, 11, 14, and 15.

Summary

Our ability to reduce MSDs is complicated due to the substantial variability in the size and strength of musculoskeletal tissues between individuals. Personal characteristics such as age, sex, and anthropometry would be expected to influence the fatigue failure response of musculoskeletal tissues and in some cases, these characteristics may influence the response to repetitive loading experienced by these tissues. The tremendous diversity in size, shape, strength, and quality of musculoskeletal tissues inevitably results in highly variable rates of damage accumulation, even if individuals are exposed to equivalent loading histories. The influence in terms of MSD risk can be quite marked due to variability in these factors. To the extent possible, these factors should be considered while evaluating the work demands of different individuals. For example, the decrease in tissue strength due to aging would suggest that job demands on older workers should be stepped down as they age. Conditions such as obesity may have multiple negative outcomes, including increased repetitive loading on joints, potentially leading to osteoarthritis. Therefore, it is difficult to design work that provides a semblance of equivalent risk across individuals. Methods that design jobs so that the large majority of workers can perform the job inevitably will place weaker workers at increased MSD risk compared to their stronger compatriots. Personalized risk assessment methods may one day be available to help control for the effects of personal characteristics such as age, sex, and anthropometry/body composition.

Bibliography

Abate, M., Schiavone, C., Di Carlo, L., & Salini, V. (2012). Achilles tendon and plantar fascia in recently diagnosed type II diabetes: role of body mass index. *Clinical Rheumatology, 31*, 1109–1113.

Abbate, L., Stevens, J., Schwartz, T., Renner, J., Helmick, C. G., & Jordan, J. (2006). Anthropometric measures, body composition, body fat distribution, and knee osteoarthritis in women. *Obesity, 14*, 1274–1281.

Alexanderson, K., Sydsjo, A., Hensing, G., Sydsjo, G., & Carsternsen, J. (1996). Impact of pregnancy on gender differences in sickness absence. *Scandinavian Journal of Social Medicine, 24*, 169–176.

Aloia, J., Cohn, S. H., Vaswani, A., Yeh, J., Yuen, K., & Ellis, K. (1985). Risk factors for postmenopausal osteoporosis. *The American Journal of Medicine, 78*, 95–100.

Ammann, P., & Rizzoli, R. (2003). Bone strength and its determinants. *Osteoporosis International, 14*(Suppl 3), 13–18.

Armstrong, C., & Mow, V. (1982). Variations in the intrinsic mechanical properties of human articular cartilage with age, degeneration, and water content. *The Journal of Bone and Joint Surgery, 64*, 88–94. *American volume*

Arya, S., & Kulig, K. (2010). Tendinopathy alters mechanical and material properties of the Achilles tendon. *Journal of Applied Physiology, 108*, 670–675.

Bank, R., Bayliss, M., Lafeber, F., Maroudas, A., & Tekoppele, J. (1998). Ageing and zonal variation in post-translational modification of collagen in normal human articular cartilage. The age-related increase in non-enzymatic glycation affects biomechanical properties of cartilage. *The Biochemical Journal, 330*, 345–351.

Bank, R., Krikken, M., Beekman, B., Stoop, R., Maroudas, A., Lafeber, F., & te Koppele, J. (1997). A simplified measurement of degraded collagen in tissues: Application in healthy, fibrillated and osteoarthritic cartilage. *Matrix Biology, 16*, 233–243.

Beliaeff, S., Bouchard, D., Hautier, C., Brochu, M., & Dionne, I. (2008). Association between muscle mass and isometric muscle strength in well-functioning older men and women. *Journal of Aging and Physical Activity, 16*, 484–493.

Bijur, P., Horodyski, M., Egerton, W., Kurzon, M., Lifrak, S., & Friedman, S. (1997). Comparison of injury during cadet basic training by gender. *Archives of Pediatrics & Adolescent Medicine, 151*, 456–461.

Boskey, A., & Coleman, R. (2010). Aging and bone. *Journal of Dental Research, 89*, 1333–1348.

Bougea, A., Papadimas, G., Papadopoulos, C., Paraskevas, G., Kalfakis, N., Manta, P., & Kararizou, E. (2016). An age-related morphometric profile of skeletal muscle in healthy untrained women. *Journal of Clinical Medicine, E97.*

Caramés, B., Taniguchi, N., Seino, D., Blanco, F., D'Lima, D., & Lotz, M. (2012). Mechanical injury suppresses autophagy regulators and pharmacologic activation of autophagy results in chondroprotection. *Arthritis and Rheumatism, 64*, 1182–1192.

Chen, A., Temple, M., Ng, D., Verzijl, N., DeGroot, J., TeKoppele, J., & Sah, R. (2002). Induction of advanced glycation end products and alterations of the tensile properties of articular cartilage. *Arthritis and Rheumatism, 46*, 3212–3217.

Chen, G., Liu, L., & Yu, J. (2012). A comparative study on strength between American college male and female students in Caucasian and Asian populations. *Sport Science Review, 21*, 153–165.

Chen, L., Nelson, D., Zhao, Y., Cui, Z., & Johnston, J. (2013). Relationship between muscle mass and muscle strength, and the impact of comorbidities: A population-based, cross-sectional study of older adults in the United States. *BMC Geriatrics, 13*, 74.

Choi, S. (2016). Age-related functional changes and susceptibility to eccentric-induced damage in skeletal muscle cell. *Integrative Medical Research, 5*, 171–175.

Currey, J., Brear, K., & Zioupos, P. (1996). The effects of ageing and changes in mineral content in degrading the toughness of human femora. *Journal of Biomechanics, 29*, 257–262.

Currey, J., Brear, K., & Zioupos, P. (1997). Erratum. *Journal of Biomechanics, 30*, 1001.

Daly, R., Rosengren, B., Alwis, G., Ahlborg, H., Sernbo, I., & Karlsson, M. (2013). Gender specific age-related changes in bone density, muscle strength, and functional performance in the elderly: A 10-year prospective, population-based study. *BMC Geriatrics, 71.*

Dean, D., Martel-Pelletier, J., Pelletier, J., Howell, D., & Woessner, J. J. (1989). Evidence for metalloproteinase and metalloproteinase inhibitor imbalance in human osteoarthritic cartilage. *Journal of Clinical Investigation*, *84*, 678–685.

Felson, D., Anderson, J., Naimark, A., Walker, A., & Meenan, R. (1988). Obesity and knee osteoarthritis The Framingham Study. *Annals of Internal Medicine*, *109*, 18–24.

Felson, D., Zhang, Y., Hannan, M., & Anderson, J. (1993). Effects of weight and body mass index on bone mineral density in men and women—The Framingham study. *Journal of Bone and Mineral Research*, *8*, 567–573.

Fu, S., Chan, B., Wang, W., Pau, H., Chan, K., & Rolf, C. (2002). Increased expression of matrix metalloproteinase 1 (MMP1) in 11 patients with patellar tendinosis. *Acta Orthopaedica Scandinavica*, *73*, 658–662.

Funakoshi, T., Iwasaki, N., Kamishima, T., Nishida, M., Ito, Y., Kondo, M., . . . Minami, A. (2010). In vivo visualization of vascular patterns of rotator cuff tearsising contrast-enhanced ultrasound. *American Journal of Sports Medicine*, *38*, 2464–2471.

Gaida, J., Ashe, M., Bass, S., & Cook, J. (2009). Is adiposity an under-recognized risk factor for tendinopathy? A systematic review. *Arthritis and Rheumatism*, *61*, 840–849.

Goodpaster, B., Carlson, C., Visser, M., Kelley, D., Scherzinger, A., Harris, T. B., . . . Newman, A. B. (1985). Attenuation of skeletal muscle and strength in the elderly: The Health ABC Study. *Journal of Applied Physiology*, *90*, 2157–2165.

Guccione, A., Felson, D., Anderson, J., Anthony, J., Zhang, Y., Wilson, A., . . . Kannel, W. (1994). The effects of specific mdeical condition on the functional limitations of elders in the Framingham study. *American Journal of Public Health*, *84*, 351–358.

Haizlip, K., Harrison, B., & Leinwand, L. (2015). Sex-based differences in skeletal muscle kinetics and fiber-type composition. *Physiology*, *30*, 30–39.

Hales, C., Fryar, C., Carroll, M., Freedman, D., & Ogden, C. (2018). Trends in obesity and severe obesity prevalence in US youth and adults by sex and age, 2007–2008 to 2015–2016. *JAMA*, *319*, 1723–1725.

Hanna, F., Teichtahl, A., Wluka, A., Wang, Y., Urquhart, D., English, D., . . . Cicuttini, F. (2009). Women have increased rates of cartilage loss and progression of cartilage defects at the knee than men: A gender study of adults without clinical knee osteoarthritis. *Menopause*, *16*, 666–670.

Hashimoto, S., Ochs, R., Komiya, S., & Lotz, M. (1998). Linkage of chondrocyte apoptosis and cartilage degradation in human osteoarthritis. *Arthritis and Rheumatism*, *41*, 1632–1638.

Hassager, C., & Christiansen, C. (1989). Estrogen/gestagen therapy changes soft tissue body composition in postmenopausal women. *Metabolism: Clinical and Experimental*, *38*(7), 662–665.

Hewett, T., Myer, T., & Ford, K. (2001). Prevention of anterior cruciate ligament injuries. *Current Women's Health Reports*, *1*, 218–224.

Hiol, A., von Hurst, P., Conlon, C., Mugridge, O., & Beck, K. L. (2021). Body composition associations with muscle strength in older adults living in Auckland New Zealand. *PLOS ONE*, *16*, e0250439.

Hirano, T., Turner, C., Forwood, M., Johnston, C., & Burr, D. (2000). Does suppression of bone turnover impair mechanical properties by allowing microdamage accumulation? *Bone*, *27*, 13–20.

Hudelmaier, M., Glaser, C., Englmeier, K., Reiser, M., Putz, R., & Eckstein, F. (2003). Correlation of knee-joint cartilage morphology with muscle cross-sectional areas vs. anthropometric variables. *The Anatomical Record. Part A, Discoveries in Molecular, Cellular, and Evolutionary Biology*, *270*, 175–184.

Hyldstrup, L., Andersen, T., McNair, P., Breum, L., & Transbol, I. (1993). Bone metabolism in obesity—Changes related to severe overweight and dietary weight reduction. *Acta Endocrinologica*, *129*, 393–398.

Jager, M., & Luttmann, A. (1991). Compressive strength of lumbar spine elements related to age, gender, and other influencing factors. *Journal of Electromyography and Kinesiolology*, 291–294.

Johnson, V., & Hunter, D. (2014). The epidemiology of osteoarthritis. *Best Practice & Research. Clinical Rheumatology*, *28*, 5–15.

Jones, B., Bovee, M., Harris, J., III, & Cowan, D. (1993). Intrinsic risk factors for exercise-related injuries among male and female army trainees. *The American Journal of Sports Medicine*, *21*, 705–710.

Jones, B., Thacker, S., Gilchrist, J., Kimsey, C., & Sosin, D. (2002). Prevention of lower extremity stress-fractures in athletes and soldiers: A systematic review. *Epidmiology Review*, *24*, 228–247.

Josza, L., & Kannus, P. (1997). *Human tendons: Anatomy, physiology, and pathology*. Champaign, IL: Human Kinetics.

Kanis, J. (2002). Diagnosis of osteoporosis and assessment of fracture risk. *Lancet*, *359*, 1929–1936.

Kannus, L., Jozsa, L., Renstrom, P., Jarvinen, M., Kvist, M., Lehto, M., . . . Vuori, I. (1992). The effects of training, immobilization, and remobilization on musculoskeletal tissue. I. Training and immobilization. *Scandinavian Journal of Medicine and Science in Sports*, *2*, 100–118.

Kannus, P., Paavola, M., & Józsa, L. (2005). Aging and degeneration of tendons pages. In N. Maffulli, P. Renström, & W. Leadbetter (Eds.), *Tendon injuries: Basic science and clinical medicine* (pp. 25–31). London: Springer-Verlag London Limited.

Kirkwood, T. (2005). Understanding the odd science of aging. *Cell*, *120*, 437–447.

Kleerekoper, M., Peterson, E., Nelson, D., Tilley, B., Phillips, E., Schork, M., & Kuder, J. (1989). Identification of women at risk for developing postmenopausal osteoporosis with vertebral fractures: Role of history and single photon absorptiometry. *Bone*, *7*, 171–186.

Klein, E., Weil, L. J., Weil, L. S., & Fleischer, A. (2013). Body mass index and achilles tendonitis: a 10-year retrospective analysis. *Foot & Ankle Specialist*, *6*, 276–282.

Knight, J., Nigam, Y., & Hore, N. (2017). Anatomy and physiology of ageing 10: The musculoskeletal system. *Nursing Times*, *113*, 60–63.

Lau, A., & Adachi, J. (2011). Bone aging. In Y. Nakasato & R. Yung (Eds.), *Geriatric rheumatology: A comprehensive approach*. New York, NY: Springer.

Lavagnino, M., & Arnoczky, S. (2005). In vitro alterations in cytoskeletal tensional homeostasis control gene expression in tendon cells. *Journal of Orthopaedic Research*, *23*, 1211–1218.

Liu, S., Al-shaikh, R., Panossian, V., Finerman, G., & Lane, J. (1997). Estrogen affects the cellular metabolism of the anterior cruciate ligament: A potential explanation for female athletic injury. *American Journal of Sports Medicine*, *25*, 704–709.

Longo, U., Franceschi, F., Ruzzini, L., Rabitti, C., Morini, S., Maffulli, N., & Denaro, V. (2008). Histopathology of the supraspinatus tendon in rotator cuff tears. *American Journal of Sports Medicine*, *36*, 533–538.

Lotz, M., & Loeser, R. F. (2012). Effects of aging on articular cartilage homeostasis. *Bone*, *51*, 241–248.

Magnusson, S., Hansen, M., Langberg, H., Miller, B., Haraldsson, B., Westh, E., . . . Kjaer, M. (2007). The adaptability of tendon to loading differs in men and women. *International Journal of Experimental Pathology*, *88*, 237–240.

Malliaras, P., Cook, J., & Kent, P. (2007). Anthropometric risk factors for patellar tendon injury among volleyball players. *British Journal of Sports Medicine*, *41*, 259–263.

Maroudas, A. (1990). Different ways of expressing concentration of cartilage constituents with special reference to the tissue's organization and functional properties. In A. Maroudas & K. Kuettner (Eds.), *Methods in cartilage research* (pp. 211–219). New York, NY: Academic Press.

McCarthy, M., & Hannafin, J. (2013). The mature athlete: Aging tendon and ligament. *Sports Health*, *6*(1), 41–48.

Melton, L. (1996). Epidemiology of hip fractures: Implications of the exponential increase with age. *Bone*, *18*(3 Suppl), 121S–125S.

Miller, A., MacDougall, J., Tarnopolsky, M., & Sale, D. (1993). Gender differences in strength and muscle fiber characteristics. *European Journal of Applied Physiology, 66*, 254–262.

Miller, B., Olesen, J., Hansen, M., Døssing, S., Crameri, R., Welling, R., . . . Rennie, M. (2005). Coordinated collagen and muscle protein synthesis in human patella tendon and quadriceps muscle after exercise. *The Journal of Physiology, 567*(Pt 3), 1021–1033.

Muraoka, T., Muramatsu, T., Fukunaga, T., & Kanehisa, H. (2005). Elastic properties of human Achilles tendon are correlated to muscle strength. *Journal of Applied Physiology, 99*, 665–669.

Murgia, M., Toniolo, L., Nagaraj, N., Ciciliot, S., Vindigni, V., Schiaffino, S., . . . Mann, M. (2017). Single muscle fiber proteomics reveal fiber-type-specific features of human muscle aging. *Cell Reports, 19*, 2396–2409.

Myers, D., Gebhardt, D., Crump, C., & Fleishman, E. (1983). *Validation of the military enlistment physical strength capacity test. Technical Report 610*. Natick, Mass: U.S. Army Research Institute for the Behavioral Sciences.

National Institutes of Health. (2021). *Osteoporosis: Peak bone mass in women*. Retrieved from https://www.bones.nih.gov/health-info/bone/osteoporosis/bone-mass

Noyes, F., & Grood, E. (1976). The strength of the anterior cruciate ligament in humans and rhesus monkeys. *Journal of Bone and Joint Surgery (American), 58*, 1074–1082.

O'Brien, F., Brennan, O., Kennedy, O., & Lee, T. (2005). Microcracks in cortical bone: How do they affect bone biology? *Current Osteoporosis Reports, 3*, 39–45.

Pepper, M., Akuthota, V., & McCarty, E. (2006). The pathophysiology of stress fractures. *Clinics in Sports Medicine, 25*, 1–16.

Pluijm, S., Visser, M., Smit, J., Popp-Snijders, C., Roos, J., & Lips, P. (2001). Determinants of bone mineral density in older men and women: Body composition as mediator. *Journal of Bone and Mineral Research, 16*, 2142–2151.

Poole, A. (2005). Cartilage in health and disease. In W. Koopman (Ed.), *Arthritis and allied conditions*. Philadelphia: Williams and Wilkins.

Power, G., Dalton, B., & Rice, C. (2013). Human neuromuscular structure and function in old age: A brief review. *Journal of Sport and Health Science, 2*(4), 215–226.

Pritzker, K., Gay, S., Jimenez, S., Ostergaard, K., Pelletier, J., Revell, P., . . . Van den Berg, W. (2006). Osteoarthritis cartilage histopathology: Grading and staging. *Osteoarthritis and Cartilage, 14*, 13–29.

Punnett, L., & Bergqvist, U. (1999). Musculoskeletal disorders in visual display unit work: Gender and work demands. *Occupational Medicine, 14*, 113–124.

Punnett, L., & Herbert, R. (2000). Work-related musculoskeletal disorders: Is there a gender differential, and if so, what does it mean? In M. Goldman & M. Hatch (Eds.), *Women and health*. San Diego: Academic Press.

Rechardt, M., Shiri, R., Karppinen, J., Jula, A., Heliövaara, M., & Viikari-Juntura, E. (2010). Lifestyle and metabolic factors in relation to shoulder pain and rotator cuff tendinitis: A population-based study. *BMC Musculoskeletal Disorders, 11*, 165.

Reid, I. (2002). Relationships among body mass, its components and bone. *Bone, 31*, 547–555.

Ricci, T., Heymsfield, S., Pierson, R., Stahl, T., Chowdhury, H., & Shapses, S. (2001). Moderate energy restriction increases bone resorption in obese postmenopausal women. *The American Journal of Clinical Nutrition, 73*, 347–352.

Rollman, G., & Lautenbacher, S. (2001). Sex differences in musculoskeletal pain. *The Clinical Journal of Pain, 17*, 20–24.

Rudzki, J., Adler, R., Warren, R., Kadrmas, W., Verma, N., Pearle, A., . . . Fealy, S. (2008). Contrast-enhanced ultrasound characterization of the rotator cuff tendon: Age- and activity-relatedchanges in the intact asymptomatic rotator cuff. *Journal of Shoulder and Elbow Surgery, 17*(1 Suppl), 96S–100S.

Ruff, C. B. (1994). Morphological adaptation to climate in modern and fossil hominids. *American Journal of Physical Anthropology, 37*(19 S), 65–107.

Ruff, C. (2002). Variation in human body size and shape. *Annual Review of Anthropology, 31*, 211–232.

Schaffler, M., Choi, K., & Milgrom, C. (1995). Aging and matrix microdamage accumulation in human compact bone. *Bone, 17*, 521–552.

Schechtman, H., & Bader, D. (1997). In vitro fatigue of human tendons. *Journal of Biomechanics*, 829–835.

Seeman, E. (2001). Sexual dimorphism in skeletal size, density, and strength. *The Journal of Clinical Endocrinology & Metabolism, 86*, 4576–4584.

Srikanth, V., Fryer, J., Zhai, G., Winzenberg, T., Hosmer, D., & Jones, G. (2005). A meta-analysis of sex differences prevalence, incidence and severity of osteoarthritis. *Osteoarthritis and Cartilage, 13*, 769–781.

Stokinger, J., Maxwell, N., Shapiro, D., deCabo, R., & Valdez, G. (2017). Caloric restriction mimetics slow aging of neuromuscular synapses and muscle fibers. *The Journals of Gerontology, Series A, 73*, 21–28.

Svensson, R., Heinemeier, K., Couppé, C., Kjaer, M., & Magnusson, S. (2016). Effect of aging and exercise on the tendon. *Journal of Applied Physiology, 121*, 1353–1362.

Teves, M., Wright, J., & Vogel, J. (1985). *Performance on selected candidate screening test procedures before and after Army basic and advanced individual training. Technical Report T13-85*. Natick, Mass.: U.S. Army Research Institute of Environmental Medicine.

Treaster, D., & Burr, D. (2004). Gender differences in prevalence of upper extremity musculoskeletal disorders. *Ergonomics, 47*, 495–526.

Tuite, D., Renstrom, P., & O'Brien, M. (1997). The aging tendon. *Scandinavian Journal of Medicine and Science in Sports, 7*, 72–77.

Vashishth, D. (2007). Hierarchy of bone microdamage at multiple length scales. *International Journal of Fatigue, 29*, 1024–1033.

Wang, Y., Wluka, A., English, D., Teichtahl, A., Giles, G., O'Sullivan, R., & Cicuttini, F. (2007). Body composition and knee cartilage properties in healthy, community-based adults. *Annals of the Rheumatic Diseases, 66*, 1244–1248.

Wentz, L., Liu, P.-Y., Haymes, E., & Ilich, J. (2011). Females have a greater incidence of stress fractures than males in both military and athletic populations: A systematic review. *Military Medicine, 176*, 420–430.

West, C. (2014). Genetic susceptibility and predictive assays. In A. Brahme (Ed.), *Comprehensive biomedical physics* (pp. 143–156). Amsterdam: Elsevier.

Wijnhoven, H., de Vet, H., & Picavet, H. (2006). Prevalence of musculoskeletal disorders is systematically higher in women than in men. *The Clinical Journal of Pain, 22*, 717–724.

Woo, S., Hollis, J., Adams, F., Lyon, R., & Takai, S. (1991). Tensile properties of the human femur-anteriorcruciate ligament-tibia complex. The effects of specimen age and orientation. *American Journal of Sports Medicine, 19*, 219–225.

Yates, L., Karasik, D., Beck, T., Cupples, L., & Kiel, D. (2007). Hip structural geometry in old and old-old age: Similarities and differences between men and women. *Bone, 41*, 722–732.

Yu, W., Panossian, V., Hatch, J., Liu, S., & Finerman, G. (2001). Combined effects of estrogen and progesterone on the anterior cruciate ligament. *Clinical Orthopaedics, 383*, 268–281.

Zhang, Y., & Jordan, J. (2010). Epidemiology of osteoarthritis. *Clinics in Geriatric Medicine, 26*, 355–369.

13

Using Fatigue Failure Principles to Assess MSD Risk

Introduction

Previous chapters have provided substantial evidence that musculoskeletal tissues experience fatigue failure when exposed to repeated stress, both *ex vivo* and *in vivo*. Evidence has also shown that the damage to tissues from *in vivo* animal studies involving repeated stress demonstrates damage patterns that mirror those observed in MSDs involving tendons, cartilages, ligaments, and bones (Barbe et al., 2013; Shepherd et al., 2014; Shepherd & Screen, 2013; Sun et al., 2010). If fatigue failure is indeed a causal mechanism in the development of MSDs, it would seem sensible to use validated fatigue failure methods to estimate the development of cumulative damage in tissues experiencing repeated stress. As will be described in this chapter, numerous benefits can accrue from the application of fatigue failure principles to MSD risk assessment. Further, when fatigue failure principles are applied to MSD risk assessment, strong associations are demonstrated between fatigue-based cumulative damage model estimates and MSD outcomes.

Chapter 9 described several principles of fatigue failure analysis and showed how these principles have been used to assess the development of cumulative damage in normal (non-biological) materials. The current chapter describes how some of these very same techniques can be applied to the assessment of the damage development in musculoskeletal tissues, specifically in the context of occupational MSDs. We will describe three recently developed assessment tools to assess the risk of MSDs for various regions of the body, including the low back, shoulders, and the distal upper extremity (DUE). We will begin, however, with a brief discussion of the application of fatigue failure principles with respect to risk assessment, and describe criteria that have guided the development of the fatigue failure-based risk assessment tools.

Application of Fatigue Failure Principles to MSD Risk Assessment

Fatigue failure theory provides several key insights that are helpful in assessing cumulative damage development in materials exposed to repeated stress. As will be seen, some of these techniques can be readily implemented in easy-to-use MSD risk assessment tools. Other fatigue failure techniques hold great promise for application as future developments in risk assessment emerge. Examples include the use of rainflow analysis (or other related techniques) once methods of assessing continuous joint loads are developed; and combining the effects of creep loading and cyclic loading in estimates of MSD risk. However, well before these (and other) more advanced

Musculoskeletal Disorders: The Fatigue Failure Mechanism, First Edition. Sean Gallagher and Mary F. Barbe.

techniques can be applied, there are several fundamental fatigue assessment techniques available to develop straightforward and easy-to-use tools to evaluate MSD risk.

A key insight of fatigue failure theory is that there is an exponential increase in damage caused by each repetition as the stress level intensifies. The cumulative damage associated with each high-force repetition can be several hundred times greater than a low-force repetition. This is a fundamental relationship that is critical to MSD risk assessment. Another major benefit is that fatigue failure provides a validated method to determine the development of cumulative damage when highly variable loading is experienced, such as in the performance of multiple tasks with different physical demands (Miner, 1945; Palmgren, 1924; Post, Case, & Lesko, 2008). Loading of musculoskeletal tissues in humans tends to be highly variable in nature; thus, it is quite helpful to have validated methods for assessing variable loading readily available for use (Manson, Freche, & Ensign, 1967; Post, Case, & Lesko, 2008). As will be seen later, not only can the total cumulative damage be estimated for highly variable multi-task jobs, but the fatigue failure methodology allows the determination of the proportion of the total damage associated with each task.

This chapter will describe the development, use, and validation of three fatigue failure-based risk assessment tools. The Lifting Fatigue Failure Tool or "LiFFT", is a tool designed to assess the risk of low back injuries due to manual lifting; the second tool (the Distal Upper Extremity Tool, or DUET) is employed to assess the risk of distal upper extremity injuries due to hand intensive work; lastly, the third tool (The Shoulder Tool) is used to assess the risk of shoulder outcomes resulting from shoulder intensive work. We will provide the logic underlying the development of these tools, describe proper methods of use, interpret the results, and present the results of validation studies that demonstrate the efficacy of these tools in assessing a wide range of MSD outcomes.

General Principles of Fatigue Failure Theory

Fatigue failure theory states that cumulative damage development in a material is the result of repetitive stress experienced by that material. Thus, to develop a risk assessment tool for MSDs, one would ideally require direct knowledge of the magnitude of stress (and/or the resultant strain) experienced by the material at issue. Unfortunately, direct stress and strain measurements are not easily obtained from living biological tissues at the current time. Fortunately, there are several surrogate measures that can be used in place of stress, which includes estimates of load, moment, torque, or strain (Stephens et al., 2001).

Once a measure representing stress for a particular task has been determined, an accurate count of the number of daily repetitions performed for that task will be needed. Several methods can be used to derive such estimates, including data from video analysis, production counts, etc. Obviously, methods having higher degrees of accuracy are preferable. Recent advances in technology have provided new techniques that may be able to provide excellent estimates of the number of cycles performed by workers, as well as continuous estimates of loading on joints of interest. These include the use of wearable sensors such as inertial measurement units (IMUs) and/or use of video-based exposure assessment methods (Radwin, 2011; Robert-Lachaine, Mecheri, Larue, & Plamondon, 2017; Schall Jr., Fethke, Chen, & Gerr, 2015; Schall Jr., Fethke, & Chen, 2016; Wang, Hu, Lu, & Radwin, 2019).

Suggested Criteria for Risk Assessment Tools

When developing or assessing MSD risk assessment tools, it is helpful to consider what the desirable features of a risk assessment tool might be. Clearly, the tool should be able to demonstrate a

Table 13.1 Criteria for Assessment of MSD Risk Assessment Tools

- The tool should have a sound basis in the scientific literature
- The tool should be quick to use and easily administered
- The tool should be applicable in a wide variety of occupations/settings
- The tool should be able to handle complex jobs as well as relatively straightforward jobs without undue difficulty
- The tool should be able to demonstrate criterion-related validity (concurrent and/or prospective) with respect to MSD outcomes
- Risk estimates provided by the tool should demonstrate a dose-response relationship to the prevalence or incidence of the MSD outcome in cross-sectional or prospective epidemiology studies.
- The tool should provide an estimate of the cumulative load exposure when a worker performs multiple tasks.
- The tool results should be consistent when a single practitioner evaluates a specific task on more than one occasion (intra-observer reliability) or when two separate practitioners measure the same task (inter-observer reliability).

strong relationship between the score obtained and the risk of developing some MSD outcome. In addition, the tool should be reasonably quick and easy to use and should be applicable across a wide variety of jobs. That is, the *applicability* and *usability* of the tool should be considered so that the assessment of jobs is not too onerous for the analyst. In addition, the tool should be able to demonstrate that the tool scores are generally repeatable for different raters and for the same rater evaluating the same job multiple times (i.e., the tool should show suitable inter-rater and intra-rater reliability).

The preceding paragraph suggests certain criteria that musculoskeletal risk assessment tools should strive to achieve. To formalize such an assessment, we suggest the eight criteria be considered when assessing MSD risk assessment tools, as shown in Table 13.1.

Fatigue-Failure Based Risk Assessment Tools

The following sections will discuss three recently developed MSD risk assessment tools based on fatigue failure theory. These tools were developed by a team of professors and students at Auburn University from 2016 to 2020. For each of these tools, the model logic will be presented, along with guidance regarding the tool's use and interpretation. In addition, criterion-related validation studies demonstrating the relationship between the cumulative damage estimates of these tools and various MSD outcomes will be presented for each of the tools.

The Lifting Fatigue Failure Tool (LiFFT)

The LiFFT tool provides a new method of assessing the risk of low back outcomes associated with manual lifting and lowering tasks. This tool assumes that the development of low back disorders (LBDs) is the result of cumulative damage development due to a fatigue failure process in spinal or para-spinal tissues resulting from the repeated stresses experienced in lifting/lowering tasks. Benefits associated with this tool include quick assessment for each lifting task (only three pieces of information are required); an approach that provides estimates of the cumulative effects associated with a variety of lifting tasks; and identification of tasks or tasks responsible for the greatest proportion of risk (i.e., those most in need of task redesign) in multitask jobs.

Model logic

The LiFFT model uses a measure known as the Peak Load Moment (PLM) of the lifting or lowering task along with the number of daily lifting repetitions of the task to generate a risk assessment (Marras, Fine, Ferguson, & Waters, 1999). The PLM is simply the product of the object weight times the maximum horizontal distance from the spine to the object experienced during the lifting or lowering task. A measuring tape can be used to obtain the horizontal distance. The PLM has been demonstrated to be highly predictive of low back disorders, one large study showed a higher association (i.e., an odds ratio (OR) of 5.2) with low back disorders (LBDs) than either the 1981 or 1993 NIOSH Lifting Guides (ORs of 4.3 and 4.6, respectively) (Marras et al., 1999). Thus, the PLM has been found to compare favorably to other (more complicated) procedures in assessing the risk of LBDs.

Estimates of cumulative damage in LiFFT were developed by estimating the spinal compression associated with each load moment and then comparing these estimates to the ultimate compressive strength of an "average" person (approximately 6 kN; Jager & Luttmann, 1991). Damage per cycle (DPC) estimates for different levels of loading were derived from studies of fatigue failure of spinal motion segments (Brinckmann, Biggemann, & Hilweg, 1988; Gallagher et al., 2007). Data from these two studies were analyzed using Weibull analyses to estimate the probability of spine failure at varying levels of estimated ultimate strength (US) of motion segments, where predicted US was calculated using the procedure outlined by Brinckmann et al. (1988). The resulting relationship is characterized by the following equation:

$$Cycles\ to\ Failure = 902{,}416 * e^{-0.162*\%US}$$

where e is Euler's number (approximately 2.71828), and $\%US$ is the percentage of the ultimate strength for a motion segment. From this relationship, it was possible to estimate the expected number of cycles to failure at different percentages of US, and the inverse—the expected DPC at each level of US.

The compressive load associated with a wide range of PLMs was obtained using a static biomechanical model (Bloswick & Villnave, 2000). Analyses were performed in an upright posture using an individual of average anthropometry (blended male and female). Regression techniques were used to develop an equation defining this relationship. These steps allowed each PLM to be associated with an estimated spine compressive load, which is, in turn, related to the ultimate compressive strength of an average spine. The DPC associated with each estimated compressive load was then multiplied by the number of repetitions performed to obtain the total cumulative damage (CD) associated with each given task (Gallagher, Sesek, Schall Jr, & Huangfu, 2017). If multiple lifting or lowering tasks are performed during the workday, the CD associated with each is summed to provide the total CD for the day—effectively a "daily dose" of exposure.

Using LiFFT

In the development of LiFFT, considerable attention was paid to developing a tool that not only demonstrated significant associations with low back outcomes but was also easy to use by a practitioner. This is the reason that the choice was made to use the PLM as the primary measure of loading on the low back, as described earlier. All that is needed to use the LiFFT tool are three pieces of information for each lifting task, namely (a) the weight of the load; (b) a measurement of the greatest horizontal distance from the spine (or hip) to the center of the load during the lift, and

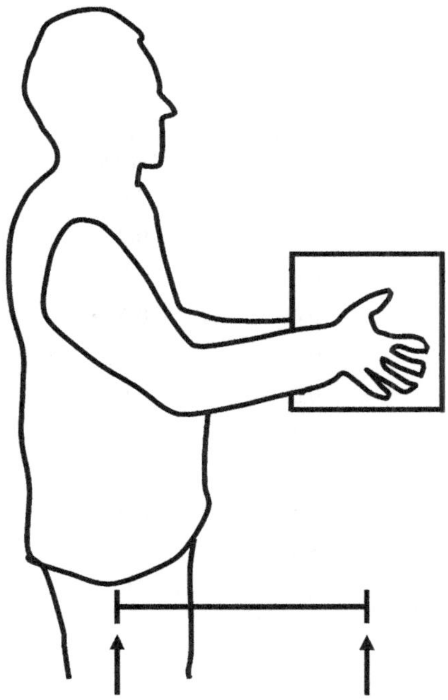

Figure 13.1 Proper measurement of the maximum horizontal distance during a sagittal lift.

(c) the number of repetitions of this task during the workday. If the worker performs several lifting tasks throughout the workday, the same variables need to be collected for each task. Both one-handed and two-handed lifts can be analyzed using LiFFT. Figure 13.1 demonstrates how the maximum distance from the hip joint to the center of the load should be measured during the lifting or lowering task.

As with all the fatigue-failure based risk assessment tools discussed here, LiFFT comes in two versions: a web-based version that can be accessed by computer, tablet, or smartphone, or a computer-based Excel version that allows saving of analyses in a database (Excel versions for all tools freely available from https://eng.auburn.edu/occupational-safety-ergonomics-injury-prevention/risk-assessment/index.html). Figure 13.2 shows the graphical user interface for the web-based version of the LiFFT tool (freely available at http://lifft.pythonanywhere.com). Several features can be observed. On the right-hand header above the tool, on the upper right-hand side, one can see a "Home" link, an "Instructions" link, and links to "DUET" and "The Shoulder Tool" (the other fatigue failure-based risk assessment tools). The "Home" link simply takes you back to the main page should you visit the "Instructions" page. The "Instructions" link takes you to a page providing guidance regarding the use and interpretation of the LiFFT tool. Underneath this header on the right-hand side, either English or Metric units can be selected for the analysis. Data input consists of providing a lever arm, a load, and the repetitions performed per day for each lifting/lowering task being analyzed.

The simplest example of using LiFFT to analyze tasks involving lifting demands is that of a mono-task job (i.e., a job in which the same lifting task is performed throughout an entire shift). In the following example, the job involves lifting a 30-pound load that is performed 325 times during the workday, involving a maximal horizontal distance of 24 in. Figure 13.3 shows the LiFFT tool analysis for this mono-task job, which indicates this job has about a 43% probability of being a high-risk job.

LiFFT 1.4.1 Home Instructions DUET The shoulder tool

The lifting fatigue failure tool

Unit: English | Metric

Task #	Lever arm (in.)	Load (lb)	Moment (ft.lb)	Repetitions (per work day)	Damage (cumulative)	% Total (damage)
1			0.0		0.0	0.0
2			0.0		0.0	0.0
3			0.0		0.0	0.0
4			0.0		0.0	0.0
5			0.0		0.0	0.0
6			0.0		0.0	0.0
7			0.0		0.0	0.0
8			0.0		0.0	0.0
9			0.0		0.0	0.0
10			0.0		0.0	0.0
			Total cumulative damage:		0	
			Probability of high risk job *(%):		0	

Reset Calculate

Figure 13.2 Graphical user interface for the LiFFT.

The lifting fatigue failure tool

Unit: English | Metric

Task #	Lever arm (in.)	Load (lb)	Moment (ft.lb)	Repetitions (per work day)	Damage (cumulative)	% Total (damage)
1	24	30	60.0	325	0.0106	100.0
2			0.0		0.0	0.0
3			0.0		0.0	0.0
4			0.0		0.0	0.0
5			0.0		0.0	0.0
6			0.0		0.0	0.0
7			0.0		0.0	0.0
8			0.0		0.0	0.0
9			0.0		0.0	0.0
10			0.0		0.0	0.0
			Total cumulative damage:		0.0106	
			Probability of high risk job *(%):		42.6	

Reset Calculate

Figure 13.3 A screenshot of a LiFFT analysis for a mono-task job.

Notice that the cumulative damage score for this mono-task job is a little > 0.01. Jobs exhibiting this level of cumulative damage should be considered strong candidates for ergonomic design methods to reduce the risk of injury. For example, if the job could be redesigned (for example, a barrier removed) such that the maximum lever arm was just 12 in., the high-risk probability would drop to 27%.

The lifting fatigue failure tool

Unit: English | Metric

Task #	Lever arm (in.)	Load (lb)	Moment (ft.lb)	Repetitions (per work day)	Damage (cumulative)	% Total (damage)
1	18	5	7.5	420	0.001	4.7
2	16	27	36.0	240	0.0023	10.9
3	22	45	82.5	80	0.008	37.9
4	24	35	70.0	180	0.0098	46.4
5			0.0		0.0	0.0
6			0.0		0.0	0.0
7			0.0		0.0	0.0
8			0.0		0.0	0.0
9			0.0		0.0	0.0
10			0.0		0.0	0.0
				Total cumulative damage:	0.0211	
				Probability of high risk job *(%):	50.2	

Reset Calculate

Figure 13.4 An example of a multi-task lifting job analysis using LiFFT.

For jobs that require multiple lifting tasks during the workday, each lifting task should be analyzed using the methods described earlier. The CD associated with each lift will be summed by the LiFFT tool to determine the daily dose of cumulative spine loading. An example is provided in Figure 13.4.

The preceding example shows that the combination of these four tasks leads to a combined probability of 50% that this would be a high-risk job, which should cause significant concern to the analyst. Further, note that tasks 3 and 4 account for about 84% of the total damage accumulated for the workday. These two tasks would be prime candidates for redesign. For example, if the lever arm for tasks 3 and 4 were reduced to 12 in., the probability that the overall job is high risk would be reduced to 37%, indicating a significant risk reduction.

If many highly variable lifting tasks are performed (e.g., warehouse picking), we recommend the use of the Excel-based LiFFT which allows adding up to 100 additional lines for additional lifting/lowering task analyses. Alternatively, a "binning" procedure can be used in which lifts within the same range of peak moments are summed up and the cumulative damage score is developed using the number of lifts within each "bin". For example, one might have 130 lifts between 0 and 10 ft.-lbs., 75 lifts between 11 and 20 ft.-lbs., and so forth. These can then be entered into the tool using the top load moment of the range (10, 20 ft.-lbs., etc.), and the cumulative damage for the workday can be determined.

Validation of the LiFFT tool

If fatigue failure is indeed an important mechanism associated with the development of LBDs, we would expect that tools employing fatigue failure techniques to demonstrate significant associations with the prevalence or incidence of these disorders. This requires criterion-related validation of the assessment tool estimates of risk against adverse low back outcomes in epidemiological studies. There are two types of criterion-related validity typically utilized in such comparisons. The first is concurrent criterion-related validity, which is when tool predictions are compared to outcomes in a cross-sectional epidemiology study. This type of validity demonstrates the association between the tool risk estimates and injury prevalence. Because the cross-sectional study is a snapshot of injury prevalence at one point in time, it does not demonstrate the ability to predict future injury occurrence. The second type of validity is prospective criterion-related validity, in which tool predictions are made at the beginning of the study and these estimates are compared to the incidence of adverse outcomes in the future. This provides a stronger degree of evidence related to the utility of the tool predictions (i.e., the risk tool may be able to predict future injury).

LiFFT was validated against two separate cross-sectional epidemiology studies to evaluate concurrent criterion-related validity. The first was a study examining the efficacy of the Lumbar Motion Monitor (LMM), which examined the low back disorder risk associated with monotask jobs (Marras et al., 1993). A database from this study was published by Zurada and colleagues, which contained the peak load moment, the lifting frequency (per hour), and whether the job was high-risk (defined as a job having 12 or more low back disorders per 200,000 man-hr) or not (no low back disorders and no turnover), all the necessary information for validation of LiFFT (Zurada, Karwowski, & Marras, 1997). Logistic regression was performed to determine the association between LiFFT's estimate of cumulative damage and the probability that the job in question was a high-risk one.

Results of the analysis demonstrated that the log of LiFFT's cumulative damage measure (Log CD) was significantly associated with jobs defined as high risk of LBDs. The cumulative damage measure was treated as a continuous variable in this analysis and showed a continuous OR of 2.78 (95% CI: 2.02, 3.83). This indicates that for every unit increase in the log of LiFFT's CD (Log CD) score, the odds of the job being classified as high risk would increase by a factor of 2.78. Figure 13.5 illustrates the dose-response relationship between the Log CD metric and the probability that the job is high risk (Gallagher, Sesek, Schall Jr, & Huangfu, 2017).

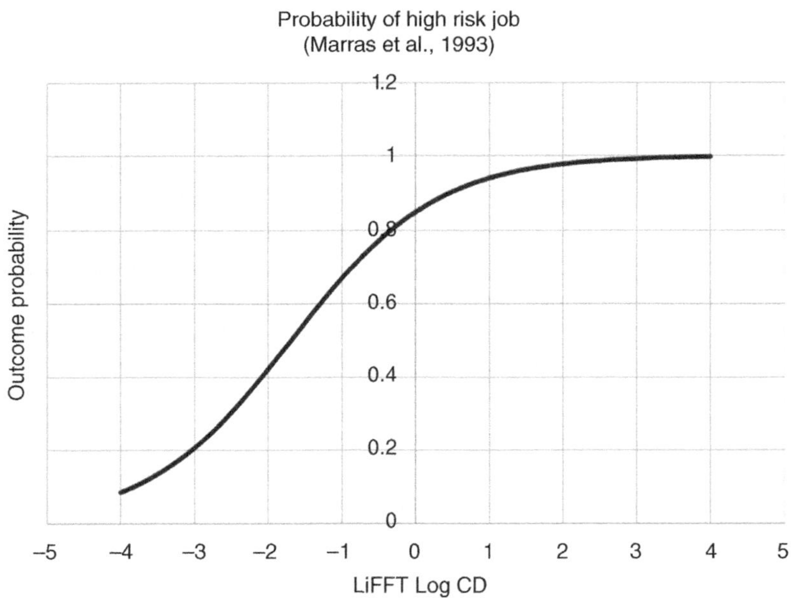

Figure 13.5 Probability of high-risk job for low back disorders (Zurada et al., 1997) as a function of LiFFT Log CD (Gallagher, S., Sesek, R., Schall Jr, M., & Huangfu, R. (2017). Development and validation of an easy-to-use risk assessment tool for cumulative low back loading: The lifting fatigue failure tool (LiFFT). *Applied Ergonomics, 63,* 142–150/with permission of Elsevier).

Table 13.2 Crude and Adjusted Odds Ratios for the LiFFT Log CD Measure Versus Low Back Pain Outcomes in the Epidemiology Study by Sesek (1999).

Outcome	Analysis	Variable	*df*	Chi-sq	*P*	OR	95% CI
Low back pain today (1 v. 5)	Crude	Log CD	1	5.82	0.016	1.621	(1.068, 2.460)
	Adjusted	Log CD	1	4.29	0.038	1.513	(1.008, 2.272)
		Site	5	9.44	0.93	Var	Var
		Gender	1	0.20	0.656	0.839	(0.389, 1.809)
		Age	1	1.66	0.198	1.584	(0.785, 3.195)
		BMI	1	0.84	0.360	0.726	(0.363, 1.453)

Note. Var = various.

As stated previously, the study by Marras et al. (1993) examined only monotask jobs. However, a major benefit of the fatigue failure approach to risk assessment is that it can evaluate the total cumulative damage associated with multiple lifting tasks performed during a workday. Thus, the validation of the LiFFT risk assessment tool was performed against an additional epidemiology database which evaluated low back outcomes for jobs comprised of multiple lifting tasks (up to six separate lifting tasks) (Sesek, 1999). The Log CD measure was calculated by summing the cumulative damage estimates calculated for each lifting task. The PLM for each task was calculated by multiplying the horizontal distance to the load (measured according to the revised NIOSH lifting equation method) and the known load mass. Repetitions for each task were available and were multiplied by the DPC to get the Log CD on a task-by-task basis.

Several low back outcomes were evaluated from this database, all of which demonstrated significant dose-response relationships to the log of the LiFFT CD metric. We will focus on the outcome of job-related back pain (a positive case) versus no back symptoms (a negative case). Table 13.2 provides the crude and adjusted ORs for the outcome cited earlier. As seen in this table, adjusted analyses controlled for the plant site (six plants were included in the study), along with the sex, age, and BMI of the workers. Both crude and adjusted odds ratios for the Log CD measure were significant and indicated a dose-response relationship between Log CD and low back pain outcomes. This relationship is visually represented in Figure 13.6.

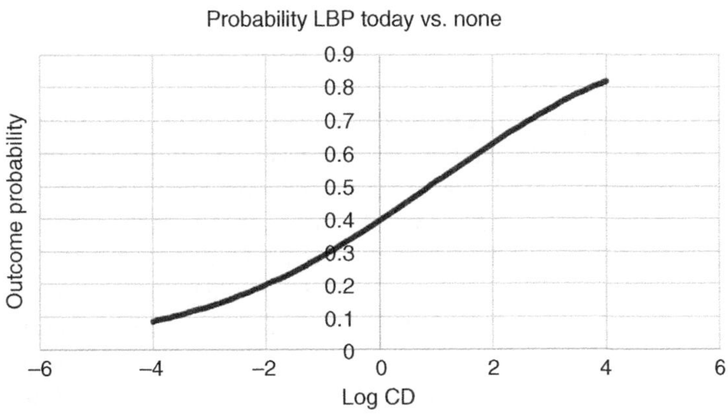

Figure 13.6 Dose-response relationships between the LiFFT Log CD measure and low back pain prevalence in the Sesek (1999) study. Data from Sesek, R. (1999). *Evaluation and refinement of ergonomic survey tools to evaluate worker risk of cumulative trauma disorders* (Dissertation).

Results of this analysis demonstrate that the LiFFT Log CD measure is significantly associated with both low back outcomes in these studies. Since the Log CD measure is a continuous measure relating to risk, the adjusted odds ratios in the latter study can be interpreted as follows: for every unit increase in Log CD, there is a 51.3% increase in the prevalence of current back pain.

LiFFT summary

LiFFT, an easy-to-use risk assessment tool for manual lifting and lowering tasks, is based on fatigue failure techniques and is designed to estimate cumulative damage development in materials exposed to repeated stress. All that is needed to assess the risk for a task is a measuring tape, the weight of the load, and the number of repetitions performed per day. Stress on the low back due to lifting and lowering activities is estimated by ascertaining the PLM experienced during lifting and lowering tasks. The tool easily combines the cumulative damage associated with multiple lifting/lowering tasks, the sum of which has shown significant associations with numerous low back outcomes. Due to the relationships established by the validation studies, probabilities of experiencing various low back outcomes can be provided. By evaluating the proportion of cumulative damage associated with each task, it can be determined which tasks are driving the risk to the worker (and should be candidates for job redesign). If high cumulative damage jobs are redesigned, reanalysis can provide an estimate of the decreased probability of a low back outcome. Validation studies indicate that LiFFT cumulative damage measure demonstrates significant dose-response associations with low back outcomes for mono-task lifting jobs as well as multi-task jobs.

The Distal Upper Extremity Tool

A second risk assessment tool based on fatigue failure theory is the Distal Upper Extremity Tool, or "DUET" (Gallagher, Schall Jr, Sesek, & Huangfu, 2018). This tool is designed to assess the likelihood of upper extremity outcomes due to repeated stress associated with hand-intensive tasks. All that is needed to assess the risk associated with a task is a rating of perceived exertion and the number of daily repetitions performed for the task. Based on this information, a cumulative damage score is developed. As with the LiFFT tool, if multiple hand-intensive tasks are performed, DUET sums the cumulative damage for each to get a total cumulative damage score. Once again, the proportion of cumulative damage for each task can be examined to determine which tasks are responsible for the greatest proportions of risk (and are most in need of ergonomic interventions).

Model logic

Whenever possible, it is preferable to have a quantitative method of estimating stress or a surrogate measure for stress. In the LiFFT tool, for example, the PLM was used as a quantitative measure related to the stress on the low back due to lifting and lowering tasks. However, due to the difficulties associated with obtaining quantitative force measures from the fingers, hands, and wrists, the developers of the DUET tool opted to use a perceived exertion scale to obtain information related to loading for distal upper extremity tasks. Several such scales exist; however, the DUET developers decided to use the OMNI Resistance Exercise Scale (OMNI-RES), due to its linear and symmetric nature (Lagally & Robertson, 2006; Robertson, et al., 2003). As illustrated in Table 13.3, the ratings on the scale go from 0 to 10, and the verbal anchors range from "very easy" (0) to "very hard" (10).

To assign DPC values to the various ratings of perceived exertion ratings, we used data on the fatigue failure of tendons. As many distal upper extremity MSDs are tendon-related, we used an *S–N* curve developed in a study of *ex vivo* tendon fatigue failure to estimate cumulative damage

Table 13.3 OMNI-Res Scale Damage per Cycle (DPC) Estimates from an *In Vitro* Study on Fatigue Failure of Human Tendons

OMNI-res scale	Estimated cycles to failure (extensor digitorum longus)	Damage per cycle
0 = very easy	3,842,605	0.00000026
1	2,231,607	0.00000045
2 = easy	729,651	0.00000137
3	242,301	0.00000413
4 = somewhat easy	79,223	0.00001262
5	26,308	0.00003801
6 = somewhat hard	8,602	0.00011625
7	2,856	0.00035014
8 = hard	949	0.00105374
9	310	0.00322581
10 = very hard	103	0.00970874

development (Schechtman & Bader, 1997). As discussed earlier, this study provided data regarding fatigue failure of 90 human extensor digitorum longus tendons at 10–90% of the ultimate tensile stress (UTS) of the tendon (i.e., 100 MPa). The stress associated with a peak perceived exertion (100% MVC) is not the same as the ultimate failure stress of the tendon. Thus, the *ex vivo* fatigue failure test results were scaled according to data on tendon strain at different percentages of MVC (Kubo, Teshima, Ikebukuro, Hirose, & Tsunoda, 2014). Data from this study suggested that the failure strain of tendons was approximately 1.4 times the strain observed at 100% MVC.

Thus, cycles to failure were scaled so that one cycle failure value (i.e., ultimate stress) was 1.4 times the maximum exertion force on the OMNI-RES scale (Gallagher et al., 2018). Table 13.3 provides the estimated cycles to failure at different levels of perceived exertion used by the DUET cumulative damage model, along with the DPC (the reciprocal of the estimated cycles to failure).

The DUET cumulative damage model works as follows. Let us say a worker has a job composed of three upper extremity tasks. The first task is judged to be a "very easy" exertion and involves 2,500 cycles per day. The second task requires a "somewhat hard" exertion and must be performed 150 times a day. Finally, the third task is considered 'easy' and has 575 repetitions per day. The number of cycles for each task is then multiplied by the DPC associated with the specific level of perceived exertion assigned to each task:

$$\begin{aligned} DUET\,CD &= 2{,}500 * 0.00000026 + 150 * 0.00011625 + 575 * 0.00000137 \\ &= 0.00065 + 0.0174375 + 0.00078755 = 0.01887505 \end{aligned}$$

The proportion of damage associated with each task can also be calculated. For example, the proportion of damage associated with the second task would be as under:

$$\frac{0.0174375}{0.01887505} = 92.4\%$$

So even though the second task has the fewest exertions, it accounts for the vast majority of cumulative damage.

Using DUET

Figure 13.7 provides an example of a mono-task analysis performed by DUET. In this example, the job involves an upper extremity task with an exertion intensity rating of "Somewhat Easy" (4 on the OMNI-RES scale), which is performed 1,350 times during the workday. Figure 13.7 shows a screenshot of the DUET tool for this mono-task job, which demonstrates that this job has approximately a 32.1% probability of experiencing distal upper extremity symptoms.

For jobs involving multiple exertions during the workday, each task should be analyzed using the methods described earlier. The cumulative damage associated with each task is summed by the DUET tool to determine the daily dose of cumulative upper extremity damage. An example is provided in Figure 13.8.

The example shows that the combination of these three tasks leads to a combined probability of 48.2% for distal upper extremity symptoms. Further, task #3 accounts for approximately 92.5% of the total damage for the workday. This task would be a prime candidate for redesign. For example, if the task #3 exertion level were reduced to "Somewhat Easy", the probability that the overall job is high risk would be reduced to 29.5%.

Finally (as with the LiFFT tool), if a great many tasks need to be analyzed, the Excel-based DUET tool allows up to 100 tasks to be analyzed. Alternatively, a "binning" procedure such as the one discussed for the LiFFT tool mentioned earlier can be used.

Validation of DUET Model

The DUET cumulative damage model was validated against five distal upper extremity outcomes from a cross-sectional epidemiologic study performed in the automotive industry (Sesek, 1999), each with separate case/control definitions. These included Injury, Injury plus Pain Today, Injury plus Pain Last Year, Pain Today, and Pain Last Year. 'Injury' was defined as a job where a first-time office visit (FTOV) for distal upper extremity symptoms was reported (Gallagher et al., 2018).

Controls were participants on jobs not having had a reported injury (FTOV) during the past year. Outcomes involving injury plus pain were treated similarly. In these circumstances, participants

The distal upper extremity tool

Task #	OMNI-RES Scale	Repetitions (per work day)	Damage (cumulative)	% Total (damage)
1	4: Somewhat easy	1350	0.01704	100.0
2	Please select ...	0	0.0	0.0
3	Please select ...	0	0.0	0.0
4	Please select ...	0	0.0	0.0
5	Please select ...	0	0.0	0.0
6	Please select ...	0	0.0	0.0
7	Please select ...	0	0.0	0.0
8	Please select ...	0	0.0	0.0
9	Please select ...	0	0.0	0.0
10	Please select ...	0	0.0	0.0
			Total cumulative damage:	0.01704
			Probability of distal upper extremity outcome (%):	32.1

Reset | Calculate

Figure 13.7 A screenshot of the DUET tool analysis of a mono-task job.

The distal upper extremity tool

Task #	OMNI-RES Scale	Repetitions (per work day)	Damage (cumulative)	% Total (damage)
1	2: Easy	1000	0.00137	1.0
2	4: Somewhat easy	700	0.00883	6.5
3	8: Hard	120	0.12645	92.5
4	Please select ...	0	0.0	0.0
5	Please select ...	0	0.0	0.0
6	Please select ...	0	0.0	0.0
7	Please select ...	0	0.0	0.0
8	Please select ...	0	0.0	0.0
9	Please select ...	0	0.0	0.0
10	Please select ...	0	0.0	0.0
			Total cumulative damage:	0.13665
			Probability of distal upper extremity outcome (%):	48.2
Reset				Calculate

Figure 13.8 A screenshot of the DUET tool for analyzing a multi-task job.

on jobs having a recorded FTOV during the past year-plus participant-reported pain (>15 mm VAS current or past year) were considered cases, and individuals on jobs without an FTOV and no current pain or pain last year (<15 mm VAS) were controls. Outcomes "Pain Today" or "Pain Last Year" were considered positive if participants reported pain >15 mm on a 100 mm Visual Analogue Scale (VAS) over the relevant time period. Controls for "pain only" outcomes were those not reporting pain >15 mm VAS over those time periods. Due to the exponential relationship between cumulative damage and the outcome, Log CD was used to assess the DUET cumulative damage model (Gallagher et al., 2018).

Crude and adjusted logistic regression analyses were performed on all five outcomes. Crude analyses assessed the Log CD measure alone, while adjusted analyses controlled for covariates known to have an influence on MSDs including plant site (six sites), age, gender (sex), and BMI. Results demonstrated that the DUET Log CD measure demonstrated significant dose-response relationships for all five outcomes investigated. Adjusted ORs ranged from 1.36 to 2.11 depending on the specific outcome (Gallagher et al., 2018). These ratios suggest that for every unit increase in the Log CD measure, the increase in the prevalence of the DUE outcomes ranged from 36 to 211%, depending on the specific outcome. In general, outcomes that included the FTOV in their definition had higher odds ratios than those assessing pain alone. Figure 13.9 presents the relationship of the DUET Log CD metric against each of the five outcomes studied.

In addition, the DUET tool has been validated against prevalent cases of carpal tunnel syndrome (CTS) as diagnosed by occupational health physicians (Bandekar et al., 2021). This analysis evaluated workers who had no CTS (control) versus those who had diagnosed cases that were ascribed by workers to their current job (case). Both crude and adjusted logistic regression analyses were performed. The crude analysis examined the log of the DUET tool's cumulative damage metric was entered as a continuous variable in an analysis of 403 workers (94 females, 309 males). The adjusted analysis included 395 participants (91 females, 304 males) and included adjustments for the following factors: age and BMI (continuous variables), and sex and plant (both categorical variables).

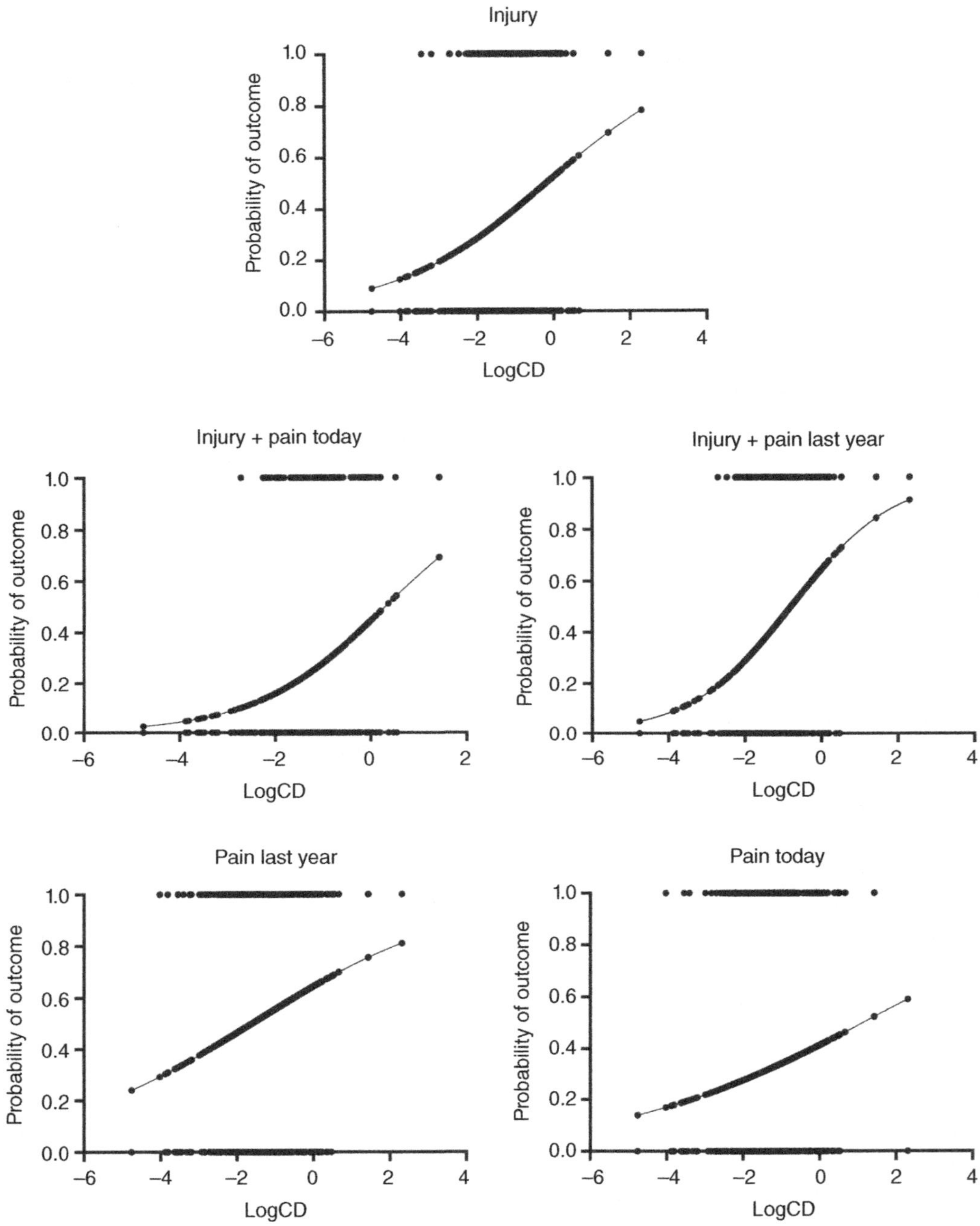

Figure 13.9 Dose-response relationships observed between DUET's Log CD measure and for five distal extremity outcomes (Adapted from Gallagher, S., Schall Jr, M., Sesek, R., & Huangfu, R. (2018). An upper extremity risk assessment tool based on material fatigue failure theory: The distal upper extremity tool (DUET). *Human Factors, 60*, 1146–1162.).

As shown in Table 13.4, results of both crude and adjusted analyses revealed significant associations between the log of the DUET CD measure and occupational physician-diagnosed CTS. In the crude analysis, the odds ratio for the DUET log CD was 1.75 (95% CI: 1.25, 2.45). In the adjusted analysis, the OR was 1.79 (95% CI: 1.18, 2.71).

Table 13.4 Summary of Crude and Adjusted Logistic Regression Analysis for DUET Log CD and Physician-diagnosed CTS

Outcome	Analysis	Cases	*N*	Variable	*df*	Chi-sq	*P*	OR	95% CI
Carpal tunnel syndrome	Crude	65	403	Log CD	1	12.17	<0.001	1.75	1.25, 2.45
	Adjusted	65	395	Log CD	1	7.55	0.006	1.79	1.18, 2.71
				Site	5	42.14	<0.001	Var	Var
				Age	1	0.07	0.788	1.00	0.97, 1.04
				Sex	1	6.07	0.014	0.45	0.23, 0.85
				BMI	1	0.43	0.510	0.98	0.91, 1.05

Note. Var = various.

These results demonstrate that the DUET CD measure is not only associated with pain symptoms and first-time office visits for hand/wrist injury complaints, but it also demonstrates a significant association with prevalent CTS cases. These consistently significant results suggest that the use of fatigue failure techniques works well in assessing distal upper extremity pain reports, clinic visits for hand complaints, as well as occupational physician differential diagnoses for CTS.

DUET summary

DUET is a fatigue failure-based risk assessment tool that evaluates the risk associated with hand-intensive tasks. The tool requires only two pieces of information for each task examined: an estimate of perceived exertion and the number of repetitions for the task. If multiple tasks are performed by a worker, these can be summed to assess the total estimated cumulative damage. Total cumulative damage estimates for workers have been shown to demonstrate dose-response relationships to numerous MSD outcomes of the distal upper extremity, including physician-diagnosed CTS cases.

The Shoulder Tool

A third fatigue failure-based risk assessment tool developed at Auburn University was designed to assess the risk of shoulder MSDs associated with shoulder intensive tasks (Bani Hani et al., 2021). This tool, named “The Shoulder Tool”, evaluates stressful shoulder tasks by the type of exertion performed (handling loads, pushing/pulling), estimates the PLM experienced by the shoulder, and the number of repetitions performed for a given task. If multiple tasks are performed during the workday, the cumulative damage estimated for each task can be summed, as with the tools described earlier. The tool is designed to analyze the stresses of one shoulder at a time.

Model logic

As with the LiFFT tool, the surrogate measure of stress used by “The Shoulder Tool” is the moment about the shoulder. This is obtained by measuring the lever arm from the shoulder joint (acromion) to the line of action of force exerted by the hands. Tendons are the tissues of primary concern for the shoulder, thus data gathered for tendon *ex vivo* fatigue failure studies are used to obtain DPC for different levels of stress and force. As with DUET, the Schechtman and Bader

(1997) fatigue data for the extensor digitorum longus (EDL) tendon to estimate the fatigue failure behavior in human tendons were used. When a worker is performing multiple tasks the DPC for each task is multiplied by its corresponding repetitions. The summation of the cumulative damage for the tasks will give an estimate for the daily dose, as described for the LiFFT and DUET tools.

Using the shoulder tool

To analyze a shoulder intensive task, all that is needed for The Shoulder Tool are four pieces of information for each shoulder being analyzed: (a) the type of task performed, (b) the weight of the load lifted (or force exerted by) the hand(s), (c) a measurement of the greatest horizontal distance from the shoulder joint (from the acromion) to the center of the hand or load during the task (using a measuring tape), and (d) the number of repetitions completed of the task being analyzed during the workday. Figures 13.10–13.12 demonstrate how to measure the maximum distance from the shoulder joint to the load.

In analyzing the risk for both shoulders, measuring the maximum lever arms for each shoulder during the task is important. The maximum lever arm for the left shoulder may occur at a different time than the maximum lever arm for the right shoulder.

The simplest application of 'The Shoulder Tool' is for mono-task shoulder intensive jobs (i.e., jobs involving repetition of the same shoulder intensive task throughout the workday). Assume a job involves handling a 9 N load with the right shoulder having a lever arm of 41 cm repeated 2,880 times during the workday. Figure 13.13 shows a screenshot of The Shoulder Tool for this mono-task job, which demonstrates this job's probability for a right shoulder outcome is 21% (fairly low risk).

Now, let us assume another monotask job involves an operator requiring a 45 N force to lift a panel from a conveyor to a rack using both hands (with even weight distribution). Assuming equal loads on both shoulders, this task will require a force of 22.5 N from both hands. This task

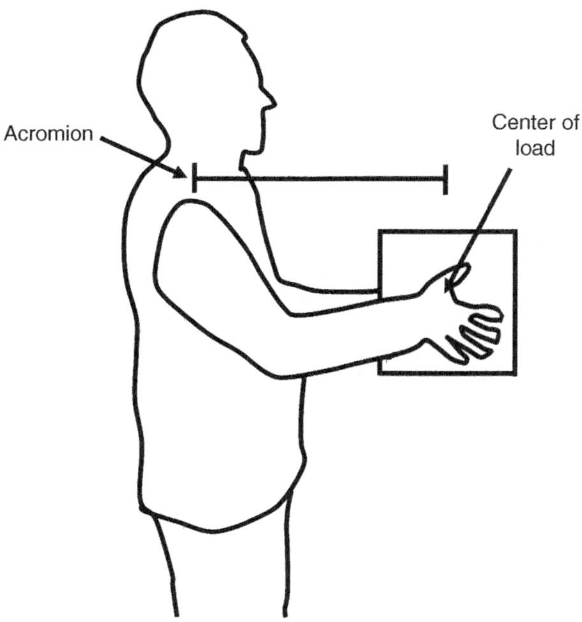

Figure 13.10 Proper measurement of the distance from the shoulder joint to the hand/load. Note that the tape measure should be held horizontally.

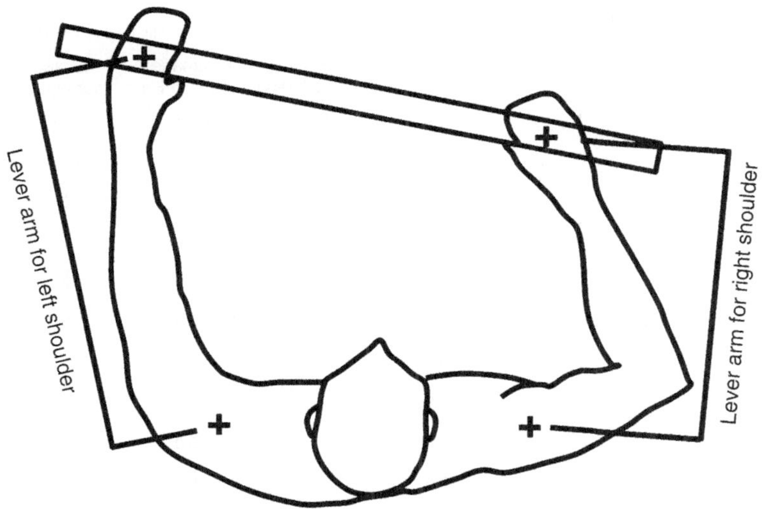

Figure 13.11 Illustration of measuring the lever arm for the left and right shoulders for a manual handling activity. The weight of the item should be divided between the hands. In many cases, the weight may be evenly divided, but there will also be cases where the analyst should divide the weight unevenly if one shoulder is bearing more of the weight of the object. This may have to be estimated by the analyst.

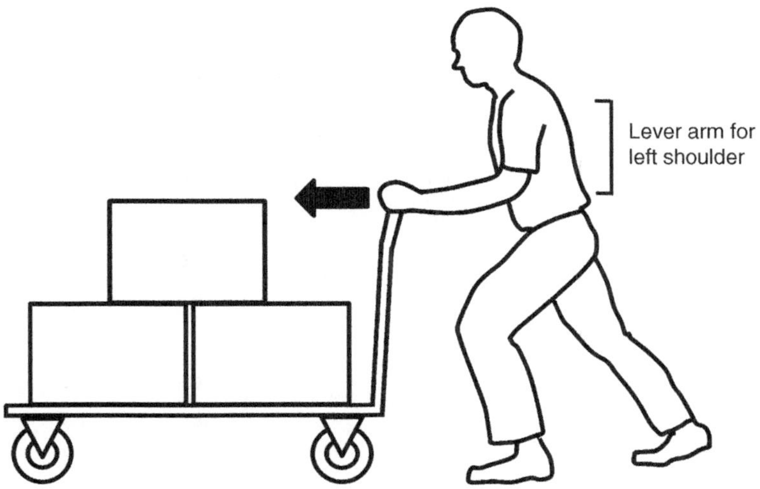

Figure 13.12 For pushing and pulling tasks, the lever arm may be a vertical measurement as in pushing the cart shown earlier. Forces may be obtained using force gauges and should represent the *peak* force observed during the exertion, for example, the initial force required to get a cart moving.

is performed 4,800 times per shift. Note that since the weight is evenly distributed and the lever arms are the same, the risk to each shoulder should be similar. The analysis is shown in Figure 13.14:

For jobs involving multiple exertions during a workday, each task should be analyzed using the same methods illustrated earlier. The cumulative damage associated with each task will be summed by 'The Shoulder Tool' to determine the "daily dose" of cumulative damage for both left and right shoulders. An example is provided in Figure 13.15.

The shoulder tool

Unit: English | Metric

Task #	Type of task	Lever arm (cm)	Load (N)	Moment (N.m)	Repetitions (per work day)	Damage (cumulative)	% Total (damage)
1	Handling loads	41	9	11.5	2880	0.00441	100.0
2	Handling loads			0.0		0.0	0.0
3	Handling loads			0.0		0.0	0.0
4	Handling loads			0.0		0.0	0.0
5	Handling loads			0.0		0.0	0.0
6	Handling loads			0.0		0.0	0.0
7	Handling loads			0.0		0.0	0.0
8	Handling loads			0.0		0.0	0.0
9	Handling loads			0.0		0.0	0.0
10	Handling loads			0.0		0.0	0.0
					Total cumulative damage:	0.00441	
					Probability of shoulder outcome (%):	21.0	

Reset Calculate

Figure 13.13 A screenshot of 'The Shoulder Tool' for analyzing a monotask job.

The shoulder tool

Unit: English | Metric

Task #	Type of task	Lever arm (cm)	Load (N)	Moment (N.m)	Repetitions (per work day)	Damage (cumulative)	% Total (damage)
1	Handling loads	46	22.5	19.3	4800	0.03495	100.0
2	Handling loads			0.0		0.0	0.0
3	Handling loads			0.0		0.0	0.0
4	Handling loads			0.0		0.0	0.0
5	Handling loads			0.0		0.0	0.0
6	Handling loads			0.0		0.0	0.0
7	Handling loads			0.0		0.0	0.0
8	Handling loads			0.0		0.0	0.0
9	Handling loads			0.0		0.0	0.0
10	Handling loads			0.0		0.0	0.0
					Total cumulative damage:	0.03495	
					Probability of shoulder outcome (%):	38.0	

Reset Calculate

Figure 13.14 Analysis of a monotask two-handed lift with even weight distribution.

The shoulder tool validation

The Shoulder Tool was initially validated against epidemiological data from a large automotive manufacturer (using several shoulder MSD outcomes). One hundred randomly selected jobs were examined in the video analysis. For each job, the job description and its corresponding tasks

The shoulder tool

Unit: English I Metric

Task #	Type of task	Lever arm (cm)	Load (N)	Moment (N.m)	Repetitions (per work day)	Damage (cumulative)	% Total (damage)
1	Handling loads	46	22	19.0	1920	0.01335	31.7
2	Handling loads	38	33	19.8	480	0.00384	9.1
3	Handling push or pull	41	89	36.5	96	0.02247	53.3
4	Handling loads	46	4	10.8	1920	0.00251	6.0
5	Handling loads			0.0		0.0	0.0
6	Handling loads			0.0		0.0	0.0
7	Handling loads			0.0		0.0	0.0
8	Handling loads			0.0		0.0	0.0
9	Handling loads			0.0		0.0	0.0
10	Handling loads			0.0		0.0	0.0
					Total cumulative damage:	0.04217	
					Probability of shoulder outcome (%):	39.8	

Reset | Calculate

Figure 13.15 A screenshot of The Shoulder Tool for analyzing a multi-task job.

description were available from the automotive dataset (Sesek, 1999). Most jobs comprised multiple tasks (up to 6 tasks) and the total number of tasks analyzed was 250. Information about the repetitions per minute for each task was obtained from the video analysis. Posture analysis was performed for the most awkward shoulder posture observed, where the neutral posture was defined as arms by side of torso hanging straight down. Postural changes for the shoulder were considered when the angle between the upper arm and torso increases when the arm was flexed, abducted, adducted, or extended. Sustained or repeated postures with load were also defined for cases where the upper arm was unsupported. The analysis involved torso angle, lateral bending, and axial rotation of the torso and head angle. To make sure that the estimates for the postures were accurate, the digital human in the University of Michigan 3D Static Strength Prediction Program (3DSSPP version 6.0.6) was used to simulate the task being analyzed. To get the required inputs for the shoulder model, postural data and the loads carried (magnitude and direction) were used to obtain the moment at each shoulder joint. Loads lifted in the calculations for the moments were retrieved from the automotive dataset. Moments for both right and left shoulders were calculated. The ultimate strength was estimated by considering the shoulder strength estimates from 3DSSPP and the calculated shoulder moments for each task. The number of cycles to failure for right and left shoulders was then obtained.

The DPC was then calculated using the reciprocal of the number of estimated cycles to failure, and the CD was determined by multiplying the DPC by the repetitions per day. The job cumulative damage for the left and right shoulders was then calculated. An assumption was made that the highest value for the cumulative damage between left and right shoulders was responsible for a higher probability for the development of shoulder outcomes.

Several shoulder outcomes were used in the initial validation of The Shoulder Tool. These included: first-time office visits (FTOV) for shoulder symptoms in the past year, current shoulder pain, and shoulder pain in the last year. Additional outcomes included: (a) having an

FTOV for shoulder symptoms in the past year and experiencing current shoulder pain, and (b) having an FTOV and also experiencing shoulder pain during the past year. Reports of discomfort, injury reports, and self-reported symptoms were collected on the day of the interview and were reported retrospectively for the previous year and included subject attribution of the impact of the current job on the development (or amelioration) of symptoms. A VAS was used to rate their pain for different body parts including the shoulder. The FTOV was recorded if any worker on a subject job reported shoulder symptoms to the clinic during the past year. It should be noted that workers experiencing the FTOV might not be the same ones used for exposure assessment in the study. Jobs analyzed included up to six tasks, for which cumulative damage was summed.

Since multiple tasks were often performed in the same job, a cumulative damage summation was used to get an overall estimate for the damage for a job (a daily dose of exposure). Outcomes for shoulder pain today and shoulder pain last year were only considered a case if VAS ratings were >15 mm. Once the cumulative damage was calculated for each task and summed, crude and adjusted binary logistic regression was used to test model significance and get estimates of the odds ratios associated using the log of the continuous CD. When multiple workers performed the job, the worst outcome was used for the analysis. Covariates included plant site, gender, age, and BMI. Age and BMI and gender were dichotomized, with 1 M, 0 F for gender, 40 years for age and >30 for BMI.

Figure 13.16 shows the fitted logistic regression line for all five outcomes studied in the initial validation. In all cases, it was found that higher values of log CD are associated with an increase in the probability of shoulder outcomes. Adjusted odds ratios ranged from 2.12 to 5.20, and all of them demonstrated probabilities at or lower than the 0.001 value.

Additional validation of The Shoulder Tool was recently reported in which the tool was evaluated against occupational physician definitive diagnoses of bicipital tendinosis in the shoulder (Bandekar et al., 2021). A total of 293 subjects were evaluated using The Shoulder Tool, 35 of whom were diagnosed as having bicipital tendinosis. Fifty-three percent of workers were > 40 years of age, 72% were male and the percentage of workers having a BMI over 30 was 21%. Data were analyzed using logistic regression. In both crude and adjusted analyses, The Shoulder Tool's Log CD metric was treated as a continuous measure, while in adjusted analyses age and BMI were treated as continuous variables, and sex and plant were treated as categorical variables.

Results showed that The Shoulder Tool's log CD metric was significantly associated with bicipital tendinosis in both crude and adjusted analyses. As can be seen in Table 13.5, the crude analysis of the log CD metric revealed a significant odds ratio of 1.64 (95% CI: 1.13, 2.38). When adjusted for site, sex, age, and BMI, the odds ratio was 1.80 (95% CI: 1.16, 2.82). Thus, The Shoulder Tool's cumulative damage measure has demonstrated concurrent criterion-related validity for office visits for shoulder complaints, shoulder pain reports, worker attribution of shoulder symptoms to their current job, and definitive diagnosis of bicipital tendinosis in the shoulder.

Summary of The Shoulder Tool

The Shoulder Tool is a quantitative risk assessment tool based on fatigue failure principles. The tool assesses the risk associated with shoulder outcomes based upon the type of task performed, the peak moment associated with the performance of the task, and the number of repetitions of the task. If multiple tasks are performed the cumulative damage associated with each can be summed to assess the cumulative risk associated with all tasks. The tool was validated against multiple outcomes including office visits for shoulder symptoms, current shoulder pain or pain in the last year, and physician-diagnosed shoulder tendinitis. All outcomes demonstrated dose-response relationships with The Shoulder Tool's cumulative damage measure.

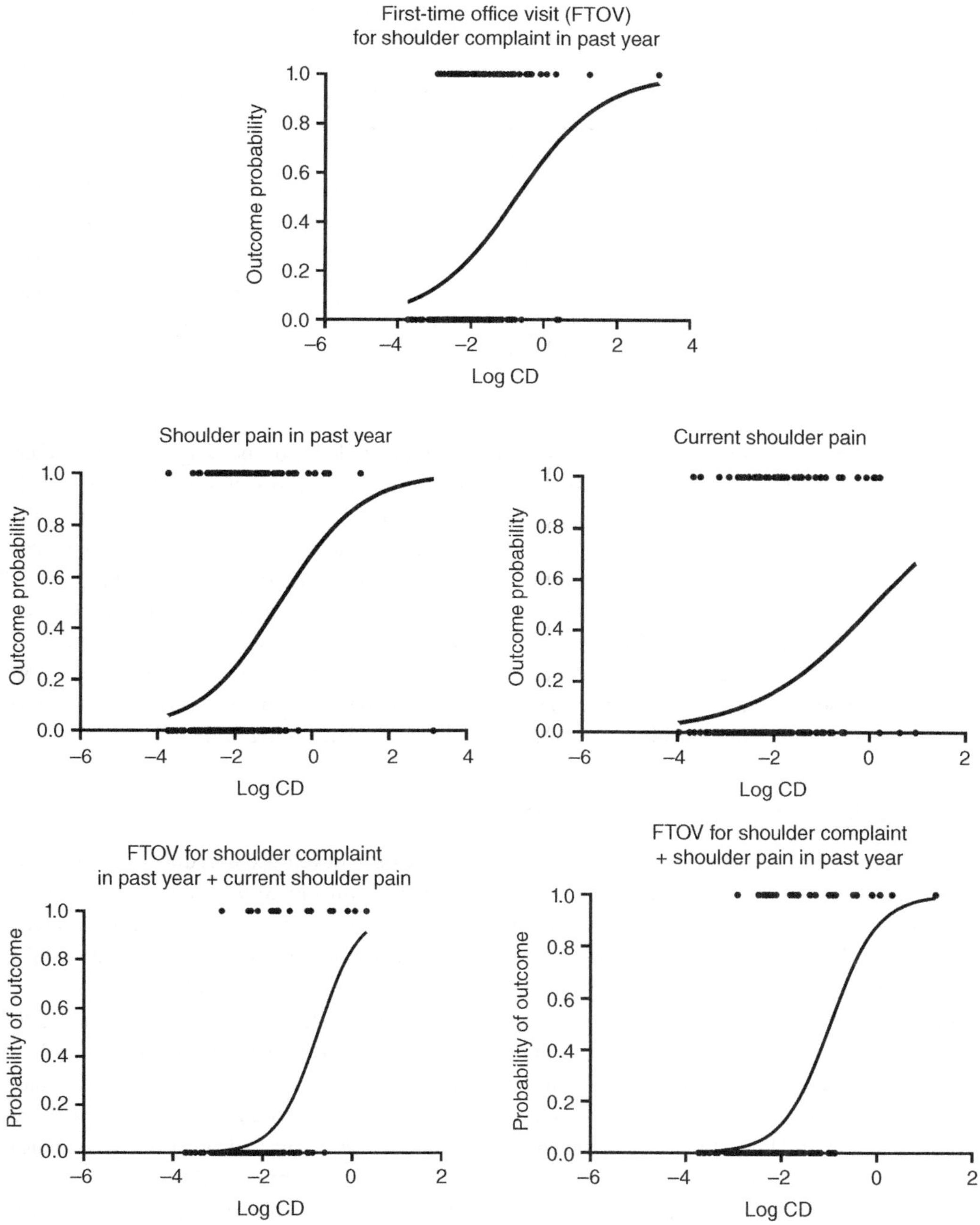

Figure 13.16 Logistic regression models for The Shoulder Tool Log CD measure and several shoulder outcomes.

Current and Future Developments

The fatigue failure tools described earlier have been designed for ease of use and have each shown strong and consistent dose-response relationships to numerous MSD outcomes of the low back, distal upper extremity, and shoulder. The tools described earlier can be performed by almost any safety and

Table 13.5 Summary of Crude and Adjusted Logistic Regression Analysis Relating Log CD Estimates from The Shoulder Tool and Physician-diagnosed Bicipital Tendinosis

Outcome	Analysis	Cases	*N*	Variable	*df*	Chi-sq	*P*	OR	95% CI
Bicipital tendinosis	Crude	35	293	Log CD	1	6.65	0.010	1.64	1.13, 2.38
	Adjusted	35	293	Log CD	1	6.74	0.009	1.80	1.15, 2.82
				Site	5	10.07	0.073	Var	Var
				Age	1	0.05	0.823	1.00	0.96, 1.05
				Sex	1	1.02	0.312	0.66	0.29, 1.48
				BMI	1	3.09	0.079	1.07	0.99, 1.15

Note. Var = various.

health professional with only the use of a tape measure and knowledge of the weight being handled (or force exerted). However, these tools are also well-positioned for forthcoming advances in risk assessment; for example, those that promise acquisition of real-time exposure estimates of the loads and repetitions experienced by workers. These include inertial measurement units (IMUs), video-based methods of capturing kinematic and force data, and a variety of other new wearable sensors and devices. The fatigue failure tools also are well-positioned to adapt to improvements in our knowledge of factors affecting the remodeling and healing capacities of musculoskeletal tissues. As described in the following section, these risk assessment models can also be employed to estimate the reduction in MSD risk associated with the use of exoskeletons. The following sections describe current and potential applications of fatigue failure methods to current and forthcoming MSD-related issues.

Evaluating the Effectiveness of Exoskeletons (ExoLiFFT)

In the past couple of decades, a variety of exoskeletons have been developed to reduce musculoskeletal stresses experienced by workers. These exoskeletons are considered wearable assist devices, and come in a wide variety of models, ranging from fully-powered varieties to passive (non-powered) versions. Exoskeletons are considered by some to represent personal protective equipment (PPE); however, others believe them to be better described as engineering controls (Zelik et al., 2021).

One of the important research issues regarding the use of exoskeletons is establishing their efficacy. Until recently, many researchers examining the effect of exoskeletons designed to reduce low back stress have used electromyography (EMG) to demonstrate a reduction in trunk muscle contraction associated with exoskeleton use. However, while EMG is an extremely useful research tool, there are several issues and limitations associated with EMG that limit its ability to determine (or estimate) an actual decrease in low back risk. For example, EMG is time-consuming and requires someone with specialized expertise to collect and interpret the data. In addition, not all relevant muscles are accessible for measurement and the effects of passive tissues (ligaments and tendons) are not generally accounted for. Moreover, while EMG studies can demonstrate decreases in muscle activity associated with exoskeleton use, the conclusion in terms of its effect on low back risk (for example) is less apparent, especially when dealing with multiple manual handling tasks having complex loading histories. Certainly, EMG use and interpretation are beyond the capabilities of many safety professionals that might have an interest in assessing the effectiveness of a low-back exoskeleton.

However, researchers have found that employing the LiFFT risk assessment tool provides a straightforward method of assessing the decrease in cumulative damage development (and associated decrease in the probability of low back disorders) associated with exoskeleton use. A new tool (Exo-LiFFT) uses the LiFFT model to estimate the reduction in low back disorder risk based upon the moment reduction provided by the exoskeleton (Zelik et al., 2021). The estimated reduction in risk is easily calculated by reducing the cumulative damage associated with exoskeleton use (with its reduced moment) from the original task performed without an exoskeleton. As with the original LiFFT tool, the cumulative damage associated with multiple tasks can be summed and the overall difference in risk can be estimated (Zelik et al., 2021). Exo-LiFFT is the first tool to assess exoskeleton efficacy; however, a similar approach could be used with 'The Shoulder Tool'.

Using Fatigue Failure Techniques to Evaluate Real-Time Exposure Assessment Data

The advent of risk assessment methods allowing the collection of continuous real-time exposure data comes with the added complexity of the highly variable loading patterns experienced by humans performing occupational tasks. Many current methods of assessing MSD risk would have difficulty interpreting the effects of complex service histories. Fortunately, fatigue failure theory has several validated methods that can break down complex loading histories into stress reversals and eventually cycles with a given stress range and mean stress that can be analyzed using standard fatigue failure cumulative damage models. An example of this is the rainflow analysis technique, an example of which is provided in Chapter 9. Thus, fatigue failure tools have the benefit of available techniques to deal with complexities inherent with the development of new methods of exposure assessment. Additional fatigue failure techniques may also prove helpful in risk assessment.

Assessment of the Effects of Job Rotation

As discussed in Chapter 12, fatigue failure tools can also provide insight into the impact of job rotation schemes. Many companies use job rotation as a method to try to balance the biomechanical demands associated with a group of jobs (some high stress and some low). However, the exponential nature of the fatigue failure process indicates that such a practice may be detrimental as opposed to beneficial with respect to overall injury risk for the cohort in the job rotation pool (Mehdizadeh et al., 2020). For example, if there are three low-risk jobs and one high-risk job in a rotation pool, the increase in risk to the low-risk workers (not originally exposed to the high-risk job) would be greater than the decrease in risk to the high-risk worker. This result would be expected to also occur with rotating workers through the jobs stressing different parts of the body, for example, back intensive jobs versus hand intensive jobs. This result suggests that job rotation is not an effective method for reducing injury risk for workers who have varying job demands. It appears that the best method to reduce injury risk is to intervene to reduce the stresses associated with jobs having high cumulative damage values as assessed by the fatigue failure risk assessment tools.

Accounting for Personal Factors and Healing

Fatigue failure theory informs us that material strength is a critical factor in the development of fatigue failure. Specifically, if two materials of unequal strength are loaded at the same stress level, the weaker material will develop cumulative damage more quickly. An individual's personal characteristics can have a large influence on the strength of musculoskeletal tissues, including anthropometry, and age. Fatigue failure tools have the potential to account for such factors, potentially allowing personalized risk assessment incorporating such factors.

As discussed previously, the fatigue failure process in musculoskeletal tissues can be thought of as a "modified" fatigue failure process in which damage is incurred by the tissues; however, a healing process is available to help repair the fatigue damage. As suggested many decades ago, the fatigue failure approach can incorporate the healing response if sufficient information is available (Nash, 1966). While details associated with the damage and healing kinetics of different tissues are not well established currently, fatigue failure-based risk assessment tools are well-positioned to incorporate advances in our understanding of these dynamic processes as our knowledge in this area becomes better developed.

Summary

This chapter has discussed principles of fatigue failure and their use in the development of MSD risk assessment tools. Three tools were introduced: one to evaluate the risk associated with lifting and lowering tasks (LiFFT), one to assess the risk of distal upper extremity disorders due to hand intensive tasks (DUET), and one to assess the risk of shoulder outcomes resulting from shoulder intensive tasks (The Shoulder Tool). Each of these tools has been designed for ease of use and allows one to easily obtain the cumulative risk associated with multiple tasks. This is easily accomplished using a standard fatigue failure cumulative damage model. Evaluation of the cumulative damage associated with individual tasks compared to the total cumulative damage can provide insight into those tasks responsible for the greatest proportions of total damage and which should be candidates for job redesign.

Validation of these tools against existing databases has demonstrated strong and consistent dose-response relationships to MSDs in each region of the body studied. The LiFFT tool was validated against two cross-sectional studies (one examining monotask lifting jobs and the other comprised of multiple lifting tasks) and in both cases it demonstrated strong associations with prevalent low back outcomes. The DUET tool has been validated against cross-sectional studies (against multiple DUE outcomes) and has demonstrated a significant dose-response relationship to physician-diagnosed CTS. Finally, 'The Shoulder Tool' was validated against multiple shoulder outcomes and, again, exhibited strong dose-response relationships with multiple shoulder outcomes, including physician diagnosed shoulder tendinitis. These strong and consistent relationships to MSD outcomes in three distinct musculoskeletal regions using fatigue failure principles provide additional evidence that fatigue failure plays an important role in the etiology of MSDs.

These tools are freely available by visiting https://eng.auburn.edu/occupational-safety-ergonomics-injury-prevention/risk-assessment/index.html. From this location, you can link to web-based tool versions (allowing quick analysis of jobs), or downloadable Excel-based versions (which allow you to save analyses on a spreadsheet). Spanish versions of the Excel-based tools are also downloadable at this website address.

Bibliography

Armstrong, T. (2006). The ACGIH TLV for hand activity level. In W. Marras & W. Karwowski (Eds.), *Fundamentals and assessment tools for occupational ergonomics* (pp. 41-1–41-14). Boca Raton, FL: CRC Press.

Bandekar, A., Sesek, R., Schall, M., Jr., Huangfu, R., Bani Hani, D., & Gallagher, S. (2021). Validation of Fatigue Failure Risk Assessment Tools Against Physician-Diagnosed Outcomes. In *HFES 65th International Annual Meeting* (p. TBD). Washington, DC: Human Factors and Ergonomics Society.

Bani Hani, D., Huangfu, R., Sesek, R., Schall, M., Davis, G., & Gallagher, S. (2021). Development and validation of a cumulative exposure shoulder risk assessment tool based on fatigue failure theory. *Ergonomics*, *64*, 39–54.

Barbe, M., Gallagher, S., Massicotte, V., Tytell, M., Popoff, S., & Barr-Gillespie, A. (2013). The interaction of force and repetition on musculoskeletal and neural tissue responses and sensorimotor behavior in a rat model of work-related musculoskeletal disorders. *BMC Musculoskeletal Disorders*, *14*, 303.

Bloswick, D., & Villnave, T. (2000). Ergonomics (chap 54). In R. Harris (Ed.), *Patty's industrial hygiene and toxicology* (5th ed.). New York, NY: Wiley.

Brinckmann, P. B., Biggemann, M., & Hilweg, D. (1988). Fatigue fracture of human lumbar vertebrae. *Clinical Biomechanics*, *3*(Suppl. 1), S1–S23.

Dale, A., Harris-Adamson, C., Rempel, D., Gerr, F., Hegmann, K., Silverstein, B., . . . Merlino, L. (2013). Prevalence and incidence of carpal tunnel syndrome in US working populations: Pooled analysis of six prospective studies. *Scandinavian Journal of Work, Environment, and Health*, *39*, 395.

Dempsey, P., Burdorf, A., Fathallah, F., Sorock, G., & Hashemi, L. (2001). Influence of measurement accuracy on the application of the 1991 NIOSH equation. *Applied Ergonomics*, *32*, 91–99.

Gallagher, S., Marras, W., Litsky, A., Burr, D., Landoll, J., & Matkovic, V. (2007). A comparison of fatigue failure responses of old versus middle-aged lumbar motion segments in simulated flexed lifting. *Spine*, *32*, 1832–1839.

Gallagher, S., Schall, M., Jr., Sesek, R., & Huangfu, R. (2018). An upper extremity risk assessment tool based on material fatigue failure theory: The distal upper extremity tool (DUET). *Human Factors*, *60*, 1146–1162.

Gallagher, S., Sesek, R., Schall, M., Jr., & Huangfu, R. (2017). Development and validation of an easy-to-use risk assessment tool for cumulative low back loading: The lifting fatigue failure tool (LiFFT). *Applied Ergonomics*, *63*, 142–150.

Garg, A., Moore, J., & Kapellusch, J. (2017). The composite strain index (COSI) and cumulative strain index (CUSI): Methodologies for quantifying biomechanical stressors for complex tasks and job rotation using the revised strain index. *Ergonomics*, *60*, 1033–1041.

Garg, A., Moore, J., & Kapellusch, J. (2017). The revised strain index: An improved upper extremity exposure assessment model. *Ergonomics*, *60*, 912–922.

Harris-Adamson, C., Eisen, E., Kapellusch, J., Garg, A., Hegmann, K., Thiese, M., . . . Silverstein, B. (2015). Biomechanical risk factors for carpal tunnel syndrome: A pooled study of 2474 workers. Occupation. *Occupational and Environmental Medicine*, *72*, 33–41.

Jager, M., & Luttmann, A. (1991). Compressive strength of lumbar spine elements related to age, gender, and other influencing factors. *Journal of Electromyography and Kinesiolology*, *17*, 291–294.

Kubo, K., Teshima, T., Ikebukuro, T., Hirose, N., & Tsunoda, N. (2014). Tendon properties and muscle architecture for knee extensors and plantar flexors in boys and men. *Clinical Biomechanics*, *29*, 506–511.

Lagally, K., & Robertson, R. (2006). Construct validity of the OMNI resistance exercise scale. *The Journal of Strength and Conditioning Research*, *20*, 252–256.

Latko, W., Armstrong, T., Foulke, J., Herrin, G., Rabourn, R., & Ulin, S. (1997). Development and evaluation of an observational method for assessing repetition in hand tasks. *American Industrial Hygiene Association Journal*, *58*, 278–285.

Lowe, B., Dempsey, R., & Jones, E. (2019). Ergonomics assessment methods used by ergonomics professionals. *Applied Ergonomics*, *81*, 8.

Manson, S., Freche, J., & Ensign, S. (1967). *Application of a double linear damage rule to cumulative fatigue*. Conshohocken, PA: American Society for Testing and Measurement (ASTM).

Marras, W., Fine, L., Ferguson, S., & Waters, T. (1999). The effectiveness of commonly used lifting assessment methods to identify industrial jobs associated with elevated risk of low-back disorders. *Ergonomics, 42*, 229–245.

Marras, W., & Hamrick, C. (2006). The ACGIH TLV for low back risk. In W. Marras & W. E. Karwowski (Eds.), *The occupational ergonomics handbook: Fundamentals and assessment tools for occupational ergonomics* (2nd ed., pp. 50-1–50-15). Boca Raton, FL: CRC Press.

Marras, W., Lavender, S., Leurgans, S., Rajulu, S., Allread, W. G., Fathallah, F., & Ferguson, S. (1993). The role of dynamic three-dimensional motion in occupationally-related low back disorders: The effects of workplace factors, and trunk motion characteristics on risk of injury. *Spine, 18*, 617–628.

McAtamney, L., & Corlett, N. (1993). RULA: A survey method for the investigation of work-related upper limb disorders. *Applied Ergonomics, 24*, 91–99.

Mehdizadeh, A., Vinel, A., Hu, Q., Schall, M., Jr., Gallagher, S., & Sesek, R. (2020). Job rotation and work-related musculoskeletal disorders: a fatigue-failure perspective. *Ergonomics, 63*, 461–476.

Miner, M. A. (1945). Cumulative damage in fatigue. *Journal of Applied Mechanics, 16*, A159–A164.

Moore, J., & Garg, A. (1995). The strain index: A proposed method to analyze jobs for risk of distal upper extremity disorders. *American Industrial Hygiene Association Journal, 56*, 443–458.

Nash, J. C. (1966). *Fatigue of self-healing structure: a generalized theory of fatigue failure*. New York: American Society of Mechanical Engineers.

National Institute for Occupational Safety and Health (NIOSH) (1981). *Work practices guide for manual lifting*. Cincinnati, OH: Department of Health and Human Services.

Palmgren, A. (1924). Die Lebebsdaue rvon Kugellagern. *Zeitschrift des Vereines Deutscher Ingenieure, 68*, 339–341.

Post, N., Case, S., & Lesko, J. (2008). Modeling the variable amplitude fatigue of composite materials. *International Journal of Fatigue, 30*, 2064–2086.

Radwin, R. G. (2011). Automated video exposure assessment of repetitive motion. In *Proceedings of the Human Factors and Ergonomics Society Annual Meeting* (Vol. 55, pp. 995–996). Los Angeles, CA: SAGE Publications.

Rempel, D. (2018). 1631c recent changes to the ACGIH hand activity level TLV. *Occupational and Environmental Medicine, 75*, A258.

Robert-Lachaine, X., Mecheri, H., Larue, C., & Plamondon, A. (2017). Validation of inertial measurement units with an optoelectronic system for whole-body motion analysis. *Medical & Biological Engineering & Computing, 55*, 609–619.

Robertson, R., Goss, F., Rutkowski, J., Lenz, B., Dixon, C., Timmer, J., . . . J. (2003). Concurrent validation of the OMNI perceived exertion scale for resistance exercise. *Psychobiology and Behavioral Sciences., 35*, 333–341.

Russell, S., Winnemuller, L., Camp, J., & Johnson, P. (2007). Comparing the results of five lifting analysis tools. *Applied Ergonomics, 38*, 91–97.

Schall, M. C., Jr., Fethke, N. B., & Chen, H. (2016). Working postures and physical activity among registered nurses. *Applied Ergonomics, 54*, 243–250.

Schall, M. C., Jr., Fethke, N. B., Chen, H., & Gerr, F. (2015). A comparison of instrumentation methods to estimate thoracolumbar motion in field-based occupational studies. *Applied Ergonomics, 48*, 224–231.

Schechtman, H., & Bader, D. (1997). In vitro fatigue of human tendons. *Journal of Biomechanics*, 829–835.

Sesek, R. (1999). *Evaluation and refinement of ergonomic survey tools to evaluate worker risk of cumulative trauma disorders* (Dissertation).

Sesek, R., Gilkey, D., Drinkaus, P., Bloswick, D., & Herron, R. (2003). Evaluation and quantification of manual material handling risk factors. *International Journal of Occupational Safety and Ergonomics, 9*, 271–287.

Shepherd, J., & Screen, H. (2013). Fatigue loading of tendon. *International Journal of Experimental Pathology, 94*, 260–270.

Shepherd, J. H., Legerlotz, K., Demirci, T., Klemt, C., Riley, G., & Screen, H. (2014). Functionally distinct tendon fascicles exhibit different creep and stress relaxation behaviour. *Proceedings of the Institution of Mechanical Engineers. Part H, Journal of Engineering in Medicine, 228*(1), 49–59.

Stephens, R., Fatemi, A., Stephens, R., & Fuchs, H. (2001). *Metal Fatigue in Engineering* (2nd ed.). New York: John Wiley & Sons.

Sun, H., Andarawis-Puri, N., Li, Y., Fung, D., Lee, J., Wang, V., . . . Flatow, E. L. (2010). Cycle-dependent matric remodeling gene expression response in fatigue-loaded rat patellar tendons. *Journal of Orthopaedic Research, 28*, 1380–1386.

Takala, E.-P., Pehkonen, I., Forsman, M., Hansson, G.-Å., Mathiassen, S., Neumann, W. S., . . . Winkel, J. (2010). Systematic evaluation of observational methods assessing biomechanical exposures at work. *Scandinavian Journal of Work, Environment & Health, 36*, 3–24.

Wang, M., Garg, A., Chang, Y., Shih, Y., Yeh, W., & Lee, C. (1998). The relationship betweevn low back discomfort ratings and the NIOSH lifting index. *Human Factors, 40*, 509–515.

Wang X., Hu, Y. H., Lu, M. L., & Radwin, R. G. (2019). The accuracy of a 2D video-based lifting monitor, *Ergonomics, 68*(8), 1043–1054.

Waters, T., Baron, S., Piacitelli, L., Anderson, V., Skov, T., Haring-Sweeney, M., . . . Fine, L. J. (1999). Evaluation of the revised NIOSH lifting equation: A cross-sectional epidemiologic study. *Spine, 24*, 386–395.

Waters, T., Putz-Anderson, V., & Garg, A. (1994). *Applications manual for the revised NIOSH lifting equation*. Cincinnati, OH: National Institute for Occupational Safety and Health.

Waters, T., Putz-Anderson, V., Garg, A., & Fine, L. (1993). Revised NIOSH equation for the design and evaluation of manual lifting tasks. *Ergonomics, 36*, 749–776.

Zelik, K. E., Nurse, C. A., Schall, M. C. Jr, M. C., Sesek, R. F., Marino, M. C., & Gallagher, S. (2022). An ergonomic assessment tool for evaluating the effect of back exoskeletons on injury risk. *Applied Ergonomics, 99*, 103619.

Zurada, J., Karwowski, W., & Marras, W. (1997). A neural network-based system for classification of industrial jobs with respect to risk of low back disorders due to workplace design. *Applied Ergonomics, 28*, 49–58.

14

Implications for MSD Prevention

Introduction

The picture of musculoskeletal disorder (MSD) development provided by the fatigue failure model is one in which musculoskeletal tissues exposed to repeated stress eventually experience a small microfailure, and that the initial site of failure will propagate through the tissue with continued loading (Gallagher & Schall, 2017). Eventually, this process will lead to damage significant enough to lead to the development of pain and disability (and sometimes frank rupture or fracture). The rate of damage accumulation will depend on the ultimate strength of the tissues involved and the level(s) of stress imposed. Personal factors such as anthropometry, age, and gender (sex) may all influence the strength of tissues and thus the rate at which MSDs develop.

However, the picture is not complete without consideration of other key processes involved in the maintenance of musculoskeletal health, especially the remodeling and healing processes that act to maintain tissue health and repair damage (Gallagher & Barbe, 2021). The remodeling and healing processes employed by the body are unfortunately time-consuming and imperfect, and often unable to keep pace with fatigue damage development. These processes clearly provide critical assistance in extending the fatigue life of musculoskeletal tissues. However, the healing process can be negatively impacted by several factors, including (but not limited to) psychological stress, obesity, gender, aging, and poor sleep quality. A reduction in the effectiveness (or rate) of healing would be expected to permit damage to accrue more quickly, thereby reducing the fatigue life of musculoskeletal tissues (Gallagher & Barbe, 2021).

If one wishes to assess risk and/or prevent MSDs, the fatigue failure model provides numerous insights into factors that should be considered for MSD prevention presently and consideration of how to develop more comprehensive risk analyses and prevention methods going forward. The following sections detail some of the insights and methods that may be useful in both assessing risk and preventing MSD development. The topics in this chapter are not exhaustive; however, they provide a sampling of the insights and benefits provided by the fatigue failure mechanism that is not always available from other existing techniques.

The importance of Assessing Cumulative Damage

Most researchers in the ergonomics field have subscribed to the concept that the cumulative impact of loading on tissues is of high importance on the development of MSD risk (Armstrong et al., 1993; Norman et al., 1998). In spite of this widely held belief, historically many risk

Musculoskeletal Disorders: The Fatigue Failure Mechanism, First Edition. Sean Gallagher and Mary F. Barbe.

assessment tools have not provided a means with which to assess the cumulative load associated with the performance of multiple tasks (e.g., NIOSH, 1981). Even when risk assessment tools have provided methods of assessing cumulative loading, these have often been accompanied by rather vague rationales for the techniques recommended to assess cumulative load. Even now, several MSD risk assessment tools are limited to the assessment of mono-task jobs, without methods to capture the cumulative loading necessary to obtain the full breadth of worker exposure.

Fatigue failure theory clearly underscores the importance of obtaining the cumulative load on material to fully appreciate the extent of cumulative damage development (Stephens, Fatemi, Stephens, & Fuchs, 2001). It follows that estimation of the cumulative load experienced by a musculoskeletal tissue is essential for the process of MSD risk assessment and prevention. Not only does the theory demonstrate the importance of cumulative loading, but it also provides validated methods of calculating the cumulative effects of loading (even with highly variable loading histories) (Miner, 1945; Palmgren, 1924). As opposed to the rather vague rationales sometimes provided, fatigue failure offers a specific mechanism of cumulative damage development that has been well validated (Stephens et al., 2001), and shown to occur in musculoskeletal tissues (Andarawis-Puri, Flatow, & Soslowski, 2015; Barbe et al., 2013; Sun et al., 2010).

In terms of MSD prevention, one goal is clearly to minimize the cumulative load experienced by a worker to an acceptable level of risk for both mono-task and multi-task jobs. As discussed in the following text, multi-task jobs should be analyzed using methods that can obtain the cumulative damage for each individual task.

Identifying and Managing Risky Tasks

The ability of fatigue failure tools to estimate the extent of damage associated with each task of a multitask job can help to identify and prioritize jobs in need of redesign attention. It is not uncommon to find that a large proportion of the risk associated with a particular job is associated with one specific task out of several tasks performed during a workday. It should be apparent that the task accounting for the bulk of cumulative damage should be a top priority for intervention by the ergonomist. This allows the ergonomist to fix the most hazardous task first.

Establishing an effective intervention for a task exhibiting the greatest cumulative damage would be expected to be quite effective in terms of MSD risk reduction and the requisite information is easily obtained from the fatigue failure risk assessment tools discussed in Chapter 13. Once an intervention has been put in place, a reanalysis using the risk assessment tools can be performed to determine how effective the job change has been (i.e., how much the probability of an MSD outcome has been reduced). If the decrease in risk is not sufficient, alternative job design changes can be considered and other tasks exhibiting substantial proportions of overall risk should be evaluated for redesign.

Stress Reduction/Cycle Reduction

An essential truth of the fatigue failure process is that reducing the stress experienced by a material will lead to an exponential increase in the number of cycles that can be tolerated prior to failure. This effect can be dramatic. For example, *ex vivo* tests on tendons suggest that at 40% US, failure will occur in approximately 10,000 cycles. However, if one is able to reduce the repeated stress to 10% US, the tendon will be able to experience approximately a million cycles (two orders of magnitude greater) before failure occurs (Schechtman & Bader, 1997). Thus, anything that can be done to reduce the stress associated with a task should provide significant benefits in reducing MSD risk.

Of course, fatigue damage can also be reduced by limiting the number of loading cycles to which a tissue is exposed. The degree to which damage will be reduced by limiting loading cycles will be a function of the level of stress to which the individual is exposed. Limiting high-stress exertions will be much more impactful on cumulative damage development than limiting low-stress exertions. Thus, when considering job redesign options, anything that can reduce the number of high-stress exertions will have the most beneficial impact on risk reduction, while reducing lower stress repetitions will have a more modest effect on risk.

The Load/Repetition Trade-off

In a discussion with a prominent ergonomics expert many years ago, the trade-off between the weight of the load being handled and the number of repetitions performed was brought up. If one wanted to move a given amount of material, was it better to lift heavier weights using fewer repetitions, or lighter weights with more repetitions? His answer: "That is the 64-billion-dollar question!" At the time there was little basis with which to answer this question with certainty. However, fatigue failure theory provides a clear answer to this fundamental question. Due to the exponential decrease in cycles to failure with increasing stress, if moving the same amount of overall load, it will be better to lift lighter loads more frequently than to lift heavier weights less frequently if one wants to prevent cumulative damage development in musculoskeletal tissues. The same will hold true for any task involving the application of force.

An example using the Lifting Fatigue Failure Tool (LiFFT) provides an illustration of this principle. If one had a lifting task in which a worker was lifting 50 pounds 100 times with a maximum lever arm from the spine to a load of 16 in., the cumulative damage developed would be *nearly three times greater* than if one lifted 25 pounds 200 times with the same lever arm (0.0044 versus 0.0017). This basic principle will hold true for any exertions stressing the shoulder, the hands and wrists, or other body parts.

Unfortunately, lifting lighter weights more frequently is not the most time-efficient method of handling materials, and may incur increased physiological demands, depending on the particulars of the task. It is common to see workers (and others) increase the load they choose to carry so they do not need to make as many trips (minimizing energy expenditure at the expense of the increased biomechanical load). It may also be noted that this principle may conflict with the desire of businesses to be time efficient in the handling of materials. Thus, there are several factors that may play into the trade-off between load and repetition. However, if one wants to reduce the risk of injury to musculoskeletal tissues, when lifting the same total load, lifting less weight more often will lead to less tissue damage than lifting more weight less frequently. Wherever feasible, jobs should be designed accordingly. It should be understood that the decision to have workers lift heavier weights less frequently as opposed to lighter weights more frequently will come with a hidden cost—a cost of increased injury risk. In economic terms, this might be considered a factor that may lead to diminishing returns in spite of a perceived increase in productivity.

The Central Role of Tissue Strength

Variability in the strength of musculoskeletal tissues between individuals is substantial and will have a significant impact on their susceptibility to fatigue damage and MSD risk. An example is shown in Table 14.1. The table provides an estimated spinal compressive strength of human lumbar motion segments for males and females of different age ranges (Jager & Luttmann, 1991),

Table 14.1 Average Ultimate Compressive Strength for Male and Female Spines for Different Age Ranges (Jager & Luttmann, 1991), and Predicted Fatigue Life if Exposed to a Repeated 2,000 N Compressive Load.

Sex	Age	Average ultimate compressive strength	Predicted fatigue life (cycles) given 2 kN compressive load
Males	20–30	7,800	43,769
	30–40	7,700	42,053
	40–50	6,000	17,134
	50–60	5,000	7,597
Females	20–30	5,900	15,993
	30–40	5,400	10,905
	40–50	4,700	5,564
	50–60	3,600	1,139

(Adapted from Gallagher, S., Marras, W., Litsky, A., Burr, D., Landoll, J., & Matkovic, V. (2007). A comparison of fatigue failure responses of old versus middle-aged lumbar motion segments in simulated flexed lifting. *Spine, 32*, 1832–1839; Brinckmann, P., Biggemann, M., & Hilweg, D. (1988). Fatigue fracture of human lumbar vertebrae. *Clinical Biomechanics, 3* (Suppl. 1): S1–S23; Huber, G., Nagel, K., Skrzypiec, D., Klein, A., Püschel, K., & Morlock, M. (2016). A description of spinal fatigue strength. *Journal of Biomechanics, 49*, 875–880; and Jager, M., and A. Luttmann. 1991. *Compressive Strength Of Lumbar Spine Elements Related To Age, Gender, And Other Influences*. In: Electromyographical Kinesiology, Proceedings of the 9th Congress of the International Society of Electrophysiological Kinesiology, 291–294.)

and an estimate of the fatigue life (number of cycles) that would be expected given a repeated compressive load of 2,000 N based on prior studies on fatigue failure of spine motion segments (Brinckmann et al., 1988; Gallagher et al., 2007; Huber et al., 2016).

As can be seen in this table, the ultimate compressive strength of the spine is highly affected by both the age and the sex of the individual. As a result, if subjected to a repeated 2,000 N load, it will represent a different percentage of the estimated ultimate strength of each spine depending on the age and sex of the individual. As can be seen from Table 14.1, greater fatigue life is predicted (on average) for males as opposed to females and for younger individuals as opposed to older ones.

This example highlights an unfortunate disparity in fatigue failure risk that flows directly from material strength differences in individuals of different sex and age. In considering the ramifications of this difference in musculoskeletal tissue strength, several observations can be made. If we look at this result from the perspective of injury prevention, these differences suggest that females and elderly workers would enjoy decreased injury risk if the stress imposed were reduced in accordance with the reduced US of the spine. On the flip side, this same relationship suggests that younger individuals and those of the male gender would be capable of withstanding higher repetitive loads than those having the characteristics mentioned earlier.

Understanding the critical role of tissue strength on fatigue life can help to shed some light on the setting of standards with respect to acceptable loads. A method that has been commonly used in establishing acceptable loads is to design tasks such that the load can be safely handled by 75% of women (Snook, 1978), a level generally acceptable to approximately 90% of males. This is certainly a rational method of establishing acceptable loads. However, it should be recognized that establishing load limits in this manner will result in highly variable risks for individuals with different tissue strengths. Individuals with weaker tissues will assume a higher relative risk of injury (i.e., they will accrue damage more quickly) when handling loads established by this criterion, while those with stronger tissues will accrue damage more slowly and enjoy considerably lower levels of MSD risk.

The tremendous variability of tissue strength among humans provides an unfair playing field in terms of injury risk. To develop a more egalitarian approach to injury risk would require an understanding of the individual's tissue strength and its relationship to the repeated loading they are experiencing, something that is currently not realistic. However, fatigue failure theory clearly indicates that tissue strength is of vital importance in the assessment of injury risk. It is important to have a sensitivity to this tremendous variance, especially for certain individuals on the low side of the tissue strength range, who may be well served to have the loads they are exposed to stepped down, for example, with increased age.

Impaired Healing and the Fatigue Life of Musculoskeletal Tissues

As discussed in Chapter 10, fatigue failure in the biological setting can be considered a *modified* fatigue failure process due to the ability of musculoskeletal tissues to self-heal when damage occurs. This capacity for self-repair would be expected to increase the fatigue life of these tissues, and evidence from controlled studies of engineered self-healing materials (which mimic the features of biological systems) demonstrate greatly increased fatigue life with faster healing rates. However, if the healing rate is diminished, data from self-healing materials suggest that fatigue life will be substantially reduced (Jones, Rule, Moore, Sottos, & White, 2007).

Psychological (psychosocial) stress, obesity, increasing age, and sex have consistently demonstrated significant relationships to increased rates of MSD (National Research Council—Institute of Medicine, 2001; NIOSH, 1997). One attribute that these factors have in common is that each has been demonstrated to result in a reduced rate of healing (Gallagher & Barbe, 2021; Gosain & DiPietro, 2004; Gouin & Kiecolt-Glaser, 2011; Miller et al., 2005). The suppressed healing rate would be expected to reduce tissue fatigue life, thereby increasing MSD risk. Of course, if the healing response is suppressed in the presence of a high level of repeated stress (both factors acting to reduce fatigue life), MSD risk would be expected to increase substantially. Certain factors (such as obesity) may have multiple influences on MSD risk. For example, the increased weight associated with obesity may result in increased repeated stress on a variety of body structures. The combination of increased loading and suppressed healing would seem to be a recipe for the rapid development of MSDs (Gallagher & Barbe, 2021).

The presence of conditions that suppress the body's ability to heal may be a significant contributor to the effort to reduce the risk of MSDs at the workplace and in other settings. Efforts to reduce factors such as psychosocial stress and obesity may pay substantial dividends in an effort to reduce MSDs. In addition, if an employee is experiencing significant psychological stress, for example, it may be helpful to reduce the psychological stress and/or the physical loading to which they are being exposed. One should also be cognizant of the effects of sex and age in this regard. As Nash proposed in 1966, the fatigue failure model is capable of modeling both damage accumulation and the effect of self-healing processes on musculoskeletal health (Nash, 1966). However, a great deal more needs to be understood regarding the damage-healing relationship in the biological setting to fully realize this capability.

Rest

Rest is clearly an important factor in maintaining musculoskeletal health; however, at present, the influence of rest on musculoskeletal health is far from being fully understood. If one considers rest to be a period during which musculoskeletal tissues are relatively unloaded, it seems that the length of time that rest is provided will play a substantial role in how effective rest is in (a) decreasing the cumulative damage experienced by tissues and/or (b) how much healing can be achieved.

In terms of maintenance of musculoskeletal health, good quality sleep may well be the most important form of rest. As discussed previously, sleep provides an ideal platform for the healing of tissues. Not only is the musculoskeletal system is largely unloaded during this period, but the body also initiates anabolic (tissue healing processes), as opposed to the catabolic processes that predominate in the waking state. Growth factors are released in deep sleep that serve to repair musculoskeletal structures and other tissues (Adam & Oswald, 1984), the rate of which is higher when damaged tissues are present in the body. The benefits of good quality sleep can thus help to counter the adverse effects of cumulative damage incurred during the day. As a result, it would seem important that individuals who experience significant musculoskeletal loading during waking hours should be encouraged to obtain a sufficient amount of good quality sleep.

Short-term rest (such as the seconds of rest that may be available during a work cycle) is unlikely to be of much benefit with respect to the healing of tissues. Healing is a time-consuming process and brief periods of rest (e.g., between loading cycles) is unlikely to significantly help the healing process. Damage kinetics would likely predominate in cyclic loading, as opposed to any healing that could be accomplished during this process. However, short-term rest may be helpful in terms of reducing the cumulative damage incurred during a workday and may have physiological benefits (e.g., reducing physiological muscle fatigue). For example, the greater the rest time per cycle the better the blood perfusion would likely be for the tissues involved with the activity.

Job Rotation

As discussed in Chapter 8, many companies have used job rotation as a means of trying to control MSD risk in the workplace. The idea is to try to balance biomechanical (and/or physiological) demands between the workers. However, evidence regarding the effectiveness of this approach has been equivocal. A recent systematic review found that studies examining this matter were generally of poor quality and provided weak evidence regarding the effectiveness of job rotation as a method to control MSD risk (Padula, Comper, Sparer, & Dennerlein, 2017).

One issue with quantifying the risk associated with different jobs making up a rotation is that many risk assessment tools make it difficult to combine the likelihood of MSDs associated with each individual task, as well as that of the combined tasks. Fatigue failure tools provide a straightforward method of calculating these effects. In this example, we use the Shoulder Tool, (described in Chapter 13) to assess the efficacy of a job rotation strategy to balance the shoulder risks associated with three tasks: a low-risk task, a moderate-risk task, and a high-risk task (Bani Hani et al., 2021). In this example, we will use three “mono-task” shoulder intensive jobs, having probabilities of being a high-risk job for low back disorders of approximately 20% (low risk), 40% (medium risk), and 60% (high risk). Each mono-task job requires 1,800 repetitions during the workday. Table 14.2 provides the details for the three individual monotask jobs.

Let’s assume that the job rotation seeking to balance the risk of a shoulder outcome is designed such that each worker rotates through each task and performs 600 repetitions at each workstation (low, medium, and high-risk tasks). Table 14.3 provides the risk assessment of the job rotation scheme. As can be seen in this table, the job rotation method ends up with a total cumulative damage of 0.12224, which is associated with a 50.4% probability of a shoulder injury for each worker. Thus, the worker on the original low-risk job has their shoulder injury probabilities increase from 20 to 50.4%. The worker originally on the medium-risk job sees shoulder injury probability increase

Table 14.2 Estimates of Cumulative Damage Derived from the Shoulder Tool

Task	Peak moment (Nm)	Repetitions	Cumulative damage	Probability of shoulder injury
Low risk	13.1	1,800	0.00377	20%
Medium risk	25.1	1,800	0.04275	40%
High risk	35.1	1,800	0.32020	60%

Table 14.3 Results of the Cumulative Damage Estimates for The Job Rotation Scheme. Each Worker Would Experience the Total Cumulative Damage Score Presented in the Table. The Probability of a Shoulder Outcome Associated with the Cumulative Damage Score (0.12224) is 50.4%

Task	Peak moment	Repetitions	Cumulative damage	Percent of total damage
Low risk	13.1	600	0.00126	1.0
Medium risk	25.1	600	0.01425	11.7
High risk	35.1	600	0.10673	87.3
Total		1,800	0.12224	100

from 40 to 50.4%, and the worker on the high-risk job sees the probability of a shoulder injury decrease from 60 to 50.4%. Thus, in this attempt to "balance" the MSD risk of these jobs, two workers have had their risk increased and one has had their risk decrease (with increases being more substantial than the decrease). Thus, the job rotation results in an overall increase in MSD risk for this rotation pool.

The results of this example demonstrate that the exposure to the high-risk task substantially increases the risk to those workers originally in the low- and medium-risk jobs. In fact, the high-risk task accounts for 87.3% of the total damage incurred by each worker in the job rotation. This result is due to the exponential decrease in cycles to failure associated with exposure to increased stress. Exposing those in lower-risk tasks to this high-risk task substantially increases the cumulative damage they experience, thus increasing shoulder outcome risk. The worker in the original high-risk task does get some relief; however, the result is that the overall risk for the three workers is increased due to this job rotation scheme.

A comprehensive simulation analysis has been performed to assess a wide range of potential job rotation schemes on MSD risk using the fatigue failure model (Mehdizadeh et al., 2020). In this paper, it was demonstrated that the concavity of the fatigue risk function guarantees that any reductions in MSD risk obtained by persons with high-risk jobs will be more than offset by increases in risk experienced by those in the rotation pool having lower risk, leading to an overall increase in MSD risk to the group. However, the magnitude of the increase will be highly dependent on the makeup of the pool of jobs involved in the rotation. In fact, if all jobs are relatively low risk, to begin with, the increase in MSD risk will be modest. In such a situation, the relatively modest effect on MSD risk may allow certain other benefits of job rotation (such as relief from boredom, skill acquisition, and motor variation) to be appreciated. However, if even one high-risk job is included in the job rotation pool, the overall increase in MSD risk for others in the pool may be substantial and will intensify as the magnitude of the difference in MSD risk among jobs increases (Mehdizadeh et al., 2020).

The data in this example shows that job rotation is unlikely to be a useful MSD prevention method if one tries to use it to try to "balance" the physical demands associated with a group of tasks. If an ergonomist finds themselves in a situation in which there is one high risk job that is problematic, it would be advisable not to institute a job rotation including this job. Instead, an ergonomic redesign of the high-risk task should be performed to reduce risk. Similarly, rotation used in an attempt to balance the risks of tasks with high spine demands versus those with high upper extremity demands will result in the same finding. That is, the *overall* risk for the rotation pool will be higher for both low back and upper extremity disorders (Mehdizadeh et al., 2020).

Exoskeletons and MSD Prevention

In the early 1990s, there was a substantial increase in the use of back belts in an attempt to reduce the risk of low back injuries associated with manual lifting. Various claims were made regarding these devices including that they reduced spinal forces, supported the spine through increased intra-abdominal pressure, reduced bending motions, and that these factors decreased the risk of back injuries. However, systematic reviews of the literature and controlled epidemiology studies ultimately showed a lack of scientific support regarding the effective use of back belts in reducing injuries. Ultimately, studies were unable to demonstrate that back belts significantly reduced loading on the spine during the performance of lifting tasks (NIOSH, 1994).

More recently, externally worn devices having the capability of decreasing loads on joints of the body during manual work tasks have been developed. These devices, known as *exoskeletons*, are wearable devices designed to reduce the load experienced by an individuals' musculoskeletal system due to the performance of physical tasks. These devices can be passive or powered and have been shown to reduce musculoskeletal forces during physical task performance (Bär, Steinhilber, Rieger, & Luger, 2021; Howard, Murashov, Lowe, & Lu, 2020; Kermavnar, Vries, & de Looze, 2021). Previous assessments of the efficacy of low-back exoskeletons have generally relied on electromyography (EMG) to estimate the decreased load experienced by the low back (Bär et al., 2021; Howard et al., 2020; Kermavnar et al., 2021). While this approach is useful in establishing that muscular loads are decreased, there are some downsides associated with the use of EMG as a measure of the effectiveness of low-back exoskeletons. For example, EMG requires specialized training, equipment, and expertise to properly interpret. These qualities are not generally available to the average safety and health professional who may want to evaluate exoskeleton efficacy in a workplace setting (Zelik et al., 2021).

However, the LiFFT risk assessment tool (a fatigue failure-based tool discussed in Chapter 13) has been shown to provide the ability to estimate the decrease in low back disorder risk due to exoskeleton use. The LiFFT tool risk calculation is based upon the low-back load moment, and since low back exoskeletons act to counterbalance the moment about the lumbar spine, the LiFFT risk equation can be used to estimate the decrease in risk associated with the use of an exoskeleton during a lifting task. As mentioned in Chapter 8, the new exoskeleton efficacy tool is called "Exo-LiFFT" and provides an estimate of the degree to which the low back is offloaded by the exoskeleton. The decrease in the low-back moment can be plugged into LiFFT's risk assessment equation to provide an estimate of the decreased risk associated with the offloading of the spine due to exoskeleton use (Zelik et al., 2021).

Summary

Having a likely causal mechanism for the development of MSDs can provide several important benefits. In the current context, the tenets of fatigue failure can be used to evaluate and prescribe practices that would be of benefit to MSD prevention efforts. Furthermore, the theory can, in some cases, be used to demonstrate that certain methods used to try to prevent MSDs may not be of benefit (Mehdizadeh et al., 2020).

One clear message from the fatigue failure mechanism is that the cumulative damage associated with the entirety of the work exposure is of critical importance to understanding MSD risk (Gallagher & Schall, 2017). Risk assessment methods that do not allow for assessment of the totality of exposure may underestimate the true risk experienced by the worker. Fatigue failure methods not only provide the benefit of assessing the totality of risk but also can break down the risk on a task-by-task basis, identifying the tasks associated with the greatest proportion of risk which can then be prioritized for intervention (fixing the most hazardous jobs first).

The fatigue failure model indicates that reduction of stress should be a major goal of the ergonomist and will usually reduce risk to a greater degree than the reduction of repetitions. While both actions will be of benefit in reducing risk, the decrease in stress brings with it an exponential increase in the number of cycles that can be tolerated. For example, if given the choice of reducing the stress by 25% or reducing the repetition by 25%, the stress reduction option will provide the greatest decrease in MSD risk.

In the past, many companies have adopted practices purported to reduce injuries such as stretching, use of back belts, and other methods that have ultimately been shown to lack scientific evidence in terms of their effectiveness (NIOSH, 1994). Job rotation is another method used in industry to attempt to reduce MSD risk. The goal associated with job rotation is to try to "balance" jobs with high job demands to those with low job demands. However, fatigue failure theory shows that such attempts to balance physical demands between workers are not likely to be successful, especially if even one high-risk job is in the job rotation pool (Mehdizadeh et al., 2020). Exoskeletons provide another approach to MSD risk reduction and are becoming more popular. In contrast with previous approaches, exoskeletons appear to show promise at reducing joint loading, thereby reducing risk. A new tool (Exo-LiFFT) based on the LiFFT fatigue failure risk assessment method has been developed to estimate the reduction in risk associated with low back exoskeleton use (Zelik et al., 2021).

The topics covered in this chapter provide a sampling of the implications associated with the fatigue failure model and MSD risks. As advancements in technology and understanding occur, many more benefits would be expected to accrue from this approach, including real-time risk assessment and assessment of loading resulting from different modalities (e.g., cumulative damage for both whole-body vibration and manual lifting effects on the low back), which should also provide support in the prevention of MSD risk.

Bibliography

Adam, K., & Oswald, I. (1984). Sleep helps healing. *British Medical Journal*, *289*, 1400–1401.

Andarawis-Puri, A., Flatow, E., & Soslowski, L. (2015). Tendon basic science: Development, repair, regeneration, and healing. *Journal of Orthopaedic Research*, *33*, 780–784.

Armstrong, T., Buckle, P., Fine, L., Hagberg, M., Jonsson, B., Kilbom, A., . . . Viikari-Juntura, E. (1993). A conceptual model for work-related neck and upper-limb musculoskeletal disorders. *Scandinavian Journal of Work, Environment & Health*, *19*, 73–84.

Bani Hani, D., Huangfu, R., Sesek, R., Schall, M., Davis, G., & Gallagher, S. (2021). Development and Validation of a Cumulative Exposure Shoulder Risk Assessment Tool Based on Fatigue Failure Theory. *Ergonomics*, *64*(1), 39–64.

Bär, M., Steinhilber, B., Rieger, M., & Luger, T. (2021). The influence of using exoskeletons during occupational tasks on acute physical stress and strain compared to no exoskeleton – a systematic review and meta-analysis. *Appl. Ergon.*, *94*, 103385.

Barbe, M., Gallagher, S., Massicotte, V., Tytell, M., Popoff, S., & Barr-Gillespie, A. (2013). The interaction of force and repetition on musculoskeletal and neural tissue responses and sensorimotor behavior in a rat model of work-related musculoskeletal disorders. *BMC Musculoskeletal Disorders*, *14*.

Brinckmann, P., Biggemann, M., & Hilweg, D. (1988). Fatigue fracture of human lumbar vertebrae. *Clinical Biomechanics*, *3*(Suppl. 1), S1–S23.

Gallagher, S., & Barbe, M. (2021). The impaired healing hypothesis: A mechanism by which psychosocial stress and personal characteristics increase MSD risk? *Ergonomics*, 1–14. https://doi.org/10.1080/00140139.2021.1974103

Gallagher, S., Marras, W., Litsky, A., Burr, D., Landoll, J., & Matkovic, V. (2007). A comparison of fatigue failure responses of old versus middle-aged lumbar motion segments in simulated flexed lifting. *Spine*, *32*, 1832–1839.

Gallagher, S., & Schall, J. M. (2017). Musculoskeletal disorders as a fatigue failure process: Evidence, implications and research needs. *Ergonomics*, *60*, 255–269.

Gallagher, S., Sesek, R., Schall, M., Jr., & Huangfu, R. (2017). Development and validation of an easy-to-use risk assessment tool for cumulative low back loading: The Lifting Fatigue Failure Tool (LiFFT). *Applied Ergonomics*, *63*, 142–150.

Gosain, A., & DiPietro, L. (2004). Aging and wound healing. *World Journal of Surgery*, *28*, 321–326.

Gouin, J.-P., & Kiecolt-Glaser, J. (2011). The impact of psychological stress on wound healing. *Immunology and Allergy Clinics of North America*, *31*, 81–93.

Howard, J., Murashov, V., Lowe, B., & Lu, M.-L. (2020). Industrial exoskeletons: Need for intervention effectiveness research. *American Journal of Industrial Medicine*, *63*, 201–208.

Huber, G., Nagel, K., Skrzypiec, D., Klein, A., Püschel, K., & Morlock, M. (2016). A description of spinal fatigue strength. *Journal of Biomechanics*, *49*, 875–880.

Jager, M., & Luttmann, A. (1991). Compressive strength of lumbar spine elements related to age, gender, and other influencing factors. In *Electromyographical kinesiology, proceedings of the 9th congress of the international society of electrophysiological kinesiology* (pp. 291–294).

Jones, A., Rule, J., Moore, J., Sottos, N., & White, S. (2007). Life extension of self-healing polymers with rapidly growing fatigue cracks. *Journal of the Royal Society, Interface*, *4*, 395–403.

Kermavnar, T., Vries, A., & de Looze, M. O. (2021). Effects of industrial back-support exoskeletons on body loading and user experience: An updated systematic review. *Ergonomics*, *64*, 685–711.

Mehdizadeh, A., Vinel, A., Hu, Q., Schall, M., Jr., Gallagher, S., & Sesek, R. (2020). Job rotation and work-related musculoskeletal disorders: A fatigue-failure perspective. *Ergonomics*, *63*, 461–476.

Miller, B., Olesen, J., Hansen, M., Døssing, S., Crameri, R., Welling, R., . . . Rennie, M. (2005). Coordinated collagen and muscle protein synthesis in human patella tendon and quadriceps muscle after exercise. *The Journal of Physiology*, *567*(Pt 3), 1021–1033.

Miner, M. A. (1945). Cumulative damage in fatigue. *Journal of Applied Mechanics*, *16*, A159–A164.

Nash, J. C. (1966). *Fatigue of self-healing structure: A generalized theory of fatigue failure*. New York, NY: American Society of Mechanical Engineers.

National Institute for Occupational Safety and Health (1994). *Applications manual for the revised NIOSH lifting equation*. Cincinnati, OH: DHHS.

National Research Council—Institute of Medicine (2001). *Musculoskeletal disorders and the workplace: Low back and upper extremities*. Washington, DC: National Academy Press.

NIOSH. (1981). *Work practices guide for manual lifting* (NIOSH Technical Report No. 81-122). Cincinnati, OH: US Department of Health and Human Services.

NIOSH (1994). *Back belts: Do they prevent injury?* Cioncinnati, OH: DHHS (NIOSH). Publication Number 94-127

NIOSH (1997). *Musculoskeletal disorders and workplace factors*. Cincinnati, OH: National Institute for Occupational Safety and Health.

Norman, R., Wells, R., Neumann, P., Frank, J., Shannon, H., Kerr, M., & Group, T. (1998). A comparison of peak vs cumulative physical work exposure risk factors for the reporting of low back pain in the automotive industry. *Clinical Biomechanics, 13*, 561–573.

Padula, R., Comper, M., Sparer, E., & Dennerlein, J. (2017). Job rotation designed to prevent musculoskeletal disorders and control risk in manufacturing industries: A systematic review. *Applied Ergonomics, 58*, 386–397.

Palmgren, A. (1924). Die Lebebsdaue rvon Kugellagern. *Zeitschrift des Vereines deutscher Ingenieure, 68*, 339–341.

Schechtman, H., & Bader, D. (1997). In vitro fatigue of human tendons. *Journal of Biomechanics*, 829–835.

Sekkay, F., Imbeau, D., Chinniah, Y., Dubé, P.-A., de Marcellis-Warin, N., Beauregard, N., & Trépanier, M. (2018). Risk factors associated with self-reported musculoskeletal pain among short and long distance industrial gas delivery truck drivers. *Applied Ergonomics, 72*, 69–87.

Snook, S. (1978). The design of manual handling tasks. *Ergonomics, 21*, 963–985.

Stephens, R., Fatemi, A., Stephens, R., & Fuchs, H. (2001). *Metal fatigue in engineering* (2nd ed.). New York, NY: Wiley.

Sun, H., Andarawis-Puri, N., Li, Y., Fung, D., Lee, J., Wang, V., . . . Flatow, E. L. (2010). Cycle-dependent matric remodeling gene expression response in fatigue-loaded rat patellar tendons. *Journal of Orthopaedic Research, 28*, 1380–1386.

Zelik, K., Nurse, C., Schall, M., Jr., Sesek, R., Marino, M., & Gallagher, S. (2021). An ergonomic assessment tool for evaluating the effect of back exoskeletons on injury risk. *Applied Ergonomics, 99*, 103619.

15

Optimizing Musculoskeletal Health

Introduction

In previous chapters, we have covered numerous aspects related to damage development and healing of the musculoskeletal tissues. While a great deal has been learned regarding these topics, we still wallow in ignorance regarding crucial aspects of this immensely complicated system. One thing that is very clear is that the musculoskeletal system is highly dynamic and continuously responds and adjusts to the magnitude and repetition of the loads it experiences. The influence of stress (or its absence) on tissues can be either negative or positive depending on the specific magnitude and duration of the loading experienced. The dynamic balance required to maintain the optimal functioning of this system is such that some loading is beneficial (but too much is detrimental) and some rest is beneficial (but too much is detrimental). What appears to be needed to maintain musculoskeletal health is to achieve a happy middle ground involving a certain amount of stress (but not too much) and a certain degree of rest (but not too much). The amount of stress (or rest) acceptable to any particular individual will undoubtedly depend on personal characteristics that will vary widely in the population.

As suggested by the previous paragraph, optimization of the health of the musculoskeletal system seems to depend (in large part) on managing its exposure to stress as well as to sufficient rest (allowing healing to occur). Due to the dynamic nature of the system (and its remodeling and healing capacity), a limited amount of high-stress exposure (along with sufficient rest) can lead to beneficial remodeling resulting in increased tissue strength and capacity. However, there appears to be a threshold beyond which remodeling and healing processes cannot cope effectively, leading to the development of cumulative damage. As we will discuss in this chapter, there are several clear implications regarding fatigue failure that are important with respect to optimizing musculoskeletal health, but clearly, attention to healing and remodeling aspects of the system are also very important.

In addition to damage and healing, there are additional aspects to be considered in optimizing musculoskeletal health. For example, proper nutrition and avoidance of certain substances that might negatively impact the functioning of the musculoskeletal system important in maintaining musculoskeletal health need to be discussed. Finally, despite our best efforts to prevent musculoskeletal disorders (MSDs), it is almost certain that MSDs will be experienced by all of us at some point during our lives. When they do occur, proper treatment and management of musculoskeletal injuries and diseases will be necessary. We will discuss basic principles that appear to be useful in the treatment and rehabilitation of musculoskeletal injuries.

Musculoskeletal Disorders: The Fatigue Failure Mechanism, First Edition. Sean Gallagher and Mary F. Barbe.

We will begin by discussing actions recommended to improve the overall musculoskeletal health and will then provide some specific advice for reducing the risk of developing musculoskeletal disorders in the occupational setting. Finally, we will describe procedures that may help reduce the pain and promote the healing process when an injury does occur.

General

There are certain procedures that would appear to be beneficial for most people to help maintain (or potentially improve) the functioning of the musculoskeletal system. This section will focus primarily on some of the lifestyle habits that have been shown to be of benefit to musculoskeletal health.

Avoid a Sedentary Lifestyle

Although intense physical/occupational activity can increase the risk for MSDs, a major challenge to musculoskeletal health in the present day is the lack of sufficient physical activity in the general population. Even a modest amount of activity appears to have a significant impact in reducing the risk of death ascribed to sedentary activities (as summarized in Table 15.1), such as sitting 8 hr/day (Ekelund et al., 2016). For example, the World Health Organization (WHO) recommends 2 hr per week of physical activity sufficient to moderately increase heart rate. Such activity has been shown to significantly reduce the lifetime risk of cardiovascular disease according to a 25-year longitudinal study of 13,000 adults (Kubota et al., 2017).

Management of mechanical stress on the musculoskeletal system does not only involve the reduction of stress but also may sometimes require mechanical stress enhancement. We live in a dynamic age where the needs required for living have been made much easier to attain than those in the past, and this (along with the popularity of various technologies such as television, computer, and gaming) has promoted a sedentary lifestyle that can be deleterious to the musculoskeletal system. It has been estimated that nearly half of the United States (US) population fails to obtain even the barest minimum of recommended aerobic activity levels (Centers for Disease Control and Prevention (CDC), U.S. Department of Health & Human Services, 2017). Similar findings are

Table 15.1 Effects of a Sedentary Lifestyle Versus Active Lifestyle on Musculoskeletal Tissues

Sedentary lifestyle	Moderate exercise/resistance training
↓ Tendon collagen synthesis, organization, vascularity	↑ Tendon healing
↓ Muscle capillary density, ATP productivity, myofiber cross-sectional area; ↓ force production	↑ Muscle strength, mass, myofiber hypertrophy, capillary density
↓ Bone mass and quality	↑ Bone mass and quality
Hyaline cartilage may convert to stiffer fibrocartilage	↑ Cartilage healing, presumedly through ↑ the diffusion of nutrients
	Axon regeneration
	↓ Cardiovascular risk
	↓ Effects of aging on tissues

reported in the United Kingdom, where only 36% of adults perform 30 min of moderate exercise at least once per week (Office for National Statistics, 2019).

A sedentary lifestyle can have numerous adverse impacts on musculoskeletal health. It has been demonstrated, for example, that decreased physical activity adversely affects structural and mechanical properties of tendons, as well as their metabolism (Frizziero et al., 2016). Tendon morphology, collagen synthesis and organization, and vascularity are all negatively impacted. Similar adverse changes occur in muscle. Detraining leads to decreased capillary density in muscle, along with reduced ATP production, reductions of muscle cross-sectional areas, and force production (Mujika & Padilla, 2001). Hyaline cartilage can convert into stiffer and less pliable fibrocartilage with prolonged joint immobility (Coq et al., 2008). Similar declines are seen with other musculoskeletal tissues. As has been mentioned previously, musculoskeletal tissues need to experience a certain degree of mechanical stress to maintain optimal performance, and therefore, inactivity results in adverse effects on the system.

Sedentary behavior can result in adverse effects on other body systems that can also impact the musculoskeletal system. A clear example is the role of a sedentary lifestyle in the development of obesity and type II diabetes. These disorders are associated with increased joint degeneration, and the development and progression of osteoarthritis (Felson, Anderson, Naimark, Walker, & Meenan, 1988). From the fatigue failure perspective, the additional stress experienced by the knee joint in walking due to excess adiposity in obese individuals would be expected to result in much more rapid joint degeneration compared to that if this additional stress was absent. Obesity is also associated with impaired healing (Guo & DiPietro, 2010); therefore, obesity would be expected to both increase cumulative damage development and decrease the capacity to heal (a "double whammy" on the musculoskeletal system). Increased levels of physical activity would be expected to both maintain the health of individual tissues of the musculoskeletal system and decrease the likelihood of developing obesity and type-2 diabetes.

It should also be noted that chronic musculoskeletal pain may play an important role in causing individuals to avoid physical activity. In this way, chronic musculoskeletal pain or disability may have a large negative impact on the health of other important systems (e.g., cardiovascular, respiratory). Thus, avoidance of chronic musculoskeletal pain is not just important from an orthopedic perspective but may also pose a significant and lasting health risk to many other essential systems in the body. Table 15.1 provides some of the changes that result from a sedentary lifestyle juxtaposed with a lifestyle that includes moderate exercise and resistance training.

Moderate Exercise

Improved ligament healing has been observed with controlled early resumption of activity after injury (Hauser & Dolan, 2011), which seems to stimulate repair and restore ligament function. A delay in activity may postpone recovery and adversely impact tissue repair. Although there is some controversy, and it remains debatable if acute exercise has any effects on tendon properties, optimal tendon properties differ between activities: more compliant tendons seem to benefit from slow stretch-shortening cycle (SSC) activities, such as countermovement jumps, whereas stiffer tendons seem to benefit from fast SSC movements, such as sprinting (Tardioli, Malliaras, & Maffulli, 2012). Although symptoms of pain improved with exercise in athletes with tendon patellar pathology, no improvement of tendon structure or dimensions are seen using ultrasound tissue characterization (van Ark et al., 2018).

Controlled passive motion and early weight-bearing have become a staple of knee rehabilitation protocols and have shown some benefit for articular cartilage healing, likely by increasing diffusion of nutrients through the cartilage. Early active motion shows no detrimental effect on the cartilage in basic science or clinical reports and has been shown to safely improve pain, function, and activity while also maintaining bone mass, which declines rapidly with prolonged immobilization (Howard, Mattacola, Romine, & Lattermann, 2010).

Axonal regeneration can be accelerated by various forms of exercise with as little as 3–7 days of exercise (Molteni, Zheng, Ying, Gomez-Pinilla, & Twiss, 2004; Teodori et al., 2011; Udina, Puigdemasa, & Navarro, 2011). Exercise results in axonal outgrowth, higher numbers of axons in a nerve, Schwann cell proliferation, as well as better regeneration as evaluated by recovery of compound motor action potentials and larger myofiber size in the nerve's target muscles (Cooper, Kluding, & Wright, 2016; Park & Hoke, 2014; Wood et al., 2012). These effects appear to be related to increased production of neurotrophic factors in dorsal root ganglion neuronal cells bodies (e.g., brain-derived neurotrophic factor, nerve growth factor and growth-associated protein 43) that then stimulate axonal growth (Lopez-Alvarez, Modol, Navarro, & Cobianchi, 2015; Molteni et al., 2004). Interestingly, there are sex-related requirements for exercise in enhancing peripheral axonal regeneration (Sabatier, Redmon, Schwartz, & English, 2008; Wood et al., 2012), in that male mice need 1 hr of continuous treadmill walking per day, at a slow speed for ensuring the effective promotion of axon outgrowth. This treatment was not effective in female mice. Instead, female mice needed interval training (2 min of fast running followed by 5 min of the rest period, which was repeated four times) for enhanced axonal regeneration. The interval training was not effective in the male mice.

Resistance Training

The fatigue failure model of MSD development indicates that excessive exposure to repeated stress is associated with cumulative damage in musculoskeletal tissues, leading to damage, pain, and discomfort. However, high stress exposure of limited duration can be beneficial to tissues. Musculoskeletal tissues respond positively to a limited number of high-stress exertions performed 2–3 times per week, typically through resistance training. Resistance training can significantly improve the strength of musculoskeletal tissue and morphology of system components and may thereby provide a certain degree of protection to repetitive stress injuries. Such exercise, while it cannot prevent aging of the neuromuscular system, does appear to have the potential to reduce the degree of adverse changes due to aging (Frontera & Bigard, 2002).

A recent systematic review examined various aspects of resistance training such as the training period, frequency, intensity, and volume of exercise leading to the best outcomes in older adults (Borde, Hortobágyi, & Granacher, 2015). A meta-regression of data from 25 studies indicated that best muscle strength gains were associated with a training period of 50–53 weeks, a training intensity of 70–79% of the individual's one-repetition maximum strength, a training frequency of two sessions per week consisting of 2–3 sets per exercise with each set consisting of 7–9 exertions. The optimal time under tension was found to be 6 s with a rest between exertions of 4 s. The optimal rest period between sets was 60 s.

Effects on resistance training on muscle morphology were less pronounced than strength gain; however, different variables have been shown to improve tissue morphology. In fact, the optimal training period, training volume, and repetitions per set were the same for both muscle strength and morphology changes. However, while the best training frequency for morphology improvement was 3 times per week, optimal training intensity was reduced (51–69% of one-repetition maximum), and increased rest periods between sets (120 s) were suggested (Borde et al., 2015).

Many positive changes are associated with a limited number of high-stress exertions and appropriate rest. This is clearly the case for individuals who are otherwise sedentary or who experience modest amounts of stress in everyday life. However, it is doubtful that high-stress weight training exercises should be recommended for those who also experience a high degree of stress in the performance of their normal occupational duties. In this case, additional weightlifting may prove detrimental—increasing exposure to stress and exacerbating cumulative damage that may have developed on the job.

Nutrition

Dietary factors also appear to be important with respect to musculoskeletal health (Table 15.2). Proper nutrition is critical in maintaining a healthy weight and in improving the health of the components of the musculoskeletal system (Lewis et al., 2019). Simply maintaining a healthy weight can help to reduce stresses experienced by musculoskeletal structures and reduce the risk of injury. For example, a diet high in potassium (from fruits and vegetables) has been associated with a reduction in muscle loss in adults over the age of 65 (Dawson-Hughes, Harris, & Ceglia, 2008). Bone mineral density and bone resorption in post-menopausal women have been correlated with the intake of flavonoids, compounds common in many fruits and vegetables (Hardcastle, Aucott, Reid, & Macdonald, 2011). Bone health has been shown to improve with adequate intake of protein, calcium, and vitamin D (Daly, 2017; Meyer, Pedersen, Loken, & Tverdal, 1997). Calcium and vitamin D work in tandem to improve both bone and muscle health. Their absence from our diet leads the body to pilfer stores of these substances from bone and other tissues, leading to bones that are brittle and weak (Lawrence University, 2021). A diet rich in fruits and vegetables can decrease the effects of metabolic acidosis on the kidneys associated with increased protein intake by decreasing renal acid load (Heaney & Layman, 2008; Remer & Manz, 1995).

Table 15.2 Dietary Factors Necessary for Musculoskeletal Health

Nutrient	Source	Health value
Potassium	Fruits and vegetables	Reduction of muscle loss
Flavonoids	Fruits and vegetables	Bone anabolic activity: higher levels correlate with greater bone mineral density
Protein	Beans, meats, poultry, seafood, and more	Improved bone health, although too much can increase renal load; increases muscle mass in patients with sarcopenia
Calcium	Milk products, green leafy greens, supplements, and others	Improved bone health
Vitamin D	Sunlight, eggs, supplements	Improved bone health, increases muscle mass in patients with sarcopenia
Antioxidants	Multiple food sources, supplements	Improve tissue repair
Glucocorticoids, chondroitin	Shark and bovine cartilage; synthesized in a lab	Short-term benefits in pain reduction; low long-term clinical efficacy
Curcumin, collagen hydrolysate, Boswellic acid	Turmeric, multiple food sources, and plants in the genus *Boswellia*, respectively	Short-term benefits in pain reduction; low long-term clinical efficacy

There is some evidence that appropriate nutritional supplements to the diet may result in short-to-medium-term benefits for certain musculoskeletal conditions. For example, supplemental antioxidants appear to improve tissue repair; however, the optimal dosage remains unclear (Sen, 2001). Individuals with sarcopenia may benefit from increased muscle mass and strength from supplements containing whey protein fortified with vitamin D (Molnar et al., 2016). Glucosamine (often given with chondroitin) is a supplement that was initially recommended by certain medical societies for the treatment of knee osteoarthritis; however, while recent evidence has shown some short-term benefits in pain reduction, there does not appear to be much evidence of long-term clinical efficacy (Liu, Machado, Eyles, Ravi, & Hunter, 2018). Other nutritional supplements, including curcumin, collagen hydrolysate, and boswellic acid provided more significant short-term pain reduction than glucosamine and chondroitin; however, in the long term supplements have not demonstrated effectiveness in reducing pain and improving joint function (Liu et al., 2018).

Avoid Obesity

The sedentary lifestyle experienced by many individuals has unfortunately led to a significant rise in obesity, often resulting in Type II diabetes (Lewis et al., 2019). As mentioned previously, obesity is associated with an impaired healing response (Guo & DiPietro, 2010); however, obesity is also associated with several musculoskeletal disorders, most notably knee joint osteoarthritis (OA) (Figure 15.1) (Driban et al., 2020; Mobasheri & Batt, 2016). In the knees, this may result from the repeated exposure of increased stress due to the increased body weight on the knee joint (i.e., a local risk factor). Fortunately, it appears that exercise and weight loss can be helpful in the treatment of knee OA (Messier et al., 2004).

However, obesity is also a systemic risk factor for knee and hand OA, as are age, female gender, and various genetic factors (Figure 15.1). Obesity is also a risk factor for MSDs in general, as shown in Figure 10.10 (Gallagher & Barbe, 2021). The fact that obesity is also a risk factor for hand

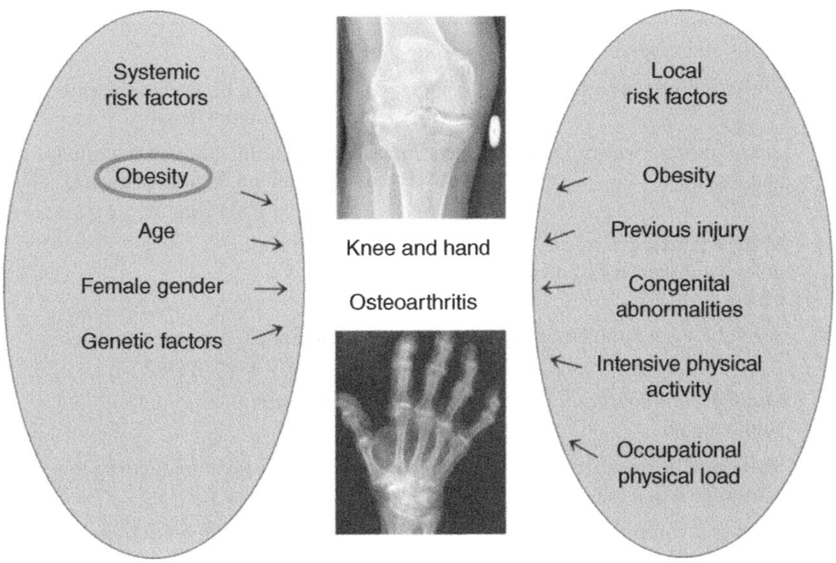

Figure 15.1 Systemic and local risk factors for osteoarthritis. Vuolteenaho et al. (2014).

osteoarthritis (OA) cannot be explained only by increased load on joints. Rather, it points to an obesity-related systemic factor contributing to the inflammation in the OA joints, thereby linking obesity to OA. Systemic leptin levels have been suggested as a systemic factor since leptin levels in synovial fluid are increased in obese patients (Vuolteenaho, Koskinen, & Moilanen, 2014). The underlying mechanism is thought to be that leptin receptor Ob-R is expressed in cartilage, and leptin induces the production of matrix metalloproteinases (MMPs), pro-inflammatory mediators, and nitric oxide in chondrocytes. Figure 15.1 also depicts several local risk factors for joint OA, including prior injury, genetic factors, intensive physical activity, and occupational physical load. When these factors are combined, the risk of joint OA is likely compounded.

Sleep

A great deal of attention has been paid recently to the important benefits of sleep on general health and well-being. Unfortunately, there are many aspects of the modern world that serve to interfere with getting a good night's sleep, which can lead to wide-ranging adverse consequences. For example, inadequate sleep has been shown to substantially impair physical performance, neurocognitive function, increase injury risk, increase illness susceptibility, and decrease pain tolerance (Simpson, Gibbs, & Matheson, 2017).

Sleep is an important factor in the tissue healing and remodeling processes, and indeed there is substantial and growing evidence that getting a prolonged amount of high-quality sleep is beneficial to the healing of wounds and remodeling of musculoskeletal tissues (Figure 15.2) (Klyne, Barbe, James, & Hodges, 2021). When one examines the sleep process, it would appear to create a set of conditions highly conducive to the repair of musculoskeletal tissues. During the sleep process, the musculoskeletal system is also generally at rest, as the tissues experience a prolonged

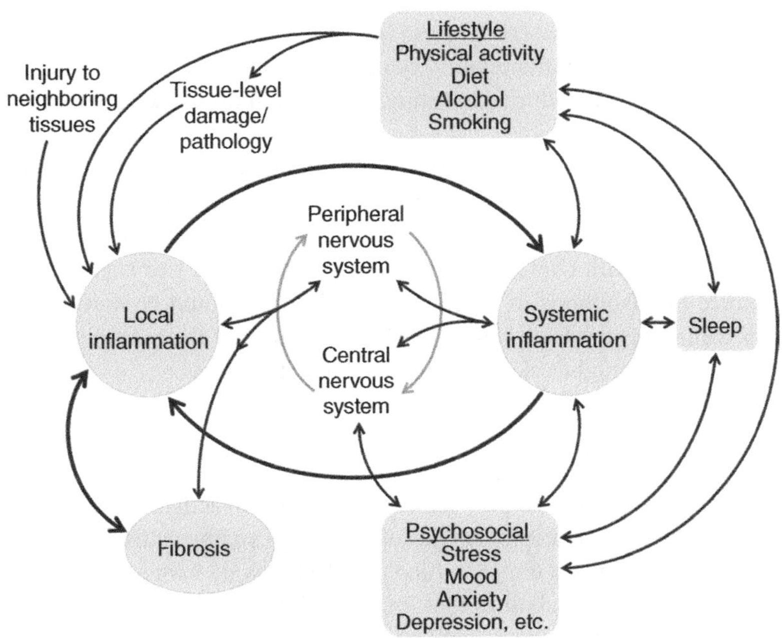

Figure 15.2 Conceptual model of the factors that impact tissue health in musculoskeletal conditions. Klyne et al. (2021) / MDPI / CC BY 4.0.

state of decreased loading. The decreased loading state greatly reduces the chance of additional damage accrual due to exposure to repeated stress and helps to assure that additional physical damage to tissues will be unlikely. This state also allows for uninterrupted healing to take place. Interestingly, studies of non-biologic self-healing materials indicate that fatigue life of materials increases in proportion to the length of rest periods (Jones, Rule, Moore, Sottos, & White, 2007), likely due to providing additional time for the healing process to take place. Having an extended period of rest may confer the same benefit to the repair process in biological materials as well.

Several processes take place during sleep that are favorable to healing, including protein synthesis, cell division, and growth hormone secretion, which are all substantially increased during sleep (Adam & Oswald, 1984; Mostaghimi, Obermeyer, Ballamudi, Martinez-Gonzolez, & Benca, 2005).

A general daily cycle appears to occur in which the activities performed during wakefulness lead to catabolism (or degradation) of tissues, while in sleep, the body appears to engage in processes that foster anabolic (renewal) processes that assist in healing (Adam & Oswald, 1984). For example, deep sleep (Stage 4) is the primary stimulus for the secretion of growth hormones. This substance increases the synthesis of protein and helps mobilize free fatty acids for energy requirements associated with this process. Growth hormone and insulin-like growth factor-I (IGF-1) have been shown to enhance the synthesis of bone (Isaksson, Jansson, & Gause, 1982), as well as collagen synthesis in human tendon and skeletal muscle (Doessing et al., 2010). When tissues have been damaged, the rate of repair in sleep is accelerated compared to normal (Adam & Oswald, 1984). Sleep also appears to suppress the secretion of substances that favor catabolism, including cortisol and catecholamines.

Not surprisingly, sleep deprivation has been found to result in changes to many processes that may negatively affect the healing process. For example, lack of sleep serves to inhibit the secretion of growth hormone (Van Cauter et al., 1992). In addition, sleep deprivation leads to increased activation of the sympathetic nervous system (Irwin, Thompson, Miller, Gillin, & Ziegler, 1999), activation of the hypothalamic-pituitary-adrenal (HPA) axis (Leproult, Copinschi, Buxton, & Van Cauter, 1997), and increased secretion of proinflammatory cytokines such as TNF-alpha and IL-1 beta (Krueger et al., 1998), all of which act to reduce the healing process in musculoskeletal tissues (Figure 15.2).

The findings noted earlier indicate that it is important that steps should be taken to ensure that sufficient sleep is obtained so that healing can be maximized. It is generally recommended that adults should get between 7 and 9 hr of sleep per night (Hirshkowitz et al., 2015). Table 15.3 provides recommendations that can assist with obtaining an appropriate amount of sleep, as well as potential factors that can reduce the likelihood of a good night's sleep. It should be noted that psychological stress as well as commonly used substances (such as caffeine and alcohol) can negatively impact the ability to obtain a good night's sleep, as described in detail below.

Reduce Alcohol Consumption and Smoking

It has been known for decades that alcohol consumption and smoking are two activities that negatively affect the body's healing processes. A conceptual model of how they can impact tissue health in musculoskeletal conditions is depicted in Figure 15.2. Alcohol affects a wide variety of healing pathways through the production of toxic metabolites that impact cellular mechanisms required for efficient repair (Jung et al., 2011). Exposure to alcohol has been shown to alter systemic and local inflammatory processes, such as decreased neutrophil function and decreased macrophage recruitment (Fitzgerald et al., 2007). These effects impact the early stages of the inflammation

Table 15.3 Recommended Sleep Durations

Age	Recommended, hr	May be appropriate, hr	Not recommended, hr
Infants	12–15	10–11	Less than 10, more than 18
Toddlers	11–14	9–10	Less than 9, more than 16
Preschoolers	10–13	8–9	Less than 8, more than 14
School-aged children and teenagers (6–18 years)	8–11	7–8	Less than 7, more than 12
Adults (18–64 years)	7–9	6	Less than 6, more than 10
Older adults (≥65 years)	7–8	5–6	Less than 5, more than 9

Hirshkowitz et al. (2015).

process and lead to increased wound healing time (Radek et al., 2005). Alcohol has also been demonstrated to reduce angiogenesis in wounds (resulting in a more hypoxic wound environment) and decreases the stimulation of fibroblasts leading to decreased collagen production (Stephens, Al-Khateeb, Davies, Shepherd, & Thomas, 1996), also hindering the healing response.

Though alcohol resides in a class of drugs known as sedatives, it can be quite disruptive to the sleeping process (Walker, 2017). Alcohol affects several neurotransmitter systems that control the sleep process. While alcohol consumption will lead to decreased sleep onset latency early in the process (when blood alcohol levels are high), it will later result in sleep disruption and poor-quality sleep (Colrain, Nicholas, & Baker, 2014). Alcohol abuse and dependence can lead to chronic sleep disturbance, decreased slow-wave sleep, and more rapid eye movement sleep than normal (Colrain et al., 2014). Of importance to optimizing the fatigue life-enhancing healing process in musculoskeletal tissues, alcohol administration has been shown to reduce the secretion of growth hormone by up to 70–75% (Prinz, Roehrs, Vitaliano, Linnoila, & Weitzman, 1980). This reduction would be expected to severely curtail the restorative healing process in these tissues, leading to slower healing of injured tissue and increased likelihood of injured tissues sustaining additional damage, as previously discussed.

Smoking can lead to a number of adverse impacts on the musculoskeletal system, both in terms of injury susceptibility and recovery. Smokers are more susceptible to sprain and strain injuries as a result of the decreased vascularity that is inherent with smoking. Osteoporosis is also more common among smokers as it appears to affect the balance between osteoblasts (which deposit new bone) and osteoclasts (which resorb bone). Smoking also causes the body to break down estrogen more quickly, which is an important hormone for bone health.

Due to decreased blood flow associated with smoking, the healing process is adversely impacted in those who smoke. This leads to an inability for the body to perform adequate maintenance on the musculoskeletal tissues, reducing the ability to completely repair areas of microdamage, allowing damage in these areas to further propagate, resulting in a more significant injury. The impacts of smoking on healing may also affect the ability to recover completely from surgery, such as from rotator cuff surgery. Due to the poorer quality of both the tendon and the bone in smokers, a surgical repair may fail to heal completely or tear again after surgery. The rate of post-surgical infection for a smoker is three times greater than a non-smoker. The good news is that quitting smoking can lead to a reversal of these adverse effects on the musculoskeletal system.

Combatting the Effects of Aging

The degenerative changes in the musculoskeletal system that occur due to aging are not, unfortunately, reversible at present. However, it is clear that physical exercise and healthy nutritional habits can continue to positively impact system components throughout the aging process (Figure 15.3) (Lewis et al., 2019). Appropriate mechanical loading of musculoskeletal tissues appears to continue to provide significant positive effects on the health of several system components, including tendons (Zhang, Yuan, & Wang, 2016), cartilage (Figure 15.1) (Guilak, 2011), and bone (Grabowski, 2009). For example, tendons exposed to physical exercise demonstrate increased tendon collagen synthesis and improved tissue quality compared to those lacking the stimulus of beneficial mechanical loading (Svensson, Heinemeier, Couppé, Kjaer, & Magnusson, 2016).

Another significant change that occurs with aging is the development of muscle sarcopenia, which is the loss of primarily type II (fast twitch) muscle fibers that lead to decreased muscle mass and strength (Beaudart et al., 2017). This decrease in muscle strength has ancillary effects, as tendon and bone will be deprived of the magnitude of stress stimulus that may be useful in maintaining their structural integrity. Exposure to appropriate mechanical loading has been shown

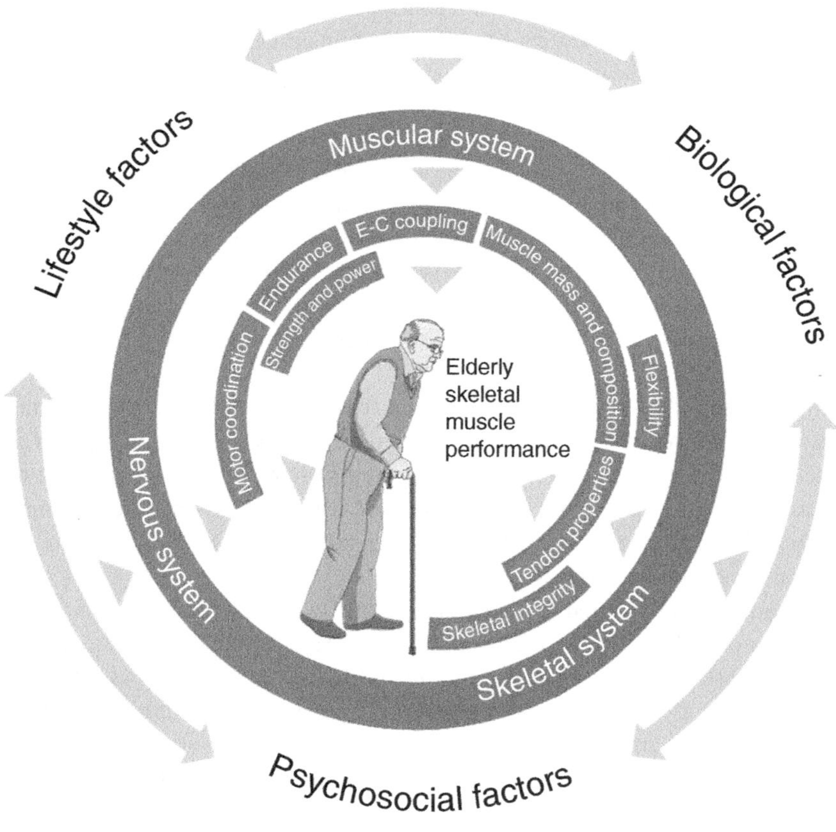

Figure 15.3 The multifactorial determinants of elderly nerve and musculoskeletal system performance. *Journal of Cachexia, Sarcopenia, and Muscle*, 9(1), 3–19. First published: 19 November 2017. https://onlinelibrary.wiley.com/doi/full/10.1002/jcsm.12238.

to have a beneficial impact on muscle mass and muscle function and can increase the ratio of type I to type II fibers and can result in an increase in the cross-sectional area of type II fibers (Lundberg & Nader, 2008).

Reducing MSD Risk in Occupational Settings

Avoid Cumulative Damage Development from Repeated Stress

We have noted previously that a limited amount of high stress activity can lead to beneficial remodeling of musculoskeletal tissues. Normally when a person performs an exercise routine for their general health, the amount of activity is self-regulated. However, in the occupational environment, an individual will often lack the ability to stop whenever one wants (that is, if one wants to maintain employment). Most occupational tasks are going to require 8 (or more) hrs of activity, often performing repetitive tasks that may lead to cumulative damage accrual beyond the ability of the healing processes to repair.

Fatigue failure theory makes it clear that it is the sum total of stress experienced by a tissue during the workday that is critical in determining the damage development (and risk of injury) for that tissue. There are many ways in which cumulative damage may accrue. The cumulative damage development might be the result of a mono-task job, or more often, jobs comprised of multiple tasks. Thus, methods of assessing risk should be able to sum the total cumulative damage associated with all tasks comprising a job. Fortunately, validated methods of assessing cumulative damage resulting from variable loading tasks are provided in fatigue failure theory, which has been utilized in recent risk assessment tools, as discussed in Chapter 13.

A fundamental principle of fatigue failure theory is that high-stress loading can only be tolerated for a limited number of loading cycles. As stress is decreased, the number of cycles necessary to inflict damage will increase in an exponential manner. Thus, to reduce cumulative loading on a worker performing a highly repetitive job, it is an important principle to reduce the stress range experienced during the performance of physical tasks to the extent possible (even at the cost of a modest increase in repetition). As mentioned previously, it is apparent that a limited number of high-stress exertions can be beneficial to musculoskeletal tissues, it is also clear that exposure to excessive repeated loading at a high-stress level can lead to the rapid development of cumulative damage in musculoskeletal tissues.

Duty Cycles and Work Break Schedules

Current equations for repetitive occupational task thresholds were developed from 69 short-term psychophysical data tasks (each <4 weeks in duration) using physiological data from six studies demonstrating muscle fatigue after only 1 hr (Potvin, 2012). The duty cycle is the proportion of time worker is active (i.e., exerts force) during a work cycle in a repetitive task. Decreasing the duty cycle may increase the allowable maximum acceptable forces and enhance tissue recovery (Potvin, 2012). Increasing periods of complete relaxation between work cycles also reduce health risks (Sjogaard, Lundberg, & Kadefors, 2000), supporting the need for further exploration of rest periods in loading models.

Relatively few studies have examined the effects of changing work break scheduling, frequency, and duration. A recent systematic review examining the results of six studies comprising 373 total workers found low-quality evidence that different work-break frequencies may have no effect on musculoskeletal pain, discomfort, or fatigue (Luger, Maher, Rieger, & Steinhilber, 2019). Very low-quality evidence indicated that work-break frequencies might have a positive effect on productivity and work performance. Low-quality evidence suggested that there may not be an effect of the type of work break (active versus passive) on pain, discomfort, or fatigue (Luger et al., 2019). Work break duration was not examined by any of the studies in this review. Results of this review indicate the need for high-quality studies with large sample sizes to better evaluate the efficacy of work break scheduling, the type of break (active or passive), and frequency and duration of work breaks (Luger et al., 2019).

Avoid Job Rotation to Balance Biomechanical Demands

As we have described, several lines of evidence suggest that MSDs are the result of a fatigue failure process. An important ramification of this result relates to the attempt to control MSD occurrence by rotating workers through stressful jobs. For example, consider an employer that has workers performing three jobs with the same repetition rate - one worker has a job highly stressful to the low back and two other workers have low back stress jobs. It might seem reasonable to rotate three workers through those jobs for equal portions of time, to decrease the stress on the worker performing the highly stressful job. However, in doing so it needs to be recognized that the two other workers will experience higher cumulative loading when the high-stress job is performed. Because the relationship between stress and repetition is exponential in nature, it turns out that the increase in stress for the two low-stress workers will be much greater than the decrease in stress for the high-stress worker. As a result, the overall likelihood of an injury for these three workers will be higher *with* the job rotation than without it (Mehdizadeh et al., 2020). A much better approach would be to decrease the demands of the high-stress job through job design, which would clearly lower the risk of back injury for the worker in the high-stress job and would not increase the stress experienced for the other workers.

Fatigue failure theory indicates that the same phenomenon will occur if one tries to balance jobs having high stress on the low back (but low stress on the upper extremities) versus jobs having high upper extremity stress (but little back stress). Rotating workers through this arrangement will result in an overall higher risk of injury for both regions (Mehdizadeh et al., 2020). However, it should be noted that if jobs possess relatively equivalent stresses, job rotation may be useful in providing workers with varied work tasks, cross-training, and decreased boredom and monotony, which may provide some psychosocial benefits.

Avoid Non-neutral Postures

Adoption of non-neutral postures may have an important role in increasing stress on musculoskeletal tissues, which has an important impact on the fatigue life of tissues. Clearly, awkward postures can have other impacts such as impeding blood flow (Chaffin, 1999) or increasing ligament laxity (Solomonow et al., 2003), which may affect tissue health and/or injury potential. However, a major reason why awkward postures emerge as a risk factor for MSDs may simply be due to the increased tissue loads that result from the adoption of awkward or non-neutral postures, and the effects of these increased loads in the fatigue failure paradigm.

Maximize Fatigue Life

As discussed in Chapters 10 and 11, it would be expected that the self-healing capability of musculoskeletal tissues would serve to significantly extend fatigue life. Thus, the fatigue life is going to be dependent on the ultimate strength (US) of the tissue, the cumulative damage experienced as the result of exposure to repeated stress, and the efficacy of the healing process. Longer fatigue lives will ensue when cumulative damage accrual is low and the healing process is functioning optimally. On the other hand, the fatigue life of these tissues will be adversely affected when (a) cumulative damage accrual is increased, (b) the healing process is adequate or impaired, or (c) a combination of (a) and (b). Thus, optimization of the fatigue life of musculoskeletal tissues requires both minimizing cumulative damage accrual and maintaining robust remodeling and healing processes (a process sufficient to maintain or increase fatigue life).

This model would suggest that it would be advisable to decrease cumulative damage exposure in individuals that are exposed to factors that might impair the healing process. For example, workers in jobs having high psychosocial stress (potentially impairing the healing process) might be well served to have their physical exposure to repeated stress reduced. Similarly, workers with high BMIs and of older age (both associated with increased healing times) might benefit from a reduction in exposure to repeated stress. Of course, a combination of high cumulative damage due to repeated stress in concert with a condition that leads to impaired healing (such as psychosocial stress) would be a recipe for rapid MSD development.

Reduce Psychological Stress

General psychological conditions such as depression, anxiety, and job-related psychosocial factors including job satisfaction, social support at work, monotonous work, and psychological stress on the job, and perceived job demands have been associated with the development of many MSDs (NRC-IOM, 2001). As discussed previously psychological stress may lead to impaired healing due to the significant impact it has on sleep disruption, and increased secretion of glucocorticoid compounds which affect the immune healing response. The impairment of the healing process will likely decrease the fatigue life of musculoskeletal tissues undergoing repetitive stress, leading to an increased likelihood of MSD development as shown in Figure 10.8 (Gallagher & Barbe, 2021).

In discussing psychosocial work factors, it may be apparent that there may be several linkages between physical risk factors and psychosocial ones. For example, having a physically stressful job would likely lead to a concomitant increase (in all likelihood), psychological stress. The observation has also been made that design of the workplace and work processes may affect both the physical load patterns (work pace, repetitiveness, rest breaks) as well as psychosocial exposures like job demands (work pace) and monotony (Punnett & Wegman, 2004). The entanglement of these two factors has made it difficult to determine whether specific musculoskeletal outcomes are the result of physical factors, psychosocial factors, or both.

It should be evident that an individual's psychological state is the result of a complex combination of factors and stresses, many of which may be due to home and family life and perhaps beyond the ability of the work organization to control. However, there is some evidence to suggest that improvement of psychosocial factors at work can be beneficial in helping to control MSD development. Based on the factors mentioned earlier, it would seem apparent that controlling psychological stress will be to improve job satisfaction and social support at work, decrease monotonous work and psychological stress at work, and decrease job demands. Recommendations made by the National Research Council suggest that modification of psychosocial factors may lead to substantial risk reductions for low back and upper extremity MSDs (NRC-IOM, 2001). Reducing conflict and/or other stressful situations at work may be helpful in the control of psychosocial stressors, and in many cases can be done in a manner that also can make the company and/or its production processes more efficient (Roquelaure, 2017).

A summary of these suggested means to reduce MSD risk in occupational settings is listed in Table 15.4.

Table 15.4 Suggested Means to Reduce MSD Risk in Occupational Settings

Factor	Means to implement
• Avoid repeated high-stress loading levels • Maximize tissue fatigue life • Avoid job rotation that increases the higher risk of injury • Avoid non-neutral postures • Reduce psychological stress	• Limit the number of loading cycles at high-stress levels. • Reduce cofounders that might impair the healing process. • Job rotation might be useful if work task is varied and if boredom and monotony are decreased. • Strive to maintain neutral postures • Improve job satisfaction and social support at work; reduce conflict and other stressful situations at work.

Treatment of Injuries

Despite our best efforts to prevent musculoskeletal injuries, there can be little doubt that a great many injuries will still occur. When they do happen, there are several methods that have demonstrated the ability to promote healing and facilitate a more rapid return to normal function (Malanga, Yan, & Stark, 2015). A surprising number of persons never seek treatment for musculoskeletal pain, even though they may be experiencing chronic pain (Woolf et al., 2004). Early treatment of acute pain can potentially avoid the transition to chronic pain and its adverse long-term consequences (Walsh et al., 2008). Depending on the duration and severity of the chronic pain, consequences may include changes to the neuronal cytoarchitecture and the loss of inhibitory neurons leading to secondary hyperalgesia and protracted sensitization of spinal neurons (Voscopoulos & Lema, 2010).

The goals of treatment for injured musculoskeletal tissue should include reducing pain and edema and facilitation of the healing process so that normal function can be quickly regained. Treatment can include both pharmacological and nonpharmacological methodologies (many of which are summarized in Table 15.5). Nonpharmacological approaches typically include the application of heat and/or cold therapy to the injured site after the initial injury, and subsequent manual therapy to reduce pain and improve healing. Pharmaceuticals used in the treatment of musculoskeletal pain may include nonsteroidal anti-inflammatory drugs (NSAIDs), skeletal muscle relaxants, antidepressants, corticosteroid injections (e.g., cases of back pain with radiculopathy), and opioids (for intractable pain) (Malanga et al., 2015).

RICE

The "RICE" principle (Rest, Ice, Compression, Elevation) is generally accepted as the best initial treatment for acute soft-tissue injuries, although it seems less effective in the case of chronic overuse MSDs. The goal of this combination of actions is primarily to reduce the amount of bleeding experienced at the injury site (Järvinen, Järvinen, & Kalimo, 2014). It is somewhat surprising that such a widely employed procedure lacks the validation of even a single randomized clinical trial. However, evidence is available for individual components of the RICE principle from various experimental studies (Järvinen et al., 2014). Studies of rest immediately after trauma have shown that further damage can be avoided, hematoma size reduced, and the amount of scar tissue after repair reduced—if rest is provided early. The application of ice has also been shown to decrease the hematoma, inflammation, tissue necrosis, and leads to an acceleration of the

Table 15.5 A Review of Common Pharmacological and Nonpharmacological Treatments

Treatment	Time point after injury	Effect
"RICE" (Rest, Ice, Compression, Elevation)	Acute	Unconfirmed effect; thought to reduce the amount of bleeding
Rest alone	Acute	Further damage avoided, hematoma size reduced, amount scar tissue after repair reduced
Rest alone	Acutely and then sustained	Delayed recovery and poorer outcomes
Rest alone	Late—weeks after onset of injury symptoms	Reduces persistent inflammation, partially reduction in some sensorimotor declines, less effective in reducing all attributes of fibrosis
Compression alone	Acute	Reduces bleeding; any other contribution is debated
Exercise/loading	Early after injury	Application of controlled stress early on promotes better restoration of function by aligning matrix cells in direction of forces applied to the tissues
Ice alone	Acute	Decreased hematoma, inflammation, tissue necrosis; accelerated regenerative process
Cold therapy	Acute	Decreases threshold of pain receptors and blood flow, yet can induce frostbite and neuropathy; other findings show conflicting efficacy
Heat therapy (superficial or deep)	Acute	Decreases pain, increases blood flow and healing, increases the elasticity of soft tissue
Manual therapy	Acute, or acutely and then sustained	Reduces sensorimotor declines, reduces tissue inflammation and connective tissue fibrosis, although increases collagen in tendons beneficially
Manual therapy	Late—weeks after onset of injury symptoms	Partially reduced sensorimotor declines, tissue inflammation, and connective tissue fibrosis (not as well as preventive).
NSAID (e.g., ibuprofen)	After pain onset	Short-term use effectively reduces inflammation; long term use has potential negative side-effects
Anti-TNF-α (anti-tumor necrosis factor-alpha)	After pain onset	Reduces pain; partially reduces cartilage degeneration. Negative immunosuppressive effects if used long-term.
Glucocorticoids	After pain onset	Many negative consequences with respect to the healing (e.g. necrosis of muscle tissues).

regenerative process. Of the four recommended RICE procedures, compression is the most debated. While it has been shown to reduce blood flow into the area of damage, it is not clear that this step improves the healing time (Thorsson, Lilja, Nilsson, & Westlin, 1997). Elevation of the injured area above the level of the heart reduces hydrostatic pressure in the damaged area and reduces interstitial fluid buildup (Järvinen et al., 2014).

After a few days of rest (assuming recovery proceeds uneventfully), progressive remobilization and controlled introduction of stress to the injured area may be undertaken. In years past, there was a debate as to whether complete rest or a return to activity was the best method of treatment for healing of musculoskeletal tissues (Buckwalter, 1987). This issue has been resolved and it is now clear that while some rest may be necessary at the start of the healing process, application of controlled stress early on promotes better restoration of function. Treatment consisting of total rest (with no stress application) may lead to delayed recovery and poorer outcomes. In addition, exercises focused on the eccentric lengthening of the injured tissue have recently been demonstrated to provide a more rapid return to activity compared to traditional strengthening exercises (Askling, Tengvar, & Thorstensson, 2013). Measures (obtained 3–5 days after injury) that appear predictive of the long-term recovery from injury include the degree of bruising/hematoma, tenderness on palpation, range of motion, and pain on limb lengthening (Guillodo, Bouttier, & Saraux, 2011).

Yet, rest has its limits. With repetitive strain/motion injuries, the exact point of injury can be unclear. In studies using an animal model of repetitive motion injury in which rats perform a high repetition high force lever pulling task, forepaw mechanical hypersensitivity is evident immediately after the initial training to high force (55% of the rats" maximum pulling force, 10–15 min/day during the training period) (Xin et al., 2017), indicating that the injury occurred during the initial training to high force. Rest for 12 weeks partially improved this mechanical hypersensitivity in young adult animals (Xin et al., 2017). Yet, aged animals (14–18 months of age) showed no recovery even after 12 weeks of rest (Elliott, Barr, Clark, Wade, & Barbe, 2010). Persistent pain and dysfunction were associated with persistently maintained high TNF-α levels in the muscles and median nerve of the aged task rats, compared to age-matched control rats and young adult task rats (Elliott et al., 2010; Xin et al., 2017). These results are suggestive of lowered healing capacity in musculoskeletal tissues and nerve systems in aged animals. In this same model, rest as an intervention was also examined later, after the establishment of fibrosis and sensorimotor declines (14–18 weeks after their onset in adult rats performing a high intensive task for 18 weeks). Six weeks of rest alone after cessation of the repetitive task successfully reduced inflammation, partially restored grip strength declines, but failed to restore mechanical hypersensitivity, to control rat levels (Barbe, Hilliard, Amin, Harris, Hobson, Cruz, Dorotan, et al., 2020; Barbe, Hilliard, Amin, Harris, Hobson, Cruz, & Popoff, 2020; Barbe et al., 2019). Rest alone has also been reported as ineffective in reducing collagen and other non-contractile tissue in skeletal muscles by 6 weeks of repeated chronic strain injury in rats (50 strains daily, five times weekly for 6 weeks to hyperactive soleus muscles in which hyperactivity was induced by tetanus toxin) (Stauber, Smith, Miller, & Stauber, 2000). In that study, 3 months of ambulation only (with no induced strains and cessation of tetanus induced hyperactivity) did not lower muscle levels of collagen, which remained 18% above control levels. Thus, rest alone is not enough to allow recovery from established muscle fibrogenic changes induced in chronically strained or overloaded muscles. In humans, Silverstein et al. have shown that more than half of human workers (55.6%) with overuse-induced median mononeuropathy do not recover even after 1 year of rest (Silverstein et al., 2010).

Heat and Cold Therapy

Despite their common use, the efficacy of heat and cold treatments is still not well understood (Malanga et al., 2015). However, available clinical evidence suggests that the application of cold therapy is effective at reducing pain for acute strain and sprain injuries. Cold therapy has been shown to result in a local anesthetic effect by decreasing the threshold of pain receptors (nociceptors) and results in decreasing blood flow to the site leading to reduced edema and decreased inflammation. Cold treatment may decrease the metabolism of hypoxic tissues which may prevent secondary hypoxic damage to tissues that have sustained damage (Merrick, Rankin, Andres, & Hinman, 1999) and may reduce the likelihood of muscle spasm (Lee, Bang, & Han, 2002). Care must be taken with cryotherapy not to have the treatment lead to cold-induced injuries including frostbite, neuropathy of superficial nerves, pain, and burns. Certain conditions (such as hypertension, vascular compromise, cold hypersensitivity, and Raynaud's disease) should rule out the use of cryotherapy. Short-term adverse effects may also result, such as decreased joint position sense (Costello & Donnelly, 2010), muscle strength (Bleakley, Costello, & Glasgow, 2012; Raicinais & Oksa, 2010), and substandard motor task performance (Bleakley et al., 2012). The literature is somewhat conflicting regarding the efficacy of cold therapy; however, some studies have found a significant reduction of pain (Bleakley, McDonough, Macauley, & Bjordal, 2006) and improved return to work and sports (Hubbard, Aronson, & Denegar, 2004). In addition, short-term ankle function was improved when cryotherapy was combined with compression and therapeutic exercise (Bleakley et al., 2007)

Therapy with heat (heat wraps, heating pads, hot water bottles, etc.) is another common method of treating musculoskeletal injuries. In addition to the superficial methods listed earlier, it is also possible to perform heat therapy using deep-heating methods, such as ultrasound, microwave diathermy, and shortwave diathermy (Nadler, Weingand, & Kruse, 2004). The application of heat has been found to decrease pain, increase blood flow and healing and increase the elasticity of soft tissue (Malanga et al., 2015). The latter may explain why heat therapy shows efficacy in an increasing range of motion (Bleakley & Costello, 2013). Heat therapy has been shown to be therapeutic in reducing low back pain and in treating the effects of delayed onset muscle soreness (DOMS) (Malanga et al., 2015).

Manual Therapies

Manual therapy (MT) is any therapy that is applied by using the hands, including massage therapy and manipulative therapy. The effects of various types of massage or manual therapy on inflammation have been examined for centuries in human subjects and in animal models. In studies using a cyclic loading roller, muscles that underwent immediate treatment after highly intense exercise (continued every 24 hr for 4 days) exhibited only minimal disruption of myofibers and lower inflammatory cell infiltration than muscles that received the same treatment 48 hr later (Haas et al., 2013). A robot-assisted mechanical therapy resembling deep tissue therapy was shown to prevent behavioral and histological markers of muscle damage following experimental stroke (Sen et al., 2017). In mice, active stretching has been shown to reduce the number of neutrophil and inflammatory macrophages in subcutaneous connective tissues after carrageenan injection, as well as the thickness of the lesioned subcutaneous tissue (carrageenan is a seaweed extract used in the food industry that can induce inflammation after injection) (Berrueta et al., 2016; Corey, Vizzard, Bouffard, Badger, & Langevin, 2012). Using a method designed to emulate cross-fiber massage, treatment augmented pain induced by experimental subcutaneous inflammation (Loghmani, Tobin, Quigley, & Fennimore, 2021).

Manual therapy of the entire upper extremity (involving forearm skin rolling, gentle mobilization, upper extremity traction, deeper massage, and wrist joint mobilization) has also been used in a rat model of work-related MSDS (Bove, Harris, Zhao, & Barbe, 2016). Early administration of this manual therapy treatment prevented the development of work task-induced tissue inflammation (macrophage density and pro-inflammatory cytokine production), fibrosis (excessive fibroblast-like cell density and collagen deposition in nerves, muscles, and tendons), and reduced the development of sensorimotor declines that correlated with these various tissue changes (Bove et al. 2016, 2019). This treatment also prevented or at least reduced the development of forearm nerve and musculotendinous fibrosis (collagen deposition and cell density) and motor declines (Barbe et al., 2021; Barbe, Harris, et al., 2021). A similar reduction in connective tissue fibrosis has been observed after manual mobilization or brief active stretching of the back after injury (it reduced subcutaneous connective tissue fibrosis induced by subcutaneous microsurgical injury) (Altomare & Monte-Alto-Costa, 2018). In contrast, in tendons, massage therapy provided after injury increased the number of collagen fibrils in tendon regions, suggestive of a beneficial effect of this therapy on tenocyte metabolite activity (Kassolik et al., 2013).

Yet, avoiding repetitive work is not always possible, and preventive treatment is not routinely available. The manual therapy of the entire upper extremity described earlier (forearm skin rolling, gentle mobilization, upper extremity traction, deeper massage, and wrist joint mobilization) was used in another study using the rat model of MSDs (Barbe, Panibatla, et al., 2021). The effectiveness of manual therapy with rest to treat the inflammation and fibrosis after it already had developed (specifically, the manual therapy was provided for 7 weeks after 14 weeks of work). Manual therapy in conjunction with rest improved many but not all of the behavioral and tissue pathologies that had developed during 14 weeks of a repetitive work task. The 7-week rest treatment alone also improved several of the functional and neuromuscular pathologies, although the manual therapy combined with rest ameliorated cold sensitivity and elevated muscle IL-10 levels more than rest alone (Barbe, Panibatla, et al., 2021). These findings stand in contrast to the more robust preventive effects of manual therapy in this animal model (Barbe, Harris, et al., 2021; Bove et al., 2016, 2019).

Several clinical studies have shown that pain symptoms associated with median neuropathies can improve after massage/manual therapies (De-la-Llave-Rincon et al., 2012; Elliott & Burkett, 2013; Field, Diego, Hernandez-Reif, Schanberg, & Kuhn, 2004; Tsao, 2007; Wolny, Saulicz, Linek, Shacklock, & Mysliwiec, 2017). Yet, the literature is mixed on the effectiveness of manual therapy as a treatment, perhaps due to differences in treatment type, time of administration, assessment tools, and high variability in diagnoses (Ballestero-Perez et al., 2017; Tsao, 2007). Further studies are needed in future to fully determine the efficacy of this treatment.

Medications

While few randomized controlled trials exist, there is some evidence to support the use of non-steroidal anti-inflammatory drugs (NSAIDs) in the treatment of musculoskeletal injuries in humans (Järvinen et al., 2014). For example, in minor muscle injuries, short-term use of NSAIDs has shown some benefit in exercise-induced muscle injury (O'Grady et al., 2000). NSAIDs are clearly effective in reducing inflammation, and in early short-term use has been found to result in no adverse effects on healing of muscle, nor on tensile strength or muscle fiber generation (Järvinen, Lehto, & Sorvari, 1992). Early treatment with selective or non-selective cyclooxygenase inhibitor drugs (nonsteroidal anti-inflammatory drugs, such as ibuprofen and meloxicam, are non-selective types) may also attenuate some tissue histopathological changes, although they may only attenuate periarticular trabecular bone loss and bone marrow lesion formation (Driban, Barr, Amin, Sitler, & Barbe, 2011; Jones et al., 2010). Steroid injections and NSAIDs have been used to reduce ligament pain and inflammation, although long-term or repeated treatment may inhibit healing, perhaps by reducing the inflammatory clearance process or mitochondrial function. Anti-TNF-α drugs are used to reduce pain in the patients and may partially slow advancing cartilage degeneration (Fernandes, Martel-Pelletier, & Pelletier, 2002). Yet, the negative immunosuppressive effects of long-term use of any anti-TNFα drug are substantial. On the other hand, the use of glucocorticoids appears to have many negative consequences with respect to the healing of musculoskeletal injuries. These include increased necrosis in skeletal muscle tissue, delayed elimination of the hematoma, slower regeneration of the muscle tissue, and reduced biomechanical strength at the end of the healing process (Beiner, Jokl, & Cholewicki, 1999; Järvinen et al., 1992).

Other Regenerative Treatments

Due to the high incidence of tendon and ligament damage as a consequence of sports injuries, aging and overuse, and the poor healing status of these tissues, there is a strong need for improved regenerative therapy. There is no adequate method of treatment for the extensive tendon defects observed after rotator cuff tears, and direct repair of anterior cruciate ligaments is mostly unsuccessful. Autologous bone marrow aspirate concentrate, platelet-rich plasma, autografting, and autologous stromal vascular fraction therapies have been used to improve tendon and ligament regeneration, with varying success. These treatments are not specific for these particular tissues, and there are significant differences in the methods of administration and dosing that has led to controversy in the field of regeneration/orthopedics.

Over the past thirty years, several cartilage repair strategies have been developed for the treatment of cartilage lesions. Contemporary clinical treatment includes reconstructive cartilage surgery that comprises bone marrow stimulation techniques by microfractures (that enhances blood supply from subchondral bone), autologous chondrocyte implantation, osteochondral autograft, and allograft transplantation, provision of exogenous recruitment signals, as well as implantation of scaffolds designed to aid endogenous cartilage regeneration that allow migration into and "temporary homes" for MSPCs (Hu et al., 2021; Stampoultzis, Karami, & Pioletti, 2021; Wei & Dai, 2021). Although each method still has limitations and challenges, the increasing understanding of the poor self-repair mechanisms in articular cartilage is aiding researchers in exploring problem-solving approaches for the successful repair of damaged cartilage.

Summary

The musculoskeletal system is complex and maintaining an optimal level of system health is therefore dependent on a number of factors. The manner in which stress is applied to musculoskeletal tissues appears to be a fundamental factor in the maintenance of musculoskeletal health. Musculoskeletal tissues need a certain amount of stress simply to maintain musculoskeletal health, and the health of the tissue can often be enhanced by exposure to a limited number of high-stress exertions. However, there is a limit to the cumulative stress that can be endured by a tissue, which can be the cumulative result effect of loading at highly variable stress levels. This may lead to damage accumulation, pain, and disability.

Keeping the musculoskeletal system healthy requires attention to other factors as well. For example, healthy nutrition, avoiding a sedentary lifestyle with moderate and appropriate exercise, avoiding obesity, obtaining sufficient high-quality sleep, and reducing or eliminating smoking, and alcohol consumption can lead to improved musculoskeletal health. A healthy lifestyle should include adequate amounts of recovery time, hydration, and stress management. Rest, anti-inflammatory medications, a change in biomechanics, and good ergonomics can also be effective intervention strategies. Note, the nonsteroidal anti-inflammatory drugs should be used judiciously for pain management while also avoiding interference of the healing process. Occupationally, it is important to avoid excessive exposure to cumulative damage in tissues, minimize psychosocial stresses, and avoid job rotation whose intent is to evenly distribute biomechanical exposures, and avoid the adoption of non-neutral postures (which increase stress on musculoskeletal tissues).

Finally, when musculoskeletal tissues do get injured, there are some procedures that can help minimize the pain and facilitate the healing response. The RICE procedure can help reduce bleeding and fluid accumulation at the injury site and thus reduce the hematoma. Finally, it is becoming clearer that excessive rest is detrimental to the healing process. While a few days' rest can be useful, musculoskeletal tissues seem to heal best when they are exposed to controlled exercise as soon as practicable.

Bibliography

Adam, K., & Oswald, I. (1984). Sleep helps healing. *British Medical Journal, 289*, 1400–1401.

Altomare, M., & Monte-Alto-Costa, A. (2018). Manual mobilization of subcutaneous fibrosis in mice. *Journal of Manipulative and Physiological Therapeutics, 41*(5), 359–362. https://doi.org/10.1016/j.jmpt.2017.10.011

Ark, M., Rio, E., Cook, J., Akker-Scheek, I., Gaida, J. E., Zwerver, J., & Docking, S. (2018). Clinical improvements are not explained by changes in tendon structure on ultrasound tissue characterization after an exercise program for patellar tendinopathy. *American Journal of Physical Medicine & Rehabilitation, 97*(10), 708–714. https://doi.org/10.1097/PHM.0000000000000951

Askling, C., Tengvar, M., & Thorstensson, A. (2013). Acute hamstring injuries in Swedish elite football: A prospective randomized con- trolled clinical trial comparing two rehabilitation protocols. *British Journal of Sports Medicine, 47*, 953–959.

Ballestero-Perez, R., Plaza-Manzano, G., Urraca-Gesto, A., Romo-Romo, F., Atin-Arratibel, M. L. A., Pecos-Martin, D., & Romero-Franco, N. (2017). Effectiveness of nerve gliding exercises on carpal tunnel syndrome: A systematic review. *Journal of Manipulative and Physiological Therapeutics, 40*(1), 50–59. https://doi.org/10.1016/j.jmpt.2016.10.004

Barbe, M. F., Harris, M. Y., Cruz, G. E., Amin, M., Billett, N. M., Dorotan, J. T., & Bove, G. M. (2021). Key indicators of repetitive overuse-induced neuromuscular inflammation and fibrosis are prevented by manual therapy in a rat model. *BMC Musculoskeletal Disorders, 22*(1), 417. https://doi.org/10.1186/s12891-021-04270-0

Barbe, M. F., Hilliard, B. A., Amin, M., Harris, M. Y., Hobson, L. J., Cruz, G. E., . . . Popoff, S. N. (2020). Blocking CTGF/CCN2 reverses neural fibrosis and sensorimotor declines in a rat model of overuse-induced median mononeuropathy. *Journal of Orthopaedic Research, 38*(11), 2396–2408. https://doi.org/10.1002/jor.24709

Barbe, M. F., Hilliard, B. A., Amin, M., Harris, M. Y., Hobson, L. J., Cruz, G. E., & Popoff, S. N. (2020). Blocking CTGF/CCN2 reduces established skeletal muscle fibrosis in a rat model of overuse injury. *The FASEB Journal, 34*(5), 6554–6569. https://doi.org/10.1096/fj.202000240RR

Barbe, M. F., Panibatla, S. T., Harris, M. Y., Amin, M., Dorotan, J. T., Cruz, G. E., & Bove, G. M. (2021). Manual therapy with rest as a treatment for established inflammation and fibrosis in a rat model of repetitive strain injury. *Frontiers in Physiology, 12*(1925). https://doi.org/10.3389/fphys.2021.755923

Barbe, M. F., White, A. R., Hilliard, B. A., Salvadeo, D. M., Amin, M., Harris, M. Y., & Popoff, S. N. (2019). Comparing effects of rest with or without a NK1RA on fibrosis and sensorimotor declines induced by a voluntary moderate demand task. *Journal of Musculoskeletal and Neuronal Interactions, 19*(4), 396–411.

Beaudart, C., Dawson, A., Shaw, S., Harvey, N., Kanis, J., Binkley, N., & Group, I.-E. S. (2017). Nutrition and physical activity in the prevention and treatment of sarcopenia: Systematic review. *Osteoporosis International, 8*, 1817–1833.

Beiner, J., Jokl, P., & Cholewicki, J. (1999). The effects of anabolic steroids and corticosteroids on healing of muscle contusion injury. *The American Journal of Sports Medicine, 27*, 2–9.

Berrueta, L., Muskaj, I., Olenich, S., Butler, T., Badger, G. J., Colas, R. A., & Langevin, H. M. (2016). Stretching impacts inflammation resolution in connective tissue. *Journal of Cellular Physiology, 231*(7), 1621–1627. https://doi.org/10.1002/jcp.25263

Bleakley, C., & Costello, J. (2013). Do thermal agends affect range of movement and mechanical properties in soft tissues? A systematic review. *Archives of Physical Medicine and Rehabilitation, 94*, 149–163.

Bleakley, C., Costello, J., & Glasgow, P. (2012). Should athletes return to sport after applying ice? A systematic review of the effect of local cooling on functional performance. *Sports Medicine, 42*, 69–87.

Bleakley, C., McDonough, S., Macauley, D., & Bjordal, J. (2006). Cryotherapy for acute ankle sprains: A randomized controlled study of two different icing protocols. *British Journal of Sports Medicine, 40*, 700–705.

Bleakley, C., O'Connor, S., Tully, M., Rocke, L., Macauley, D., & McDonough, S. (2007). The PRICE study (Protection Rest Ice Compression Elevation): Design of a randomized controlled trial comparing standard versus cryokinetic ice applications in the management of acutel ankle sprain. *BMC Musculoskeletal Disorders, 8*, 125.

Borde, R., Hortobágyi, T., & Granacher, U. (2015). Dose–response relationships of resistance training in healthy old adults: A systematic review and meta-analysis. *Sports Medicine, 45*, 1693–1720.

Bove, G. M., Delany, S. P., Hobson, L., Cruz, G. E., Harris, M. Y., Amin, M., & Barbe, M. F. (2019). Manual therapy prevents onset of nociceptor activity, sensorimotor dysfunction, and neural fibrosis induced by a volitional repetitive task. *Pain, 160*(3), 632–644. https://doi.org/10.1097/j.pain.0000000000001443

Bove, G. M., Harris, M. Y., Zhao, H., & Barbe, M. F. (2016). Manual therapy as an effective treatment for fibrosis in a rat model of upper extremity overuse injury. *Journal of the Neurological Sciences, 361*, 168–180. https://doi.org/10.1016/j.jns.2015.12.029

Buckwalter, J. (1987). Activity vs. rest in the treatment of bone, soft tissue and joint injuries. *The Iowa Orthopaedic Journal, 15*, 29–42.

Centers for Disease Control and Prevention. (2017). *Behavioural risk factors surveillance system (BRFSS)*. https://www.cdc.gov/brfss/index.html

Chaffin, D. A. (1999). *Occupational biomechanics* (3rd ed.). New York: John Wiley & Sons, Inc.

Colrain, I., Nicholas, C., & Baker, F. (2014). Alcohol and the sleeping brain. *Handbook of Clinical Neurology, 125*, 415–431.

Cooper, M. A., Kluding, P. M., & Wright, D. E. (2016). Emerging relationships between exercise, sensory nerves, and neuropathic pain. *Frontiers in Neuroscience, 10*, 372. https://doi.org/10.3389/fnins.2016.00372

Coq, J. O., Strata, F., Russier, M., Safadi, F. F., Merzenich, M. M., Byl, N. N., & Barbe, M. F. (2008). Impact of neonatal asphyxia and hind limb immobilization on musculoskeletal tissues and S1 map organization: Implications for cerebral palsy. *Experimental Neurology, 210*(1), 95–108. https://doi.org/10.1016/j.expneurol.2007.10.006

Corey, S. M., Vizzard, M. A., Bouffard, N. A., Badger, G. J., & Langevin, H. M. (2012). Stretching of the back improves gait, mechanical sensitivity and connective tissue inflammation in a rodent model. *PLoS One, 7*(1), 29831. https://doi.org/10.1371/journal.pone.0029831

Costello, J., & Donnelly, A. (2010). Cryotherapy and joint position sense in healthy participants: A systematic review. *Journal of Athletic Training, 45*, 306–316.

Daly, R. (2017). Exercise and nutritional approaches to prevent frail bones, falls and fractures: An update. *Climacteric, 20*, 119–124.

Dawson-Hughes, B., Harris, S., & Ceglia, L. (2008). Alkaline diets favor lean tissue mass in older adults. *The American Journal of Clinical Nutrition, 87*, 662–665.

De-la-Llave-Rincon, A. I., Ortega-Santiago, R., Ambite-Quesada, S., Gil-Crujera, A., Puentedura, E. J., Valenza, M. C., & Fernandez-de-las-Penas, C. (2012). Response of pain intensity to soft tissue mobilization and neurodynamic technique: A series of 18 patients with chronic carpal tunnel syndrome. *Journal of Manipulative and Physiological Therapeutics, 35*(6), 420–427. https://doi.org/10.1016/j.jmpt.2012.06.002

Doessing, S., Heinemeier, K., Holm, L., Mackey, A., Schjerling, P., Rennie, M., & Kjaer, M. (2010). Growth hormone stimulates the collagen synthesis in human tendon and skeletal muscle without affecting myofibrillar protein synthesis. *The Journal of Physiology, 588*(Pt 2), 341–351.

Driban, J. B., Bannuru, R. R., Eaton, C. B., Spector, T. D., Hart, D. J., McAlindon, T. E., & Arden, N. K. (2020). The incidence and characteristics of accelerated knee osteoarthritis among women: The Chingford cohort. *BMC Musculoskeletal Disorders, 21*(1), 60. https://doi.org/10.1186/s12891-020-3073-3

Driban, J. B., Barr, A. E., Amin, M., Sitler, M. R., & Barbe, M. F. (2011). Joint inflammation and early degeneration induced by high-force reaching are attenuated by ibuprofen in an animal model of work-related musculoskeletal disorder. *Journal of Biomedicine & Biotechnology, 691412*. https://doi.org/10.1155/2011/691412

Ekelund, U., Steene-Johannessen, J., Brown, W., Fagerland, M., Owen, N., Powell, K., & Group, L. S. (2016). Does physical activity attenuate, or even eliminate, the detrimental association of sitting time with mortality? A harmonised meta-analysis of data from more than 1 million men and women. *Lancet, 388*, 1302–1310.

Elliott, M. B., Barr, A. E., Clark, B. D., Wade, C. K., & Barbe, M. F. (2010). Performance of a repetitive task by aged rats leads to median neuropathy and spinal cord inflammation with associated sensorimotor declines. *Neuroscience, 170*(3), 929–941. https://doi.org/10.1016/j.neuroscience.2010.07.041

Elliott, R., & Burkett, B. (2013). Massage therapy as an effective treatment for carpal tunnel syndrome. *Journal of Bodywork and Movement Therapies, 17*(3), 332–338. https://doi.org/10.1016/j.jbmt.2012.12.003

Felson, D., Anderson, J., Naimark, A., Walker, A., & Meenan, R. (1988). Obesity and knee osteoarthritis The Framingham Study. *Annals of Internal Medicine, 109*, 18–24.

Fernandes, J. C., Martel-Pelletier, J., & Pelletier, J. P. (2002). The role of cytokines in osteoarthritis pathophysiology. *Biorheology, 39*(1–2), 237–246.

Field, T., Diego, M. A., Hernandez-Reif, M., Schanberg, S., & Kuhn, C. (2004). Massage therapy effects on depressed pregnant women. *Journal of Psychosomatic Obstetrics and Gynaecology, 25*(2), 115–122. https://doi.org/10.1080/01674820412331282231

Fitzgerald, D. J., Radek, K., Chaar, M., Faunce, D., DiPietro, L., & Kovacs, E. (2007). Effects of acute ethanol exposure on the early inflammatory response after excisional injury. *Alcoholism, Clinical and Experimental Research, 31*, 317–323.

Frizziero, A., Salamanna, F., Della Bella, E., Vittadini, F., Gasparre, G., Nicoli Aldini, N., & Fini, M. (2016). The role of detraining in tendon mechanobiology. *Frontiers in Aging Neuroscience, 8*, 43.

Frontera, W., & Bigard, X. (2002). The benefits of strength training in the elderly. *Science & Sports, 17*, 109–116.

Gallagher, S., & Barbe, M. F. (2021). The impaired healing hypothesis: A mechanism by which psychosocial stress and personal characteristics increase MSD risk? *Ergonomics*, 1–14. https://doi.org/10.1080/00140139.2021.1974103

Grabowski, P. (2009). Physiology of bone. *Endocrine Development, 16*, 32–48.

Guilak, F. (2011). Biomechanical factors in osteoarthritis. *Best Practice & Research. Clinical Rheumatology, 25*, 815–823.

Guillodo, Y., Bouttier, R., & Saraux, A. (2011). Value of sonograpphy combined with clinical assessment to evaluate muscle injury sever- ity in athletes. *Journal of Athletic Training, 46*, 500–504.

Guo, S., & DiPietro, L. (2010). Factors affecting wound healing. *Journal of Dental Research, 89*, 219–229.

Haas, C., Butterfield, T. A., Abshire, S., Zhao, Y., Zhang, X., Jarjoura, D., & Best, T. M. (2013). Massage timing affects postexercise muscle recovery and inflammation in a rabbit model. *Medicine and Science in Sports and Exercise*, *45*(6), 1105–1112. https://doi.org/10.1249/MSS.0b013e31827fdf18

Hardcastle, A., Aucott, L., Reid, D., & Macdonald, H. (2011). Associations between dietary flavonoid intakes and bone health in a Scottish population. *Journal of Bone and Mineral Research*, *26*, 941–947.

Hauser, R. A., & Dolan, E. E. (2011). Ligament injury and healing: An overview of current clinical concepts. *Journal of Prolotherapy*, *3*(4), 836–846.

Heaney, R., & Layman, D. (2008). Amount and type of protein influences bone health. *The American Journal of Clinical Nutrition*, *87*, 1567–1570.

Hirshkowitz, M., Whiton, K., Albert, S. M., Alessi, C., Bruni, O., DonCarlos, L., & Adams Hillard, P. J. (2015). National Sleep Foundation's sleep time duration recommendations: Methodology and results summary. *Sleep Health*, *1*(1), 40–43. https://doi.org/10.1016/j.sleh.2014.12.010

Howard, J. S., Mattacola, C. G., Romine, S. E., & Lattermann, C. (2010). Continuous passive motion, early weight bearing, and active motion following knee articular cartilage repair: evidence for clinical practice. *Cartilage*, *1*(4), 276–286. https://doi.org/10.1177/1947603510368055

Hu, H., Liu, W., Sun, C., Wang, Q., Yang, W., Zhang, Z., & Wang, B. (2021). Endogenous repair and regeneration of injured articular cartilage: A challenging but promising therapeutic strategy. *Aging and Disease*, *12*(3), 886–901. https://doi.org/10.14336/AD.2020.0902

Hubbard, T., Aronson, S., & Denegar, C. (2004). Does cryotherapy hasten return to participation? A systematic review. *Journal of Athletic Training*, *39*, 88–94.

Irwin, M., Thompson, J., Miller, C., Gillin, J., & Ziegler, M. (1999). Effects of sleep and sleep deprivation on catecholamine and interleukin-2 levels in humans: Clinical implications. *The Journal of Clinical Endocrinology and Metabolism*, *84*, 1979–1985.

Isaksson, O., Jansson, J.-O., & Gause, I. (1982). Growth hormone stimulates longitudinal bone growth directly. *Science*, *216*, 1237–1239.

Järvinen, M., Lehto, M., & Sorvari, T. (1992). Effect of some anti-inflammatory agents on the healing of ruptured muscle. An experimental study in rats. *Journal of Sports Traumatology*, *14*, 19–28.

Järvinen, T., Järvinen, M., & Kalimo, H. (2014). Regeneration of injured skeletal muscle after the injury. *Muscles, Ligaments and Tendons Journal*, *3*, 337–345.

Jones, A., Rule, J., Moore, J., Sottos, N., & White, S. (2007). Life extension of self-healing polymers with rapidly growing fatigue cracks. *Journal of the Royal Society, Interface*, *4*, 395–403.

Jones, M. D., Tran, C. W., Li, G., Maksymowych, W. P., Zernicke, R. F., & Doschak, M. R. (2010). In vivo microfocal computed tomography and micro-magnetic resonance imaging evaluation of antiresorptive and antiinflammatory drugs as preventive treatments of osteoarthritis in the rat. *Arthritis and Rheumatism*, *62*(9), 2726–2735. https://doi.org/10.1002/art.27595

Jung, M., Callaci, J., Lauing, K., Otis, J., Radek, K., Jones, M., & Kovacs, E. (2011). Alcohol exposure and mechanisms of tissue injury and repair. *Alcoholism, Clinical and Experimental Research*, *35*, 392–399.

Kassolik, K., Andrzejewski, W., Dziegiel, P., Jelen, M., Fulawka, L., Brzozowski, M., & Podhorska-Okolow, M. (2013). Massage-induced morphological changes of dense connective tissue in rat's tendon. *Folia Histochemica et Cytobiologica*, *51*(1), 103–106. https://doi.org/10.5603/FHC.2013.0014

Klyne, D. M., Barbe, M. F., James, G., & Hodges, P. W. (2021). Does the interaction between local and systemic inflammation provide a link from psychology and lifestyle to tissue health in musculoskeletal conditions? *International Journal of Molecular Sciences*, *22*(14). https://doi.org/10.3390/ijms22147299

Krueger, J. M., Fang, J., Taishi, P., Chen, Z., Kushikata, T., & Gardi, J. (1998). Sleep. A physiologic role for IL-1 beta and TNF-alpha. *Annals of the New York Academy of Sciences*, *856*, 148–159.

Kubota, Y., Evenson, K., MacLehose, R., Roetker, N., Joshu, C., & Folsom, A. (2017). Physical activity and lifetime risk of cardiovascular disease and cancer. *Medicine and Science in Sports and Exercise, 49*, 1599–1605.

Lawrence University. (2021). Musculoskeletal health. Retrieved from https://www.lawrence.edu/conservatory/about/health_wellness/musculoskeletal_health

Lee, S., Bang, M., & Han, T. (2002). Effect of cold therapy in relieving spasticity: Applied to spinalized rabbit. *Spinal Cord, 40*, 167–173.

Leproult, R., Copinschi, G., Buxton, O., & Van Cauter, E. (1997). Sleep loss results in an elevation of cortisol levels the next evening. *Sleep, 20*, 865–870.

Lewis, R., Alvarez, C., Rayman, M., Lanham-New, S., Woolf, A., & Mobasheri, A. (2019). Strategies for optimising musculoskeletal health in the 21st century. *BMC Musculoskeletal Disorders, 20*, 164.

Liu, X., Machado, G., Eyles, J., Ravi, V., & Hunter, D. (2018). Dietary supplements for treating osteoarthritis: A systematic review and meta-analysis. *British Journal of Sports Medicine, 52*, 167–175.

Loghmani, M. T., Tobin, C., Quigley, C., & Fennimore, A. (2021). Soft tissue manipulation may attenuate inflammation, modulate pain, and improve gait in conscious rodents with induced low back pain. *Military Medicine, 186*(Suppl 1), 506–514. https://doi.org/10.1093/milmed/usaa259

Lopez-Alvarez, V. M., Modol, L., Navarro, X., & Cobianchi, S. (2015). Early increasing-intensity treadmill exercise reduces neuropathic pain by preventing nociceptor collateral sprouting and disruption of chloride cotransporters homeostasis after peripheral nerve injury. *Pain, 156*(9), 1812–1825. https://doi.org/10.1097/j.pain.0000000000000268

Luger, T., Maher, C., Rieger, M., & Steinhilber, B. (2019). Work-break schedules for preventing musculoskeletal symptoms and disorders in healthy workers. *Cochrane Database of Systematic Reviews, 7*, 70.

Lundberg, I., & Nader, G. (2008). Molecular effects of exercise in patients with inflammatory rheumatic disease. *Nature Clinical Practice. Rheumatology, 4*, 597–604.

Malanga, G., Yan, N., & Stark, J. (2015). Mechanisms and efficacy of heat and cold therapies for musculoskeletal injuries. *Postgraduate Medicine, 127*, 57–65.

Mehdizadeh, A., Vinel, A., Hu, Q., Schall, M., Jr., Gallagher, S., & Sesek, R. (2020). Job rotation and work-related musculoskeletal disorders: A fatigue-failure perspective. *Ergonomics, 63*, 461–476.

Merrick, M., Rankin, J., Andres, F., & Hinman, C. (1999). A preliminary examination of cryotherapy and secondary injury in skeletal muscle. *Medicine & Science in Sports & Excercise, 31*, 1516–1521.

Messier, S., Loeser, R., Miller, G., Morgan, T., Rejeski, W., Sevick, M., & Williamson, J. (2004). Exercise and dietary weight loss in overweight and obese older adults with knee osteoarthritis: The arthritis, diet, and activity promotion trial. *Arthritis and Rheumatism, 50*, 1501–1510.

Meyer, H., Pedersen, J. I., Loken, E., & Tverdal, A. (1997). Dietary factors and the incidence of hip fracture in middle-aged Norwegians. A prospective study. *American Journal of Epidemiology, 145*, 117–123.

Mobasheri, A., & Batt, M. (2016). An update on the pathophysiology of osteoarthritis. *Annals of Physical and Rehabilitation Medicine, 59*, 333–339.

Molnar, A., Jonasne Sztruhar, I., Csontos, A., Ferencz, C., Várbíró, S., & Szekacs, B. (2016). Special nutrition intervention is required for muscle protective efficacy of physical exercise in elderly people at highest risk of sarcopenia. *Physiology International, 103*, 368–376.

Molteni, R., Zheng, J. Q., Ying, Z., Gomez-Pinilla, F., & Twiss, J. L. (2004). Voluntary exercise increases axonal regeneration from sensory neurons. *Proceedings of the National Academy of Sciences of the United States of America, 101*(22), 8473–8478. https://doi.org/10.1073/pnas.0401443101

Mostaghimi, L., Obermeyer, W., Ballamudi, B., Martinez-Gonzolez, D., & Benca, R. (2005). Effects of sleep deprivation on wound healing. *Journal of Sleep Research, 14*, 213–219.

Mujika, I., & Padilla, S. (2001). Muscular characteristics of detraining in humans. *Medicine and Science in Sports and Exercise, 33*, 1297–1303.

Nadler, S. F., Weingand, K., & Kruse, R. (2004). The physiological basis and clinical applications of cryotherapy and thermotherapy for the pain practitioner. *Pain Physician, 7*, 395–399.

National Research Council – Institute of Medicine [NRC-IOM] (2001). *Musculoskeletal disorders and the workplace: low back and upper extremities.* The National Academies Press.

O'Grady, M., Hackney, A., Schneider, K., Bossen, E., Steinberg, K., Douglas, J., Jr., . . . Watkins, W. (2000). Diclofenac sodium (Voltaren) reduced exercise-induced injury in human skeletal muscle. *Medicine and Science in Sports and Exercise, 32*, 1191–1196.

Office for National Statistics (UK), (2019). Measuring national well-being in the UK: international comparisons. https://www.ons.gov.uk/peoplepopulationandcommunity/wellbeing/articles/measuringnationalwellbeing/internationalcomparisons2019.

Park, J. S., & Hoke, A. (2014). Treadmill exercise induced functional recovery after peripheral nerve repair is associated with increased levels of neurotrophic factors. *PLoS One, 9*(3), 90245. https://doi.org/10.1371/journal.pone.0090245

Potvin, J. R. (2012). Predicting maximum acceptable efforts for repetitive tasks: An equation based on duty cycle. *Human Factors, 54*(2), 175–188. https://doi.org/10.1177/0018720811424269

Prinz, P., Roehrs, T., Vitaliano, P., Linnoila, M., & Weitzman, E. (1980). Effect of alcohol on sleep and nighttime plasma growth hormone and cortisol concentrations. *The Journal of Clinical Endocrinology and Metabolism, 51*, 759–764.

Punnett, L., & Wegman, D. (2004). Work-related musculoskeletal disorders: The epidemiologic evidence and the debate. *Journal of Electromyography and Kinesiology, 14*, 13–23.

Radek, K., Matthies, A., Burns, A., Heinrich, S., Kovacs, E. J., & Dipietro, L. (2005). Acute ethanol exposure impairs angiogenesis and the proliferative phase of wound healing. *American Journal of Physiology. Heart and Circulatory Physiology, 289*, 1084–1090.

Raicinais, S., & Oksa, J. (2010). Temperature and neuromuscular function. *Scandinavian Journal of Medicine & Science in Sports, 20*, 1–18.

Remer, T., & Manz, F. (1995). Potential renal acid load of foods and its influence on urine pH. *Journal of the American Dietetic Association, 95*, 791–797.

Roquelaure, Y. (2017). *Musculoskeletal disorders and psychosocial factors at work—Report 142.* European Trade Union Institute.

Sabatier, M. J., Redmon, N., Schwartz, G., & English, A. W. (2008). Treadmill training promotes axon regeneration in injured peripheral nerves. *Experimental Neurology, 211*(2), 489–493. https://doi.org/10.1016/j.expneurol.2008.02.013

Sen, C. (2001). Antioxidants in exercise nutrition. *Sports Medicine, 31*, 891–908.

Sen, C. K., Khanna, S., Harris, H., Stewart, R., Balch, M., Heigel, M., & Rink, C. (2017). Robot-assisted mechanical therapy attenuates stroke-induced limb skeletal muscle injury. *The FASEB Journal, 31*(3), 927–936. https://doi.org/10.1096/fj.201600437R

Silverstein, B. A., Fan, Z. J., Bonauto, D. K., Bao, S., Smith, C. K., Howard, N., & Viikari-Juntura, E. (2010). The natural course of carpal tunnel syndrome in a working population. *Scandinavian Journal of Work, Environment & Health, 36*(5), 384–393. https://doi.org/10.5271/sjweh.2912

Simpson, N., Gibbs, E., & Matheson, G. (2017). Optimizing sleeep to maximize performance. *Scandinavian Journal of Medicine & Science in Sports, 27*, 266–274.

Sjogaard, G., Lundberg, U., & Kadefors, R. (2000). The role of muscle activity and mental load in the development of pain and degenerative processes at the muscle cell level during computer work. *European Journal of Applied Physiology, 83*(2–3), 99–105. https://doi.org/10.1007/s004210000285

Solomonow, M., Baratta, R., Banks, A., Freudenberger, C., & Zhou, B. (2003). Flexion–relaxation response to static lumbar flexion in males and females. *Clinical biomechanics, 18*, 273–279.

Stampoultzis, T., Karami, P., & Pioletti, D. P. (2021). Thoughts on cartilage tissue engineering: A 21st century perspective. *Current Research in Translational Medicine*, *69*(3), 103299. https://doi.org/10.1016/j.retram.2021.103299

Stauber, W. T., Smith, C. A., Miller, G. R., & Stauber, F. D. (2000). Recovery from 6 weeks of repeated strain injury to rat soleus muscles. *Muscle & Nerve*, *23*(12), 1819–1825.

Stephens, P., al-Khateeb, T., Davies, K., Shepherd, J., & Thomas, D. (1996). An investigation of the interaction between alcohol and fibroblasts in wound healing. *International Journal of Oral and Maxillofacial Surgery*, *25*, 161–164.

Svensson, R., Heinemeier, K., Couppé, C., Kjaer, M., & Magnusson, S. (2016). Effect of aging and exercise on the tendon. *Journal of Applied Physiology*, *121*, 1353–1362.

Tardioli, A., Malliaras, P., & Maffulli, N. (2012). Immediate and short-term effects of exercise on tendon structure: Biochemical, biomechanical and imaging responses. *British Medical Bulletin*, *103*(1), 169–202. https://doi.org/10.1093/bmb/ldr052

Teodori, R. M., Betini, J., Oliveira, L. S., Sobral, L. L., Takeda, S. Y., & Lima Montebelo, M. I. (2011). Swimming exercise in the acute or late phase after sciatic nerve crush accelerates nerve regeneration. *Neural Plasticity*, *783901*. https://doi.org/10.1155/2011/783901

Thorsson, O., Lilja, B., Nilsson, P., & Westlin, N. (1997). Immediate external compression in the management of an acute muscle injury. *Scandinavian Journal of Medicine & Science in Sports*, *7*, 182–190.

Tsao, J. C. (2007). Effectiveness of massage therapy for chronic, non-malignant pain: A review. *Evidence-based Complementary and Alternative Medicine*, *4*(2), 165–179. https://doi.org/10.1093/ecam/nel109

Udina, E., Puigdemasa, A., & Navarro, X. (2011). Passive and active exercise improve regeneration and muscle reinnervation after peripheral nerve injury in the rat. *Muscle & Nerve*, *43*(4), 500–509. https://doi.org/10.1002/mus.21912

Van Cauter, E., Caufriez, A., Kerkhofs, M., Van Onderbergen, A., Thorner, M., & Copinschi, G. (1992). Sleep, awakenings, and insulin-like growth factor-I modulate the growth hormone (GH) secretory response to GH-releasing hormone. *The Journal of Clinical Endocrinology and Metabolism*, *74*, 1451–1459.

Voscopoulos, C., & Lema, M. (2010). When does acute pain become chronic? *British Journal of Anaesthesia*, *105*, 69–85.

Vuolteenaho, K., Koskinen, A., & Moilanen, E. (2014). Leptin—A link between obesity and osteoarthritis. Applications for prevention and treatment. *Basic & Clinical Pharmacology & Toxicology*, *114*(1), 103–108. https://doi.org/10.1111/bcpt.12160

Walker, M. (2017). *Why we sleep*. New York: Scribner.

Walsh, N., Brooks, P., Hazes, R. J., Walsh, M., Dreinhöfer, K., Woolf, A., & Pain, B. a. (2008). Standards of care for acute and chronic musculoskeletal pain. *The Bone and Joint Decade*, *89*, 1830–1845.

Wei, W., & Dai, H. (2021). Articular cartilage and osteochondral tissue engineering techniques: Recent advances and challenges. *Bioactive Materials*, *6*(12), 4830–4855. https://doi.org/10.1016/j.bioactmat.2021.05.011

Wolny, T., Saulicz, E., Linek, P., Shacklock, M., & Mysliwiec, A. (2017). Efficacy of manual therapy including neurodynamic techniques for the treatment of carpal tunnel syndrome: A randomized controlled trial. *Journal of Manipulative and Physiological Therapeutics*, *40*(4), 263–272. https://doi.org/10.1016/j.jmpt.2017.02.004

Wood, K., Wilhelm, J. C., Sabatier, M. J., Liu, K., Gu, J., & English, A. W. (2012). Sex differences in the effectiveness of treadmill training in enhancing axon regeneration in injured peripheral nerves. *Developmental Neurobiology*, *72*(5), 688–698. https://doi.org/10.1002/dneu.20960

Woolf, A., Zeidler, H., Haglund, U., Carr, A., Chaussade, S., Cucinotta, D., & Martin-Mola, E. (2004). Musculoskeletal pain in Europe: Its impact and a comparison of population and medical perceptions of treatment in eight Eurpoean countries. *Annals of the Rheumatic Diseases*, *63*, 342–347.

Xin, D. L., Hadrevi, J., Elliott, M. E., Amin, M., Harris, M. Y., Barr-Gillespie, A. E., & Barbe, M. F. (2017). Effectiveness of conservative interventions for sickness and pain behaviors induced by a high repetition high force upper extremity task. *BMC Neuroscience*, *18*(1), 36. https://doi.org/10.1186/s12868-017-0354-3

Zhang, J., Yuan, T., & Wang, J. (2016). Moderate treadmill running exercise prior to tendon injury enhances wound healing in aging rats. *Oncotarget*, *7*, 8498–8512.

16

Status of Knowledge and Unanswered Questions

Introduction

This book has presented multiple lines of evidence indicating that fatigue failure is a mechanism fundamental to the development of MSDs. The evidence includes musculoskeletal tissue fatigue failure responses to repeated stress in both *ex vivo* and *in vivo* studies (e.g., Andarawis-Puri, Flatow, & Soslowski, 2015; Barbe et al., 2013; Brinckmann, Biggemann, & Hilweg, 1988; Carter & Hayes, 1976; Cyron & Hutton, 1978; Fung et al., 2010; Schechtman & Bader, 1997; Shepherd & Screen, 2013; Sun et al., 2010; Thornton, Schwab, & Oxland, 2007), a consistent pattern of force-repetition interaction predicted by the fatigue failure theory across a variety of MSD outcomes (Gallagher & Heberger, 2013; Barbe et al., 2013), and validation studies of risk assessment tools employing fatigue failure principles (Bani Hani et al., 2021; Gallagher, Schall Jr, Sesek, & Huangfu, 2018; Gallagher, Sesek, Schall Jr, & Huangfu, 2017). Fatigue failure theory can explain how and why certain physical risk factors (force, repetition, posture, and vibration exposure), long associated with MSD outcomes, have emerged (Gallagher & Schall, 2017). However, the fatigue failure mechanism in the biological environment is modified by the presence of remodeling and healing processes that function to repair the damage, extending the service life of these tissues. Yet, this healing process can be impaired by certain conditions (e.g., psychological stress, age, obesity, inadequate sleep, alcohol use, and/or smoking), which may help to explain why these factors are associated with MSD incidence (Gallagher & Barbe, 2021).

The biological environment adds considerable complexity to the assessment of musculoskeletal health and damage development due to fatigue. In the biological setting, the fatigue failure process is modified by the presence of mechanoreceptors that can sense the applied stress and adapt accordingly. Systems are available to continuously remodel musculoskeletal tissues based on stress exposures (Duncan & Turner, 1995) and to undergo healing when these tissues experience significant damage. If we are to optimize our ability to intervene to prevent cumulative trauma development in our tissues, we need to understand a great deal more about the process itself and the complex system in which our musculoskeletal tissues reside. Increasing our understanding will require a significant investment in research to acquire the necessary knowledge and techniques to improve our understanding. While the evidence that fatigue failure is happening in musculoskeletal tissues is consistent and convincing, at the current time, we are lacking the knowledge fundamental to our understanding of the specifics of the process as it occurs in living tissues.

In an ideal world, the risk of an MSD for an individual could be accurately predicted given knowledge of the strength of the individual's tissues and the magnitude, distribution, and frequency of loading of these tissues. We would have accurate knowledge of the healing rate of the

Musculoskeletal Disorders: The Fatigue Failure Mechanism, First Edition. Sean Gallagher and Mary F. Barbe.

involved tissues and would understand the proper balance in terms of activity and rest for healing to be optimized. We would understand how the adoption of different postures changes the stress distribution in the involved tissues. We would understand the effects of aging, sex, anthropometry, and relevant disease processes. The impact of prior tissue damage would be wholly appreciated. The understanding of how psychological stresses and personal characteristics impact tissue loading and healing would also be fully comprehended.

It is likely that advances in research and technology will eventually provide methods that allow a better understanding of these issues, though, for some aspects, it may be in a rather distant future. At the current time, we find ourselves lacking a great deal of basic information necessary to fully comprehend the modified fatigue failure process in musculoskeletal tissues that occurs *in vivo*. The following sections highlight some of the areas where research is needed to better understand fatigue failure processes in the human body, which will hopefully lead not only to better design of jobs but also to better overall musculoskeletal health through life.

Improved Characterization of Musculoskeletal Tissue Properties

In the world of engineering materials, a great deal of effort has been put into characterizing material characteristics critical to the development of fatigue failure. Factors such as tensile properties, monotonic, cyclic, and strain-life properties, and fatigue crack thresholds are well tabled for a wide range of engineering alloys (Stephens, Fatemi, Stephens, & Fuchs, 2001). Conversely, data on fatigue life properties of musculoskeletal tissues remain rather sparse and disorganized. Thus, a more comprehensive exploration of the responses of musculoskeletal tissues to repeated stress would seem warranted (*ex vivo*, *in vitro*, and *in vivo*). For example, there is scant evidence evaluating long cycle fatigue (>10,000 loading cycles) for many musculoskeletal tissues (Gallagher & Schall, 2017). An improved understanding of long cycle responses of these tissues would be important in developing *S–N* curves that better define fatigue life at lower loading conditions. Knowledge of the effects of load rate, variable loading amplitudes, residual stress effects, creep stress, and damage nucleation and propagation are not sufficient. Viscoelastic responses are also not well understood, especially the effects associated with variable load rates that may be experienced during a loading process. Our knowledge of the load sharing of tissues is very poor at the present time, as well as how and where stress concentrations develop in various tissues.

Statistical variability is an important issue with respect to fatigue testing and using an appropriate sample size is a critical aspect of developing *S–N* curves. The classic study by Schechtman and Bader (1997) is instructive as a model of how the relationship between loading and cycles to failure is necessary for constructing an *S–N* curve. As these authors demonstrate, testing of specimens at several stress levels is needed to properly define the *S–N* curve for a tissue. Obviously, the development of a complete *S–N* curve (especially when including long cycle fatigue) is tedious; however, understanding of the fatigue responses of all musculoskeletal tissues is critical to improved modeling of the fatigue process and MSD prevention efforts. For many tissues involved with specific MSDs, we have little to no fatigue data at all (Gallagher & Schall, 2017).

It should be recognized that damage to viscoelastic tissues may result from a combination of fatigue failure and creep loading. The former mode of damage seems to lead to more rapid tissue damage than the latter (Thornton et al., 2007); however, these loading modes are expected to have an additive effect on damage development. The nature of the relationship between these two loading modalities in musculoskeletal tissues remains unknown at the current time, including what the nature of potential carryover effects might be when experiencing combinations of creep and cyclic loading.

Quantifying tissue strength is of crucial importance in terms of assessing MSD risk, and it would be useful to better understand tissue strength in the living human, as well as factors that influence this metric. Fortunately, there are technologies that may be very helpful in estimating tissue strengths *in vivo*. An example is dual-energy x-ray absorptiometry (DEXA), which can provide information on bone densitometry that may be extremely helpful in understanding, for example, the risk of vertebral end-plate fractures in the spine. Bone mineral content has been shown to be highly correlated with the ultimate strength (Biggemann, Hilweg, & Brinckmann, 1988) and fatigue life (Gallagher et al., 2007) of spinal motion segments *ex vivo*, a relationship that is likely present *in vivo* as well. Such measures may be helpful when comparing demands of the job to worker capacity and establishing the associated risk. Of course, other useful imaging techniques include MRI, ultrasound, and others that can establish the dimensions and estimated strength of tissues, critical to the determination of stress experienced *in vivo*.

Improved Characterization of the Damage Response to Repeated Stress of Musculoskeletal Tissues *In Vivo*

As described previously in Chapter 7, results of both *ex vivo* and *in vivo* studies of musculoskeletal tissues make it abundantly clear that musculoskeletal tissues are susceptible to fatigue failure. To date, most of the studies examining fatigue failure responses in musculoskeletal tissues have been *ex vivo* in nature, with relatively few *in vivo* studies. While these *ex vivo* studies provide valuable information about material characteristics, we need to know a great deal more about how (and why) the tissues respond differently to repeated stress in the biological setting.

Relatively few studies have examined differences in loading response in tissues among *ex vivo*, *in vitro*, and *in vivo* loading conditions. This may be partially explained by complications and ethical considerations associated with *in vivo* testing (Ramo et al., 2018). However, there are clearly limitations to *ex vivo* and *in vitro* studies regarding their ability to reproduce the loading conditions that are present *in vivo*. *In vitro* studies can answer certain fundamental research problems in a more controlled environment; however, these will lack the ability to assess longer-term effects that can be obtained with *in vivo* testing (Nickien, Heuijerjans, Ito, & van Donkelaar, 2018). Each mode of testing can provide important knowledge regarding the effects of repeated stress on musculoskeletal tissues, though it may be difficult to reconcile certain difference in results due to methodological differences in the different testing approaches (Nickien et al., 2018). Clearly, we should continue to press forward to understand the loading responses of musculoskeletal tissues *in vivo* more fully so that we can improve our ability to prevent the development of MSDs.

Characterization of the Remodeling and Healing Responses in Musculoskeletal Tissues

The most fundamental research issue related to MSDs is the tug of war between the rate of fatigue damage in tissues and the rate of the remodeling/healing processes that aim to repair damaged tissues. Thus, the effort to better define musculoskeletal tissue characteristics should include a better understanding of the rate of healing in various tissues and factors that can influence this process. It is also important to understand the healing kinetics associated with specific injuries. For example, how long does it take to heal a tendon lesion that is 1 mm in diameter versus a lesion that is 3 mm in diameter? Currently, there is little information on the rate of healing in different musculoskeletal tissues subject to repeated stress and influences that affect the rate of healing.

Most studies that have focused on healing times have involved *acute* injury and the influences that may affect the healing process after a single damaging blow, and not those involving continued repeated stress. But how does continued repetitive loading affect the healing response and the time required for healing? Obviously, the greater the repeated stress load is on an injured tissue, the longer it would be expected to take to heal (and vice versa). However, to fully understand the complex relationship between tissue damage and healing, we will need to be able to answer such questions quantitatively.

One of the few studies examining the healing of musculoskeletal tissues after controlled fatigue damage *in vivo* was a study by Wu and colleagues in which bone healing was quantified after fatigue failure microdamage was induced by loading (Wu et al., 2013). The microcracks were healed approximately 2–3 weeks post damage. There are several animal studies that have examined fatigue failure microdamage and healing time with or without persistent loading, some of which were discussed in Chapter 11. Yet our knowledge of this important relationship remains poorly developed, and the studies thus far suffer from significant shortcomings. For example, it may be difficult to project healing times in human tissues from studies of animal tissues. Nonetheless, a clear need is to develop a more robust understanding of the interplay between damage development and healing using multiple research strategies.

Musculoskeletal Stress Thresholds

Our ability to maintain (or improve) the musculoskeletal health of tissues in workers, athletes, and others requires an increased understanding of the responses of tissues to different degrees of mechanical stress. As discussed previously, musculoskeletal tissues are highly attuned to the amount of stress they experience and can display remarkable changes in structure and function based on their stress history. It is apparent that there are several stress-related thresholds that exist which alter the status of musculoskeletal tissue health; however, the processes responsible are still not well understood.

Figure 16.1 provides a model of stress-related thresholds that appear to affect musculoskeletal health. As depicted in this model, there is plainly a stress threshold that must be surpassed to prevent tissues from experiencing atrophy or loss. If tissue loading is not sufficient to maintain the current tissue health status, this stress threshold will be crossed and will trigger a catabolic response. It appears a lack of stress on musculoskeletal tissues causes the body to completely forego the implementation of processes designed to maintain or enhance tissue strength. For example, studies have demonstrated that astronauts in microgravity experience up to a 20% loss of muscle mass on spaceflights lasting 5–11 days and may lose up to 2% of their bone density per month if bone and muscle are not purposefully stressed (NASA, 2001, 2021). To maintain the health of their tissues, astronauts must exercise for 2.5 hr/day. While no other working population is subjected to the extreme microgravity condition of space, atrophy of tissues will also occur under normal gravity if individuals are not active (though at a less rapid pace) (Rudrappa et al., 2016). Thus, it is apparent that musculoskeletal tissues need a certain baseline of stress exposure to maintain their healthy functioning. If loading is sufficient (but not excessive), the tissue will invoke systems that work to maintain (or improve) its integrity.

It is also apparent that a limited number of high-stress exertions (combined with sufficient rest) can lead to significant gains in the strength of tissues, including muscle, tendons, and ligaments. For example, Arampatzis and colleagues showed that increased Achilles' tendon stiffness occurs during a 14-week exercise protocol involving strain of 4.5%, but not for an exercise involving strain of 3%, even though exercise frequency and volume were equal (Arampatzis, Karamanidis, & Albracht, 2007).

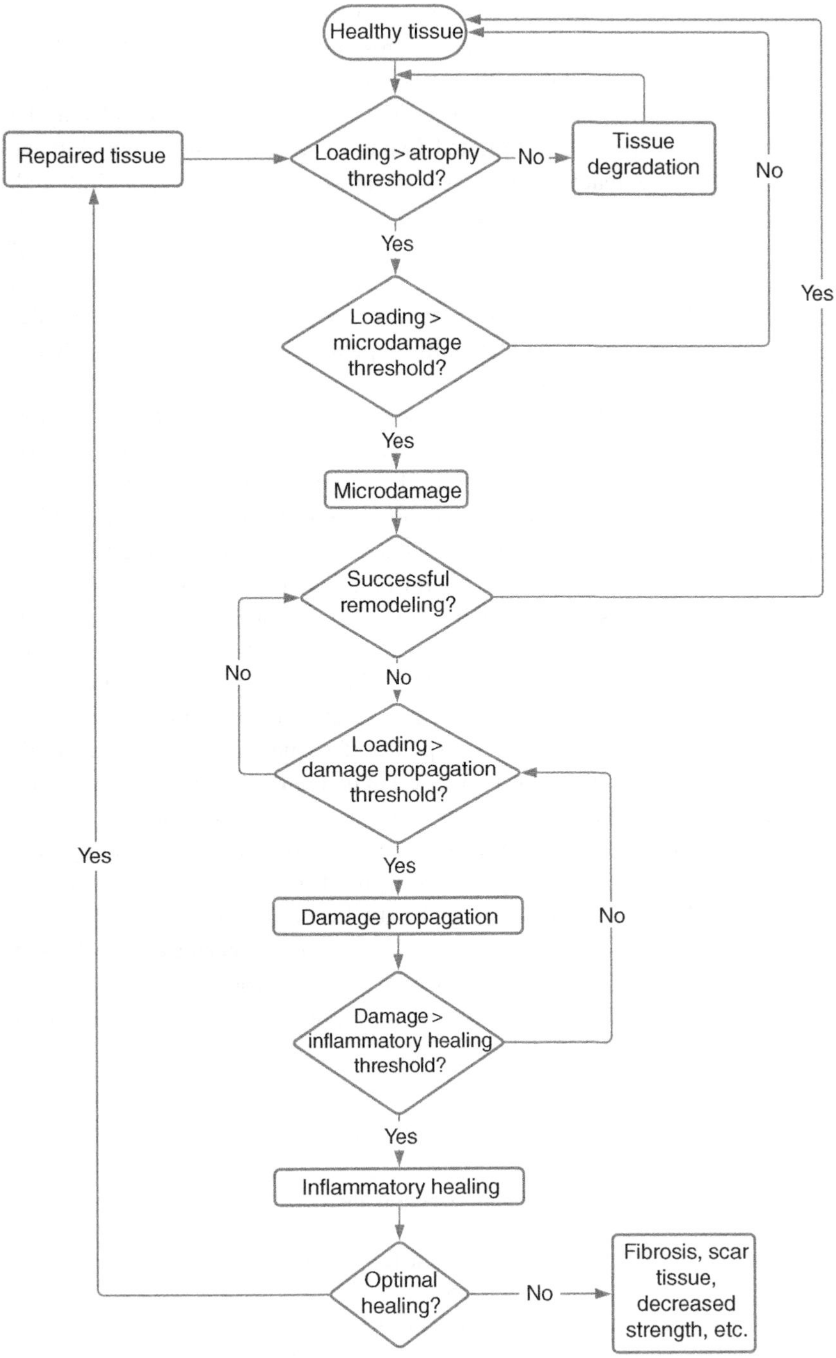

Figure 16.1 Model of musculoskeletal tissue thresholds.

It has also been demonstrated that increased tendon stiffness (in the patellar tendon) will occur with a high resistance load, but not for a light resistance regimen (Kongsgaard et al., 2007). These data suggest that a certain stress magnitude threshold must be exceeded to elicit an anabolic tissue response. However, the difference between high magnitude stress that leads to an anabolic response versus that leading to catabolic changes appears not to be tremendously different (Heinemeier &

Kjaer, 2011). Clearly, the number of cycles experienced will play into this relationship as well. Much more needs to be understood regarding the levels of repeated stress and other characteristics of loading that lead to improvements in musculoskeletal health versus those that result in negative outcomes.

If repeated stress experienced by the tissue is sufficiently great, another threshold may be crossed: the threshold where tissue damage is initiated (what we will call the "microdamage threshold"). As shown in Figure 16.1, if loading is not excessive after the microdamage is initiated, remodeling and/or healing processes may be able to repair the microdamage at an early stage leading to timely restoration of function. However, if exposure to repetitive stress is persistent and of sufficient magnitude, another threshold may be crossed in which the initial microdamage will begin to propagate through the tissue (i.e., the "propagation threshold"). As discussed in earlier chapters, the rate at which damage propagates will be highly dependent on the tissue strength and the quantity of repetitive stress experienced by the tissue.

In the presence of continued repeated stress, the tissue may cross another threshold: the "inflammatory repair" threshold. Crossing this threshold will invoke the inflammatory repair process, which will attempt to make repairs to the injured region. The success of this repair process also appears to be somewhat stress-dependent. Too much stress on the injured area may result in additional damage development and a vicious cycle of injury and inflammation, leading to a poor repair result. However, studies suggest that the careful introduction of controlled stress to an injured tissue can have important benefits and can facilitate the healing process. Controlled loading has been shown to improve the synthesis and alignment of collagen fibers, leading to an improved repair outcome (Kellet, 1986; Müller, Todorov, Heisterbach, Martin, & Majewski, 2013).

A key question to be asked is: "What factors influence the point at which the interaction of repetition, force, and duration shifts from driving a net response of tissue formation (an anabolic response) versus tissue degradation (a catabolic response)"? There are a multitude of factors that can influence the response of tissues to mechanical loading including, but not limited to, gender, age, genetic and epigenetic traits, hormonal status, serum mineral balance, nutritional status/diet, smoking status, emotional status (e.g., stress/anxiety), and the presence of co-morbidities that can affect musculoskeletal tissue health (e.g., hypertension, obesity, hypercholesterolemia, diabetes) (Romano et al., 2015; Santos, Elliott-Sale, & Sale, 2017; Wohl, Boyd, Judex, & Zernicke, 2000). Even when some factors are controlled, it is difficult to predict which factor or group of factors will prevail given their interwoven complexity. As shown in Table 16.1, for example, some contributions of

Table 16.1 Factors That Favor Bone Anabolic Versus Catabolic Responses

Pro-anabolism (accrual)	Pro-catabolism (loss)
• Sex (male > female) • Young adult • Decreased sclerostin-increased osteoblast activity • Decreased RANKL-increased osteoblast activity • Somatosensory innervation • βAR antagonists	• Sex (female > male) • Aging • Microcracks and osteocyte apoptosis • Increased sclerostin-increased osteoclast activity • Increased RANKL-increased osteoclast activity • Increased sympathetic activity • βAR agonists • Sustained inflammation—local and systemic

Barbe, M., & Popoff, S. (2020). Occupational activities: Factors that tip the balance from bone accrual to bone loss. *Exercise and Sport Sciences Rviews*, 48, 59–66.

βAR = beta-adrenergic receptor; RANKL = receptor activator of nuclear factor kappa-B ligand.

various stimuli generated by muscle on bones are known, but the process as a whole is still not well understood (Avin, Bloomfield, Gross, & Warden, 2015; Brotto & Bonewald, 2015).

Thresholds for damage development need to be better defined, as do rest and recovery allowances that enhance tissue recovery and adaptation. Current equations for repetitive occupational task thresholds were developed from 69 short-term psychophysical data tasks (each <4 weeks in duration) using physiological data from six studies demonstrating muscle fatigue after only 1 hr (Potvin, 2012). Most workers work longer than 1 hr; therefore, longer studies are needed. The duty cycle is the duration of effort (per cycle) an individual worker is engaged in a repetitive task. Decreasing duty cycles may increase the allowable maximum acceptable forces and enhance tissue recovery (Potvin, 2012). Increasing periods of complete relaxation between work cycles also reduce health risks (Sjøgaard, Lundberg, & Kadefors, 2000), supporting a need for further exploration of rest periods in loading models.

While we understand that these thresholds exist, we have a great deal to learn about the processes governing these thresholds and exactly how and why these thresholds are breached. Understanding these processes will be important to our ability to model the body's responses to stress and better define the precise nature of the modified fatigue failure process in musculoskeletal tissues. The answer to several important "threshold" questions will likely require animal studies. The effects of repetitive high-demand activities on tissues in human populations currently cannot be as well defined as in animal models. Longitudinal studies should be performed in young, mature, and aged people to capture effects of changing repair mechanisms, hormone levels, changes in metabolism and inflammaging (the increase in inflammation occurring with aging) (Salvioli et al., 2006). It has been shown that aged rats performing the same low force high repetition (LFHR) task for 12 weeks as young adult rats develop greater levels of tissue degradation, likely due to observed increases in systemic and tissue inflammatory cytokine responses occurring as a consequence of both aging and continued loading processes (Massicotte et al., 2015). Similar studies should be repeated in human populations, particularly in light of the trend of longer work times prior to retirement for workers (Welsh, Strazdins, Charlesworth, Kulik, & Butterworth, 2016).

Additionally, we need to better understand both the negative and positive impacts of loading during the tissue repair process. When the tissue becomes damaged, the damaged region becomes an area of stress concentration in the tissue and therefore becomes vulnerable to additional fatigue damage even in the presence of lower magnitude loads. A vicious cycle may thus ensue. Thus, tissue loading can be either a hindrance or a benefit in the tissue repair process. The timing and magnitude of loading that should be experienced in the repair process to (a) decrease damage and/or (b) facilitate healing is poorly known presently, but are important to the preservation of musculoskeletal tissue health.

Musculoskeletal Tissues in the Resting State

As we have discussed earlier, to understand the risk associated with musculoskeletal disorders we clearly need to develop a great deal more knowledge regarding the effects of loading on musculoskeletal tissues. However, because of the healing and remodeling processes present in the biological environment, we also need to better understand the processes that impact musculoskeletal health tissues when unloaded. A great deal remains to be learned regarding different varieties of rest and their influence on musculoskeletal health. Research in this area is particularly important, as the effects of rest are important to understanding both cumulative damage development and the repair process in musculoskeletal tissues. A deeper understanding of the role of rest on musculoskeletal tissues would help improve our ability to evaluate risk more accurately (and intervene more effectively) in the effort to reduce MSDs.

We need to understand the effect that time of unloading has on the resting tissue and the interaction between the magnitude of loading and the time necessary to recover from that loading. In addition, we need to understand the degree to which rest affects cumulative damage development on the loading side, and the amount of time necessary to heal a given amount of damage on the healing side. The roles of rest and healing appear intertwined to a degree (particularly in periods of long-term rest); however, the shorter the rest period, the smaller the benefit would be expected on the healing end. These relationships need further clarification and deserve a concentrated research effort.

Risk Assessment in Epidemiological Studies

Past epidemiological studies, including recent large multi-site efforts, have often failed to consider that MSD outcomes might be the result of a fatigue failure mechanism occurring in musculoskeletal tissues. If MSDs are indeed the result of a fatigue failure process, important modifications would be needed with respect to how physical MSD risk factors are quantified by epidemiologists. For example, it would be critically important to evaluate repetition as a function of force level experienced by participants, due to the highly variable impact of repetition at different force levels in a fatigue process. Many current tools used to assess the effects of force and repetition do not appear to appropriately weigh the impact of repetition as force levels vary. Furthermore, as mentioned earlier, fatigue failure theory would indicate that a key element of risk assessment is the evaluation of the load experienced by an individual relative to their tissue strength, which may be highly influenced by age, gender, and anthropometry.

While evidence suggests that assessing the cumulative damage associated with repeated stress exposure provides consistently strong relationships to musculoskeletal outcomes (Bani Hani et al., 2021; Gallagher et al., 2017, 2018), it should be recognized that MSD risk is likely the result of a tug-of-war between damage accrued and the capacity to heal such damage. Factors that negatively impact healing (notably psychosocial stress, aging, obesity, and gender), and those factors leading to cumulative damage development, may ultimately be able to be modeled using a singular risk metric (cumulative damage), which would incorporate the combined impact of fatigue failure damage and healing rate, as suggested long ago by Nash (1966). A holistic approach to factors both causing and repairing damage may be useful in future epidemiological studies.

As discussed previously, new risk assessment data collection methods are currently being developed that will soon allow for continuous or "real-time" exposure assessment. These techniques will pose new challenges in terms of the analysis of highly variable (or "spectrum") loading conditions. Fatigue failure risk assessment tools are well-positioned to analyze such data, using validated methods of assessing continuous spectrum loading histories. It is hoped that in the future, epidemiological studies will collect and analyze risk assessment data in a manner that allows better assessment of the fatigue failure mechanism, as this may clarify the etiology of these disorders and lead to more comprehensive risk assessment strategies.

Assessing the Risk of Multiple Loading Modes

It is not uncommon for individuals to be exposed to different repeated stress loading modalities that may act upon the same musculoskeletal structure. For example, delivery drivers are regularly exposed to whole-body vibration (WBV) and manual handling of a variety of different loads (Okunribido,

Magnusson, & Pope, 2006). These drivers have also been found to experience significant low back pain (Boshuizen, Bongers, & Hulshof, 1992; Magnusson, Wilder, Pope, & Hansson, 1993; Miyamoto, Shirai, Nakayama, Gembun, & Kaneda, 2000). However, many of the earlier studies examining delivery drivers have been concerned with a single risk factor (usually lifting demands), as opposed to the combination of whole-body vibration exposure and manual lifting exposure (Nygard & Ilmarinen, 1990; Van der Beek, 1995). This is likely due to the lack of a method to combine the exposure of the low back to both whole-body vibration (WBV) and manual handling of loads.

One advantage of the use of fatigue failure methods to assess MSD risk is that they provide the ability to combine risks associated with diverse loading modalities such as the low back stress associated with whole-body vibration exposure and manual material handling providing a single continuous measure of risk that will provide an estimate of cumulative damage associated each individual task as well as the combined tasks (Gallagher & Schall, 2017). Whole-body vibration is known to be an exposure that imposes repeated stress on the low back (International Standards Organization, 2018) as does repetitive compressive loading due to lifting (Brinckmann et al., 1988). Since both can be expressed in terms of cumulative damage, fatigue failure techniques could be used to combine these disparate loading modalities to obtain a cumulative measure of overall risk not previously available. The use of this technique should also be able to determine the separate cumulative damage associated with WBV exposure and MMH activities (providing the proportion of total damage associated with each).

Dwell and Combination Loading

While cyclic loading is the predominant mode of stress exposure in many occupational tasks, there are many tasks in which "dwell", or creep loading, may also be a significant loading modality. As discussed earlier, the low back may often experience significant creep stress during standing or sitting activities. Cyclic stress may be superimposed on creep stress, for example when performing lifting tasks interspersed with periods of static standing. Dwell is similar to cyclic loading; however, instead of cycles to failure, it uses *time* to failure (which varies exponentially in accordance with the stress level).

Clearly both modes of stress may be present in many common work activities (and other pursuits). While models are available to assess the combined effects of cyclic loading and dwell (Wright, Carroll, Sham, Lybeck, & Wright, 2016), we have insufficient information regarding the creep characteristics of musculoskeletal tissues that would allow us to model the damage associated with dwell or due to combined exposures. A great deal remains to be learned about how dwell impacts the failure of musculoskeletal tissues, and how this loading mode interacts with cyclic loading to produce musculoskeletal tissue damage.

Summary

As we have discussed in this book, many lines of evidence indicate that fatigue failure is etiologically significant in the development of MSDs. However, as of this writing, the implications of an underlying (and likely causal) fatigue failure process in MSD development have rarely been considered in prior MSD epidemiological studies, in prior MSD risk assessment tools, ànd/or MSD prevention strategies. If fatigue is indeed an important causal mechanism, there are many important implications that need to be considered, and a great deal more to be learned. These include important interactions between MSD risk factors, the ability to develop improved cumulative loading estimates on tissues, the importance of individual characteristics and MSD risk, and an improved understanding of the relationship between tissue damage and healing. We need to better understand the thresholds that lead to anabolic versus catabolic changes in musculoskskeletal tissues, various damage thresholds and the interaction of the damage and healing processes. It is our hope that the concept that MSDs are the result of a process of fatigue failure may provide fertile ground for research in the quest to reduce the pain and disability associated with these burdensome health conditions.

Bibliography

Andarawis-Puri, A., Flatow, E., & Soslowski, L. (2015). Tendon basic science: Development, repair, regeneration, and healing. *Journal of Orthopaedic Research, 33*, 780–784.

Arampatzis, A., Karamanidis, P., & Albracht, K. (2007). Adaptational responses of the human achilles tendon by modulation of the applied cyclic strain magnitude. *Journal of Experimental Biology, 210*, 2743–2753.

Avin, K., Bloomfield, S., Gross, T., & Warden, S. (2015). Biomechanical aspects of the muscle–bone interaction. *Current Osteoporosis Reports, 13*, 1–8.

Bani Hani, D., Huangfu, R., Sesek, R., Schall, M., Jr., Davis, G., & Gallagher, S. (2021). Development and validation of a cumulative exposure shoulder risk assessment tool based on fatigue failure theory. *Ergonomics, 64*, 39–54.

Barbe, M., Gallagher, S., Massicotte, V., Tytell, M., Popoff, S., & Barr-Gillespie, A. (2013). The interaction of force and repetition on musculoskeletal and neural tissue responses and sensorimotor behavior in a rat model of work-related musculoskeletal disorders. *BMC Musculoskeletal Disorders, 14*, 303.

Barbe, M., & Popoff, S. (2020). Occupational activities: Factors that tip the balance from bone accrual to bone loss. *Exercise and Sport Sciences Reviews, 48*, 59–66.

Biggemann, M., Hilweg, D., & Brinckmann, P. (1988). Prediction of the compressive strength of vertebral bodies of the lumbar spine by quantitative computed tomography. *Skeletal Radiology, 17*, 264–269.

Boshuizen, H., Bongers, P., & Hulshof, C. (1992). Self-reported back pain in forklift truck and freight-container tractor drivers exposed to whole body vibration. *Spine, 17*, 59–65.

Brinckmann, P., Biggemann, M., & Hilweg, D. (1988). Fatigue fracture of human lumbar vertebrae. *Clinical Biomechanics, 3*(Suppl. 1), S1–S23.

Brotto, M., & Bonewald, L. (2015). Bone and muscle: Interactions beyond mechanical. *Bone, 80*, 109–114.

Carter, D., & Hayes, W. (1976). Fatigue life of compact bone—I. Effects of stress amplitude, temperature and density. *Journal of Biomechanics, 9*, 27–34.

Cyron, B., & Hutton, W. (1978). The fatigue strength of the lumbar neural arch in spondylolysis. *The Journal of Bone and Joint Surgery, British Volume, 60-B*, 234–238.

Duncan, R., & Turner, C. (1995). Mechanotransduction and the functional response of bone to mechanical strain. *Calcified Tissue International, 57*, 344–358.

Fung, D., Wang, V., Andarawis-Puri, N., Basta-Pljakic, J., Li, Y., Laudier, D., . . . Flatow, E. (2010). Early response to tendon fatigue damage accumulation in a novel in vivo model. *Journal of Biomechanics, 43*, 274–279.

Gallagher, S., & Barbe, M. (2021). The Impaired Healing Hypothesis: A mechanism by which psychosocial stress and personal characteristics increase MSD risk? *Ergonomics*, 1–14. https://doi.org/10.1080/00140139.2021.1974103

Gallagher, S., & Heberger, J. (2013). Examining the interaction of force and repetition on musculoskeletal disorder risk: A systematic literature review. *Human Factors*, *14*, 108–124.

Gallagher, S., Marras, W., Litsky, A., Burr, D., Landoll, J., & Matkovic, V. (2007). A comparison of fatigue failure responses of old versus middle-aged lumbar motion segments in simulated flexed lifting. *Spine*, *32*, 1832–1839.

Gallagher, S., & Schall, J. M. (2017). Musculoskeletal disorders as a fatigue failure process: Evidence, implications and research needs. *Ergonomics*, *60*, 255–269.

Gallagher, S., Schall, M., Jr., Sesek, R., & Huangfu, R. (2018). An upper extremity risk assessment tool based on material fatigue failure theory: The Distal Upper Extremity Tool (DUET). *Human factors*, *60*, 1146–1162.

Gallagher, S., Sesek, R., Schall, M., Jr., & Huangfu, R. (2017). Development and validation of an easy-to-use risk assessment tool for cumulative low back loading: The Lifting Fatigue Failure Tool (LiFFT). *Applied Ergonomics*, *63*, 142–150.

Heinemeier, K., & Kjaer, M. (2011). In vivo investigation of tendon responses to mechanical loading. *Journal of Musculoskeletal and Neuronal Interaction*, *11*, 115–123.

International Standards Organization (2018). *INTERNATIONAL ISO STANDARD 2631-5 Second edition 2018-07 Mechanical vibration and shock—Evaluation of human exposure to whole-body vibration — Part 5: Method for evaluation of vibration containing multiple shocks*. Geneva: International Standards Organization.

Kellet, J. (1986). Acute soft tissue injuries—a review of the literature. *Medicine and Science in Sports and Exercise*, *18*, 489–500.

Kongsgaard, M., Reitelseder, S., Pedersen, T., Holm, L., Aagaard, P., Kjaer, M., & Magnusson, S. (2007). Region specific patellar tendon hypertrophy in humans following resistance training. *Acta Physiologica (Oxford)*, *191*, 111–121.

Magnusson, M., Wilder, D., Pope, M., & Hansson, T. (1993). Investigation of the long-term exposure to whole body vibration: A 2-country study. *European Journal of Physical Medicine and Rehabilitation*, *3*, 28–34.

Massicotte, V., Frara, N., Harris, M., Amin, M., Wade, C., Popoff, S., & Barbe, M. (2015). Prolonged performance of a high repetition low force task induces bone adaptation in young adult rats, but loss in mature rats. *Experimental Gerontology*, *72*, 204–217.

Miyamoto, M., Shirai, Y., Nakayama, Y., Gembun, Y., & Kaneda, K. (2000). An epidemiologic study of occupational low back pain in truck drivers. *Journal of Nippon Medical School*, *67*, 186–190.

Müller, S., Todorov, A., Heisterbach, P., Martin, I., & Majewski, M. (2013). Tendon healing: An overview of physiology, biology, and pathology of tendon healing and systematic review of state of the art in tendon bioengineering. *Knee Surgery, Sports Traumatology, Arthroscopy*, *23*, 2097–2105.

NASA. (2001, October 1). Retrieved November 2021, from Space Bones: https://science.nasa.gov/science-news/science-at-nasa/2001/ast01oct_1

NASA. (2021). *Muscle atrophy*. Retrieved November 2021, from NASA Information: https://www.nasa.gov/pdf/64249main_ffs_factsheets_hbp_atrophy.pdf

Nash, J. C. (1966). *Fatigue of self-healing structure: A generalized theory of fatigue failure*. New York, NY: American Society of Mechanical Engineers.

Nickien, M., Heuijerjans, A., Ito, K., & van Donkelaar, C. (2018). Comparison between in vitro and in vivo cartilage overloading studies based on a systematic literature review. *Journal of orthopaedic research, 36*, 2076–2086.

Nygard, C., & Ilmarinen, J. (1990). Effects of changes in delivery of dairy products on physical strain of truck drivers. In C. Haslegrave (Ed.), *Work design in practice* (pp. 142–148). London: Taylor & Francis.

Okunribido, O., Magnusson, M., & Pope, M. (2006). Delivery drivers and low-back pain: A study of the exposures to posture demands, manual materials handling and whole-body vibration. *International Journal of Industrial Ergonomics, 36*, 265–273.

Potvin, J. (2012). Predicting maximum acceptable efforts for repetitive tasks: An equation based on duty cycle. *Human Factors, 54*, 175–188.

Ramo, N., Shetye, S., Streijger, F., Lee, J., Troyer, K., Kwon, B., . . . Puttlitz, C. (2018). Comparison of in vivo and ex vivo viscoelastic behavior of the spinal cord. *Acta Biomaterialia, 68*, 78–89.

Romano, A., Vigna, L., Belluigi, V., Conti, D., Barberi, C., Tomaino, L., . . . Andersen, A. (2015). Shift work and serum 25-OH vitamin D status among factory workers in northern Italy: Cross-sectional study. *Chronobiology International, 32*, 842–847.

Rudrappa, S., Wilkinson, D., Greenhaff, P., Smith, K., Idris, I., & Atherton, P. (2016). Human skeletal muscle disuse atrophy: Effects on muscle protein synthesis, breakdown, and insulin resistance—a qualitative review. *Frontiers in Physiology, 7*, 361.

Salvioli, S., Capri, M., Valensin, S., Tieri, P., Monti, D., Ottaviani, E., & Franceschi, C. (2006). Inflamm-aging, cytokines and aging: State of the art, new hypotheses on the role of mitochondria and new perspectives from systems biology. *Current Pharmaceutical Design, 12*, 3161–3171.

Santos, L., Elliott-Sale, K., & Sale, C. (2017). Exercise and bone health across the lifespan. *Biogerontology, 18*, 931–946.

Schechtman, H., & Bader, D. (1997). In vitro fatigue of human tendons. *Journal of Biomechanics, 30*, 829–835.

Shepherd, J., & Screen, H. (2013). Fatigue loading of tendon. *International Journal of Experimental Pathology, 94*, 260–270.

Sjøgaard, G., Lundberg, U., & Kadefors, R. (2000). The role of muscle activity and mental load in the development of pain and degenerative processes at the muscle cell level during computer work. *European Journal of Applied Physiology, 83*, 99–105.

Stephens, R., Fatemi, A., Stephens, R., & Fuchs, H. (2001). *Metal fatigue in engineering* (2nd ed.). New York, NY: Wiley.

Sun, H., Andarawis-Puri, N., Li, Y., Fung, D., Lee, J., Wang, V., . . . Flatow, E. L. (2010). Cycle-dependent matric remodeling gene expression response in fatigue-loaded rat patellar tendons. *Journal of Orthopaedic Research, 28*, 1380–1386.

Thornton, G. M., Schwab, T., & Oxland, T. (2007). Cyclic loading causes faster rupture and strain rate than static loading in medial collateral ligament at high stress. *Clinical Biomechanics, 22*, 932–940.

Van der Beek, A. F.-D. (1995). Physical workload of lorry drivers: A comparison of four methods of transport. *Ergonomics, 38*, 1508–1520.

Welsh, J., Strazdins, L., Charlesworth, S., Kulik, C., & Butterworth, P. (2016). Health or harm? A cohort study of the importance of job quality in extended workforce participation by older adults. *BMC Public Health, 16*, 885.

Wohl, G., Boyd, S., Judex, S., & Zernicke, R. (2000). Functional adaptation of bone to exercise and injury. *Journal of Science and Medicine in Sport, 3*(3), 313–324.

Wright, J., Carroll, L., Sham, T.-L., Lybeck, N., & Wright, R. (2016). Determination of the creep–fatigue interaction diagram for alloy 617. In *Proceedings of the ASME 2016 Pressure Vessels and Piping Conference (PVP2016), July 17–21, 2016*. Vancouver, BC: American Society of Mechanical Engineers.

Wu, B., Zhang, C., Chen, B., Zhang, L., Dai, R., Wu, X., . . . Liao, E. (2013). Self-repair of rat corical bone microdamage after fatigue loading in vivo. *International Journal of Endocrinology, 2013*, 21074.

Index

Musculoskeletal Disorders: The Fatigue Failure Mechanism, First Edition. Sean Gallagher and Mary F. Barbe.

d

f

o

p

Printed and bound by CPI Group (UK) Ltd, Croydon, CR0 4YY
07/01/2026
14802551-0004